Physiology and Anatomy key features

This book has been written with the reader in mind.

The **key features** shown on the accompanying sample pages make the text easy to read, quick to refer to and useful for revision.

- section title page:
  list of chapters
  introduction

- headings

- left-hand running head:
  section and part title

- bullet-point lists

- right-hand running head:
  chapter title

- page number

000

There is some reason for believing that every major attack has a local commencement in some region of the brain, and that it is in reality a local fit which rapidly becomes general. When such an attack commences with a local aura there is proof positive of local commencement. When the spread of the disturbance is so rapid as to cause instant loss of consciousness there is no memory to retain the initial event of the attack.

But epilepsy is also a social distinction; those

HEADING 1

The word 'epilepsy' does not have a single meaning, and hence it defies definition. One can define a fit, a disease causing fits, a precipitating cause of fits, and the consequences of fits, all of which contribute to the overall picture of epilepsy. A physiologist can define the parameters of abnormal electrical discharge underlying seizures. The biochemist may, in the future, define a local change responsible for generating that electrical discharge. Such events are also part of epilepsy. But epilepsy is also a social distinction; those diagnosed as having epilepsy are to a greater or lesser extent penalized both economically and socially. For this reason alone, epilepsy remains a medical diagnosis with social consequences that demand restricted use.

HEADING 2

The terminology and classification of seizures have evolved over many years, creating a variety of interchangeable and confused descriptive terms. The problem has been, and is, to create a single code to cover three basically incompatible systems of classification, namely; that according to

Diagnosed as having epilepsy are to a greater or lesser extent penalized both economically and socially.

Table 1.2 Slow spike and wave abnormality in 84 patients

Age at onset of fits*	5 or less	59
	6 - 10	16
	11 - 20	5
	No fits	2
Outcome* (in 68 cases)	Dead/custodial care	46%
	Normal intelligence	30%
	Retarded	24%
Aetiology*	Birth injury	14
	Immunization	3
	Head injury	4
	Encephalitis	2
	Family history of fits	22
	Nil	42

*Information was not available for every patient.
(After Blume, David & Gomez 1973)

Tongue

Muscle

Papilla

Epithelium

Taste buds

Lamina propria

Taste bud

Sensory neurone

Chemosensitive cell

Fig 1.1
CT at level of frontal horns. There is an extensive area of decreased density deep in the right cerebral hemispheres with thick bands of calcification in its medial part extending across the midline. The lateral ventricles are displaced to the left. Histologically a low grade glioma.

clinical symptoms and signs of the fit; that relating to the anatomical and electrophysiological evidence as to the source of the fit; and defining the aetiology of the fits. An example illustrates the conflict.

Some indication of the frequency of different types of fits, generalised and partial, in a series of representative patients, referred with a diagnosis of epilepsy to one centre, is given in Table 1.2.

HEADING 2

It is not the purpose of this chapter to describe in detail the clinical phenomena of typical fits. Rather, we will concentrate on certain aspects of fits of practical clinical significance.

000

Heading 3

A typical major motor seizure or tonic-clonic fit unmistakeable, consisting of a tonic phase, followed by a clonic phase
the whole lasting for up to two minutes, and followed by a further period of five minutes or so of unrousable coma:

- After this the patient can be awoken, but is confused and disorientated, and usually prefers to sleep for a few hours, to awake often with a headache and sore muscles, but a clear mind
- An epileptic cry at the start, cyanosis, frothing at the mouth, emptying the bladder, biting the tongue, or other injury are common but not universal. During the fit the pupils dilate
- The pulse may slow initially, then accelerate, the patient sweats profusely, the plantar responses are extensor and the tendon jerks and corneal reflexes are lost. Inevitable the patient loses consciousness and falls in a grand mal attack.

Heading 4
These do not always conform to this classical sequence, but always involve loss of consciousness and convulsion. On some occasions the seizure may cease after the tonic phase, while sometimes only a clonic seizure occurs. Such

Sympathetic nervous system Adrenal medulla

Hypothalamus Pituitary

Adrenaline Noradrenaline

Growth hormone

Liver

Glycogen

Glucose

Triglyceride

Fatty acids and glycerol

Adipose tissue

Blood

Glucose dependent tissues e.g. brain

Fatty acids

Adrenaline Noradrenaline

Glucose

Muscle

Glycogen

ATP

SEIZURES

The terminology and classification of seizures have evolved over many years, creating a variety of interchangeable and confused descriptive terms. The problem has been, and is, to create a single code to cover three basically incompatible systems of classification, namely; that according to clinical symptoms and signs of the fit; that relating to the anatomical and electrophysiological evidence as to the source of the fit; and defining the aetiology of the fits. An example illustrates the conflict. The symptom complex of a seizure in which there is an abdominal and gustatory aura followed by an impairment of consciousness.

Some indication of the frequency of different types of fits, generalised and partial, in a series of representative patients, referred with a diagnosis of epilepsy to one centre, is given in Table 1.1.

This belief that all grand mal is of focal origin is compatible with the centrencephalic concept if it is assumed that primary generalised epilepsy originate in a focal discharge in the centrencephalic system, but there is no certain evidence that this is the case. A more restricted view is that all grand mal is of focal cortical origin. This view is currently expanding along with the belief that structural lesions, such as Ammon's horn sclerosis, hitherto dismissed as the consequence, not the cause of fits, may, in fact, be the focal origin for fits in many cases (see Ch.11). Again, this is a hypothesis, attractive for its simplicity and practival consequences, but unproven.

Fig 1.2
CT at level of frontal horns. There is an extensive area of decreased density deep in the right cerebral hemispheres with thick bands of calcification in its medial part extending across the midline. The lateral ventricles are displaced to the left. Histologically a low grade glioma.

limited grand mal fits are especially common in children and infants. Grand mal seizures without muscular contractions probably do not occur. True atonic seizures with collapse of muscle tone are closely associated with absences and myoclonus, and with spike and wave discharge in the EEG (Fig.1.1).

This belief that all grand mal is of focal origin is compatible with the centrencephalic concept if it is assumed that primary generalised epilepsy originate in a focal discharge in the centrencephalic sustem, but there is no certain evidence that this is the case. A more restricted view is that all grand mal is of focal cortical origin. This view is currently expanding along with the belief that structural lesions, such as Ammon's horn sclerosis, hitherto dismissed as the consequence, not the cause of fits, may, in fact, be the focal origin for fits in many cases (see Ch.11). Again, this is a hypothesis, attractive for its simplicity and practival consequences, but unproven.The debate remains whether primary grand mal seizures are due to focal cortical le-

For this reason alone, epilepsy remains a medical diagnosis with social consequences that demand restricted use

- tables

- nursing application

- general application

Physiology
and
Anatomy

About the book

The main purpose of this book is to provide nursing and health care students with a physiology and anatomy text appropriate to their needs. It has the following distinguishing characteristics:

- emphasis on physiology, with sufficient anatomy to fulfil the needs of nursing students
- holistic approach, paying particular attention to the interaction of body systems, not just the 'bits of the body'
- emphasis on systems which interact with the external world, making the book more appropriate to nursing needs than more traditional texts
- linked to practice, by means of application boxes
- highly readable and useful for revision (see **Key Features** described on inside front cover).

Physiology and Anatomy

A BASIS FOR NURSING AND HEALTH CARE

SIGRID RUTISHAUSER BSc PhD

Lecturer in Physiology and Medical Education
School of Biological Sciences
The University of Manchester

with contributions from nursing authors

Original illustrations by Marks Creative Consultants

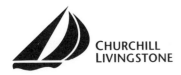

CHURCHILL
LIVINGSTONE

EDINBURGH LONDON MADRID MELBOURNE NEW YORK AND TOKYO 1994

CHURCHILL LIVINGSTONE
An imprint of Harcourt Publishers Limited

© Longman Group UK Limited 1994
© Pearson Professional Ltd 1997
© Harcourt Publishers Limited 1999

 is a registered trademark of Harcourt Publishers Limited

First published 1994
    Reprinted 1997
    Reprinted 1999

ISBN 0 443 04151 2

British Library Cataloguing in Publication Data
A catalogue record for this book is available from the British Library.

Library of Congress Cataloging in Publication Data
A catalog record for this book is available from the Library of Congress.

Note
Medical knowledge is constantly changing. As new information becomes available, changes in treatment, procedures, equipment and the use of drugs become necessary. The author and the publishers have, as far as it is possible, taken care to ensure that the information given in this text is accurate and up-to-date. However, readers are strongly advised to confirm that the information, especially with regard to drug usage, complies with latest legislation and standards of practice.

For Churchill Livingstone
Editorial Director: Mary law
Commissioning Editor: Ellen Green
Project Editors: Valerie Bain, Leigh Anne Marsden
Project Controllers: Mark Sanderson, Nancy Arnott
Design: Design Resources Unit
Sales Promotion: Hilary Brown
Editorial Assistant: Roberta Logan
Copy Editor: Susan J. Beasley
Cover design: Charles Simpson
Index: Liza Weinkove

Printed in China
GCC/02

The
publisher's
policy is to use
**paper manufactured
from sustainable forests**

Contents in brief

Contents in full

Contributors

The individuals listed below prepared the boxed applications and margin questions for the chapters cited after their names. Sue Coombes and Christopher Goodall were involved in the book from the outset; they worked with the author to develop the overall approach to the nursing input and provided advice, from the nursing perspective, on many chapters in addition to those listed after their names.

The collective work of all the nursing contributors has helped to create a book strongly linked to nursing practice and health care.

Sue Coombes BA SRN HVCert RNT DipEd
Formerly Nurse Teacher, North Yorkshire College of Health Studies, York, UK

Chapters 2, 20, 21, 22, 23, 24, 30, 31, 33, 34, 35, 36 and 37

Christopher J Goodall RGN DipN RNT
Nurse Teacher, North Yorkshire College of Health Studies, York, UK

Chapters 3, 5, 8, 12, 13, 16, 17, 18 and 19

Anne V Betts BSc(Hons) MSc RGN RNT
Senior Lecturer, Biological Sciences, Charles West School of Nursing, London, UK

Chapters 27 and 28

Cynthia B Edmond MSc GradDipEd BA RN RNT RM(Austr) CertAdmin (Austr) FRCNA MCNNSW
Freelance Lecturer/Clinical Nurse, Edinburgh, UK
Formerly Lecturer, Dept. of Health Occupations, University of Newcastle, New South Wales, Australia

Chapters 4, 11, 25 and 26

Jonathan J Sajiwandani BA MSc PhD
Senior Lecturer and Research and Development Centre Coordinator, Anglia Polytechnic University, Brentwood, UK

Chapters 10 and 29

Elizabeth M Stewart BSc(SocSci) RGN SCM RNT
Formerly Senior Lecturer, Glasgow Caledonian University, Glasgow, UK

Chapter 7

Janet M Walker PhD BSc RGN RM RHV CPsychol
Teaching Fellow, Department of Psychology, University of Southampton, Southampton, UK

Chapter 32

M C Wallington SRN RCNT DipN(A) CertEd
Lecturer in Nursing, Anglia Polytechnic University, Epping, UK

Chapter 14

Roger Watson BSc PhD RGN CBiol MIBiol
Lecturer, Department of Nursing Studies, University of Edinburgh, Edinburgh, UK

Chapters 6, 9 and 15

Preface

In developing this book I have wanted the reader to be left in no doubt at the intimate relationship between a firm grasp of the biological sciences and the intelligent practice of nursing. Many nursing students have sat in bewilderment and frustration in a physiology or anatomy class asking the question 'Why on earth am I learning *this*? How does it help me to be a better nurse? What have the intricacies of ionic movements in the nerve impulse or the names of the 12 cranial nerves got to do with the business of nursing?' It is all too easy for specialists to get carried away with their enthusiasms, or for particular elements of scientific dogma to be transmitted uncritically from year to year with only scant regard for the context in which knowledge is needed. This is a pity, as there is so much in the practice of nursing that is biology in action, and so much in biology that illuminates the practice of nursing.

The origins of this book lie in lively discussions several years ago with students of nursing in Manchester, some at the threshold of their careers, others in the thick of it. Engraved on my mind is the comment of one student, Debbie, in a tutorial: 'That may be right in theory, Sigrid, but it is not what patients complain of!' That comment and others like it have encouraged me to keep on asking questions about what I know as a bioscientist in the light of what others do and see and discover to be true in their working practice. This has been enormously interesting and illuminating. New doors and windows have opened in a house I thought I knew pretty well.

One of these 'new doors' opened as a result of contact with students of physiotherapy and speech therapy, whose professional needs dictated a greater focus on the neurosciences and an understanding of how we feel and move, think and speak. The unnatural split that has existed between physiology and psychology, whereby 'physiology' concentrated on intricacies of action potentials and synaptic mechanisms while 'psychology' dealt with the 'mind', has made it difficult for some students to see the purpose of some of the things they were learning in physiology, its relation to their own experience, as well as its significance for understanding the behaviour of patients in their care. My hope is that this book will make that less difficult. It contains more pages of neuroscience than usual, with the aim of cultivating a better understanding of the biology of people as persons, not just as bodies.

This is a new book with a new structure. Developments in understanding require always that textbooks reorder and reconstruct knowledge to reflect the changes in perspective flowing from them. For many years the structure of anatomy and physiology books for nurses was dominated by an anatomical framework in which the parts of the body were described and then their functions were explained. More recently, this traditional framework has evolved into a consideration of body systems and their relevant structure and functions. This book takes that process one stage further by going on to describe the way in which the systems of the body work together to create an inner stability as well as the capacity for us to interact with the world about us. This emphasis on integration of understanding is in line with current philosophy that seeks a holistic understanding of human life, a perspective that I share.

I hope this book may be useful at various stages of your course and future professional development. If you need a basic account of the parts and systems of the body, then you will find much of this in Section 1 and Part A of Sections 2 and 3. If you have the basics and want to move on to a broader and deeper understanding, select appropriate chapters in Parts B and C of Sections 2 and 3. Later on, Section 4, which focuses on the differences in biology between men and women, old and young, should provide an introduction to the biological basis of care of different individuals at various stages of their lives.

Whatever your specific needs, please read Chapter 1 first. It really does introduce what follows. It is not an amalgam of all those tedious but 'necessary' fundamentals that are sometimes assigned to an introductory chapter.

I hope you enjoy this book. Let us know what you like and dislike about it, what you see as its strengths as well as its shortcomings. You will then be contributing to the creation of the next edition just as other students through their probing questions and perceptive comments have contributed to this.

Macclesfield, 1994   SR

Acknowledgements

A whole host of people, knowingly and unknowingly, have contributed to the creation of this book: teachers, colleagues, students, friends and acquaintances. I am grateful to them all. Amongst them, those from a background in nursing and health care have undoubtedly played the most vital role in determining the overall shape and balance of the text. I am very pleased that so many people from different areas of practice have been involved. Early ideas grew out of interactions with staff and students of the Department of Nursing at the University of Manchester, and the then Schools of Physiotherapy at the Royal Infirmary and at Withington Hospital in Manchester. Ideas developed with the aid of feedback and encouragement from many people, including Pat Waddington, Gwen Broadhead, Jean McFarlane, Barbara Simpson, Karen Waters, Jane Merchant, Jean Minshull, Betty Oldham, Sandra Kitchen and Pat Phelps, as well as the reviewers enlisted by Churchill Livingstone. I am grateful to Moira Attree and Pat Wood, who were involved with the book in its very early stages, and Helen Bowyer who became involved for a short time later on.

The nurse contributors, whose names are listed elsewhere, have transformed ideas into reality. As well as adding their own specific contributions, their advice has been indispensable in determining the choice of material included and its presentation. The diversity of fascinating input they have injected into the text has immeasurably enriched it. I would like to record special thanks to Sue Coombes and Christopher Goodall who have borne the lion's share of the work, and whose continued enthusiasm and commitment from the first day we all signed up until now has been a source of great encouragement.

The specific content has been sharpened by the generous work of many colleagues (listed below), most from the School of Biological Sciences and the Faculty of Medicine at The University of Manchester. Each has reviewed drafts of one or more chapters linked with his/her own areas of interest, and has made many useful comments and suggestions most of which have been incorporated.

I am very grateful to all those authors and publishers, cited in the text, who have given permission to reproduce original material, particularly Churchill Livingstone the publishers of Rogers: *Textbook of Anatomy*. Where diagrams have been adapted from original work known to me, acknowledgement of their origins is made in the accompanying captions. In a few cases I have been unable to track down the original published source of an idea, and would welcome any leads that would enable due credit to be given in future.

On a personal note, I am indebted to two friends, Philip Gardner and Andrew Shackleton, whose crucial advice on the purchase of a suitable computer and software stood the test of time, multiple drafts and innumerable pages! Lastly my thanks to Sylvia James, for much conversation over many years about nursing and health care, for showing me different ways of looking and thinking, and for encouragement and patience through all the years that work on this book has invaded our home.

From *The University of Manchester*: Dr Mike Cheshire, Dr Fred Cody, Mr Blair Collister, Dr A.J.B. Emmerson, Dr David Evans, Prof Roger Green, Dr Richard Grencis, Dr Ewan Griffiths, Dr John Humpherson, Dr Ann Latham, Dr Roger Lendon, Dr Cathy McCrohan, Dr David Minors, Dr Paul O'Neill, Dr Sue Pannikker, The late Dr Derek Paul, Dr Helen Richardson, Dr Kathleen Rowsell, Dr Evelyn Russell, Dr Nancy Rothwell, Dr Colin Sibley, Dr Nalim Thakkar, Ms Janet Vale, Dr Tony Wareham, Dr James Waterhouse, Dr Peter Willan, Dr J.A.L. Yin.

From *Bournmouth University*: Dr Martyn Brimble.

From *Deakin University, Australia*: Mrs Ingrid Coles-Rutishauser.

Section 1
HUMAN BEINGS:
BIOLOGICAL PERSPECTIVES

Section Contents

Chapter 1 introduces the whole book. It explains the basis of the approach adopted and outlines the structure flowing from it. Read this chapter before delving into the rest of the book.

Chapters 2 and 3 introduce several important biological concepts including:

- cell structure and activity
- control systems and homeostasis
- endocrine and neural mechanisms.

Chapter 1
Introduction

HEALTH

'I can see purple and green spots,' said Sylvia, looking mildly euphoric. 'My legs feel odd. They feel as if they have grown longer, and they seem to have a mind of their own!' We were up in the mountains of Austria 3000 metres above sea-level, and had been walking for several hours. The village we were staying at was quite a distance away. I was worried. This was no place to become ill. Sylvia had seemed perfectly well when we set out earlier in the day. Indeed only the previous week someone had commented that she looked 'the picture of health'.

DEFINITIONS

What is meant by 'health'? What is being described when someone is said to 'look the picture of health'? Sylvia, whose experience is described above, was indeed in 'good health' back home, at 150 metres above sea-level. She not only looked healthy, she was healthy, as judged by her ability to cope with her busy round of activities in employment and at home. But whisked a few thousand metres up into the mountains, it was clear that her body was not coping fully with the unusual stresses created by high altitude.

The vivid and attractive kaleidoscope of imagined green and purple spots she saw was abnormal. Her overly carefree pattern of walking and apparent lack of concern at its riskiness on a narrow mountain path were certainly uncharacteristic. The things that she noticed, and the changes apparent to me, were *symptoms* and *signs*, respectively, of her body's reactions to the unusual stresses imposed on it.

Sylvia was experienceing *ill-health* because her body was unable to meet completely the challenges of her new environment. Usually, ill-health is experienced under normal environmental conditions when defects of body function exist or develop. However, in either case, the individual is unable to cope fully with the circumstances he or she meets.

Health may therefore be defined as a state in which someone is able to adjust to, and successfully cope with, the many and various challenges he or she encounters in daily living.

STRESSORS AND STABILITY

From the moment of conception to the time of dealth, our lives consist of challenge and change. The ability to cope with change and to adapt to it is a primary characteristic of any living thing. Any factor, internal or external, that acts on the body and disturbs it in some way acts as a *stressor*. It could be a change in room temperature, the desiccating effects of going without a drink, or simply getting out of bed in the morning.

In health, the initial disturbance, produced by the stressor, triggers a set of compensatory reactions which minimise the extent to which the internal state of the body as a whole is actually disturbed (Fig. 1.1). By this *negative feedback*, an inner stability is preserved in the face of many internal and external changes. The maintenance of this inner stability in the face of challenge is termed *homeostasis* (Ch. 3).

When we are healthy these compensatory adjustments are so effective that they usually pass unnoticed. We go about our day to day lives with relatively little awareness of the myriad biological processes contributing to our well-being. However, when a part of the body is no longer working properly, or when, as in the example above, body systems are inadequate for the circumstances faced, then we become acutely aware of

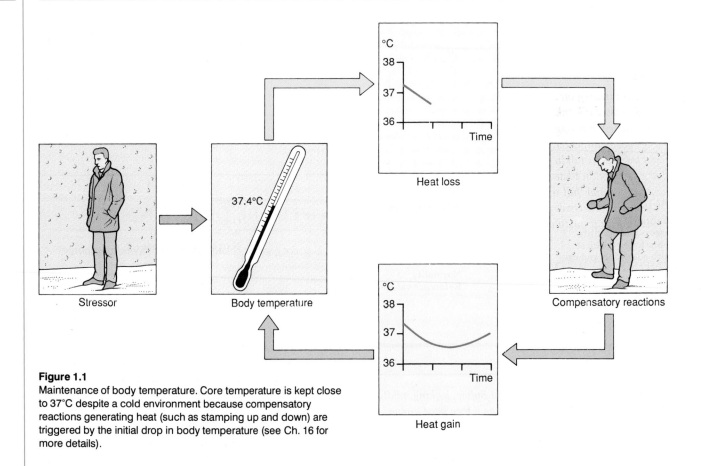

Figure 1.1
Maintenance of body temperature. Core temperature is kept close to 37°C despite a cold environment because compensatory reactions generating heat (such as stamping up and down) are triggered by the initial drop in body temperature (see Ch. 16 for more details).

some aspects of body function. At the very least we will 'feel' different (as Sylvia did), and at worst we become seriously ill.

ADAPTATION AND FITNESS

Stressors disturb body function, but they also stimulate *adaptation*. This is the long-term adjustments in biological systems whereby the body develops an increased capacity to cope with the stressors encountered. For example, after a few weeks living at high altitude an individual is much better adapted to this novel environment than on arrival (see Chs 11 and 12). Similarly, the stressors acting on the person who chooses to take up jogging are the very factors which initiate the development of improved muscular strength and endurance (see Ch. 17). By adapting to stressors we develop *fitness* appropriate to our new circumstances.

Stressors therefore should not be thought of as entirely bad. They are natural components of any normal life and vital to the development of fitness.

HEALTH EDUCATION AND CARE

To maintain good health the conditions in which we live must be kept within tolerable limits. Stressors are un-

avoidable, and even necessary, but an excess is harmful. Exercise, for example, is vital for good health, but excessive physical activity can be damaging. It is therefore important for everyone to be aware of factors contributing to health, and those that threaten it. Health professionals contribute specialised knowledge, as for example about the structure (*anatomy*) and functioning (*physiology*) of the human body, and must be able to explain its relevance for healthy living to others.

In assisting a person who is ill, the interventions of the health care team are directed towards restoring health as quickly as possible. This is achieved by working with, and not against, the body's own restorative processes. Neumann's model of health care (1982) (see also Ch. 19) identifies three elements:

● avoiding unhelpful stressors
● supplementing and supporting body function (until health is restored)
● strengthening body mechanisms (against future stressors of the same kind).

In order to provide intelligent care and therapy all members of the health care team need to understand how the human body works, its limitations, and the ways in which it reacts and adapts to stressors of different kinds.

A HOLISTIC VIEW

'My foot hurts,' said Simon, tears streaming down his face. He had been jumping off his favourite wall and had landed badly and twisted his ankle. His mother gathered him up, distress mingled with anger at the way he had ignored her warnings yet again. Later that afternoon Simon didn't feel like any tea. His foot didn't feel so bad but he felt hurt inside. He knew he shouldn't have jumped, and his guilt made him feel withdrawn and 'full up inside'. He pushed the plate of baked beans away. Usually he would have wolfed them down but today things were different.

MINDS AND BODIES

Our bodies consist of an interdependent society of cells (Ch. 2), grouped together into tissues and organs (Chs 4–10 and 20–29). If one part is injured or not working properly then the activity of other parts changes too. Restoration of health involves not only the diagnosis and treatment of the specific cause of an injury or illness (the hurt ankle in the example above) but also management of its several repercussions. These include the psychological dimensions of human living too.

Minds and bodies are not separate. The cells making up the human brain (Chs 20 and 21) are no different in their basic characteristics from any other cells in the body. Thinking, feeling and responding are all physical processes, admittedly complex and incompletely understood, but none the less subject to the same physical and chemical laws as any other parts of our bodies. To understand human health fully it is necessary therefore to be familiar with the biological basis of human experience and behaviour (Chs 20–33), as well as with the principles of homeostasis (Chs 3 and 11–19).

EXPERIENCE AND BEHAVIOUR

Disturbed thoughts and feelings are just as real as a twisted ankle and need to be treated with the same respect, objectivity, and informed care. Simon's loss of appetite and feelings of fullness were a physical expression of his guilt. He saw that his mother was angry. The pain of his hurt ankle reminded him of what had happened that morning and he remembered her words to him, telling him not to jump off that wall again. In his mind he knew he had disobeyed, and his awareness of that fact created the emotional discomfort that was putting him off his food.

Seeing, hearing, feeling, remembering and reacting all depend upon the activity of cells in the nervous system. Simon's experience of the day's events and his reactions to them would have been different if any nerve cells had functioned in a different way. If nerves carrying infor-

mation from his ankle to the brain had not transmitted signals he would not have felt pain (see Chs 23 and 32). If connections had not been forged between cells in the association areas of the cerebral cortex as a result of his experiences (see Chs 23 and 30) he would not have remembered what had happened (see Ch. 33). If parts of the autonomic nervous system (see Ch. 3) and limbic system (see Ch. 31) had been functioning differently he might have been ravenous rather than off his food.

PEOPLE ARE DIFFERENT

Ann looked a ghastly colour. Maybe a differently coloured nighty would have improved her appearance. I made a mental note that pale green was not the best choice for someone recovering from major surgery. Ann didn't hear me as I closed the door. The sedative effect of the anaesthetic had not yet worn off. I sat down alongside her, studied her features, and hoped that all had gone well. I looked curiously at the tubes 'in' and 'out' – the drip into her hand and the drain discreetly shrouded by the bedclothes. She was breathing quietly. Superimposed on the slow rhythm of her breathing was a steady throbbing of a vein in her neck. 'Heart's OK,' I thought! Later on, I thought again about that throbbing. It wasn't usual for her. It didn't look 'normal'.

NORMALITY

Just as we refer to health without necessarily stopping to define exactly what we mean, so we refer to things looking 'normal' without giving it a second thought. In popular language 'normal' means 'usual', 'customary' or 'natural'. In scientific usage 'normal' means 'conforming to the usual pattern'.

For an adult person aged 35 a blood pressure of 120/80 mmHg would be considered normal (see Ch. 5), and that was the value recorded on the chart at the bottom of Ann's bed, but it was not 'normal' for her. If note had been taken of her usual resting blood pressure in health (100/65 mmHg) it would have been recognised much sooner that her arterial blood pressure was raised, and that the throbbing in her neck (due to raised circulatory pressure) was due to fluid overload of the circulation. Later that same day her saline drip had been discontinued, her bladder had been catheterised to relieve urinary retention, and her blood pressure was reassuringly 'back to normal' (100/65 mmHg).

No two people are exactly the same. Even identical twins, though genetically identical, will have developed slightly different characteristics because their activities and experiences will not have been exactly the same. The fact that each of us is different is obvious in everyday life but textbooks of biology often make us all seem exactly the same.

REFERENCE VALUES

In describing 'normal' function, textbooks refer to the average for a large group of people (*population* in statistical terms). As at one time many data were collected by researchers from their students, it became customary to refer to the average 70 kg man (typical of a young adult male in the UK or USA). Others have used the standard of a reference man (65 kg) or woman (55 kg) (Durnin & Passmore 1967).

Sometimes *normal ranges* are quoted. This is a statistical term defining the normal range of values expected for 95% of a population (Fig. 1.2). For example, if the normal range for resting diastolic blood pressure for a woman in her 30s is stated as 72 to 87 mmHg, 95 out of 100 healthy women would have blood pressures within this range. However, 5 out of 100 healthy women would have blood pressures lower or higher than this, as Ann did. This would be entirely normal for them, though not for most women.

Knowing just one fact about a person is of course not very helpful. A shorter than average man weighing 70 kg might be obese, whereas a very tall man could be underweight for his height. Each piece of information needs to be set alongside other relevant facts and figures.

Reference values are necessary for judgement to be made about the health of an individual but always remember that:

- each person is actually unique
- there are differences at different stages of life (see Chs 34–37)

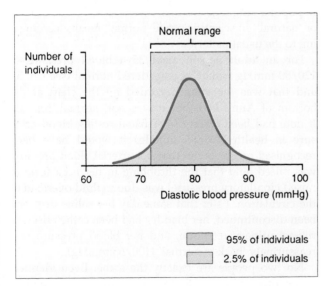

Figure 1.2
Typical distribution of diastolic blood pressures in a very large group (population) of healthy adults. In statistical terms, the values are said to follow a normal distribution. The normal range is by definition that which encompasses 95% of the population, as shown.

- there are differences between people of different gender, culture and ethnic origin
- an unexpected change for an individual is more informative than how he or she compares with someone else.

THIS BOOK

ORGANISATION

The three themes of:

- stability in the face of challenge (homeostasis)
- sensing, doing and thinking as well as existing
- variation in structure and function

form the basic framework around which this book has been structured. After introductory chapters in Section 1, describing some fundamental concepts in human biology (cells and systems of control), the three main sections (Sections 2, 3 and 4) focus in turn upon:

- systems maintaining the internal environment (homeostasis)
- systems enabling our interaction with the external environment (biological basis of experience and behaviour)
- changes in our bodies from birth to death (life cycle).

Sections 2 and 3, 'The internal environment and its maintenance' and 'Interaction with the external environment' have both been structured in the same way. The first few chapters of each section (Part A) describe the structure of relevant organs, tissues and cells, what they do and how they work. The middle chapters (Part B) show how different organs and tissues work together to achieve a particular goal, be it stabilising body temperature (Ch. 16), or enabling you to see this book (Ch. 26) or turn over its pages (Ch. 28). The last few chapters of each section (Part C) focus on particular aspects of daily living, such as exercise (Ch. 17), sleep (Ch. 31) and learning (Ch. 34), and bring together the various cells, systems and processes involved.

Sections 2 and 3 of the book concentrate on structure (*anatomy*) and function (*physiology*) in adult persons in general. Differences between men and women, and between young and old, are detailed in the final section (Section 4; Chs 34–37) which describes the process of reproduction as well as the changes occurring in our bodies from the moment of conception to the day of death.

WHERE TO BEGIN

Although the chapters of the book have been planned in a logical sequence, beginning in Section 1 with cells and ending in Section 4 with descriptions of the body as a whole at different stages of life, the chapters can be read independently of one another. Each chapter is cross-referenced to related topics in other parts of the book so that, if you need to follow up information about subjects with which you are unfamiliar, you should be able to find the information fairly easily.

There is a detailed list of contents at the beginning of each chapter. Using this, together with the index, should enable you to find material relevant to your present topic of study whether it be part of a college course in human biology or your own researches prompted by your nursing care. A basic knowledge of human biology to the equivalent of 'O' level standard has been assumed. If you want to brush up on some basic science then an excellent book to use with this text is *A textbook of science for the health professions* by Hinwood (1992).

Suggestions for further reading are listed at the end of each chapter, together with a short description of each text so that you can tell whether it is one that may be suitable for your particular needs.

NURSING APPLICATIONS

We hope that as you read this book you will apply its contents to your own situation as you seek to promote health, work with people who are disabled, and care for those who are ill. Each chapter includes some examples that have come to our minds of the ways in which physiology and anatomy relate specifically to nursing care. Some are boxed off from the text so that you can read them separately if you want to; others are included in the text if they provide a brief example of the science being described. The purpose of all the nursing applications and points is to shed light on the intimate links between the biological sciences and nursing care, to demystify science and to stimulate your own thinking. We hope that as you read this book and reflect on your own practice as a health professional you will discover many more, and will have the courage to work out and apply the implications within the scope of your daily work.

By reflecting on what you see and do, in the light of what you learn, you will improve the standard of care that you are able to offer and enhance your own job satisfaction.

KEY POINTS

What you should now begin to understand about physiology and anatomy:

- why knowledge of these subjects is essential for delivery of quality health care
- how health and fitness may be defined in biological terms
- how knowledge of physiology and anatomy helps in understanding human experience and behaviour, as well as bodily structure and function
- what standard values quoted in textbooks mean in relation to the uniqueness of every individual.

REFERENCES AND FURTHER READING

Durnin J V G A, Passmore R 1967 Energy, work and leisure. Heinemann, London

George J (ed) 1990 Nursing theories: the base for professional nursing practice, 3rd edn. Prentice-Hall International, New Jersey
(Summarises the work of 18 nurse theorists, including Betty Neumann, and describes the background to the development of their theories)

Hinwood B 1992 A textbook of science for the health professions. Chapman & Hall, London
(A comprehensive, well referenced and illustrated, easy to read book. Extremely useful as a supplementary text to follow up the basic sciences)

Jeffries P 1983 Mathematics in nursing, 6th edn. Nurses Aid Series, Baillière Tindall, London
(Ch. 16, pp 179–199, 'Statistics' provides a simple introduction to the subject and ideas for trying out the theory in practice)

Neumann B 1982 The Neumann systems model: application to nursing education and practice. Appleton-Century-Crofts, East Norwalk, Connecticut

Pearson A, Vaughan B 1991 Nursing models for practice. Butterworth-Heinemann, Oxford
(Very readable book describing what nursing models are and how they may be applied. Ch. 8, pp 105–123, describes 'The health care systems model for nursing' based on Neumann's ideas)

Chapter 2
CELLS

Each of us begins life as single cell created by the fusion of an ovum and a sperm. Contained within this cell is all the information necessary to dictate the form and function of all the other cells of which our bodies are ultimately composed.

Each cell is made up of an immense variety of molecules, including lipids, proteins and nucleic acids, whose characteristics determine the structure and activities of the different parts of the cell. Cells are dynamic self-replicating structures whose life-cycle and activities are influenced by their environment and by specific regulatory factors released by other cells. The cells of our bodies live in community, linked together to form tissues and maintained by the extracellular matrix in which they are embedded.

THE CELL AS A MOLECULAR SOCIETY

The cell can be likened to a society, the individual members of which are the atoms, molecules and ions of which it is composed (Fig. 2.1). Like people, atoms and molecules group together to form units, whose features and activities depend upon the characteristics of the members. Groupings of atoms and molecules depend, as in human society, on the affinities between individuals, and on the bonds which exist between them. The groupings are dynamic: new members are added; others are lost. Yet the basic organisation remains intact despite the turnover of individual parts. ①

① *What is the difference between affinity and bond?*

MOLECULAR ASSOCIATIONS

Affinities

Molecules can be divided into two overlapping groups (Fig. 2.2A):

- *hydrophilic* (water-loving) – those with an affinity for a water environment
- *hydrophobic* (water-hating).

Hydrophobic molecules often prefer to associate with fatty substances and are then called *lipophilic* (fat-loving).

The affinities between molecules are created by the properties of their individual atoms and the way in

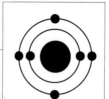

Atoms

Atoms consist of:
    protons (positively charged)
    neutrons
    electrons (negatively charged).
Number of protons = number of electrons
therefore an atom is uncharged overall.

Ions

An **atom** that gains or loses an electron is an **ion**.
Ions may have a positive charge (+) **cations**
or a negative charge (-) **anions**.

Atom	Symbol		Ion
Sodium	Na	Na minus an electron	Na^+
Chorine	Cl	Cl plus an electron	Cl^-
Hydrogen	H	H minus an electron	H^+
Carbon	C	C does not form an ion	

Molecules

A Molecule consists of atoms linked together by chemical
bonds caused by the interchange of electrons.
The type of bond formed depends on how the atoms share
their electrons.

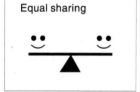

Equal sharing — produces a **covalent** bond

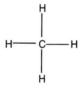

Unequal sharing 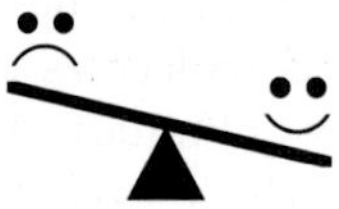 — makes the bonds **polar** e.g. oxygen has more than its fair share of the electrons in this molecule

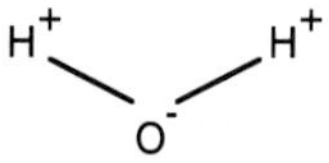

One way donation produces no sharing but irresistible attraction — two ions of opposite charge form an **ionic** bond. e.g. Na^+Cl^-

Figure 2.1 (above)
Structure of an atom and meaning of the terms ion and molecule.
The bonds formed between atoms in molecules are of several
different types: covalent, polar and ionic.

Figure 2.2 (right and facing page)
Water-loving (hydrophilic) and water-hating (hydrophobic)
molecules, and those with sympathies both ways (amphipathic):
A Characteristics and examples of each type (right)

Water molecules are polar
and are attracted towards
one another because of the
slight difference in charge
between the O of one and
the H of the other. These
bonds are termed
hydrogen bonds.
Ions have an affinity for
water molecules because
of the attractiveness of the
opposite charges. Ions are
hydrophilic.

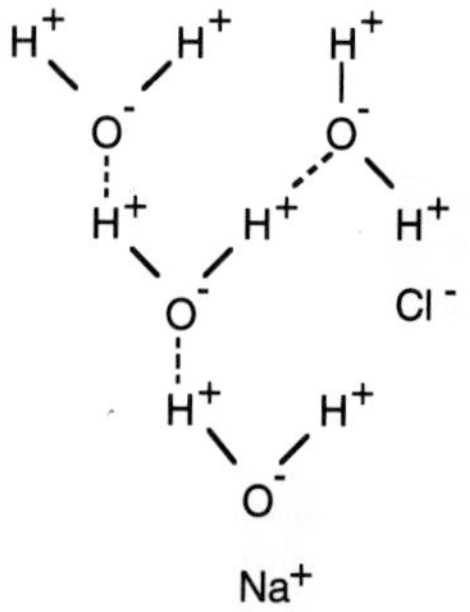

Other molecules that have
polar bonds also have an
afffinity for water.
In glucose oxygen doesn't
share equally with the other
atoms.
In ethanoic acid the
oxygens exert such a
strong pull on the electron
that hydrogen easily gives
it up and becomes a
cation.

glucose

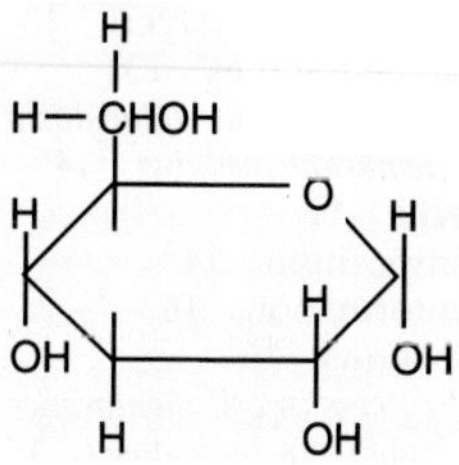

ethanoic acid (vinegar)

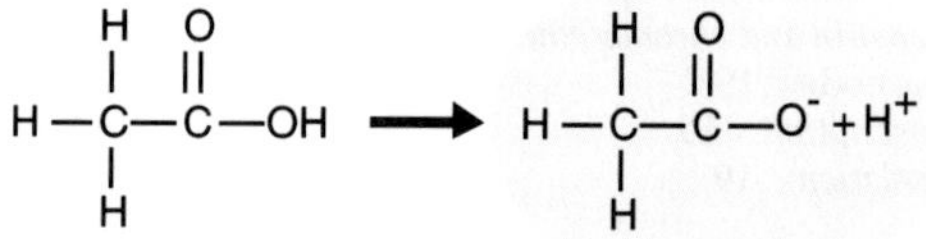

Hydrocarbons consist
solely of hydrogen and
carbon atoms. They share
electrons equally.
Therefore all the bonds are
non-polar.
There is no attraction
therefore between a
molecule of this kind and
water. It is **hydrophobic**.

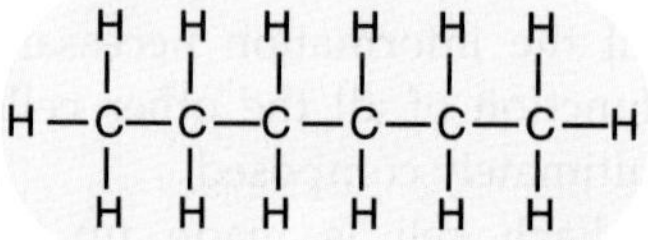

Molecules that are dominated by bonds of this kind
are also non-polar and therefore hydrophobic e.g.
triglycerides (fat).

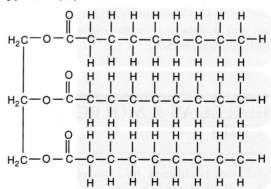

Phospholipids are **amphipathic**. Part of the molecule is hydrophilic; part is hydrophobic.

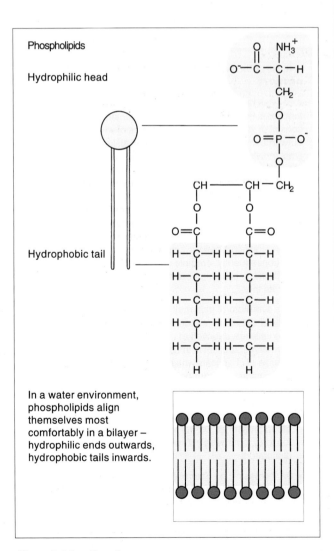

Hydrophilic   **Hydrophobic**

B

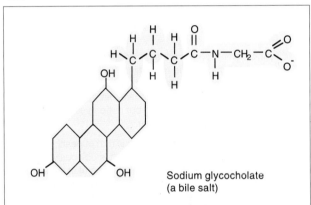

Sodium glycocholate
(a bile salt)

In its three-dimensional structure all the polar groups are on the same side of the molecule. These molecules are most comfortably arranged with their lipophilic side facing a fatty environment and their hydrophilic side facing a water environment.

lipophilic
side

hydrophilic
side

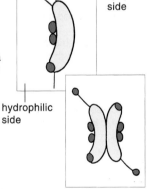

Phospholipid-bile salt **micelle**

Longitudinal section   Cross-section

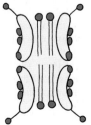   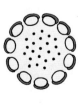

Phospholipids

Hydrophilic head

Hydrophobic tail

In a water environment, phospholipids align themselves most comfortably in a bilayer – hydrophilic ends outwards, hydrophobic tails inwards.

Figure 2.2 (*continued*)
B The way in which amphipathic molecules, such as bile salts and phospholipids, arrange themselves in a water environment to form micelles and bilayers.

which electrons are shared between them. If the sharing is unequal the molecule, such as water, is *polar* and has an affinity for other molecules with similar characteristics, such as glucose and ethanoic acid (vinegar). All these are hydrophilic.

Hydrophobic molecules, like hydrocarbons (Fig. 2.2A) have little in common with water because their atoms share electrons equally and there are no points of attraction for water. Consequently a triglyceride, which possesses three very long hydrocarbon chains, is almost completely insoluble in water. The triglyceride molecules prefer to associate with one another and separate en masse from the water molecules to form a different layer, just as oil separates from vinegar, if they are mixed together.

Amphipathic molecules

Hydrophilic and lipophilic molecules represent two extremes of affinity. In between are many molecules, such as phospholipids, which possess, *in part*, each of these characteristics (*amphipathic molecules*). These act as a 'bridge' between the two groups. Another example is sodium glycocholate (Fig. 2.2B), one of the bile salts which is used in the digestion and absorption of fats (see Ch. 6). Parts of the molecule are hydrophilic; other parts are lipophilic. Consequently sodium glycocholate is able to interact both with water molecules and with fat molecules and can promote the intermingling of the two enabling the fat to be dispersed in the water. The fat is not completely dissolved however. It is dispersed in the form of tiny droplets (*micelles*) consisting of fat molecules and bile salts.

Many amphipathic molecules in the cell associate with one another in a similar way except that their association often creates layers of molecules rather than micelles. This is true for phospholipids (Fig. 2.2B).

THE RELATIONSHIP OF THE CELL TO NURSING ACTIVITY

A cell has been defined as the basic living, structural and functional unit of all organisms. The human body is said to consist of 75 trillion cells, the activities of which are largely outwith our control. It is remarkable that, for most of the time, individual cells function normally; coping with natural wear and tear, various toxic/allergenic agents and pathogenic organisms which gain entry to the body, and our own indiscretions such as overeating. Should the cells become unable to cope, the altered body function is noticeable in the form of signs and symptoms which nurses are frequently asked by patients to explain. An understanding of cellular function makes explanation easier and, consequently, credible and reassuring to the patient. The following simplified examples have been chosen to illustrate this:

● The symptom of pain may be experienced as a result of cellular activity in response to restricted blood supply. The cells are deprived of their source of oxygen and normal metabolism is impaired. Cell damage results in the release of chemicals which stimulate pain receptors. To demonstrate this, put on a blood pressure cuff, inflate it to restrict arterial blood flow, then exercise your forearm – pain will be experienced very rapidly. This is worth remembering when difficulty is experienced in recording blood pressures. Do not maintain inflation of the cuff for too long, otherwise you will increase the patient's discomfort.

● An increasing number of people are sensitive to substances entering the bloodstream. Certain foods (shellfish, strawberries) and drugs (penicillin, aspirin) may cause skin rashes and more serious symptoms. The allergen to which the person is allergic (sensitive) causes histamine and other substances to be released from tissue mast cells (see Chs 5 and 15). A mild response may cause local dilation of blood vessels in the skin, with leakage of fluid into spaces between the cells causing signs such as redness and swelling (*hives*) and symptoms of itching and mild pain. This knowledge enables the nurse to explain why antihistamine tablets are more effective than antihistamine ointment which will temporarily relieve local itching but not prevent the more generalised release of histamine.

One of the many roles of the nurse is that of health educator for patients and their families. It is obviously not always relevant to offer detailed explanations of cellular function but the nurse should have the knowledge as a basis for her teaching. Here are two examples:

● There is a move towards the use of unleaded petrol in cars as a result of reports that high concentrations of atmospheric lead may retard mental development in young children. Think about the proximity of babies and toddlers in push chairs to exhaust fumes from cars when out shopping with adults! The organic lead alkyls which escape into the atmosphere are more toxic than the inorganic compounds (e.g. lead bromide) because their lipophilic property allows them to cross the blood–brain barrier (see Ch. 20) and enter cells within the brain. Organic lead is capable of interfering with the proper function of some cells. Fortunately, the majority of the body's unwanted lead usually accumulates in bone.

● It is well known that chronic alcoholism causes damage to the liver (*cirrhosis*). Many families support and care for heavy drinkers and consult the community nurse for advice. Liver cells require adequate protein in the diet to function properly, particularly to metabolise fat. The body is not able to synthesise all amino acids (Table 2.1) and methionine is essential to liver cells for fat metabolism. Its absence from the diet causes fat to accumulate with eventual damage to the structure of the liver. The connection with chronic alcoholism is that a high alcohol intake reduces interest in food, probably because the high calorie content of alcohol suppresses appetite. Malnutrition often results. The nurse can use this knowledge to give dietary advice to carers.

LIPID BARRIERS

Phospholipid bilayers

The hydrocarbon chains of phospholipids are lipophilic, whereas the phosphate groups at the other end of the molecule are strongly hydrophilic. The most 'comfortable' arrangement for these molecules, when they exist in a water environment, is for the phosphate groups to associate with the water molecules and for the hydrocarbon chains to face one another. A *phospholipid bilayer* is formed.

Bilayers of this kind are found in many places in the cell. Under the microscope they can be seen as boundaries (*membranes*) separating different parts of the cell.

Cell membranes

The boundary of the cell itself is the *plasma membrane*. Other membranes are organised into different structures (*organelles*) within the cell (Fig. 2.3). These organelles include:

- nucleus
- endoplasmic reticulum
- Golgi apparatus
- lysosomes
- peroxisomes.

The space between the organelles is filled with *cytosol* which consists chiefly of proteins, water and ions.

> A boundary consisting of cells or tissue is also often described as a membrane, e.g. the cells lining the mouth (mucous membrane), or the vibrating membrane of the inner ear (basilar membrane; see Ch. 25). Their composition is different.

ABSORPTION OF DRUGS

The phospholipid bilayer enables some drugs to pass through cell membranes into the cell interior. Highly liposoluble drugs like thiopentone, dicoumarol and griseofulvin diffuse rapidly though the bilayer and readily attain a high concentration inside cells. It is important to note, however, that such drugs must also be sufficiently water-soluble to dissolve in body fluids if they are to reach their target cells. Liposoluble drugs taken orally need to dissolve in the fluids of the gastrointestinal tract to be available for absorption. Controlled release drugs are designed to dissolve slowly in the gastrointestinal fluids to provide uniform absorption over a long period.

Although diagrams frequently give the impression that cell organelles are completely distinct from one another, this is not always true. The membrane surrounding the nucleus is in fact continuous with that of the endoplasmic reticulum. Also, membrane-bound vesicles are continually being incorporated into the plasma membrane, and being formed from it as a result of the twin processes of *exocytosis* and *endocytosis* (Fig. 2.4).

Exocytosis and endocytosis

In exocytosis, a vesicle fuses with the plasma membrane and its contents are released to the cell exterior. The membrane of the vesicle becomes part of the existing plasma membrane. This would grow ever larger if

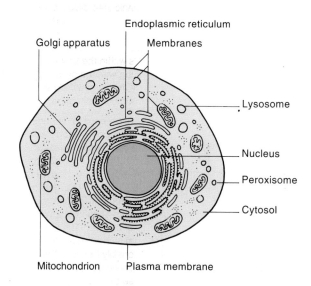

Figure 2.3
The cell and its structures.

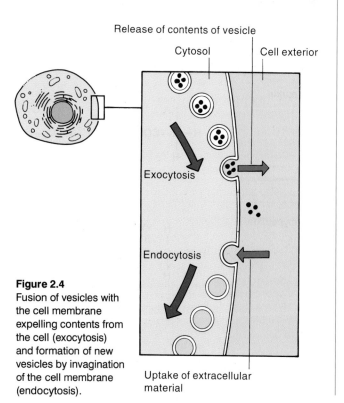

Figure 2.4
Fusion of vesicles with the cell membrane expelling contents from the cell (exocytosis) and formation of new vesicles by invagination of the cell membrane (endocytosis).

simultaneously membrane were not being removed at other sites by endocytosis.

In endocytosis a small area of plasma membrane is drawn inwards (*invaginates*) and the membranes at the mouth of the invagination fuse to form a vesicle enclosing a tiny droplet of fluid from outside the cell.

> Secretory cells in the digestive glands (see Ch. 6) secrete digestive enzymes by exocytosis. White blood cells (leucocytes; see Chs 4 and 15) are able to engulf relatively large particles, bacteria and even other cells by endocytosis (known then as *phagocytosis*).

Membrane proteins

Cell membranes do not consist just of a lipid bilayer. If they did, they would act as a very effective barrier to the movement of water-soluble substances, but they would permit very little else to happen. Inserted into and associated with the various membranes of the cell are numerous proteins. This is possible because parts of the protein molecules are lipophilic and can interact with the lipid bilayer. Proteins convert phospholipid bilayers into highly selective, sensitive, and active systems.

PROTEINS

Composition

Proteins consist of chains of *amino acids* linked by *peptide bonds* (Fig. 2.5A). 20 different amino acids are found commonly in cells and tissues (Table 2.1). They differ from one another chemically in that they may be:

- acidic, basic or neutral (see Ch. 12)
- predominantly hydrophilic or hydrophobic.

An almost infinite number of different proteins can be formed from these 20 different building blocks.

Table 2.1 Amino acids

Acidic	Basic	Neutral		
Aspartic acid	Arginine	Alanine	Valine	Phenylalanine
Glutamic acid	Histidine	Glycine	Leucine	Tryptophan
	Lysine	Serine	Isoleucine	
		Threonine	Cysteine	
		Asparagine	Methionine	
		Glutamine	Tyrosine	
		Proline		
STRONGLY HYDROPHILIC		MIXED PROPERTIES		STRONGLY HYDROPHOBIC

Following injuries, such as burns, where tissue has to be renewed, a high protein diet may be prescribed. This will supplement the body's production of amino acids.

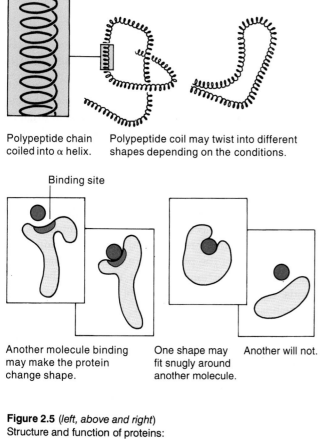

B

Polypeptide chain coiled into α helix.

Polypeptide coil may twist into different shapes depending on the conditions.

Binding site

Another molecule binding may make the protein change shape.

One shape may fit snugly around another molecule.

Another will not.

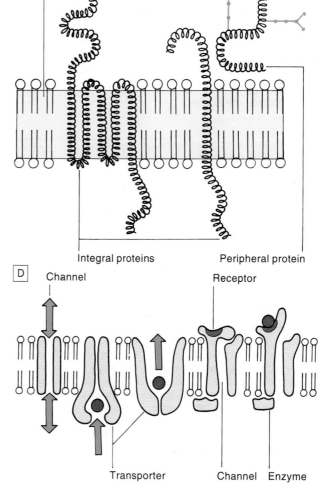

C

Hydrophobic interior

Carbohydrate

Integral proteins

Peripheral protein

D

Channel

Receptor

Transporter

Channel

Enzyme

Figure 2.5 (*left, above and right*)
Structure and function of proteins:
A Examples of different types of amino acids and how they are linked by peptide bonds to form polypeptides (*left*)
B Shapes adopted by proteins; how they change and why it matters (*above*)
C Position and arrangement of proteins in cell membranes (*right*)
D Some of the functions performed by proteins in cell membranes (*right*).

Conformation

The very long chains of amino acids can fold up into distinctive conformations (Fig. 2.5B) because of the affinity for one another of different chemical groupings on the amino acids. The shape assumed is crucial to the function of that protein in the cell. It will determine the chemical groups that are exposed to other molecules and the ones that are hidden within the interior of the protein.

The shape can change. One factor that is crucial is the concentration of hydrogen ions (H^+) in the vicinity (see Ch. 12). H^+ ions associate with chemical groupings on the amino acids, and in so doing alter their affinity for one another. As a result the protein changes its shape. This in turn will affect the way in which it is able to react with other molecules (Fig. 2.5B)

Functions

Proteins in cell membranes

The proteins which associate with cell membranes (Fig. 2.5C) are divided into two groups:

- integral
- peripheral.

The integral proteins are lodged relatively firmly within the phospholipid bilayer, anchored by lipophilic groups on the outer part of the protein. Many of these proteins span the membrane from side to side. Peripheral proteins are more loosely associated. Most are bound to integral proteins either outside or inside the cell. Some peripheral proteins are *glycoproteins* (proteins bonded to carbohydrate molecules).

②
Why do white cells move through tissues?

HOW DRUGS ACT

Some drugs act by binding to proteins. In so doing they alter the functional ability of the protein and thereby increase or decrease the processes reliant on it. The name of one group of drugs, the monoamine oxidase inhibitors (MAOIs), explains how they act. These drugs, which are used in the treatment of depression, inhibit (stop) the oxidation (a form of processing) of monoamines by binding to the enzyme monoamine oxidase (MAO). Some of the amines concerned are the neurotransmitters adrenaline, noradrenaline, serotonin and dopamine (see Chs 3 and 21). The result is an increase in the concentrations of these neurotransmitters and stimulation of their receptors; for some people there is an improvement in mood. However, excess adrenaline also causes a marked rise in blood pressure (*hypertension*), headache and abnormalities of heart activity. Other amines which are taken into the body in food and proprietary cold cures also accumulate because they too cannot be broken down. Patients for whom these drugs are prescribed are therefore given a list of 'banned' foods (e.g. cheese, yeast and meat extracts, broad beans, alcohol and proprietary cold cures) all of which contain high proportions of amines.

The proteins associated with cell membranes have many different functions (Fig. 2.5D). They can act as:

- *channels* through which small water-soluble molecules and ions can pass through the bilayer
- *transporters* that bind to molecules dissolved in the water environment on one side of the membrane and carry them through the membrane to the other side
- *enzymes* which catalyse specific chemical reactions
- *receptors* which detect hormones and neurotransmitters and control cell activity (see later)
- *markers* of cell identity.

Proteins in the cytosol

Some of these are enzymes which catalyse specific chemical reactions (e.g. glycogen synthase catalyses the formation of glycogen from glucose). Others form structures which act as a 'skeleton' for the cell (*cytoskeleton*). These include tubulin which forms *microtubules*, and actin which forms *microfilaments*. These structures are also involved in causing movement, both of the cell as a whole and of structures within the cell, in:

- cell division
- muscle contraction (see Ch. 22)
- shunting of vesicles from place to place inside the cell
- movement of white cells through the tissues (see Ch. 15).②

A pair of structures known as the *centriole pair*, formed of tubulin, is believed to be involved in organising the cytoskeleton. It is important also in cell division (see Fig. 2.10).

Formation

Amino acids are linked together to form polypeptides and proteins at *ribosomes* (see later). Ribosomes are composed of a collection of several different molecules including specific proteins and polynucleotides (see below). Some of the proteins are enzymes that catalyse the chemical reactions involved in linking the amino acids together. The sequence of amino acids in the protein is determined by a 'plan', that is fed through the ribosome and translated into protein structure. The plan is *messenger RNA* (ribonucleic acid) which is a transcript of part of the master plan (genetic code) stored in *DNA* (deoxyribonucleic acid).

NUCLEIC ACIDS

Composition

Nucleic acids such as RNA and DNA both consist of chains of *nucleotides*. A nucleotide (Fig. 2.6A) consists of three component parts:

base + sugar + phosphate

(continued on facing page)

A

Bases

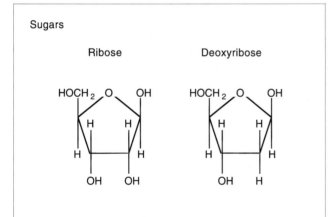

Adenine (A)   Guanine (G)   Cytosine (C)   Uracil (U)   Thymine (T)

Purines   Pyrimidines

Nucleotide

NH₂

Base

Phosphate

Sugar

Sugars

Ribose   Deoxyribose

B   Nucleotides are linked by phosphodiester bonds to form a polynucleotide (nucleic acid).

Nucleic acid (fragment of RNA)

Figure 2.6
Composition and structure of DNA and RNA:
A Basic structure of a nucleotide and the different sugars and bases of which it may be composed
B Structure of a nucleic acid

(continued from previous page)
There are five different bases:

- two purines
  - adenine (A)
  - guanine (G)
- three pyrimidines
  - cytosine (C)
  - uracil (U) (RNA only)
  - thymine (T) (DNA only).

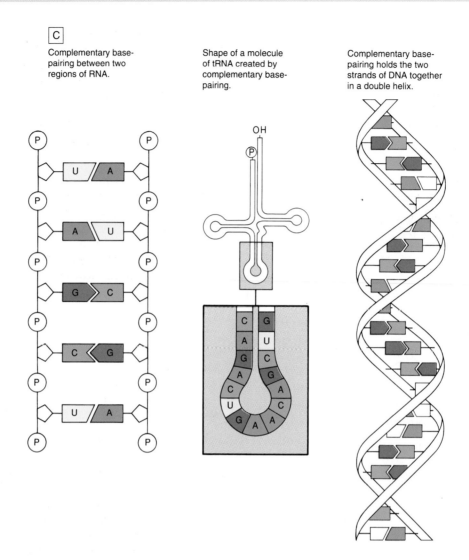

Figure 2.6 (*continued*)
C Complementary base-pairing in RNA and DNA. (Note that in DNA, adenine (A) pairs with thymine (coded white) in place of uracil (coded yellow) present in RNA)

In RNA the sugar present is *ribose*; in DNA it is *deoxyribose*. The nucleotides are linked together in different combinations by *phosphodiester bonds* to form long strands (Fig. 2.6B). Molecules of DNA are very long (up to 5 cm!) whereas those of RNA are much shorter and are of different types including:

- messenger RNA (mRNA)
- transfer RNA (tRNA)
- ribosomal RNA (rRNA).③

Conformation

Complementary base-pairing

A key feature of nucleic acids is the complementary associations that can exist between purine and pyrim-idine bases. Each purine associates most readily with one of the pyrimidines through hydrogen bonds (Fig. 2.6C):

Purine		Pyrimidine
adenine	*pairs with*	uracil or thymine
guanine	*pairs with*	cytosine

These associations between the bases of nucleic acids have important consequences. They:

- dictate the conformation of the nucleic acid
- allow nucleic acid molecules to act as templates for their own replication
- enable nucleic acids to transmit the genetic code.

Just as proteins are folded into different conformations because of the affinities that exist between dif-

③
How does 5 cm compare with the size of the cell?

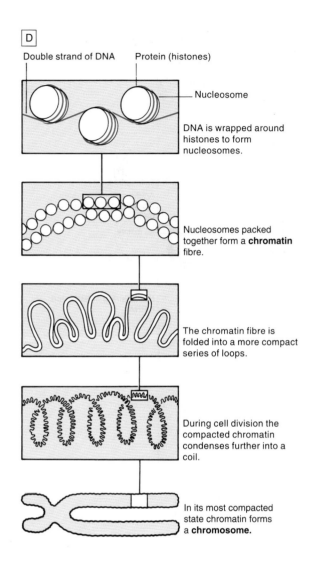

D Double strand of DNA   Protein (histones)

Nucleosome

DNA is wrapped around histones to form nucleosomes.

Nucleosomes packed together form a **chromatin** fibre.

The chromatin fibre is folded into a more compact series of loops.

During cell division the compacted chromatin condenses further into a coil.

In its most compacted state chromatin forms a **chromosome.**

Figure 2.6 (continued)
D Composition and structure of chromatin and how it is twisted and folded into a very compact form as a chromosome. (Adapted from Alberts et al 1983.)

The DNA of some bacteria (*Escherichia coli*) can be altered by adding genes from other organisms. This recombinant DNA makes the bacterial cells synthesise proteins which they do not normally produce. 'Human' insulin for people with diabetes is now produced in this way, i.e. biosynthetically, so that the amino acid sequence matches that produced by human cells. Other semi-synthetic insulin is produced by altering the amino acid sequence of porcine (pig) insulin.

ferent amino acids, so nucleic acids can fold into specific shapes depending on the base-pairing. Molecules of *transfer RNA (tRNA)*, for example, that bring amino acids to the ribosomes, have a unique shape (Fig. 2.6C) that is crucial to their function. DNA differs from RNA in being double-stranded. The two strands are held together by base-pairing to form a *double helix* (Fig. 2.6C) in which each strand exactly complements the other. ④

④
When was the 'double helix' discovered and by whom?

Chromatin and chromosomes
Each amazingly long macromolecule of DNA is usually condensed through extensive intricate folding into a form which is much more compact (Fig. 2.6D).

Each double strand of DNA is wrapped around multiple units of basic proteins (*histones*) to form *chromatin*. Chromatin is, in turn, twisted and folded to form even more compact structures. During the process of cell division (see p. 24), the chromatin is packed especially closely and is then visible under the microscope as individual *chromosomes* (literally 'chromatin bodies'). Each human cell contains 23 pairs of chromosomes, that is 46 macromolecules of DNA. Most of the time, however, chromatin is in a much less compacted state, giving the nucleus its characteristic dark-stained appearance under the light microscope. ⑤

⑤
Name one handicapping condition caused by an extra chromosome.

Genetic code
The sequence of nucleotides in DNA is the genetic code which specifies the number and order of amino acids in every protein synthesised by the cell. A *gene* is the sequence of nucleotides coding for a specific protein. A *codon* is the set of three nucleotides that codes for a single amino acid such as glycine (GGG), or alanine (GCU). There is more than one code for each amino acid but each code is specific (Fig. 2.7). For the code in DNA to be used to dictate protein synthesis it has to be:

- copied into messenger RNA (*transcription*)
- converted from sequences of nucleotides into sequences of amino acids (*translation*).

Transcription
When mRNA is being formed, the two strands of DNA separate for a small part of their length, and ribonucleotides assemble on the DNA template in the order dictated by base-pairing (Fig. 2.7). The mRNA formed then dissociates from the DNA and passes to the ribosomes in the cytosol.

Translation
As mRNA is fed through the ribosomes (Fig. 2.7), molecules of transfer RNA, bearing a specific amino acid, associate in turn with mRNA in the order dictated by base-pairing. Ribosomal enzymes then catalyse the formation of bonds between adjacent amino acids.

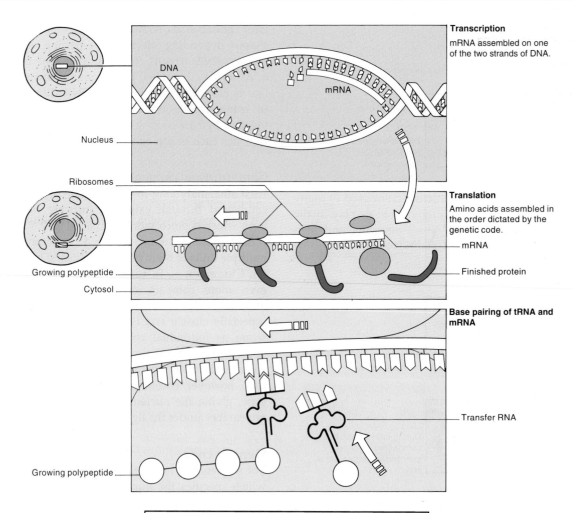

Transcription

mRNA assembled on one of the two strands of DNA.

DNA

mRNA

Nucleus

Ribosomes

Translation

Amino acids assembled in the order dictated by the genetic code.

mRNA

Growing polypeptide

Finished protein

Cytosol

Base pairing of tRNA and mRNA

Transfer RNA

Growing polypeptide

1	2				3
	Decoding the codons				
	Position				
	U	C	A	G	
U	Phe	Ser	Tyr	Cys	U
	Phe	Ser	Tyr	Cys	C
	Leu	Ser	Stop	Stop	A
	Leu	Ser	Stop	Trp	G
C	Leu	Pro	His	Arg	U
	Leu	Pro	His	Arg	C
	Leu	Pro	Gln	Arg	A
	Leu	Pro	Gln	Arg	G
A	Ile	Thr	Asn	Ser	U
	Ile	Thr	Asn	Ser	C
	Ile	Thr	Lys	Arg	A
	Met	Thr	Lys	Arg	G
G	Val	Ala	Asp	Gly	U
	Val	Ala	Asp	Gly	C
	Val	Ala	Glu	Gly	A
	Val	Ala	Glu	Gly	G

Figure 2.7 (*left*)
Transcribing and translating the genetic code. The codons in the Table relate to RNA. Phe, Ser, Tyr, etc. are abbreviations for different amino acids (phenylalanine, serine, tyrosine etc.). The codon sequence UUU codes for phenylalanine, UCU for serine etc. UAA signals the end of a polypeptide.

THE CELL IN ACTION

The living cell is an active structure composed of many parts each of which has a different role to play in the life of the whole. The cell is self-renewing and self-replicating. Its life-cycle and activities are influenced by its environment and controlled by specific regulatory factors.

COMPONENT PARTS AND FUNCTIONS

The different molecules of which the cell is composed associate with one another to form structures which can be seen under the microscope (Fig. 2.8).

Plasma membrane
This is the barrier between the cell and its environment:

- it determines what substances may enter and leave the cell
- it acts as the communication link between the inside of the cell and the outside
- it is the means by which the cell is recognised by other cells.

Endoplasmic reticulum (ER)
This consists of membranes that are engaged in the manufacture and processing of many different molecules. Numerous enzymes catalyse specific chemical reactions. The endoplasmic reticulum is the site of synthesis of some proteins, and lipids, and is the place

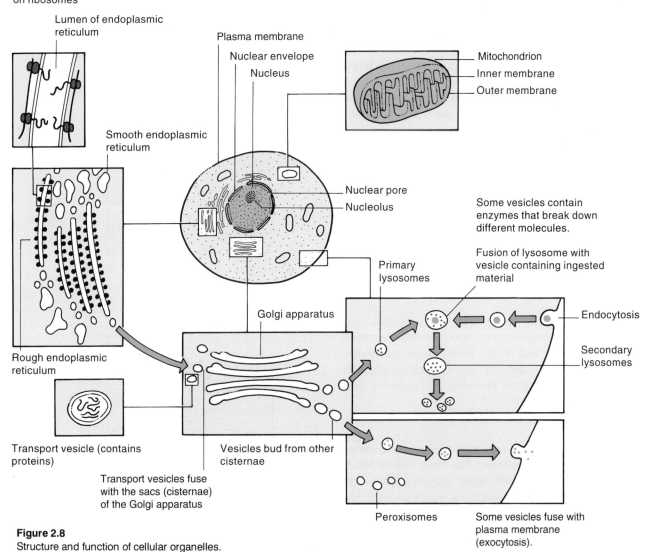

Proteins being synthesised on ribosomes

Lumen of endoplasmic reticulum

Plasma membrane

Nuclear envelope

Nucleus

Smooth endoplasmic reticulum

Mitochondrion

Inner membrane

Outer membrane

Nuclear pore

Nucleolus

Some vesicles contain enzymes that break down different molecules.

Fusion of lysosome with vesicle containing ingested material

Primary lysosomes

Endocytosis

Secondary lysosomes

Rough endoplasmic reticulum

Transport vesicle (contains proteins)

Golgi apparatus

Vesicles bud from other cisternae

Transport vesicles fuse with the sacs (cisternae) of the Golgi apparatus

Peroxisomes

Some vesicles fuse with plasma membrane (exocytosis).

Figure 2.8
Structure and function of cellular organelles.

where many waste materials are broken down and converted into products that can be excreted.

Rough and smooth

Endoplasmic reticulum is described as *rough* (RER) if it is studded with ribosomes and *smooth* (SER) if it is not. Rough endoplasmic reticulum is involved in the synthesis of proteins which are to be inserted into the membranes of the cell or exported from it. The ribosomes are not permanent features of the rough endoplasmic reticulum. They are only attracted to the endoplasmic reticulum if the protein that they are synthesising has a specific leader (signal) sequence of amino acids at the beginning of the polypeptide chain. This leader sequence has affinity for molecules of the endoplasmic reticulum, and inserts itself into the membrane. The synthesis of the protein continues, with the polypeptide chain being fed through the ER into the space within (*lumen*).

Golgi apparatus

This consists of a stack of membranous sacs. It is closely associated with the endoplasmic reticulum. It is supplied with products, such as proteins, that come off the production line of the endoplasmic reticulum in transport vesicles. It may add components to the basic product, and then packages the final item in vesicles which are either taken to the plasma membrane, so that the product can be 'exported' from the cell, or shunted to another place in the cell where it is required.

Lysosomes

These are sacs of varying sizes that contain enzymes (*acid hydrolases*) digesting intracellular macromolecules. The bigger ones (secondary lysosomes) are formed by the fusion of primary lysosomes, produced by the Golgi apparatus, with vesicles containing material to be digested (such as vesicles containing bacteria engulfed by phagocytosis).

Peroxisomes

These are similar in appearance to lysosomes but contain a different set of enzymes (*oxidative enzymes* including catalase) that break down some molecules, like fatty acids, and detoxify others such as alcohol. In the process hydrogen peroxide is produced and destroyed. ⑥

⑥
What do you understand by detoxify?

Mitochondria

Mitochondria (singular = mitochondrion) have both an outer and an inner membrane. The inner one is much folded and is studded with many enzymes. These are involved in the chemical reactions which convert the energy contained in molecules like glucose and fats into a form (*adenosine triphosphate – ATP*) that can be used to power different cellular activities (see Ch. 11), such as the synthesis of new molecules, the secretion of products, or the movement of the cell itself.

Nucleus

The nucleus consists of a collection of molecules including DNA and RNA which are enclosed by a double layer of membrane (*nuclear envelope*). The envelope is perforated by holes (*nuclear pores*). One region of the nucleus (*nucleolus*) appears different from the rest. It is here that ribosomal RNA, transcribed from DNA, is packaged together with proteins to form ribosomes which are moved through the pores in the nuclear membrane to the cytosol.

CELL SPECIALISATION

Although each nucleated cell of the body contains the same components and the same genetic material, cells differ in size (6–30 μm), form and function (Fig. 2.9).

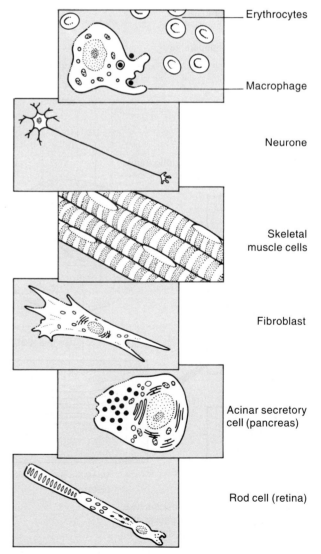

Erythrocytes

Macrophage

Neurone

Skeletal muscle cells

Fibroblast

Acinar secretory cell (pancreas)

Rod cell (retina)

Figure 2.9
Several different types of cell.

This is because each type of cell expresses different bits of the genetic code to differing extents, and consequently the amounts of different proteins formed vary. As proteins play a central role in determining the characteristics and capabilities of each cell, the structure and functions of cells will differ. ⑦

In each cell type, some structures and activities become more prominent and others become less so. In muscle cells, for example (Fig. 2.9), the actin present in all cells is developed into a sophisticated system which can develop a powerful contractile force (see Ch. 22). In enzyme secreting cells of the digestive glands (see Ch. 6), the synthesis and packaging of proteins for export dominates cell activity, and so the rough endoplasmic reticulum is particularly prominent and many secretory vesicles (*zymogen granules*) are present. Mature red cells (*erythrocytes*; see Ch. 4) in contrast have no cell organelles at all, but instead are packed full of the oxygen transporting protein *haemoglobin*.

CELL MAINTENANCE AND RENEWAL

Within all living cells there is a continual turnover of molecules: fresh nucleotides are inserted into DNA; new proteins are formed by the ribosomes; and lipids are manufactured in the endoplasmic reticulum. At the same time cellular constituents are being damaged and degraded. Many of the products of breakdown are recycled and re-used (for example amino acids derived from proteins, and iron from molecules like haemoglobin). However, a fresh supply of some materials is continually required to replace substances that are used up or which are irreversibly degraded and excreted. ⑧

Cell culture
Cells can be maintained for their natural lifespan in an artificial medium containing only amino acids, glucose, vitamins, salts, growth factors and antibiotics (Table 2.2), at 37°C, in an atmosphere of 95% air (which provides 20% oxygen) and 5% CO_2. Cells cultured in this way not only survive, but they also grow and divide to form new cells, provided a surface is available for them to adhere to and spread across.

Cell cycle
The cell cycle (Fig. 2.10) consists of two parts:

- cell growth (*interphase*)   • cell division.

In the interphase each cell has to double its constituents so that when the cell divides it contains a full complement of all its parts. Protein synthesis occurs throughout the cycle, though at varying rates. The synthesis of new DNA only occurs during part of the interphase, in the 'S' (synthesis) phase. All of the existing DNA is replicated. At the same time new nucleoproteins are synthesised.

Maintaining the genetic code
It is crucial that the genetic information carried by DNA is maintained and passed on from cell to cell without

WOUND HEALING

Wound healing is a natural, automatic process. It has been said that the body provides its own intensive care when healing is required, but this does not mean that the nurse should remain ignorant of the process. Most people experience a cut from a knife or other sharp instrument; the cut is usually made in clean conditions with straight edges similar to that made during an operation. Provided that the wound is not too deep, it usually heals very quickly because the gap is negligible, there is no irritant such as a splinter or pathogenic organisms, the supply of nutrients is uninterrupted and the temperature is unchanged. In other words, all the requirements for normal cell division and healing are being met.

⑦
How many types of cell can you name?

⑧
Can you name some materials that are continually required for replacement?

Table 2.2 Approximate composition of a medium suitable for culturing cells		
	mmol/l	
Sodium chloride	110	NaCl
Sodium hydrogen carbonate	25	$NaHCO_3$
Glucose	5	
Potassium chloride	4	KCl
Amino acids*	2	
Calcium chloride	1	$CaCl_2$
Magnesium chloride	1	$MgCl_2$
Sodium dihydrogen phosphate	1	NaH_2PO_4
Vitamins (B group)	0.005	
Plus Growth factors		
Antibiotics (penicillin, streptomycin)		
Trace elements (copper, zinc, iron)		Cu, Zn, Fe
* Total concentration: includes the essential amino acids (those the cell cannot manufacture for itself).		

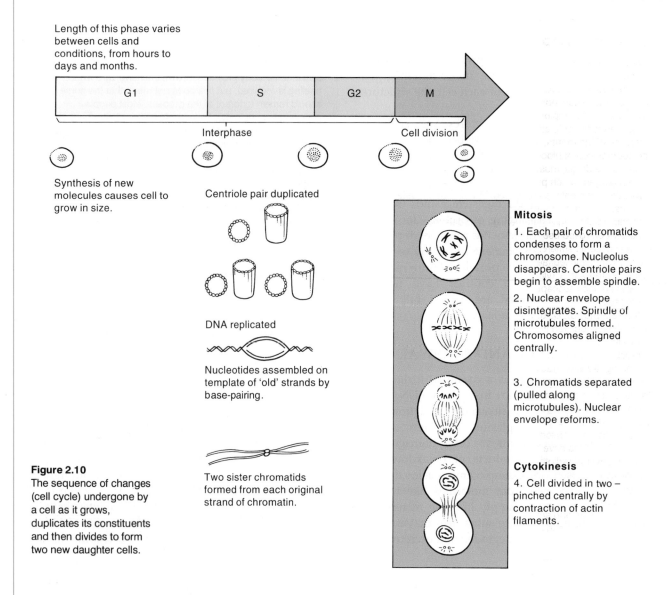

Length of this phase varies between cells and conditions, from hours to days and months.

Interphase

Cell division

Synthesis of new molecules causes cell to grow in size.

Centriole pair duplicated

DNA replicated

Nucleotides assembled on template of 'old' strands by base-pairing.

Two sister chromatids formed from each original strand of chromatin.

Figure 2.10
The sequence of changes (cell cycle) undergone by a cell as it grows, duplicates its constituents and then divides to form two new daughter cells.

Mitosis

1. Each pair of chromatids condenses to form a chromosome. Nucleolus disappears. Centriole pairs begin to assemble spindle.

2. Nuclear envelope disintegrates. Spindle of microtubules formed. Chromosomes aligned centrally.

3. Chromatids separated (pulled along microtubules). Nuclear envelope reforms.

Cytokinesis

4. Cell divided in two – pinched centrally by contraction of actin filaments.

error. If a mistake occurs and is not corrected it will be reproduced in all succeeding generations of cells (*mutation*). Changes do occur all the time in the molecules of which the genes are composed:

- bases are lost
- cytosine can be converted to uracil
- ultraviolet light (UV) can make adjacent thymines bond together.

Normally these changes are repaired by enzymes that cut out the abnormal part of the damaged DNA strand and replace it with new nucleotides, using the un-damaged strand as a template (*DNA repair*). The replication of DNA is a complex process involving the activity of several enzymes including DNA polymerase. New strands are assembled using the old strands as templates. Again, mechanisms allow checks to be made for mistakes, and errors to be corrected. Eventually duplicated sets of DNA wrapped around their nucleoproteins are formed (*chromatids*) (Fig. 2.10).

Cell division

Once all the constituents have been replicated the 'M' (mitotic) phase begins and the cell divides. This occurs in two stages (Fig. 2.10):

- *mitosis* – division of the nucleus into two halves
- *cytokinesis* – division of the rest of the cell.

A crucial role is played by components of the cell's cytoskeleton which are reorganised to form assemblies of fibres that draw the chromosomes to each pole of

All new-born babies in the UK are screened for the disease *phenylketonuria* (PKU). The abnormal DNA is unable to synthesise the enzyme phenylalanine hydroxylase which converts phenylalanine to tyrosine. As a result, phenylalanine accumulates in the blood. It is toxic to the brain cells in early life and causes mental retardation. A special diet limiting phenylalanine intake prevents retardation.

USE OF CYTOTOXIC DRUGS AND RADIATION

Cancer cells do not always form a well-defined tumour that can be removed by surgery. Diffuse malignant disease is often treated with cytotoxic drugs. These drugs are non-specific – they affect normal as well as cancerous cells. Cells which divide rapidly are most susceptible to cytotoxic drugs, hence the side effects experienced by some patients: ulceration of the mouth, irritation of the gastrointestinal tract and suppression of blood cell production.

One of the drugs, mustine, a nitrogen mustard, is an alkylating agent which prevents DNA strands from separating, thus halting replication. The nitrogen mustards were first developed as war gases to be used indiscriminately, causing immediate and delayed effects. Carefully controlled use of mustine has proved beneficial to many patients suffering from forms of cancer such as chronic lymphatic leukaemia and Hodgkin's disease. All males treated with alkylating drugs are rendered sterile; females are less susceptible but may experience an early menopause.

A group of cytotoxic drugs (e.g. vincristine and vinblastine) is derived from the periwinkle (*Vinca rosea*). They are known as plant alkaloids and act by interfering with microtubule assembly, thereby preventing mitosis.

Ionising radiation (radiotherapy) is also used to kill malignant cells and can be directed at a specific tumour. Radiation dissociates molecules causing disruption of chromosomes leading to mutation, and damaging or altering components of the cytoplasm. As with cytotoxic drugs, ionising radiation is used in carefully controlled doses. Many lives have been lost in the development of radiography and radiotherapy because, although radiation can be used to kill cancer cells, it can also cause malignant disease, genetic mutations and sterility if non-therapeutic doses are received. Adequate protection must always be given to patients and any persons involved in the use of radiation (e.g. the lead apron provided during dental X-rays).

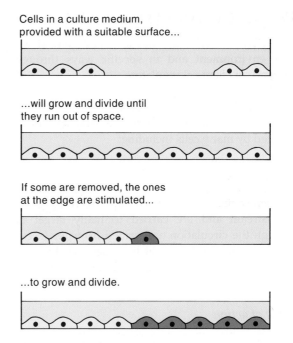

Figure 2.11
Factors controlling the growth and reproduction of cells.

the cell, and which contract around the middle of the cell to split each one into two new cells.

The time that it takes for a cell to grow and then divide varies from one cell type to another. Amongst the shortest times are taken by the surface cells of the digestive tract (see Ch. 6) These cells are continually being eroded and need to be replaced. They complete the cell cycle in about 8 hours. Others can take a couple of months, and some, like nerve cells, skeletal muscle cells and red blood cells, no longer divide at all once they are mature.⑨

Controlling factors

Two factors can affect the cycle of cell growth and division:

● cellular environment
● availability of space.

If the conditions around the cells are not optimal then the cycle of growth and division may be slowed or even completely arrested. Factors which arrest the cycle include a shortage of nutrients and lack of growth factors.

If cells are not supplied with adequate amounts of amino acids, protein synthesis will be inhibited. If there is insufficient oxygen, energy production will be limited. If the temperature of the environment is lowered, the rate at which chemical reactions occur in the cell is reduced and cells will not grow and divide as rapidly.

Cells also normally stop dividing if they run out of space (*contact inhibition*) (Fig. 2.11). If a tissue is injured, the contact between cells is broken, and the cells at the margins are stimulated to grow and divide again until the gap is repaired.

Patients who are immobile for long periods are at risk of developing pressure sores. Tissues that are compressed lack a good blood supply. Insufficient nutrients are supplied to maintain the cells and replace those that are lost.

One of the ways that cancer cells differ from normal cells is that their growth lacks 'space' control. When cultured, these cells pile up on top of one another and continue to grow and divide. Should they have acquired a good blood supply they grow exceedingly fast because of the abundance of nutrients. A growing mass of cancerous tissue makes increasing demands on the nutrient supplies available to the body as a whole. In time, other tissues are progressively starved and their growth and renewal is arrested.

⑨
Which other cells are continually being lost?

REGULATION OF CELL ACTIVITY

The activity of cells is influenced in a general way by their environment and in specific ways through the influence of chemical regulators.

Specific chemical regulators

Specific chemical regulators are manufactured and secreted by many cells including:

- endocrine cells
- nerve cells.

Chemical regulators which are secreted into the bloodstream and are carried to many target tissues through the circulation are termed *hormones* (see Chs 3 and 10), whereas those which are secreted by nerves in close contact with the target cells are *neurotransmitters* (see Chs 3 and 21).

Mode of action

Several modes of action of chemical regulators are summarised in Figure 2.12. Each regulator interacts best with a specific protein receptor present in the cell.

Many receptor molecules are embedded in the plasma membrane, where they interact with hydrophobic molecules that cannot cross the plasma membrane. Binding of the chemical regulator to the receptor may:

- open a protein channel in the membrane which allows specific ions, such as calcium, to move into the cell
- activate an enzyme located on the inner surface of the cell membrane which catalyses the formation of an intracellular regulator, such as cyclic AMP
- stimulate endocytosis (*receptor-mediated endocytosis*) and the uptake of the regulator, such as nerve growth factor into the cell
- form a complex that regulates gene transcription.

cAMP (*cyclic adenosine monophosphate*) is formed from adenosine triphosphate (ATP) by the action of the enzyme adenylate cyclase. Both calcium and cyclic AMP regulate processes inside the cell. They are termed *second messengers* because they act as secondary links between the first messengers (hormones and neurotransmitters) and the cellular processes which are being controlled.

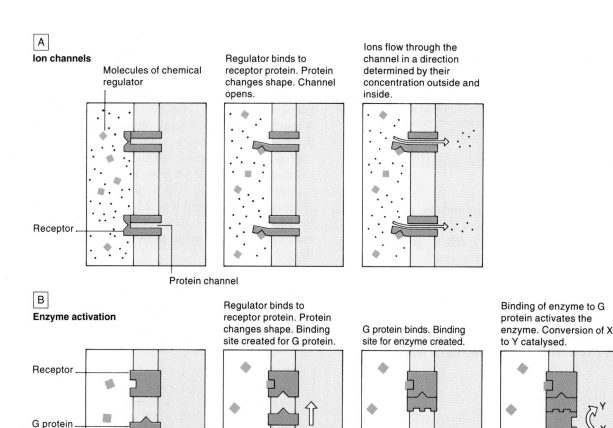

Second messengers

Calcium

Calcium acts intracellularly by binding to specific proteins, altering their conformation, and changing their activities. For example in muscle cells calcium binds to the proteins which affect the association between the contractile proteins actin and myosin. When calcium concentration in the cytosol increases, muscle cells contract. For relaxation to occur, the concentration of calcium in the cytosol has to be lowered. This is achieved by transporter proteins which remove calcium (see Ch. 22).

Cyclic AMP

Cyclic AMP activates a group of enzymes called *protein kinases* which catalyse the addition of phosphate to specific intracellular proteins. The phosphorylation of these proteins, which are often enzymes too, alters their activity. This in turn affects the rate of the chemical reactions which they catalyse. In this way cAMP, for example, regulates the breakdown of glycogen to glucose (see Ch. 14).

Other 'second messengers' are known. These include cyclic guanosine monophosphate (GMP), inositol trisphosphate (IP$_3$), and diacyl glycerol (DG).

Regulation of gene transcription

Some chemical regulators do not bind to receptors on the plasma membrane but enter the cell and bind to receptor proteins inside. Lipophilic substances, like steroid hormones, are able to pass through the cell membrane. Within the cell they bind to receptors, and the hormone receptor complex then enters the nucleus where it binds to chromatin and modifies gene transcription. This changes the balance of proteins synthesised by the cell, which, in turn, alters the capacity of the cell to perform specific functions. Anabolic steroids for example stimulate protein synthesis in muscle. The cells enlarge and are able to generate a greater force. As protein synthesis is a lengthy process, these effects, unlike those of calcium and cAMP, do not occur immediately. ⑩

⑩
Can you name any steroid hormones?

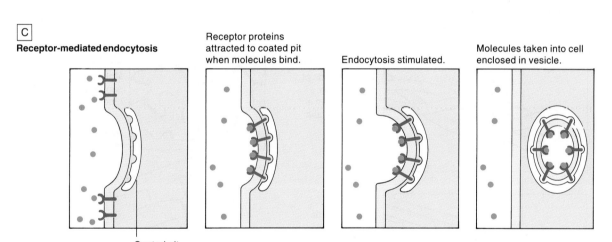

C
Receptor-mediated endocytosis

Receptor proteins attracted to coated pit when molecules bind.

Endocytosis stimulated.

Molecules taken into cell enclosed in vesicle.

Coated pit

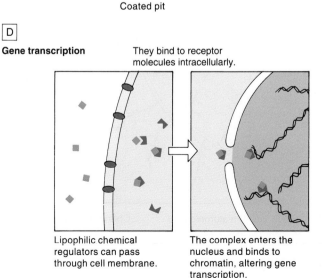

D
Gene transcription

They bind to receptor molecules intracellularly.

Lipophilic chemical regulators can pass through cell membrane.

The complex enters the nucleus and binds to chromatin, altering gene transcription.

Figure 2.12 (*facing page, above and left*)
Ways in which chemical regulators affect cell activity by controlling:
A Ion channels (*facing page*)
B Enzyme activation (*facing page*)
C Receptor-mediated endocytosis (*above*)
D Gene transcription (*left*).

CELLS IN COMMUNITY

Within the body, cells live in different communities linked together with their neighbours within a framework (*extracellular matrix*) that supports and maintains them. These organised communities of cells (*tissues*) form in different ways and are usually continually renewed as cells divide to replace those that die or are damaged.

THE EXTRACELLULAR MATRIX

Cells which are cultured readily link together to form sheets of cells if they are provided with a suitable surface to which they can adhere. Within the body, the correct environment and the right support is provided by the extracellular matrix.

Constituents

The matrix consists largely of proteins that have the form of long strands (*fibrous proteins*) embedded in a jelly-like substance composed of polysaccharides (Fig. 2.13). Proteins present in the matrix include:

- collagen (major constituent – ropelike and strong)
- elastin (can stretch and recoil)
- fibronectin (promotes cell adhesion).

The jelly-like substance (*gel*) surrounding the protein fibres consists of water and glycosaminoglycans such as:

- hyaluronic acid
- chondroitin sulphate
- heparin.

Linked to proteins they form *proteoglycans*. Glycosaminoglycans and proteoglycans are strongly hydrophilic. They attract water molecules and easily form gels. Dissolved in the water in the gel are salts and other water-soluble substances such as glucose and amino acids. The constituents of this fluid (*interstitial fluid*), which is locked into the gel like water in a jelly, and their approximate concentrations are listed in Table 2.3.

Formation

The matrix is formed chiefly by fibroblasts, though other cells, such as osteoblasts in bone and chondroblasts in cartilage (see Ch. 28), may contribute too.

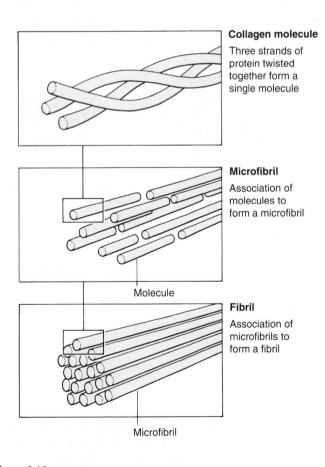

Collagen molecule
Three strands of protein twisted together form a single molecule

Microfibril
Association of molecules to form a microfibril

Molecule

Fibril
Association of microfibrils to form a fibril

Microfibril

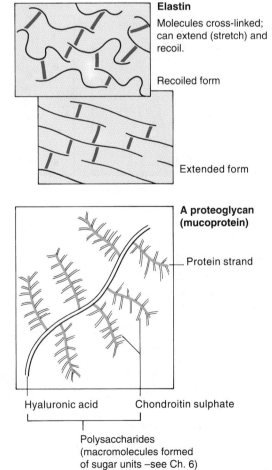

Elastin
Molecules cross-linked; can extend (stretch) and recoil.

Recoiled form

Extended form

A proteoglycan (mucoprotein)

Protein strand

Hyaluronic acid   Chondroitin sulphate

Polysaccharides (macromolecules formed of sugar units –see Ch. 6)

Figure 2.13
Composition and structure of three major constituents of the extracellular matrix: collagen, elastin and a proteoglycan.

Table 2.3	Constituents of the interstitial fluid		
	mmol/l		mmol/l
Sodium	140	Calcium	1
Chloride	115	Magnesium	1
Hydrogen carbonate	25	Phosphate	1
Glucose	5	Sulphate	0.5
Organic anions*	5	Dissolved proteins	0.3
Potassium	4	(i.e. non-fibrous)	
Amino acids	2		

* Various products of cell metabolism including: citrate, lactate, aceto-acetate, beta-hydroxybutyrate.

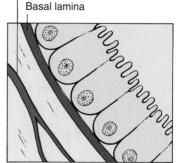

Blood capillaries
Basal lamina

Absorptive cells of the digestive tract (see Ch. 6)

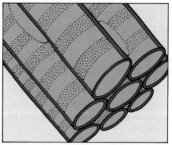

Skeletal muscle (see Ch. 22)

Basal lamina surrounds each cell. Guides the regeneration of damaged tissue.

Capillary wall   Blood

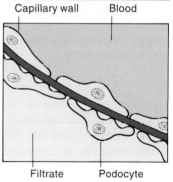

Filtration barrier: kidney glomerulus (see Ch. 8)

Substances filtered by the kidney have to pass through the basal lamina.

Filtrate   Podocyte

Figure 2.14
The basal lamina in three different tissues.

Functions

The extracellular matrix has a major influence on the cells in its locality. It helps to 'glue' cells together as well as influencing their activity and guiding their migration and development.

Connective tissue

The matrix, together with wandering cells found in it, such as fibroblasts, macrophages and mast cells (see Ch. 15), is sometimes referred to as *connective tissue*. It acts as a supporting structure for the cells which make up different organs and tissues (heart, blood vessels, liver, kidney and so on) as well as forming:

- tendons (linking muscles to bone)
- ligaments (linking bones together)
- cartilage (at the ends of bones)
- bones and teeth.

See also Chapter 28.

Variations

The composition of the matrix and its organisation varies. For example, in bones and teeth the matrix is calcified, and in tendons the collagen fibres are highly organised. Also thin layers of a distinctive form of matrix, the *basal lamina*, are found at several sites (Fig. 2.14):

- beneath sheets of cells like those lining the gut
- surrounding some individual cells such as muscle
- separating two layers of cells like those forming the kidney filter (see Ch. 8).

The basal lamina contains a unique form of collagen (type IV) and the glycoprotein laminin. It is involved in the function of the cells with which it is associated and is believed to be involved in the regeneration of tissues after injury.

JUNCTIONS BETWEEN CELLS

The factors which cause individual cells to adhere to one another instead of remaining separate are not fully understood but they include fibronectin in the extracellular matrix as well as the mutual affinity of molecules present in the outer surface of the plasma membrane.

Cells not only adhere but are linked together at discrete sites. At least three sorts of link points have been described, each composed largely of protein:

- desmosomes
- tight junctions
- gap junctions.

Each has a characteristic structure and performs distinct functions (Fig. 2.15).

TISSUE FORMATION AND RENEWAL

Formation

The various tissues of the body are usually composed of a variety of different types of cell. This mixture of types arises in one of two different ways, either by:

- *differentiation* of an unspecialised set of cells
- *migration* of cells from one place to another.

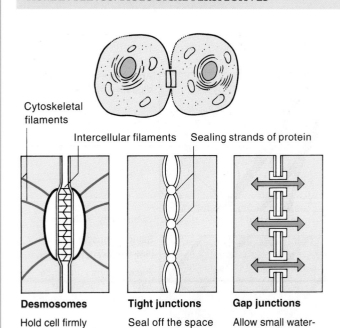

Cytoskeletal filaments

Intercellular filaments   Sealing strands of protein

Desmosomes

Hold cell firmly together.

Tight junctions

Seal off the space between two cells. Limit movement of molecules in between the cells.

Gap junctions

Allow small water-soluble molecules to pass from cell to cell.

Figure 2.15
Structure and function of three different types of linkages between cells: desmosomes, tight junctions and gap junctions.

During development, primitive sets of cells divide on site and differentiate as they do so into the variety of cells of which the tissue is composed (see Ch. 35). Although the process of differentiation is controlled genetically, the maintenance of the differentiated state depends also on the extracellular matrix.

The extracellular matrix is also believed to be important in guiding the migration of cells from one site to another. Primitive neurones, for example, migrate from nervous tissue to colonise organs and tissues at a distance forming parts of the autonomic nervous system (see Ch. 3).

Renewal

Once tissues have been formed, many undergo continual renewal. Cells are replaced in two ways, either by:

● division of the existing cells
● division and differentiation of stem cells.

Division of cells 'on site'

The cells of the liver (see Ch. 9), and those of the inner lining of the blood vessels (*endothelium*) are replaced by division of the existing cells. In both cases if cells are lost through injury some of the remaining cells are stimulated to divide and fill up the vacant space. This process in blood vessels is *angiogenesis*.

Stem cells

Blood cells (see Ch. 4) on the other hand are replaced by the division and differentiation of primitive precursor cells (*stem cells*). These can be:

● *unipotent* (giving rise to only one cell type)
● *pluripotent* (giving rise to several types as in blood cells; see Ch. 4).

Sometimes, as in muscle, stem cells may be inactive (quiescent) and are only provoked to divide in the event of damage.

Non-renewable cells

Not all cells are replaceable. Some, once formed, no longer divide. The molecules of which they are composed undergo renewal and repair, but the cell itself cannot be replaced by division of adjacent cells, or by differentiation of stem cells. This applies to nerve cells and the muscle cells of the heart. If they are irreversibly damaged they cannot be replaced.

When a person suffers a *myocardial infarction* (heart attack) the heart muscle (*myocardium*) is damaged and, as heart muscle cells cannot be replaced, there is a thinning of the heart wall which may rupture.

Tumours

The renewal and replacement of normal cells occurs in a controlled way guided by the nature and organisation of the extracellular matrix which sets boundaries for cell migration and association. Cancerous cells are not controlled in the same way and thus they are able to dominate and take over. If they remain in the same place and just grow to form a large mass of cells (*tumour*) they are referred to as *benign*. If, however, they migrate to other sites and develop there, or have the potential to do so, then they are described as *malignant*.

KEY POINTS

What you should now know and understand about cells and tissues:

- the major classes of molecules from which cells and tissues are formed
- why some molecules associate with one another and others do not, and how this relates to cell structure and function
- what is distinctive about proteins and their functions
- what DNA and RNA are and how they function as the genetic code
- what cell membranes consist of and what they do
- the structures present inside cells and what they do
- how cells reproduce and grow
- how neurotransmitters and hormones regulate cell activity
- what connective tissue is and what its functions are
- how cells are bound together to form tissues.

REFERENCES AND FURTHER READING

Alberts B, Bray D, Lewis J, Raff M, Roberts K, Watson J D 1988 Molecular biology of the cell, 2nd edn. Garland Publishing, New York & London
(A weighty but fascinating mine of information about cells)
Atkins P W 1987 Molecules. Scientific American Library, New York
(Interesting facts about molecules that matter in everyday life. A beautifully illustrated compendium for leisure-time reading as well as reference)
De Duve C 1985 A guided tour of the living cell. W H Freeman, Oxford
(Cell biology with a difference. A beautifully illustrated expedition through the intricacies and marvels of cellular life)
Gartner L P, Hiatt J L 1990 Color atlas of histology. Williams & Wilkins, Baltimore
(Very clearly presented pictures of cells and tissues)
Hinwood B 1992 A textbook of science for the health professions. Chapman & Hall, London
(Excellent book for getting to grips with the basic science of atoms and molecules)

Chapter 3
HOMEOSTASIS AND CONTROL

Every moment the environment of the cells in our bodies is threatened by cellular activity and by our own actions. Oxygen, glucose and amino acids are used up by the cells and waste products such as carbon dioxide and ammonia are produced. If you hurry along a corridor or lift bedding or people, you increase the demand for nutrients and the need to eliminate waste products. If you have also missed your lunch, because of an emergency admission, the threat posed to the cells in your body is even greater.

Our cells are able to survive these and other challenges simply because, in health, the composition of their immediate environment is stabilised. Stability (*homeostasis*) is achieved by control systems that monitor crucial factors in the cellular environment and adjust its composition accordingly. These control systems are neural or hormonal. If control breaks down, homeostasis is disturbed and illness results (see Ch. 19).

A key role in homeostasis is played by blood circulating between the tissues and organs of the body, supplying nutrients to the fluid around the cells and sweeping waste products away. Blood is also the link tissue which carries hormones secreted by endocrine cells to all tissues. ①

The neural control systems that are particularly involved in the regulation of the internal environment form the *autonomic* part of the nervous system. The neural control systems controlling our interaction with the external environment form the *somatic* nervous system. The latter will be described in Section 3.

CONTROL SYSTEMS

TYPES OF CONTROL

Stability of the internal environment (*homeostasis*) is achieved by two types of control:

- negative feedback
- open loop control.

In *negative feedback*, key constituents of the internal environment are continually monitored. If these deviate from normal, corrective adjustments are made to keep the concentration of the constituents as near normal as possible.

In *open loop control*, factors that indirectly affect the

① *List the
nutrients
carried by
blood to the
body's cells
and the waste
products it
carries away
from them.
What are these
waste products
derived from?*

② Find out the normal oxygen content of arterial and venous blood.

③ Find out the normal blood glucose level.

key constituents are monitored. If these factors alter, adjustments are made which help to prevent a change in the internal environment.

Negative feedback

Two examples of negative feedback are shown in Figure 3.1A. In the first, a decrease in the amount of oxygen in blood, such as may occur high up in the mountains, is detected by specialised cells, sensitive to oxygen. They in turn excite nerve cells stimulating the respiratory muscles, and breathing is increased. As a result the amount of oxygen taken into the body increases, which counteracts the threat to oxygen supplies and minimises

the actual change in the amount of oxygen in the blood. ②

Similarly, if your blood glucose concentration decreases because you have missed lunch, the drop in glucose excites cells in the pancreas to secrete more of the hormone glucagon. This stimulates liver cells to release glucose from their stores of glycogen and stops the blood glucose falling as much as it might. ③

The components of these systems form a complete loop (*negative feedback loop*) (Fig. 3.1B). It is so called because the disturbance in the concentration of the key constituent (*controlled variable*) brings about changes that counteract (*negate*) the disturbance itself.

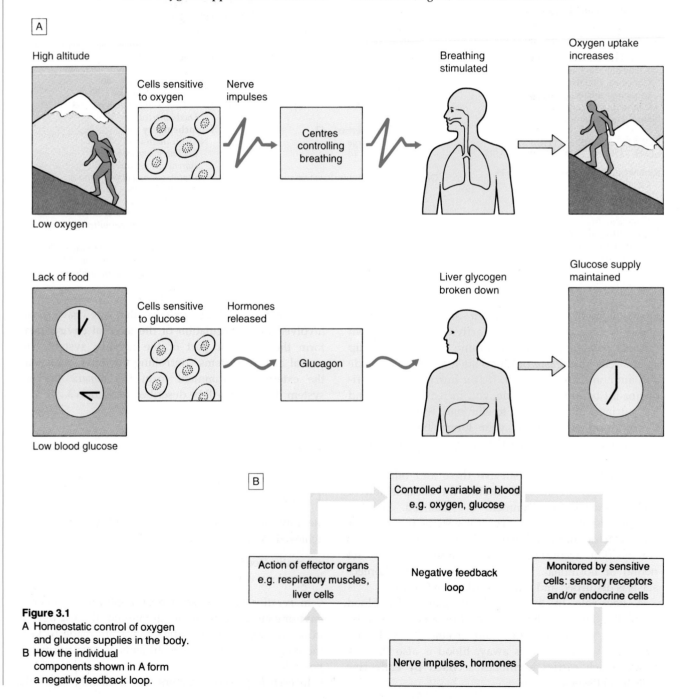

Figure 3.1
A Homeostatic control of oxygen and glucose supplies in the body.
B How the individual components shown in A form a negative feedback loop.

Open loop

An example of open loop control is shown in Figure 3.2A. Here receptors on the surface of the body detect a change in the external temperature. A series of events is set in motion that result in blood flow to the skin being cut down to reduce heat loss from the body. This protects the internal environment of the body by preventing a change in internal temperature.

This form of control is *open loop* because the original disturbance (in this case the skin temperature) is not counteracted. Indeed the decrease in the flow of warm blood to the skin makes skin temperature drop even more. The internal temperature is maintained but at the expense of cold fingers and toes.

Open loop systems work together with negative feedback systems to stabilise internal conditions (Fig. 3.2B). The open loop system provides an early warning system that triggers preventive responses, whereas the negative feedback system provides the quality control that checks that the internal environment is up to standard and makes corrective adjustments if it is not.

BASIC ELEMENTS IN THE PROCESS OF CONTROL

The various elements involved in the process of control are illustrated in Figure 3.3. In sequence, they are:

- registering relevant information
- analysing the data
- choosing a suitable strategy
- implementing the strategy
- evaluating the outcome.

These elements and their sequence apply to control systems in general whether the object of that control is physiological (e.g. control of blood pressure) or sociological (e.g. maintenance of acceptable standards of health care).

Registering relevant information

The cells in the body that have the function of registering relevant information are:

- sensory receptors
- endocrine cells.

> By reducing blood flow from the skin in chilly conditions, the body attempts to conserve heat for its important central organs – the brain and heart. Nursing intervention in such cases might include wrapping the patient in well-insulated clothing to prevent further heat loss.

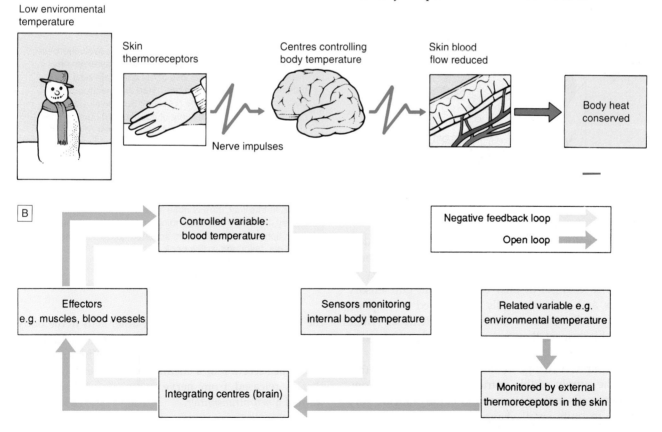

Figure 3.2
A Homeostatic control of body temperature by an open loop system.
B Negative feedback and open loop systems working together to control blood temperature.

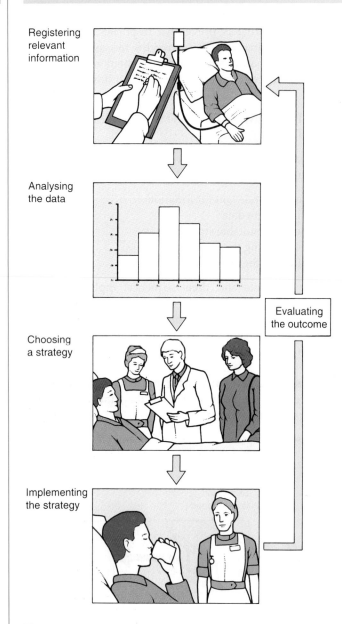

Registering
relevant
information

Analysing
the data

Choosing
a strategy

Evaluating
the outcome

Implementing
the strategy

Figure 3.3
Basic elements of a control system as applied to patient care.

Sensory receptors respond by generating nerve impulses whereas endocrine cells respond by releasing hormones into the bloodstream. All cells alter their activity in response to changes in their environment, but sensory receptors and endocrine cells are attuned to respond especially well to one or more selected features (Table 3.1). In this respect they are more *sensitive* than other cells. ④⑤

For example, a change in blood glucose concentration affects the supply of this nutrient to many cells. However, some cells in the pancreas and in the brain are very sensitive to quite small changes in glucose concentration and respond in a highly specific way.

Pancreatic cells respond by increasing or decreasing their secretion of a chemical messenger. This travels in

---

THE NURSING PROCESS AS A CONTROL SYSTEM

One of the joys of coming to physiology for the first time can be the realisation that the functions of the human body are logically ordered. One thing happens and, in response, another action occurs. The principle of homeostasis, which runs like a thread throughout this book, is perhaps the epitome of this logic in action.

Practising nurses will recognise in the basic elements of control systems features that are shared with what is called the *nursing process*. The stages of this process may be described as:

● assessing the patient (*registering relevant information*)
● planning nursing care on the basis of that assessment (*analysing the data and choosing a suitable strategy*)
● implementing nursing care (*implementing the strategy*)
● evaluating the nursing care given (*evaluating the outcome*).

Just as specialised cells monitor blood pressure and raise or lower it by adjusting the size of certain blood vessels, so the delivery of nursing care can be fine-tuned to suit a particular patient. Nursing assessment acknowledges an individual's biological, psychological, social and spiritual condition, and plans and delivers care accordingly. To give a fairly obvious example, a nurse would decide that an energetic and independent young man, now recovered from a motorcycle injury and ready for discharge from hospital, could adequately take care of his own hygiene needs. Another patient, however, might need bathing because both her arms are in plaster; and a client with a learning disability might need gently reminding to wash himself. In each case, the nurse responds appropriately and logically to an initial assessment of the patient.

The fourth stage of the nursing process – evaluation – is as logical as those that precede it. The nurse examines evidence for the effectiveness of the care delivered – is the patient now comfortable in bed? Has the injection of pethidine begun to reduce his pain? Such evaluation will necessarily affect the delivery of subsequent nursing care. It is important to note that evaluating is not described as the *last* stage of the process, which should be regarded as circular rather than linear. Assessment is continuous; so is evaluation. There is not just one period of assessment, one session of planning and delivery of care, and one evaluation. The stages continually follow on from each other. In this way, care is not a 'one-off' procedure, but day by day, hour by hour, depending on the patient's changing condition, it is monitored and adjusted; just as are the body systems described in this book.

---

the blood to affect the activity of other cells in the body, and is therefore termed a *hormone*. Cells in the brain respond by changing their firing of nerve impulses. This alters the secretion of a chemical messenger too, but one that is released from nerve endings and is therefore termed a *neurotransmitter*.

Analysing the data

When data is registered by many different sensitive cells, it is collated and compared before it is used to

Table 3.1　Examples of cells monitoring selected features of the internal environment

Detector cells		Feature monitored	Chapter reference
Sensory receptors	Endocrine cells		
Chemoreceptors			
– carotid and aortic bodies	Within the kidney	Oxygen	11
– medulla oblongata		Hydrogen ions (CSF)*	12
– hypothalamus	Alpha and beta cells (pancreas)	Glucose	14
	Chief cells (parathyroid glands)	Calcium	13
Osmoreceptors			
– hypothalamus		Osmotic pressure	13
Thermoreceptors			
– hypothalamus		Temperature	16

*CSF = cerebrospinal fluid. The hydrogen ion concentration of the CSF is directly related to the amount of carbon dioxide in the blood.

drive an appropriate response. For example, in the system controlling blood temperature (Fig. 3.2B), information from temperature receptors in the skin is combined with that from internal temperature receptors in an integrative centre in the brain known as the *hypothalamus*. Similarly, in the control of breathing, information relating to the oxygen content of blood is combined in the *medulla oblongata* of the brain with information about the carbon dioxide content of blood.

Both are important in the control of breathing (see Chs 11 and 12).

Information gathered together from different sensory receptors can be used to derive new pieces of information. For example the signals registered by each ear about a particular sound (Fig. 3.4), such as the tea trolley in the ward, are brought together in two clusters of cells (*superior olives*) deep inside the brain and compared. As each ear hears the sound slightly differently (unless the

In some patients who suffer a stroke, the hypothalamus is affected (a bleeding vessel causing damage to surrounding brain tissue). These patients lack normal temperature control and can produce a *hyperpyrexia* of 40°C or more. The prognosis is extremely poor.

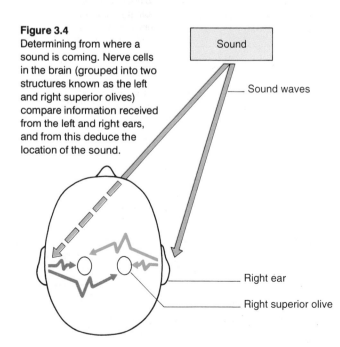

Figure 3.4
Determining from where a sound is coming. Nerve cells in the brain (grouped into two structures known as the left and right superior olives) compare information received from the left and right ears, and from this deduce the location of the sound.

Sound

Sound waves

Right ear

Right superior olive

NURSING OBSERVATIONS

Just as specialised cells are sensitive to certain changes in body state, so informed nursing care observes for changes in a patient's condition. These changes are not watched for randomly. On the contrary, the nurse plans which observations are required using her assessment of each patient.

Recordings of temperature and blood pressure are probably two of the commonest observations performed by the nurse, but their significance will depend on the nursing context. Following an operation, a rise in blood pressure may suggest that the patient is experiencing moderate pain. (There will be other important signs, such as facial expression and verbal complaints.) On the other hand, if the patient is given an injection of a strong pain killer, such as pethidine, he may experience a fall in blood pressure, one of the side effects of pethidine being vasodilation. The nurse, aware of the context in which the patient is being cared for – following an operation, or receiving a pain killer or a blood transfusion – will be alert for signs of physiological changes relevant to that nursing context.

Activity by specialised cells leads to certain body responses, and effective homeostasis depends on fully functioning neural and hormonal activity. Similarly, it could be argued that effective patient care depends on the accuracy with which the nurse carries out the required nursing observations and treatment. Accurate recording of observations (data gathering) provides information about changes in a patient's physiological state. Effective nursing and medical care help to restore homeostasis.

sound is directly in front or behind) the difference in signals received by the olives can be used to work out where the sound is coming from, and therefore where drinks are being served.

Choosing a strategy

Once data has been collected and analysed, a strategy has to be chosen. This selection depends on the balance of excitatory and inhibitory factors that are registered (Fig. 3.5A & B). An endocrine cell for example may be stimulated by one factor and inhibited by another. The secretion of the hormone depends on the *balance* of factors affecting the cell. If excitatory factors predominate the hormone is released, whereas if inhibitory factors are in the majority then secretion is prevented.

Within the nervous system too 'decisions' are made on this basis. Some neurotransmitters are excitatory. Others are inhibitory. Usually nerve cells in the brain receive a blend of both. The way in which the nerve cells respond, and therefore the strategy selected, depends on the balance of excitatory and inhibitory influences.

Implementing the strategy

The cells which perform the task required are called *effector cells*. Any cell of the body may act as an effector cell if its activity is affected by neurotransmitters or hormones. The cells usually referred to as effectors are those which:

- develop force and are concerned with movement (e.g. muscle)
- manufacture and secrete specific products (e.g. enzyme-secreting cells of the digestive tract). ⑥

The activity of effector cells is regulated by a variety of neurotransmitters and hormones (Table 3.2). These chemicals interact with specific receptor proteins on the outside or inside of the effector cells (see Ch. 2). The

action produced may be either short-lived or long-lasting. Short-lived responses include the contraction and relaxation of muscle (as when you drop a dish that is too hot) and the stimulation and inhibition of secretion as in digestion.

Longer-lasting changes in cell activity occur when the synthesis of proteins inside the cell is increased or decreased (see Ch. 2), as for example when kidney cells develop the capacity to conserve more salt (sodium chloride) in times of dietary deficiency.

Evaluating the outcome

When the task has been performed, or even while it is being performed, more information is gathered about how well the task has been or is being carried out. This data too is analysed and used to modify the original strategy and its implementation, in order to correct or improve the end result.

NEURAL AND HORMONAL SYSTEMS

Neural and hormonal systems are now recognised as representing two ends of a spectrum of intercellular communication (Fig. 3.6) instead of two completely different systems. The nature of the regulatory chemicals involved, and their mode of action on cells is similar. However, at the one extreme (*neural*) communication is selective and quick, whereas at the other (*hormonal*) it is widespread and relatively slow.

In between these two extremes lie forms of communication possessing both neural and hormonal features. Some nerves, such as those in the hypothalamus (see Ch. 10), release their regulatory chemicals into the blood-

> Note that other texts may use the term humoral rather than hormonal.

⑥
What is the definition of an enzyme?

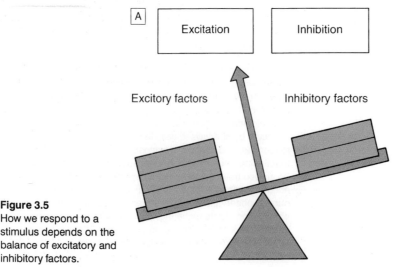
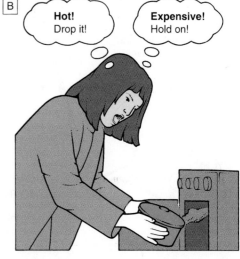

Figure 3.5
How we respond to a stimulus depends on the balance of excitatory and inhibitory factors.

Table 3.2 Examples of neurotransmitters and hormones and their actions on effector cells

Neurotransmitters	Hormones	Effector cells	Action
Acetylcholine		Skeletal muscle	Contraction
Noradrenaline		Heart	Faster, stronger beat
Opioid peptides		Gut muscle	Relaxation
VIP*		Gut secretory cells	Secretion
	Thyroxine	All cells	Stimulates metabolism
	Parathyrin	Bone, gut, kidney	Alters calcium metabolism
	Glucagon	Liver, adipose tissue	Alters glucose and fat metabolism
	Aldosterone	Kidney, gut	{ Sodium conservation { Potassium excretion

* Vasoactive intestinal polypeptide.

stream. Consequently, they are acting like endocrine cells, and the substance they secrete is termed a hormone (because it is released into the blood) even though it has been manufactured and released by nerve cells. This form of communication is termed *neuroendocrine*.

Conversely, some cells producing hormones, mainly release them locally into the surrounding tissues, rather than directly into the bloodstream. Thus, although the cell appears to be endocrine, it is acting more like a nerve cell in the scope of its activity and influence. This form of communication is typified by histamine secreted by mast cells (see Ch. 4) and is termed *paracrine*.

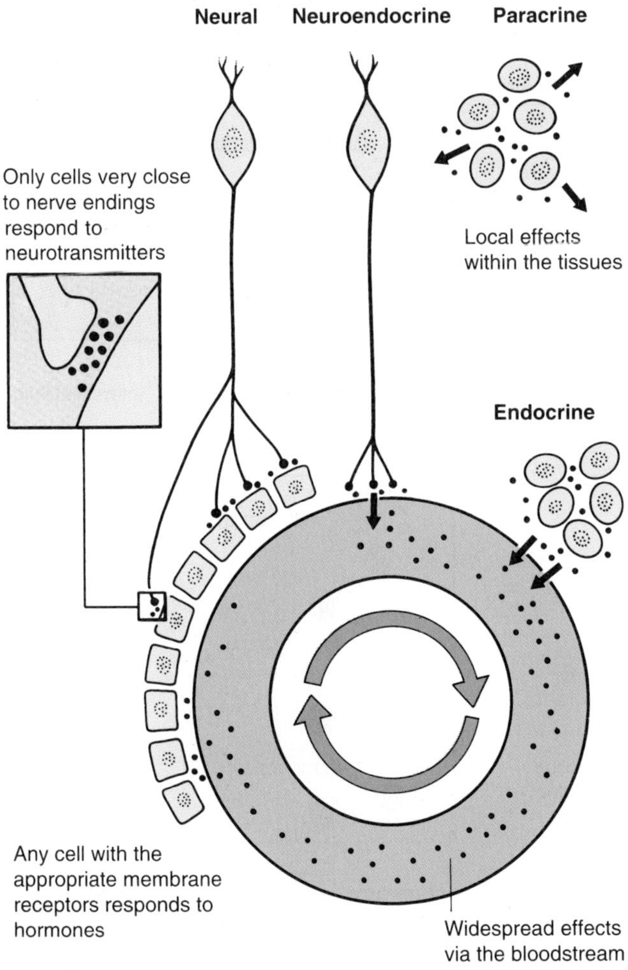

ROLE OF BLOOD IN THE MAINTENANCE OF HOMEOSTASIS

The blood circulating between the heart and the tissues plays a central role in homeostasis in:

- renewing the interstitial fluid
- representing the composition of the internal environment
- disseminating hormones.

RENEWING THE INTERSTITIAL FLUID

The interstitial fluid is the fluid held in the *extracellular matrix* (see Ch. 2). Its composition needs to be maintained in order to preserve cell function. Consequently, constituents such as glucose and oxygen that are used up by the cells need to be replaced, and waste products need to be taken away.

The interstitial fluid is separated from the blood by the walls of the tiniest blood vessels (*capillaries*) that are present in all the tissues of the body. Capillaries allow small water-soluble substances to pass across the wall in either direction with no difficulty. Substances can change places (*exchange*) freely. If the concentration of a substance differs on one side compared with the other then net movement of that substance occurs across the wall by *diffusion*.

Capillary structure

Capillaries are tiny vessels, whose walls consist of a single layer of flattish cells (*endothelial cells*) bounded by

Figure 3.6
Different forms of intercellular communication.

Neural   Neuroendocrine   Paracrine

Only cells very close to nerve endings respond to neurotransmitters

Local effects within the tissues

Endocrine

Any cell with the appropriate membrane receptors responds to hormones

Widespread effects via the bloodstream

a *basal lamina* (Fig. 3.7A & B). They are impermeable to blood cells and to many of the proteins (*plasma proteins*) present in blood (see Ch. 4). However, they are freely permeable to a variety of substances including:

- oxygen and carbon dioxide
- glucose and amino acids
- ions (hydrogen, sodium, potassium, calcium, chloride etc.)
- water.

The only exception is the capillaries in the brain which are slightly more selective (see Ch. 20).

The extra selectivity of brain capillaries in allowing only some substances to cross their walls is important in drug therapy. It is referred to as the blood–brain barrier, and its implication is that many drugs are unable to leave the bloodstream and enter brain tissue in adequate therapeutic doses (see Ch. 20).

Capillary exchange

Molecules in solution move around in all directions (*random movement*) powered simply by their own energy. If the concentration of the substance on both sides of the capillary wall is the same (Fig. 3.7B), then the random movement of molecules in all directions under their own power does not result in any *net* trans-

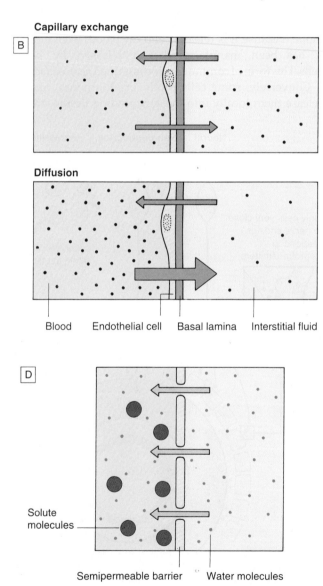

Figure 3.7
Capillaries and their function:
A Structure
B Passage of molecules across the capillary wall: difference between capillary exchange and diffusion
C Factors determining the rate at which molecules diffuse
D Osmosis: the diffusion of water from a region of high water concentration to a solution 'diluted' by the presence of dissolved substances.

fer of substance from one side to the other. Molecules cross the capillary wall, but movements in one direction are balanced by movements in the opposite direction. This interchange of molecules across the capillary wall is *capillary exchange*.

Diffusion

However, if the concentration of a substance is *not* the same in the blood and in the interstitial fluid, as is the case for oxygen or glucose, then more molecules move away from the region of higher concentration than move into it from the region of lower concentration. Consequently, there is net movement of that substance from the region of higher to the region of lower concentration (Fig. 3.7B).

The rate at which a substance is transferred between two sites depends on:

- the difference in concentration between the sites
- the distance separating the sites.

These two factors can be combined to give the *concentration gradient* (Fig. 3.7C). The steeper this is, the more *rapidly* will a substance diffuse from a region of high concentration to one of low concentration. ⑦

> This principle is used in the 'artificial kidney' (i.e. renal dialysis) where accumulated waste products cross a membrane from a high concentration – within the person's blood – to a low concentration – the dialysate or dialysing fluid (see Ch. 8).

Osmosis

When a solvent, such as water, diffuses between two solutions separated by a semipermeable barrier the process is termed *osmosis*. The barrier restricts the movement of one or more solutes, such as plasma proteins for example, but is freely permeable to water (Fig. 3.7D).

REPRESENTING THE INTERNAL ENVIRONMENT

The end result of exchange and diffusion of molecules between the blood and the interstitial fluid is that there is a close correlation between the composition of the two fluids. Substances building up in the vicinity of the cells (such as carbon dioxide produced by metabolism) flow continually into the blood and are dispersed in the bloodstream. Other substances taken up by the cells (such as oxygen) are continually replaced from the 'store' in the blood.

Arterial blood

Because blood from many different sources mixes in the large veins and in the heart, differences of composition in blood flowing from different places disappear. With the important exceptions of oxygen, carbon dioxide and pH, the composition of the blood emerging from the heart (*arterial blood*) represents an average value for the body as a whole. It is this 'average' which is monitored by cells sensitive to vital constituents of the cellular environment. If values deviate from normal, corrective adjustments are provoked bringing the composition of the arterial blood back to acceptable values. As a result, the composition of the interstitial fluid is maintained as well.

As blood pumped from the heart to the rest of the body has just passed through the lungs, the composition of arterial blood also reveals whether oxygen, carbon dioxide and pH have been brought to the correct levels by the process of breathing (see Chs 11 and 12).

DISSEMINATING HORMONES

Hormones are secreted into the blood by endocrine cells sensitive to the composition of the internal environment. Hormones differ in their chemical nature. This determines their action, the form in which they are transported in blood, and their fate.

Endocrine cells

Location

Cells which secrete hormones are found in many places in the body (Fig. 3.8, and Chs 10 and 34). Some are clustered together to form discrete endocrine glands (such as the adrenals, parathyroids, and the thyroid gland), which have their own blood supply. Others form clumps of cells sited within another organ (such as the islets of Langerhans within the pancreas). Others,

⑦
What effect might oedema (see Ch. 5) have on the diffusion of substances between sites?

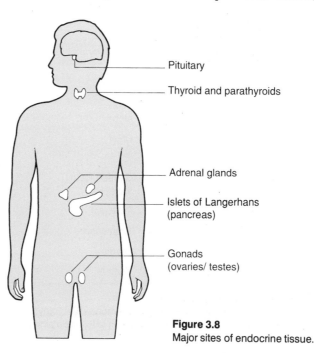

Pituitary

Thyroid and parathyroids

Adrenal glands

Islets of Langerhans (pancreas)

Gonads (ovaries/ testes)

Figure 3.8
Major sites of endocrine tissue.

⑧

Match up your list of hormones (Q. 5) with the endocrine glands shown in Figure 3.8.

such as the cells secreting gastrointestinal hormones, are scattered within a tissue (in this case the lining of the gastrointestinal tract).⑧

> Take care not to confuse the intestinal wall hormones with the digestive enzymes also produced by specialised cells in the wall of the gut (see Ch. 6).

Stimulation

Many endocrine cells are sensitive to the concentrations of key constituents of the blood, such as glucose, calcium and potassium. Others are specifically sensitive to other hormones in blood (Table 3.3).

Other cells, because of their location, may be influenced also by products secreted by cells nearby, or by the composition of other fluids to which they are exposed. For example, the β (beta) cells of the pancreas, which secrete insulin, are influenced by two other hormones, glucagon and somatostatin, secreted by endocrine cells next to them (*paracrine communication*) (see Ch. 10). In the digestive tract, endocrine cells in contact with the contents of the gut (such as the gastrin-secreting cells of the stomach; see Ch. 6) can test and respond to changes in the composition (in this case the hydrogen ion concentration) of the contents.

Hormones

Types

The majority of hormones are either *peptide* in chemical nature or *steroid* (Fig. 3.9). Whereas peptides are hydrophilic and therefore water soluble, steroids are largely lipophilic and can penetrate cell membranes.⑨

Peptide hormones usually regulate cell activity by binding to specific receptor proteins on the plasma membrane of the target cells. These in turn regulate various processes inside the cell by means of *second messengers* (see Ch. 2).

Steroid hormones, because they are lipophilic, penetrate cell membranes and bind to receptor molecules inside the cell. The steroid–receptor complex controls gene transcription and regulates protein synthesis (see Ch. 2).

Carriage in blood

Peptide hormones being water soluble are carried dissolved in the blood plasma (see Ch. 4). Steroid hormones, because of their lipophilic properties, are transported in blood in two ways:

- dissolved in plasma (*free form*)
- associated with plasma proteins (*bound form*).

The bound form cannot easily escape from the blood or pass through cell membranes. So the effective concentration of the hormone in body fluids is that of the free form.

Fate

Once secreted, hormones may leave the bloodstream, and the interstitial fluid by being:

- taken up into cells (steroids by diffusion; peptides by endocytosis; see Ch. 2)
- broken down by enzymes in blood and in the tissues.

Peptide hormones can lose their activity without being broken down if conditions cause their molecular shape to alter. This alters their ability to bind to receptors in the cell membrane (see Ch. 2).

⑨

Ensure that you can define the terms hydrophilic and lipophilic. Refer to Chapter 2 if necessary.

Table 3.3   Endocrine cells: site, sensitivity and secretion

Site	Cells	Sensitive to:	Hormone(s) secreted
Pancreas	Beta Alpha	Glucose Glucose (↓)*	Insulin Glucagon
Parathyroids	Chief	Calcium	Parathyrin
Thyroid	'C'	Calcium (↓)*	Calcitonin
Adrenal cortex	Glomerulosa Various	Potassium ACTH	Aldosterone Cortisol
Thyroid	Follicular	TSH	Thyroxine
Ovary	Granulosa	FSH and LH	Oestrogens
Testis	Leydig	LH	Testosterone
Pituitary	Various	Releasing hormones	ACTH, TSH, FSH, LH

* Sensitive to decrease in concentration.
Key: ACTH = adrenocorticotrophic hormone; TSH = thyroid stimulating hormone;
      FSH = follicle stimulating hormone; LH = luteinising hormone

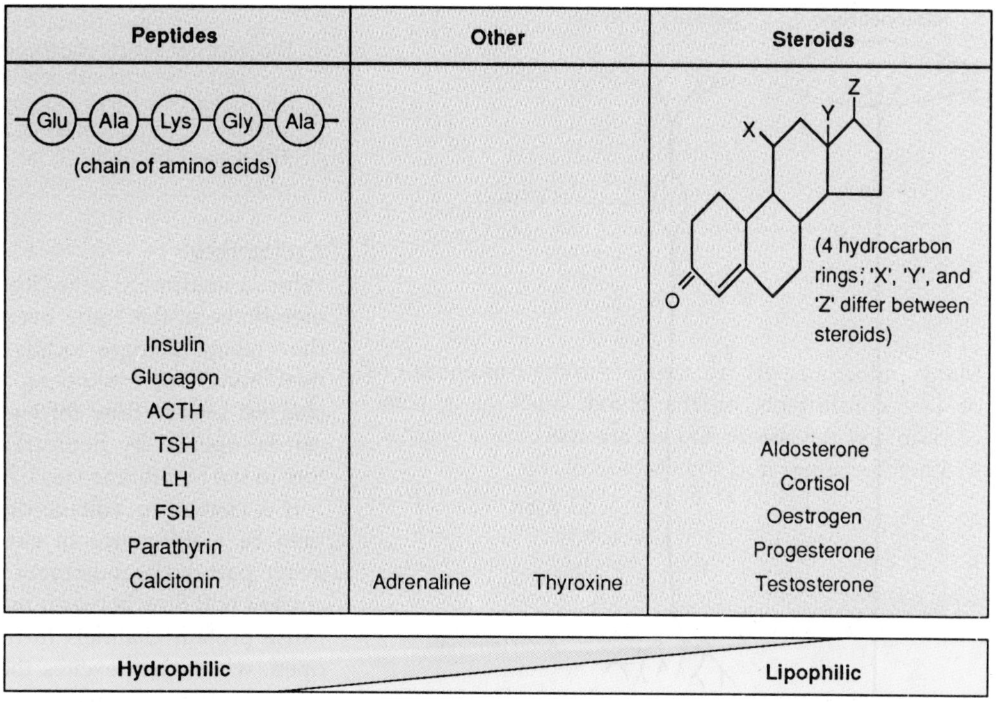

Peptides	Other	Steroids
(Glu)–(Ala)–(Lys)–(Gly)–(Ala)– (chain of amino acids)		(4 hydrocarbon rings; 'X', 'Y', and 'Z' differ between steroids)
Insulin Glucagon ACTH TSH LH FSH Parathyrin Calcitonin	Adrenaline Thyroxine	Aldosterone Cortisol Oestrogen Progesterone Testosterone
Hydrophilic		**Lipophilic**

Figure 3.9
Chemical characteristics of different hormones: peptides are soluble in water (hydrophilic) whereas steroids are less soluble in water and more soluble in fats (lipophilic) (see Ch. 2). Adrenaline and thyroxine are intermediate in properties.

NEURAL CONTROL SYSTEMS

Neural systems differ from hormonal systems of communication and control in being:

● quick
● selective.

They are quick because signals are transmitted electrically along nerve fibres rather than chemically in the blood. They are selective because nerve fibres form discrete contacts with specific cells. Neural and hormonal systems both involve the release and action of chemical messengers, but in neural systems this is restricted to specific junctions (*synapses*) between cells.

NERVE CELLS

Structure
Nerve cells (*neurones*) vary in their appearance (Fig. 3.10) depending on their location and function. All have slender branching extensions (*dendrites*) which receive and transmit electrical signals. The extent and arrangement of these many branches differs between cells. Many cells have one branch (*axon*) that differs in appearance from the rest. It is a long thin extension which acts as the route by which signals received by the nerve cell are passed on to the next cell(s) in line. The longest nerve axons extend all the way from the spinal cord within the backbone to the tips of the toes (about 1 metre). The axon branches at its end to form *axon terminals*. These make contact with the cells to which signals are being transmitted. The remaining part of the nerve cell is called the *cell body* or *soma*. It contains the nucleus and other intracellular organelles.

Electrical properties
All cell membranes are electrically charged, but nerve cells differ from other cells in that they are able to use this charge to generate and transmit signals (*nerve impulses*) rapidly over long distances.

Electrical charge
Differences in electrical charge between two points are measured in *volts*. The electrical charge existing between the inside and the outside of all cell membranes is small. In nerve cells it is about 0.07 volts ($\equiv$ 70 millivolts). This is very small in comparison with that provided by power packs and the mains (Table 3.4) but it is big enough to enable small electrical currents to flow along a nerve cell if it is excited.

Table 3.4 Comparison of several sources of electricity	
Power source	*Volts (V)*
Mains electricity (in the UK)	240
Car battery	12
Torch battery	1.5
Cell membrane	0.07

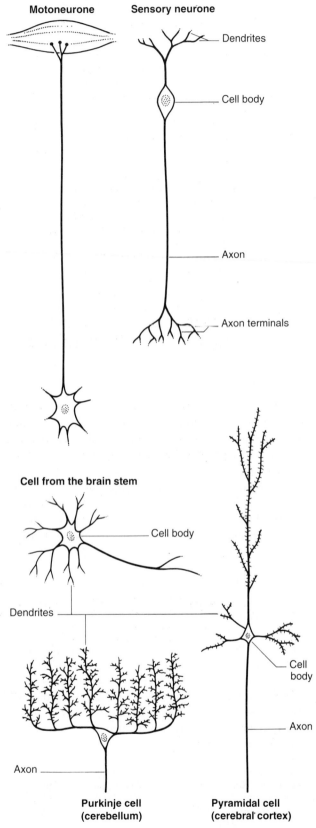

Figure 3.10
Structure of a variety of neurones (not to scale: some
motoneurones and sensory neurones can be up to 1 metre in
length whereas cells in the brain – brain stem, cerebellum and
cerebral cortex – are very much smaller).

The electrical activity of different parts of the body can be recorded by special instruments and is of great benefit in diagnosing malfunction. Examples include the electroencephalograph (EEG) and the electrocardiograph (ECG) (see Chs 5 and 23).

Excitability

When a neurone is unexcited the voltage across the cell membrane is the same everywhere (70 millivolts). But the voltage changes locally if protein channels in the membrane open allowing positively and negatively charged ions to flow through the membrane. Channels can be opened by neurotransmitters binding to receptors in the membrane (see Ch. 2).

If a change in voltage does occur locally there will then be a difference in electrical charge between this active part of the membrane and the rest and an electric current will flow between them. This flow of current can cause protein channels further along the membrane to open, which then excites the next part and so on. The result is that a wave of excitation (*nerve impulse*) is transmitted from one end of the nerve to the other. A much fuller account of this process is given in Chapter 21.

Synapses

When the nerve impulse arrives at the nerve terminals it triggers the release of neurotransmitter from small vesicles by exocytosis (see Chs 2 and 21). Most nerve terminals are in very close contact with other cells at specialised junctions known as *synapses* (Fig. 3.11). The

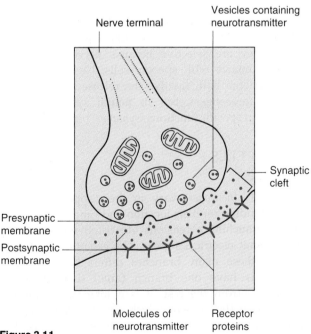

Figure 3.11
The key components of a synaptic junction between neurones (structures are not drawn to scale).

neurotransmitter diffuses across the tiny gap between the cells and binds to receptors in the membrane of the adjacent cell. This cell could be another neurone or an effector cell such as muscle.

Very little neurotransmitter escapes from the synapses into the surrounding tissue. That which does may be:

- broken down by enzymes locally (e.g. acetylcholine by acetylcholinesterase)
- taken back up into the nerve terminals (e.g. noradrenaline).

The binding of neurotransmitter to receptors in the membrane of the *postsynaptic cell* causes the membrane voltage to change. If the cell is a nerve then the change may, depending upon the neurotransmitter, either excite or suppress nerve impulses in the postsynaptic cell.

Likewise, if the cell is an effector, its activity may be stimulated or inhibited. Intracellular messengers act as a link between the postsynaptic event and cell activity. In muscle cells, for example, excitation of the cell provokes release of calcium intracellularly and this in turn triggers muscle contraction (see Ch. 22).

ORGANISATION OF NEURAL SYSTEMS

Nerve cells are linked with one another into systems of neurones, which receive and process information and activate other cells. All systems, whether simple or complex, consist of three sections (Fig. 3.12):

- sensory
- integrative
- motor.

The simplest examples of a functional system of neurones are those mediating *reflexes*. More complicated systems are involved in *voluntary* behaviour. ⑩

Basic components
The *sensory* section consists of:

- sensory receptors
- sensory neurones.

DRUG ACTIONS AND THE SYNAPSE

Knowledge of the physiology of nerve impulse transmission enables the nurse to understand more readily the action of certain drugs and their side effects. For example, some drugs have effects similar to those of neurotransmitters, such as noradrenaline or acetylcholine. Other drugs inhibit the action of neurotransmitters.

Synthetically prepared adrenaline is a *sympathomimetic* drug, enhancing the action of the naturally occurring 'messengers', noradrenaline and adrenaline. Noradrenaline, released at sympathetic nerve endings in the heart or in the smooth muscle of arterioles, causes an increase in heart rate and constriction of blood vessels (among other effects). Adrenaline injected intravenously in, for example, an emergency resuscitation, likewise increases the rate and force of the heart's contractions by stimulating β_1 adrenoceptors within the heart.

Salbutamol, another sympathomimetic drug, is more selective than adrenaline. It has a stimulant action on β_2 adrenoceptors in the bronchi, causing bronchodilation, and is of value in the treatment of asthma and other airway diseases. Salbutamol is often given in aerosol form, but even so there may be some residual β_1 adrenoceptor stimulation. Thus, if a salbutamol inhaler is used more often than is prescibed, tachycardia (increased heart rate) may occur.

Sensory receptors convert different kinds of stimuli (chemical, mechanical, thermal) into nerve impulses, whereas sensory neurones process and transmit the signals to other parts of the nervous system.

The *integrative* section consists of the interneurones upon which information from different sources converges and is the place where strategies are chosen and decisions are made about the action to be taken.

The *motor* section consists of the nerves which transmit 'commands' to the effector cells and activate them.

Damage to motoneurones may lead, for example, to paralysis of a limb. However, if sensory neurones from that limb are undamaged, the person may still be able to feel sensations in the limb, including pain.

---

⑩
List the reflexes that you can think of and state what you think is the function of each.

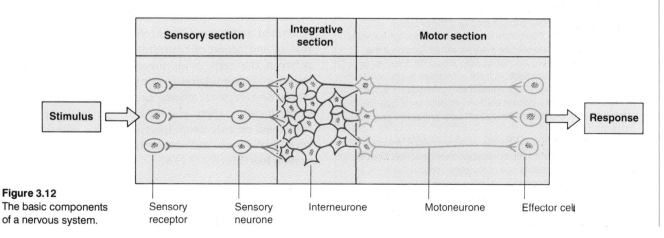

Figure 3.12
The basic components of a nervous system.

Sensory receptor — Sensory neurone — Interneurone — Motoneurone — Effector cell

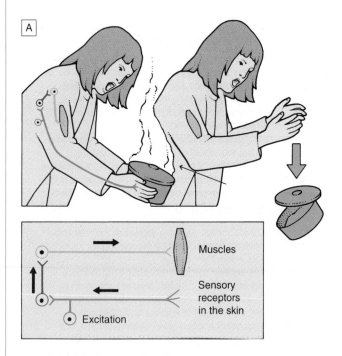

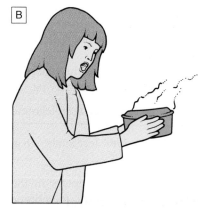

Figure 3.13
An example of a reflex response and how it can be inhibited:
A Excitation of the reflex
B Inhibition of the same reflex.

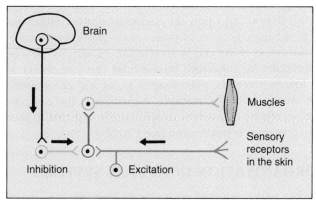

MAKING USE OF REFLEXES IN NURSING CARE

Micturition for the infant is a reflex action – as the bladder fills beyond a certain point the child passes urine. There is no 'social control' involved. This is learned during the first few years of life.

Such learned control may be interrupted when a person suffers a spinal injury because the nervous connection between the brain and lower body is lost. The person becomes paralysed (the extent of the paralysis depending on the level of the spinal injury), is no longer able to feel sensations from the lower limbs or abdomen, and has no voluntary control over movement. This loss of control includes micturition, so that passing urine becomes, once again, a reflex action.

Some 'spinal' patients are catheterised to prevent the complications that can arise from urinary incontinence. Catheterisation itself has complications, and in some cases (but not all) it is possible for the carer to utilise the patient's own reflexes in order to help maintain continence.

If pressure is applied by the carer's hands above the symphysis pubis (i.e. over the bladder) the walls of the bladder will be gently compressed and the pressure within increased. This will stimulate sensory nerve endings (*stretch receptors*) within the bladder wall, as would happen if the volume of urine were increasing, and it may be possible to bring about reflex micturition. If such pressure is applied regularly, say every 3 hours, anticipating the patient's own reflex response to his filling bladder, incontinence may be avoided, with benefits to the patient both physically and psychologically.

Similarly, in order to avoid faecal incontinence, a spinal patient can be placed on an appropriately designed bedpan after meals. This makes use of the *gastrocolic reflex* whereby the presence of food in the stomach and duodenum excites the colon through neural and hormonal mechanisms (see Ch. 6).

⑪
What reflexes can be tested by nurses, and why are they important?

Simple systems: reflex behaviour

A simple system consisting of sensory, integrative and motor components is shown in Figure 3.13A. Excitation of sensory receptors reflexly results in muscle contraction. However, this reflex can be inhibited by the system shown in Figure 3.13B. ⑪

Excitation

When sensory receptors are excited, nerve impulses are generated and passed from one cell to the next by the release and action of neurotransmitters at the synapses between the cells, with the result that one or more muscles are stimulated to contract. In this way stimulation of receptors *reflexly* causes muscle contraction. Consequently when you unwittingly pick up a hot object you reflexly drop it, because nerve impulses have been generated and transmitted through a simple system like this (Fig. 3.13A).

Inhibition

Reflexes can be inhibited by *inhibitory interneurones* which suppress the transmission of nerve impulses at synapses. The neurotransmitters released by these neurones make the cells with which they are in contact less excitable. If inhibitory interneurones are active the reflex is much less easy to evoke amd may even be suppressed (Fig. 3.13B). Reflect on the difference in behaviour of people who are very relaxed as compared with others who, through their anxiety, are very 'jumpy'. Sudden sounds easily startle anxious people but not those who are relaxed. In relaxed people reflexes are damped down by activity in inhibitory interneurones.

Complex systems: voluntary behaviour

The inhibition of the reflex response to picking up a hot object (*withdrawal reflex*; Fig. 3.13A) is achieved through a complex system of neurones that enable you to:

- see the offending object
- recognise it for what it is
- predict that if you drop it it will break
- remember that it was a special present to you
- resolve to hold on to it regardless of the pain.

This involves many more neurones than those shown in the diagram (Fig. 3.13B) and much more synaptic interaction. It is not certain whether you will hold on to the hot object, or whether you will drop it. It all depends on the balance of different signals converging on the interneurones controlling the reflex. This, in turn, depends on the balancing of 'excitatory' and 'inhibitory' signals that has gone on at synapses in your brain (Fig. 3.5).

What makes *voluntary behaviour* different from reflexes is simply that the voluntary response to a particular stimulus cannot be predicted as easily. This is because the response depends on so many different pieces of information all of which have to be integrated and 'weighed up' before action is taken.

THE AUTONOMIC NERVOUS SYSTEM

It is usual to consider the entire nervous system of the body as consisting of two parts:

- somatic
- autonomic.

The *somatic* nervous system is chiefly concerned with our interaction with the *external* environment. It monitors external events and enables the body to influence those events. This involves special sense organs, such as eyes, ears, etc. The major effector tissue is the muscle that determines movement of the trunk, limbs and hands, in the daily activities of walking, sitting, lifting etc., together with that of the face, mouth and

throat, in eating, speaking, laughing etc. This system will be described in detail in Section 3.

The *autonomic* nervous system is, in contrast, chiefly concerned with the regulation and maintenance of the *internal* environment. It therefore plays a key role in the maintenance of homeostasis. It innervates cells of the visceral systems and organs that are involved, namely those of:

- the cardiovascular system (Ch. 5)
- the digestive system (Ch. 6)
- the respiratory system (Ch. 7)
- the urinary system (Ch. 8)
- the liver (Ch. 9)
- the endocrine glands (Ch. 10).

Its organisation and neurochemistry have several distinctive and functionally important features.

ORGANISATION

Sensory components

A variety of different sensory receptors are to be found in different places within the viscera, and elsewhere (Table 3.5). They monitor:

- the composition of the blood and body fluids
- the degree of stretch of some organs and tissues (e.g. stomach, bladder)
- potentially harmful (*noxious*) stimuli.

Some of the sensory receptors are specialised endings of sensory neurones (e.g. stretch receptors, nociceptors). Others are separate receptor cells that excite sensory neurones by releasing neurotransmitters (e.g. respiratory chemoreceptors; see Ch. 11).

The impulses generated by the receptors pass along the axons of the sensory nerve fibres to nerve endings that make synaptic contact with interneurones that are situated in a number of different places.

Integrative components

The interneurones forming the integrative component of

Harmful stimuli that can excite the nerve endings of the autonomic nervous system include chemicals such as acids. For example, a peptic ulcer may perforate, spilling digestive juices including gastric acid into the peritoneal cavity (see Ch. 6). The result is severe pain. Pain can also be caused by stimulation of stretch receptors within, for example, the bladder wall. We have all experienced the discomfort of a full bladder, especially on a long bus journey! Where a patient is unable to express himself clearly – for example in severe learning disability, or following general anaesthetic – the onset of irritability may be a sign of a full bladder. Urine retention is common following many operations in the abdominal or pelvic regions and should be watched for carefully.

the autonomic nervous system are found:

- within the organ or tissue itself
- grouped into clusters of neurones (*ganglia*) at a distance from the organ or tissue
- within the spinal cord and brain stem.

Local interneurones

A good example of these are the interneurones found in the wall of the gastrointestinal tract (Fig. 3.14A). Sensory fibres make synaptic contact with interneurones present within an interlacing net of neurones (*plexus* – plural *plexi*) lying between parts of the gut wall. From these interneurones, signals are transmitted via motoneurones to local effector cells of the gut, such as secretory cells and muscle cells. Simple systems of this kind mediate a variety of *local autonomic reflexes* (see Ch. 6).

Ganglia

Some interneurones are found within clumps of nervous tissue (*ganglia*) separate from the organs and tissues innervated by the sensory neurones (Fig. 3.14B). The major ganglia of the autonomic nervous system are listed in Table 3.6. Interneurones within the ganglia receive signals from sensory neurones and pass them on to motoneurones controlling effector cells. Unlike locally sited interneurones, they are able to receive information from, and pass information to, a much wider selection of cells (Fig. 3.14B).

Spinal cord and brain stem

The largest groupings of interneurones within the autonomic nervous system are found in the spinal cord, and parts of the brain stem (medulla oblongata, pons and hypothalamus) (Fig. 3.14C and Ch. 20). Many reflex

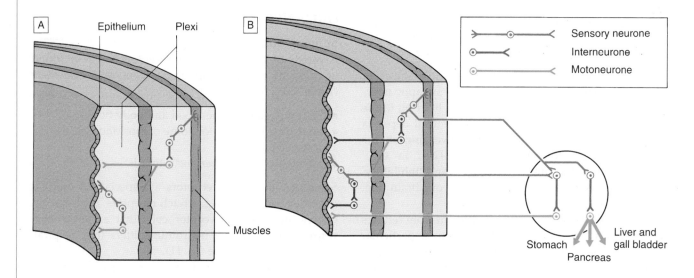

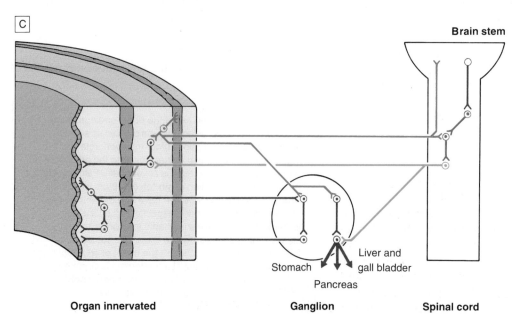

Figure 3.14
Autonomic innervation of the gastrointestinal tract:
A Arrangement of neurones in the wall of the gastrointestinal tract
B Linkages with ganglia
C Linkages with the spinal cord and brain stem.

Table 3.5 Sensory receptors of the autonomic nervous system

Type	Location	Sensitive to:	Chapter reference
Mechanoreceptors (stretch receptors)	Arteries Veins Lungs Gastrointestinal tract Bladder	Blood pressure Blood volume Inflation/deflation Volume of contents Volume of contents	5, 11 7 6 8
Chemoreceptors	Carotid and aortic arteries Hypothalamus	O_2, CO_2, H^+ Glucose	11, 12 14
Osmoreceptors	Hypothalamus	Osmotic pressure	13
Thermoreceptors	Hypothalamus	Temperature	16
Nociceptors	Most organs/tissues	Injury	32

Table 3.6 Major ganglia of the autonomic nervous system*

Superior, middle and inferior cervical ganglia
Ganglia of the sympathetic chain
Coeliac ganglion
Superior mesenteric ganglion
Inferior mesenteric ganglion

* All are at a distance from the organs/tissues innervated.

responses are mediated via groups of cells in these areas (*spinal* and *brain stem reflexes*).

The specific example shown in Figure 3.15 illustrates part of the nervous control of bladder emptying (see Ch. 8). The interneurones linking the sensory and motor parts of this system are in the lower (*sacral*) part of the spinal cord. The activity of the interneurones is influenced by impulses from sensory receptors in the bladder as well as by signals from other parts of the spinal cord and brain stem and from parts of the brain involved in voluntary behaviour (*cerebral hemispheres*; see Ch. 20). Thus the bladder emptying reflex can be inhibited by voluntary control.

The plexi, ganglia, spinal cord and brain stem also contain the cell bodies of the neurones transmitting signals back towards the effector cells (glands, muscles and endocrine cells) and which form the motor components of the autonomic nervous system.

Motor components

Some motoneurones, such as those from the plexi, contact the effector cells directly. Others, such as those coming from the spinal cord and brain stem, synapse with neurones in the ganglia or the plexi, passing their signals on to the nerve fibres (*post-ganglionic fibres*) actually innervating the effector cells.

Anatomically the motor part of the autonomic nervous system can be divided into two parts (Fig. 3.16):

- sympathetic
- parasympathetic.

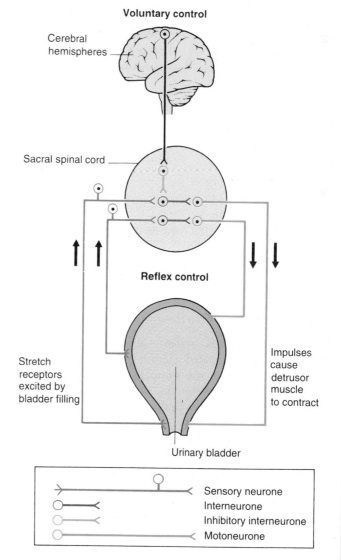

Figure 3.15
Neural control of bladder emptying (micturition).

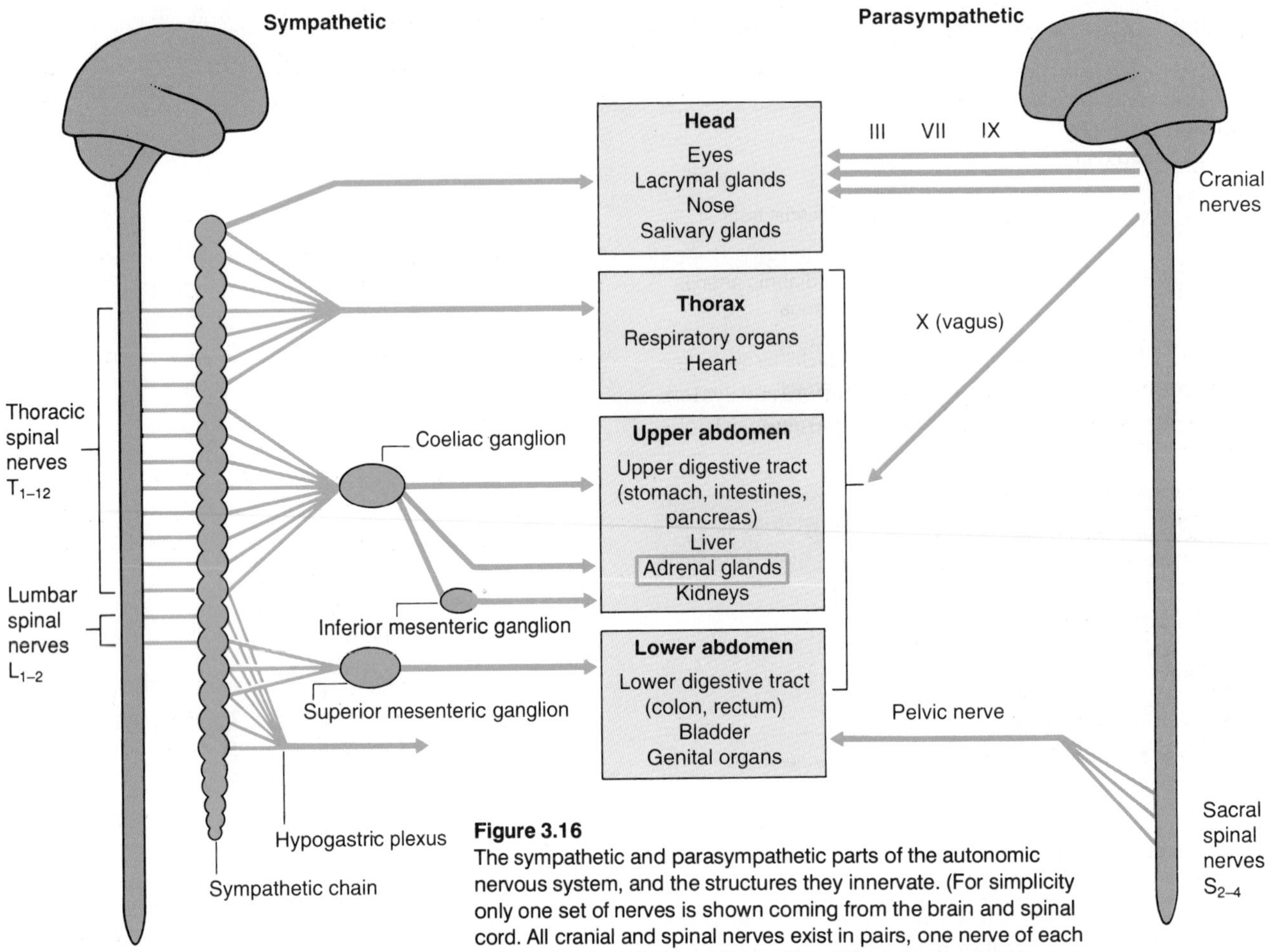

Figure 3.16
The sympathetic and parasympathetic parts of the autonomic
nervous system, and the structures they innervate. (For simplicity
only one set of nerves is shown coming from the brain and spinal
cord. All cranial and spinal nerves exist in pairs, one nerve of each
pair serving the left side of the body and the other the right.)

Sympathetic divison

The sympathetic division consists of:

- autonomic nerve fibres emerging from the *thoracic* and *lumbar* parts of the spinal cord
- interconnected ganglia of the *sympathetic chain*
- *coeliac, superior* and *inferior mesenteric ganglia*
- nerve fibres going from these ganglia to the effectors.

The ganglia in this system, allow many different effectors to be activated simultaneously, so that for example in exercise, the sympathetic nervous system simultaneously stimulates the heart, expands the airways and reduces activity in the digestive tract. ⑫

> A nervous patient can also exhibit these signs and symptoms because of increased activity in the sympathetic nervous system. Thus, a raised pulse may be psychological.

Another feature making the sympathetic nervous system exert widespread effects is that it controls secretion of hormones by the *adrenal medulla*. This endocrine gland is innervated by nerve fibres from the thoracic part of the spinal cord and secretes *adrenaline* plus a little *noradrenaline* (see Ch. 10).

Parasympathetic division

The parasympathetic division consists of the autonomic nerve fibres emerging from the *brain stem* and the *sacral spinal cord*. The autonomic fibres are bound up with the somatic fibres in:

- cranial nerves III, VII, IX, and X (see Ch. 20)
- the pelvic nerve (which arises from branches of the 2nd to 4th sacral spinal nerves).

These nerves extend directly to the organs and tissues that they supply, or to ganglia very close to them. Because ganglia are not closely interconnected, organs and tissues tend to be activated individually. ⑬

For example, the urinary bladder is reflexly excited by parasympathetic nerves in response to distension without bowel movements occurring simultaneously. Similarly, if the eyes are irritated by dust or chemicals, they water because of the reflex excitation of lacrymal glands by parasympathetic nerve fibres in cranial nerve VII, but this is not accompanied by mouth watering.

Dual innervation

Most organs and tissues are innervated by both sympathetic and parasympathetic nerves. They receive

⑫
Find out what
effect the
sympathetic
nervous
system has on
sweat glands,
salivary glands
and the eye.

⑬
The vagus
(cranial nerve
X) supplies,
among other
organs, the
stomach. What
are the effects
on the
stomach of
vagal nerve
stimulation?
What would be
the effect of
surgically
cutting the
vagus supply
to the stomach
(vagotomy)?

a *dual innervation*. Frequently the effects of the two systems are in opposition. For example the sympathetic nerves increase the heart rate whereas parasympathetic nerves slow it down; conversely, parasympathetic nerves increase the activity of the digestive glands and the contractions of the gut whereas sympathetic nerves inhibit them.

Usually there is activity in both systems simultaneously. Both are said to be *tonically active*. The activity of the cells innervated then depends upon the *balance* of activity in the two systems at any given time. This means that the heart rate can be made to increase not just by increasing activity in the sympathetic system but also by *decreasing* activity in the parasympathetic system too (Ch. 5).

If parasympathetic nerves increase gut contraction and promote defaecation, it follows that a patient who is under stress and has increased sympathetic activity may find it difficult to have a proper bowel movement. The provision of privacy and the maintenance of dignity are important in helping patients have their bowels opened. The same applies to micturition. Some people cannot pass urine in a public setting, such as a public convenience where others are present, or on a ward with others nearby.

NEUROCHEMISTRY

At one time only two neurotransmitters were believed to be of importance in the autonomic nervous system:

- acetylcholine
- noradrenaline.

It is now known that there are many more and that each neurotransmitter probably interacts with more than one type of receptor protein. Knowledge of the neurochemistry of the autonomic nervous system is important in understanding how and where some commonly used drugs act.

Neurotransmitters

The list of neurotransmitters (Fig. 3.17) grows ever larger as increasingly sophisticated techniques identify the presence of different substances within the vesicles in nerve endings. Neurones are classified according to the type of transmitter that they release:

- cholinergic (acetylcholine)
- adrenergic (noradrenaline)
- aminergic (dopamine, 5-hydroxytryptamine)
- peptidergic (peptides, of which there are many!).

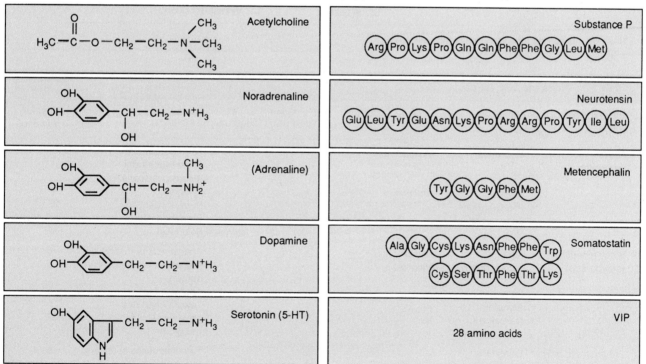

Figure 3.17
Some of the many neurotransmitters now known to be present in the autonomic nervous system. There are two major groups: monoamines (note the similarities between them in chemical structure) and peptides comprised of amino acids (Arg, Lys, Phe are abbreviations for individual amino acids; see Ch. 2). Adrenaline strictly is a hormone. (5-HT – 5-hydroxytryptamine; VIP – vasoactive intestinal polypeptide.)

Cholinergic neurones

Many of the motoneurones that are activated by locally placed interneurones (usually part of the parasympathetic nervous system) are cholinergic, as are many of the motoneurones synapsing with cells in the ganglia and plexi.

Adrenergic neurones

Most but not all of the motoneurones arising from the ganglia of the sympathetic nervous system, that control effector cells, are adrenergic. Noradrenaline is similar to the hormone adrenaline both in its chemistry (Fig. 3.17) and its actions.

Peptidergic and other neurones

Other neurones, including many sensory neurones and interneurones, release one or more peptide, or amino transmitters. Some of the peptides, such as somatostatin and VIP, are known also to be secreted by endocrine cells and can act as local hormones (see Ch. 6).

Table 3.7   Neurotransmitters and membrane receptors

Neurotransmitter	Receptor	Example		Chapter reference
		Site	Effect	
Acetylcholine	Muscarinic	Salivary glands	Mouth waters	6
	Nicotinic	Ganglia	Excited neurones	3
Noradrenaline	α_1 (alpha $_{one}$)	Iris (radial muscles)	Pupil dilates	26
		Blood vessels	Vasoconstriction	5
	α_2 (alpha $_{two}$)	Nerve cells	—	
	β_1 (beta $_{one}$)	Heart	Heart beats faster	5
	β_2 (beta $_{two}$)	Airways	Airways dilate	7
Opioid peptides	μ (mu)	Nerve cells	Analgesic effect*	32
	κ (kappa)	Nerve cells	Hallucination*	23
	δ (delta)	Nerve cells	?	
5-hydroxytryptamine	5-HT$_1$	Nerve cells	Change in mood*	31
	5-HT$_2$	Blood vessels	Vasoconstriction	5

* Involves neurones in the somatic nervous system.

Table 3.8   Drugs and their actions

General mode of action	Name	Receptors affected	Other action	Source/use	Chapter reference
Activate receptors (agonists)	Muscarine	Muscarinic	—	Toxic constituent of the mushroom *Amanita muscaria*	—
	Nicotine	Nicotinic	—	In tobacco	—
	Phenylephrine	α_1	—	Pupillary dilation	26
	Salbutamol	β_2	—	Bronchodilator	7
	Morphine	μ	—	Pain relief	32
Block receptors (antagonists)	Atropine	Muscarinic	—	Anaesthetic premedication	6
	Trimetaphan	Nicotinic	—	Lowers blood pressure in surgery	5
	Prazosin	α_1	—	Antihypertensive	5
	Atenolol	β_1	—	Lowers heart rate	5
	Naloxone	μ	—	Reverses action of morphine	32
Enhance synaptic transmission	Distigmine	—	Inhibits acetylcholinesterase	Selected cases of urinary retention	8
	Cocaine*	—	Inhibits re-uptake of noradrenaline	Promotes local vasoconstriction in nasal surgery	5

* Cocaine acts as a local anaesthetic (see Ch. 21), hence its use in nasal surgery.

Receptor proteins

Neurotransmitters work by binding to and activating receptor proteins in the cell membrane that, in turn, affect cell activity (see Ch. 2). Usually there is more than one type of membrane receptor for each neurotransmitter (Table 3.7).

For acetylcholine

The membrane receptors binding acetylcholine are of two types:

- nicotinic (activated also by nicotine)
- muscarinic (activated also by muscarine).

Muscarinic receptors are found on effector cells whereas *nicotinic receptors* are present on motoneurones of the plexi and ganglia.

For noradrenaline and adrenaline

At least four different receptors have been identified:

- α_1 and α_2 (alpha $_{one}$ and alpha $_{two}$)
- β_1 and β_2 (beta $_{one}$ and beta $_{two}$).

Noradrenaline tends to be better than adrenaline at interacting with α receptors whereas the reverse is true for β receptors. α and β receptors are found on many effector cells. Different cells may have more of one type of receptor than another. Heart muscle cells, for example, possess β receptors, whereas blood vessels have mainly α receptors.

For other neurotransmitters

Different receptors are being identified for other neurotransmitters too (Table 3.7).

Drugs

Drugs can be used in various ways to accentuate or depress activity in different parts of the autonomic nervous system. Some drugs bind to the receptors and either stimulate them or inhibit them. Others affect the release and disposal of neurotransmitters.

Mimicking natural transmitters

Drugs that are similar in structure to natural transmitters may bind to the receptors and activate them (Table 3.8). They are *agonists* as they have the same effect as the natural transmitter.

Blocking transmitter action

Substances that are similar in structure to the natural transmitters may also bind to a receptor without activating it. They are *antagonists* because they stop the neurotransmitter from getting to the receptor site and, consequently, block the transmission of nerve impulses at those synapses (Table 3.8).

DRUGS AND THE AUTONOMIC NERVOUS SYSTEM

Can drugs help us pass exams? Most of us are familiar with that mixture of excitement and anxiety as an important examination approaches. We can probably recollect some of the symptoms: a fast heart rate, a fine tremor of the hands, and sweating palms. However well we have revised, such an emotional state may prevent us from doing our best in the examination room.

Some of the drugs that work on the autonomic nervous system may be of value for people who are strongly affected by 'nerves' (although it is not suggested that they should be routinely prescribed for all examination candidates!). Propranolol is one such drug. It is one of the beta blockers, drugs that block the action of the catecholamines, adrenaline and noradrenaline, on adrenoreceptor sites in various parts of the body. Some of the principal therapeutic uses of propranolol are outlined below, but there is also some penetration of the central nervous system, causing a degree of sedation. Unfortunately, side effects, such as hallucinations, may occur. There is also a reduction in heart rate, sweating and fine tremor, which is of use in the treatment of anxiety. It is unclear whether these effects are due to the action of propranolol on the brain or more peripherally.

Propranolol is usually prescribed for the treatment of hypertension, angina and certain cardiac arrhythmias, because of its blocking action on adrenoreceptors in the heart and blood vessels. Heart rate, and force of contraction are reduced. Blood pressure falls because of the relaxation of smooth muscle in the walls of arterioles, bringing about vasodilation.

Some beta blockers are cardioselective, working only on beta receptors in the heart. Others, including propranolol, are not selective and act, for example, on the airways as well as the heart. For this reason propranolol is contraindicated for asthmatics.

Q. If adrenaline and noradrenaline have the effect of dilating the bronchioles, what side effect might propranolol have on the airways? Why might this side effect be of particular concern to an asthmatic patient?

Another drug that works on the autonomic nervous system is propantheline. It is sometimes prescribed for intestinal colic and hypermotility, and for spasm of the bladder and ureters. Like atropine (of which it is a synthetic version) propantheline reduces smooth muscle activity – for example in the intestines and urinary system – by inhibiting the action of the neurotransmitter acetylcholine released at nerve endings. It is therefore referred to as one of the *anticholinergic* drugs. Knowledge of the action of acetylcholine will assist the student in anticipating many of the side effects of the drug and explaining their occurrence to the patient. These side effects may include a dry mouth because of reduced salivary secretion and blurred vision because of reduced accommodation.

Q. Why should anticholinergics not be given to patients with glaucoma? Why might a patient taking propantheline for urethral spasm become constipated?

Enhancing synaptic transmission

Drugs can also be used to enhance synaptic transmission rather than suppress it. They may:

- facilitate the release of transmitter
- prolong the action of the transmitter.

The action of a transmitter can be prolonged either by preventing its breakdown, or by reducing its re-uptake into the nerve terminals (Table 3.8).

EXTENDING NURSING CARE – RELAXATION THERAPY AND HYPERTENSION

There is sometimes a temptation to regard the somatic and autonomic nervous systems as two entirely separate entities. After all, I can raise my arm, clench my fist, or change my posture; but I cannot influence my intestinal contractions by will power alone, or change my heart rate. Nevertheless, links may be made between the two systems: by lowering my hand into a basin of warm water I can bring about vasodilation in its surface vessels; by running up stairs I can bring about a fairly substantial increase in both my heart and respiratory rates.

Physicians and therapists have sought ways in which changes in voluntary muscle activity can produce beneficial changes in a person's autonomic nervous system. Techniques, such as biofeedback and meditation, now exist, and relaxation for relatively short periods each day is claimed to help reduce blood pressure. It is thought that regular relaxation sessions help to reduce the levels of circulating adrenaline and noradrenaline, which in turn decreases the force of contraction of the heart and, therefore, blood pressure.

Such claims are exciting for patients suffering from hypertension (raised blood pressure) and for those who care for them. Hypertension is often effectively treated with drugs, but it can only benefit the patient to feel that he is actively contributing to his own health by practising relaxation techniques. Most of such techniques pay particular attention to the respiration rate. The individual is advised to attend to his breathing, trying to ignore other stimuli, and then deliberately to slow down his respiration rate. As this occurs, it may be noticed after a time that the pulse rate reduces, blood pressure falls, and the individual feels calm and at ease.

Currently, relaxation therapy is perhaps most often used in nursing the mentally ill, but there may be scope for widening the skills of those nursing the physically ill. Might it be possible for the nurse to teach patients simple relaxation techniques, rather than reaching for the night sedation bottle? It is not suggested, of course, that such techniques would replace drug therapy. Clearly, medical and nursing skills must be regarded as complementary.

KEY POINTS

What you should now know and understand about homeostasis and control:

- what is meant by homeostasis
- the basic components of a control system and how they work together to maintain homeostasis
- why the circulation of the blood is important in the maintenance of homeostasis
- the fundamental differences between neural and hormonal control systems
- the major endocrine glands, the types of hormones produced and their fate
- the basic structure and functioning of nerve cells
- how nerve cells are linked together to form a simple nervous system
- what a reflex is and how it differs from voluntary behaviour
- what the autonomic nervous system is: its organisation, characteristics and function
- how some commonly used drugs that affect the autonomic nervous system actually work.

REFERENCES AND FURTHER READING

Most of the themes introduced in this chapter are developed in detail later in the book: the way in which the different elements of the internal environment are homeostastically controlled – Section 2, Chapters 11 to 19; blood – Chapter 4; capillaries and their function – Chapter 5; hormones – Chapter 10; neurones – Chapter 21. Further reading is listed at the ends of these chapters.

Boore J R P, Champion R, Ferguson M C (eds) Nursing the physically ill adult. Churchill Livingstone, Edinburgh, ch 12

Carson E R, Cramp D G 1985 Computers and control in clinical medicine. Plenum Publishing, New York
(Specialist text applying control systems theory and computer technology to the care and management of patients)

Hopkins S J 1992 Drugs and pharmacology for nurses, 11th edn. Churchill Livingstone, Edinburgh, chs 6 & 7

Rang H P, Dale M M 1991 Pharmacology, 2nd edn. Churchill Livingstone, Edinburgh
(Advanced student textbook. Useful for reference in following the action of drugs on the autonomic nervous system)

Trounce J 1990 Clinical pharmacology for nurses, 13th edn. Churchill Livingstone, Edinburgh
(Describes drugs commonly used in practice and explains how they work)

Section 2
THE INTERNAL ENVIRONMENT AND ITS MAINTENANCE

Human beings can survive under an amazing variety of conditions. We can live under the hot sun of desert regions, or in the thin air of the mountains. We can go all day without a drink, or we can fast for many days. We can travel from place to place and meet new threats in our environment, in the air we breathe and in the food we eat.

This freedom to live in a variety of differing environments, and to explore new ones, comes about because of the stability of our *inner* environment. This is the one in which almost all the cells of the body live. So long as this environment is preserved in the face of all the challenges that we meet from day to day, we remain well.

This section deals with the parts and systems of the body which have the primary function of creating and maintaining this inner environment.

Part A
COMPONENT PARTS AND SYSTEMS:
structure and function

The parts of the body that are chiefly concerned with creating and maintaining the internal environment are:

- blood
- heart and blood vessels
- respiratory apparatus
- digestive tract
- kidneys and bladder
- endocrine glands

and the autonomic nervous system, already described in Chapter 3.

The chapters in this part focus on different parts of the body in turn and:

- outline the relevant anatomy and histology
- explain how each part works
- show how some parts work together as a system
- describe the processes occurring in these systems.

Chapter 4
BLOOD AND RELATED TISSUES

Blood is composed of many constituents, cellular and non-cellular. The cellular components, erythrocytes, leucocytes and platelets, are formed in haemopoietic and lymphoid tissues (bone marrow, thymus gland and lymph nodes), and are disposed of by phagocytic cells mainly in the spleen and the liver. The non-cellular component (plasma) consists of water and dissolved solutes.

Blood is usually liquid. It is therefore a mobile tissue and it is this distinctive property which enables it to be circulated between all other tissues of the body. It can, however, be converted very quickly into a gel. This helps to seal off damaged blood vessels and limits the leakage of blood from the circulation.

HAEMOPOIETIC AND LYMPHOID TISSUES

Several tissues and organs are involved in the formation, and disposal of blood cells (Fig. 4.1). In the adult person, blood cells develop in the bone marrow from stem cells (see Ch. 2). Some of the cells (leucocytes; see p. 66) undergo further maturation and proliferation in lymphoid tissues such as the thymus gland and lymph nodes.

Aged and injured cells are removed from the circulation by large phagocytic cells (*macrophages*) many of which are lodged in blood vessels of the spleen and the liver.

BONE MARROW

Marrow is the soft tissue that fills the cavities present in bone (see Fig. 4.2 and Ch. 28). It consists of:

- blood cell precursors (in various stages of development)
- fat cells
- macrophages (large phagocytic cells)
- fibroblasts (which produce collagen fibres).

The blood capillaries (*sinusoids*) that supply the marrow are relatively leaky. Blood cells formed in the marrow can squeeze through spaces in the walls of the sinusoids to enter the circulatory system.

When the marrow is very active it looks red because of the huge number of developing red cells (*erythrocytes*) present. It becomes yellowish when its blood-cell-

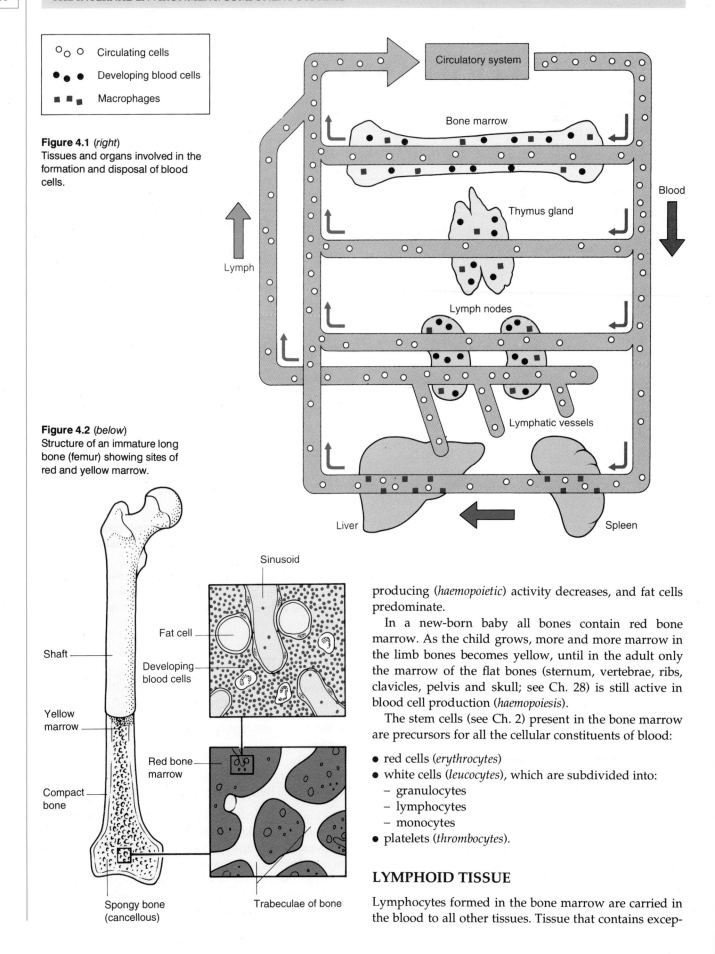

Circulating cells

Developing blood cells

Macrophages

Figure 4.1 (*right*)
Tissues and organs involved in the formation and disposal of blood cells.

Circulatory system

Bone marrow

Blood

Thymus gland

Lymph

Lymph nodes

Lymphatic vessels

Figure 4.2 (*below*)
Structure of an immature long bone (femur) showing sites of red and yellow marrow.

Liver   Spleen

Sinusoid

Fat cell

Shaft

Developing blood cells

Yellow marrow

Red bone marrow

Compact bone

Spongy bone (cancellous)

Trabeculae of bone

producing (*haemopoietic*) activity decreases, and fat cells predominate.

In a new-born baby all bones contain red bone marrow. As the child grows, more and more marrow in the limb bones becomes yellow, until in the adult only the marrow of the flat bones (sternum, vertebrae, ribs, clavicles, pelvis and skull; see Ch. 28) is still active in blood cell production (*haemopoiesis*).

The stem cells (see Ch. 2) present in the bone marrow are precursors for all the cellular constituents of blood:

- red cells (*erythrocytes*)
- white cells (*leucocytes*), which are subdivided into:
  - granulocytes
  - lymphocytes
  - monocytes
- platelets (*thrombocytes*).

LYMPHOID TISSUE

Lymphocytes formed in the bone marrow are carried in the blood to all other tissues. Tissue that contains excep-

In certain *dyscrasias* (blood disorders) specimens of red bone marrow are obtained by needle biopsy from the sternum or iliac crest. The number, size, shape and characteristics of cells in the various developmental and maturational phases are noted. This procedure can be a valuable diagnostic aid but is an unpleasant experience for the patient because of the pressure needed to penetrate the hard bony cortex, although the use of local anaesthetic ensures there is no actual pain.

tionally large congregations of lymphocytes is termed *lymphoid*. Examples include:

- thymus gland
- lymph nodes
- tonsils.

Lymphoid tissue is also present in the spleen.

Thymus gland

The thymus is a small bi-lobed gland (10–20 g in an adult) situated at the top of the chest underneath the breast bone (*sternum*) and on top of the major vessels entering and leaving the heart (Fig. 4.3A).

The thymus consists of a framework of epithelial cells housing an enormous population of developing *lymphocytes*. The outer (*cortical*) parts are more densely populated than the inner (*medullary*) parts (Fig. 4.3B). Immature lymphocytes from the bone marrow migrate into the cortex of the thymus, mature and proliferate there. Most of the cells live for only a short while and are disposed of by macrophages within the thymus. Some leave the gland and enter the bloodstream (T-lymphocytes).

The thymus secretes hormones (*lymphopoietin, thymosins*) which regulate the production and activity of lymphocytes in the thymus, other lymphoid tissues and the circulation.

The thymus is most active early in life but continues to function, to a decreasing extent, into old age.

Lymph nodes

Lymph nodes are similar in structure to the thymus in that they each consist of an encapsulated supporting framework of cells packed full of developing lymphocytes (Fig. 4.4). However, lymph nodes are much smaller than the thymus gland. They are permeated by *lymph*, which is tissue fluid carried away from the tissue spaces in *lymphatic vessels*. Lymphatic vessels are blind-ending tubes originating in the tissue spaces, which act as an overflow for interstitial fluid, and carry it back

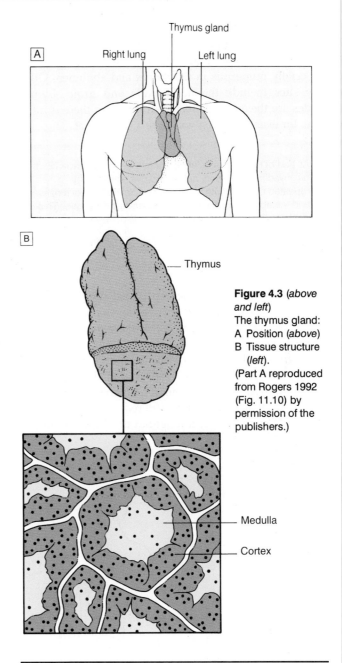

Figure 4.3 (*above and left*) The thymus gland: A Position (*above*) B Tissue structure (*left*). (Part A reproduced from Rogers 1992 (Fig. 11.10) by permission of the publishers.)

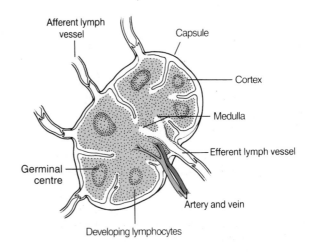

Figure 4.4 (*right*)
Structure of a lymph node. (Reproduced from Rogers 1992 (Fig. 11.2) by permission of the publishers.)

into the circulatory system (see Ch. 5 and Fig. 5.29). Lymph nodes occur at intervals along these vessels.

Lymph nodes are found throughout the body but are especially numerous in the thorax and abdomen. Other key sites include the neck, axilla and groin. Lymph nodes are the 'glands' that swell up when there is infection, for example when you have a sore throat. ①

> As part of the body's defence system, lymphoid tissue filters out invading organisms but can be overwhelmed by repeated or very acute infections and, in the case of tonsils and the appendix, may have to be removed surgically. This depletes the body defenses and is only done when essential.

Tonsils

Tonsils are clumps of unencapsulated lymphoid tissue lying just below the surface covering (*epithelium*) of the digestive tract. The uppermost of these are the *adenoids* (*nasopharyngeal tonsils*), which are prominent in young children (Fig. 4.5). Other tonsils are found at the back of the mouth (*palatine tonsils*) and around the base of the tongue (*lingual tonsils*). Similar lymphoid tissue is also found in the *appendix*, and scattered in small and large clumps (*Peyer's patches*) throughout the digestive tract.

SPLEEN

The spleen is a sizeable organ, weighing about 200 to 250 g, which filters out damaged or abnormal cells in the blood, including red cells and bacteria. In the neonate (see Ch. 35) it is one of the sites of red cell production. The spleen is situated to the left in the abdomen, tucked between the stomach and the left kidney (Fig. 4.6). It is enclosed by a capsule of connective tissue and is richly supplied with blood, which gives it its dark red appearance. Blood seeps through the tissue (*pulp*) of the spleen rather like water through a sponge. The leaky splenic capillaries (*sinusoids*) allow blood cells to pass out of the circulation into the tissue spaces, and then to move back again via different sinusoids.

The splenic pulp consists largely of blood cells and macrophages, and fibroblasts. The macrophages have the important function of phagocytosing any damaged or abnormal cells and cell debris that gets trapped in the pulp. Also scattered throughout the pulp are small clumps of lymphoid tissue, which to the naked eye look like small white spots.

① *What causes lymph glands to swell when there is infection and why are they painful?*

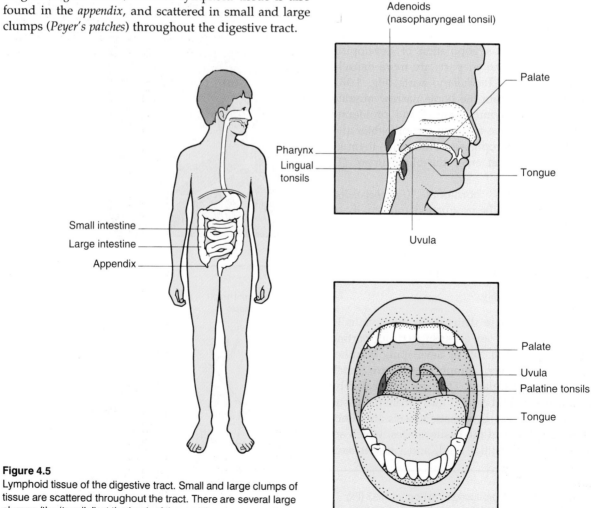

Figure 4.5
Lymphoid tissue of the digestive tract. Small and large clumps of tissue are scattered throughout the tract. There are several large clumps (the 'tonsils') at the back of the mouth.

A Position

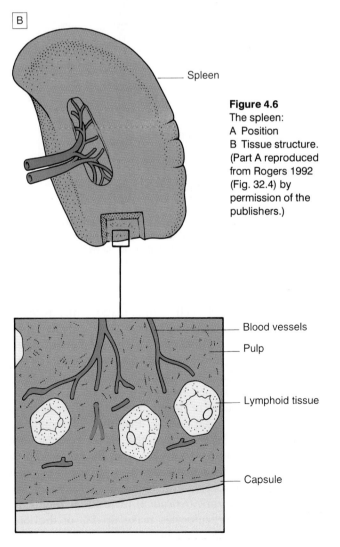

Figure 4.6
The spleen:
A Position
B Tissue structure.
(Part A reproduced
from Rogers 1992
(Fig. 32.4) by
permission of the
publishers.)

BLOOD

COMPOSITION

The circulatory system normally contains about 5 litres of blood (8% of the body weight). About 3 litres of this is plasma, a water-based solution of proteins, electrolytes and other dissolved constituents. The remainder is cellular, and consists of:

- erythrocytes (red cells)
- leucocytes (white cells)
- thrombocytes (platelets).

If a sample of blood is spun in a tube in a centrifuge, the heavier constituents (the cellular components), are driven to the bottom of the tube leaving most of the plasma as a clear area at the top (Fig. 4.7). If the tube is the same diameter all the way up, the lengths of the cellular and plasma components can be measured, and the percentage of the total blood volume occupied by each can be calculated. The cellular fraction (*packed cell volume* or PCV, sometimes also called the *haematocrit*) is between 40 and 54% in men and 36 and 47% in women. It consists almost entirely of erythrocytes. Leucocytes and platelets form a very small fraction of the blood in health (no more than 1% of the total blood sample). They can be seen as the small white band at the top of the packed red cells.

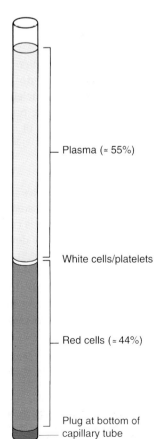

Figure 4.7
Appearance of a
sample of blood in a
capillary tube which
has been centrifuged
at high speed for 3
minutes.

BLOOD COMPONENTS AND THEIR USES

Blood can be separated into a variety of components each with qualities that can be used to treat a particular blood deficiency. The following are some examples:

- Red blood cells (packed frozen) – whole blood with 80% of the plasma removed; used to:
  - correct red blood cell deficiency and improve oxygen carrying capacity of the blood
  - transfuse organ transplant patients who have repeated *febrile* (feverish) reactions to blood transfusions containing active white cells. (In packed frozen RBCs white cells have been destroyed by freezing.)
- White blood cells (leucocyte concentrate) – whole blood with all red cells and 80% of the plasma removed; used to treat patients with life-threatening *granulocytopenia* (decreased granulocytes) when infections do not respond to antibiotics.
- Plasma (fresh or fresh frozen) – uncoagulated plasma separated from whole blood; used to:
  - treat a clotting factor deficiency when that factor is unknown
  - maintain normal clotting ability following massive intravenous infusions of stored blood.
- Platelets – platelets sedimented out from platelet-rich plasma and resuspended in 30 to 50 ml of plasma; used to treat the patient with *thrombocytopenia* (decreased platelets) whose bleeding is caused by decreased platelet production, increased platelet destruction, functionally abnormal platelets or massive transfusion of stored blood (*dilutional thrombocytopenia*).

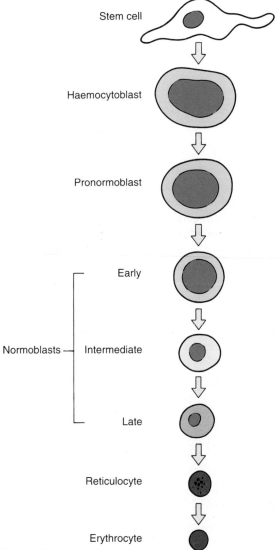

Figure 4.8
Stages in the development of the red cell from stem cells in the bone marrow to mature erythrocytes in the circulation. Cell division (mitosis; see Ch. 2) occurs at each stage as far as the late normoblast so that each pronormoblast gives rise to very many erythrocytes. (Based on McDonald, Paul & Cruickshank 1988.)

ERYTHROCYTES

Erythrocytes are quite different from any other cells in the body in that they do not possess any cellular organelles, not even a nucleus. Instead, they contain a very large amount of the protein *haemoglobin* which is involved in the transport of oxygen and carbon dioxide between the lungs and the tissues (see Ch. 7).

Development

In the adult, erythrocytes are formed in the bone marrow from pluripotent stem cells (see Ch. 2). The rate of production of red cells is controlled by erythropoietin (see Chs 10 and 11). Many developmental changes occur as red cells mature (Fig. 4.8). Each time the cells divide the daughter cells are slightly smaller than the parent cells. The synthesis of DNA for the nucleus requires the presence of vitamin B_{12} and folic acid. If these vitamins are deficient the erythrocytes formed are larger than normal (*macrocytic*).

During development the cell begins to manufacture one protein, *haemoglobin*, in very large amounts, so that eventually a large proportion of the cell is occupied by this substance. Each molecule of haemoglobin (see Fig. 7.21) consists of four units each of which is made up of:

- a polypeptide chain   • a haem unit   • an iron atom.

If iron is deficient, the cells cannot manufacture as much haemoglobin, and the cells tend to be smaller than normal in size (*microcytic*). As haemoglobin makes erythrocytes red in colour, cells that contain less of this protein look paler (*hypochromic*) than normal cells, when viewed through a microscope. ②

In the later stages of development cellular organelles disintegrate and disappear so that the cells emerging from the bone marrow into the blood contain only residual fragments, which also soon disappear. These fragments stain in a distinctive way giving these first immature erythrocytes the name of *reticulocytes* because of the network (*reticulum*) of residual fragments that is visible. Reticulocytes make up 1% of the total numbers of red cells in the blood.

② *What dietary advice would you give someone who has iron deficiency anaemia?*

Table 4.1   Red cell characteristics: normal and abnormal

	Normal	Megaloblastic anaemia	Iron deficiency anaemia
Mean cell volume (MCV)	86 ± 10 fl	High	Low
Mean cell haemoglobin (MCH)	29.5 ± 2.5 pg	High	Low
Mean cell haemoglobin concentration (MCHC)	325 ± 25 g/l	Normal	Low

Normal values

There are about 5×10^{12} red cells and 150 g haemoglobin per litre of blood (average in women: 4.8×10^{12} and 140 g/l; average in men: 5.5×10^{12} and 155 g/l). An increase in cell numbers above normal is *polycythaemia*, a decrease is *anaemia*. Clinically, anaemia is said to exist if the haemoglobin concentration in blood is less than an agreed reference value, usually 130 g/l in men and 115 g/l in women.

Using the figures for red cell count, haemoglobin concentration and PCV (42–45%) a few other values (*derived indices*) can be calculated, which are used in distinguishing between different types of anaemia (Table 4.1). The derived indices, and their normal values are:

$$\begin{aligned} \text{Mean cell volume (MCV)} &= \frac{\text{PCV}}{\text{Red cell count}} \\ &= \frac{45}{100} \times \frac{1}{5 \times 10^{12}} \\ &= 90 \times 10^{-15} \text{ litres} \\ &= 90 \text{ femtolitres (fl)} \end{aligned}$$

$$\begin{aligned} \text{Mean cell haemoglobin (MCH)} &= \frac{\text{Haemoglobin}}{\text{Red cell count}} \\ &= \frac{150}{5 \times 10^{12}} \\ &= 30 \times 10^{-12} \text{ g} \\ &= 30 \text{ picograms (pg)} \end{aligned}$$

$$\begin{aligned} \text{Mean cell haemoglobin concentration (MCHC)} &= \frac{\text{Haemoglobin}}{\text{PCV}} \times 100 \\ &= \frac{150 \times 100}{45} \\ &\approx 330 \text{ g per litre} \end{aligned}$$

Nature and metabolic activity

The mature erythrocyte is shaped like a flexible, biconcave disc (diameter 7μ). Its two major intracellular constituents, other than water, are haemoglobin and the enzyme carbonic anhydrase (see Ch. 7).

Although the erythrocyte has no mitochondria it can manufacture ATP by the process of *anaerobic glycolysis* (see Ch. 11) using enzymes of the cytosol, which generate ATP from glucose. Energy, in the form of ATP, is needed to maintain cell structure and normal conditions inside the cell. For example the high internal oxygen content, caused by the binding of oxygen by haemoglobin (see Ch. 7), threatens to oxidise some of the other molecular

ANAEMIAS

In anaemia there is a reduction in the number of circulating erythrocytes in the blood or a decrease in the concentration of haemoglobin. This results in a reduction in the capacity of the blood to carry oxygen. There are three ways in which anaemias can arise.

Anaemias secondary to decreased erythropoiesis:

- Nutritional deficiency anaemias – essential nutrients for erythrocyte production, such as iron, vitamin B_{12}, folic acid or protein, may be lacking due to dietary insufficiency or defective absorption. Treatment depends on cause and includes making good the deficit by dietary advice or supplement, or by injection.
- Aplastic anaemia – due to depressed bone marrow activity and usually involving decreased production of leucocytes and thrombocytes as well as red cells. The condition is caused by toxins from various drugs, chronic infection, excessive radiation or invasion by malignant cells. Treatment includes removal of the cause, transfusion of packed cells and platelets and possibly bone marrow transplant.

Anaemias secondary to increased destruction of red cells (haemolytic anaemias):

- Haemolytic anaemias resulting from intrinsic congenital defects where the cells do not have the ability to survive for their normal life span. These include hereditary spherocytosis, sickle cell anaemia and thalassaemia. Treatment may be removal of the spleen to reduce the excessive destruction of abnormal blood cells, and frequent blood transfusions.
- Haemolytic anaemias due to extrinsic factors, such as acquired antibodies, some infections and certain drugs and chemicals. Treatment is to remove or avoid the cause.

Anaemias secondary to blood loss:

- The loss of blood from the circulation through haemorrhage reduces the number of erythrocytes and therefore the oxygen carrying capacity of the blood. Bone marrow normally responds quickly to the hormone erythropoietin whose production is stimulated by tissue hypoxia (see Ch. 11), and blood loss can be replaced in 2 to 4 weeks. However, if over 20% of circulating volume is lost, it must be replaced by blood transfusion in order to avoid renal and cardiac failure.

components of the red cell. This chemical damage caused by oxygen has to be continually repaired.

Like other cells of the body, the red cell contains a protein in its plasma membrane, the *sodium–potassium*

ATPase, which ejects sodium from the cell. As sodium is moved against its natural concentration gradient, the transporter protein is referred to as a *pump*. The pump is important in maintaining the normal intracellular concentration of sodium. If the pumping activity decreases, sodium accumulates inside the cell, and one of the consequences of this is that water is drawn in too and the cell swells (see Ch. 13).

Fate

Eventually, erythrocyte metabolism declines, defects begin to appear, swelling occurs and the cells become less flexible. As a result, cells are more likely to get stuck in tight places, particularly in the capillaries and pulp of the spleen, and to be phagocytosed by macrophages (see Ch. 15). On average, the life span of a red cell is 120 days.

The cells that have been engulfed by the macrophages are digested by them, and the products are either recycled and re-used (for example amino acids and iron) or excreted (bilirubin) (Fig. 4.9) (see Chs 9 and 15).

Recycling of iron

This is very efficient. Only 1 to 2 mg of iron are lost from the body each day (from cells lost from the lining of the gut and from the skin). Yet about 20 mg are released daily from the breakdown of red cells. Iron in blood binds to a specific plasma protein, *transferrin*. This is a convenient way of carrying a lot of iron in the blood as well as ensuring that iron is targeted to the tissues most in need of it. Membrane receptors for transferrin are present in large numbers on the immature erythrocytes in the bone marrow.

Blood groups

Antigens and antibodies

Cells from different individuals are not exactly the same. They differ in the precise structure of some of the molecules, such as glycoproteins, projecting from the cell membrane (see Ch. 2). Some molecules occur in many individuals. Others are limited to a small family group. These variations create an enormous number of different *blood groups*, a few of which are listed in Table 4.2. The incidence of different blood groups varies between people of different ethnic origin (Table 4.3).

The fact of there being different blood groups is of no real consequence unless cells from one person are

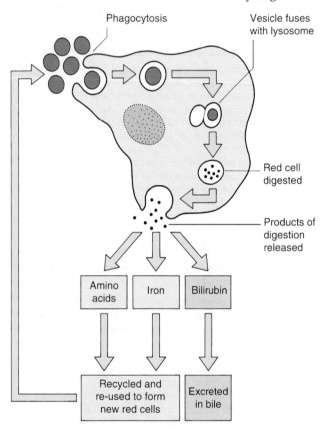

Figure 4.9
Fate of red cells and their constituents.

Table 4.2 Several blood group systems	
ABO	Lutheran
Rhesus	Kell
MNS	Lewis
P	Duffy

Table 4.3 Distribution of blood groups in different populations				
Blood group	UK*	Japan†	Indian sub-continent†	Basque region of Spain†
Rhesus positive	83%	98%	90%	69%
Rhesus negative	17%	2%	10%	31%
O	47%	31%	31%	57%
A	42%	38%	24%	42%
B	9%	22%	35%	1%
AB	3%	9%	9%	0%

* Compiled from Race & Sanger 1975.
† Compiled from Federation of American Societies for Experimental Biology publication 1971.

First pregnancy   **Second pregnancy**   **Third pregnancy**

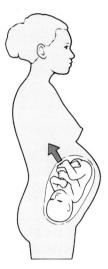
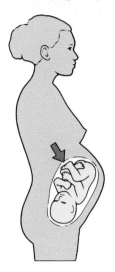
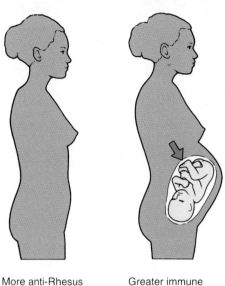

Some Rh+ cells from the baby enter the mother's circulation at birth.

Antibodies develop to the Rh+ cells.

Antibodies cross the placenta and destroy some of the baby's cells.

More anti-Rhesus antibodies develop in the mother.

Greater immune response and greater damage to the baby's red cells.

Figure 4.10
The sequence of events occurring when a mother whose blood group is Rhesus negative bears children who are Rhesus positive.

given to another, as for example in a blood transfusion. If the cells differ the recipient responds by developing an *immune* response: the molecules that are different (*antigens*) cause some white cells (*lymphocytes*) to proliferate and to secrete specific proteins (*antibodies*) targeted against the intruding cells (see Ch. 15 for details).

The first exposure to a brand new antigen elicits only a modest immune response. However, if the antigen is encountered again, the antibodies are ready and waiting, and react swiftly and powerfully to destroy the foreign cells.

A good example of this series of events is that of a pregnant mother who is *Rhesus negative* (does not possess the D Rhesus antigen) and who carries a baby who has inherited this antigen from its father, and who is therefore *Rhesus positive* (Rh+). Rhesus positive cells from the baby trigger the production of anti-D antibodies (anti-D immunoglobulin; see Ch. 15) an immune response in the mother, which can create serious difficulties for subsequent pregnancies (Fig. 4.10).

RHESUS INCOMPATIBILITY

About one in ten babies born to Rhesus negative mothers has Rh+ blood. Although the first such pregnancy usually results in a healthy baby, the antibodies that the mother develops have potentially fatal consequencies for any Rh+ babies of subsequent pregnancies when the maternal antibodies will cross the placenta and destroy fetal red blood cells. This condition is known as *erythroblastosis fetalis* and requires constant monitoring. The fetus becomes anaemic and hypoxic, and development is compromised. Brain damage and death may occur. Intrauterine exchange blood transfusion is often done to replace the Rh+ blood with Rh– and this may be repeated in the perinatal period.

In order to prevent this condition, the following measures are taken:

- Routine antenatal screening and blood grouping of all pregnant women.
- When a woman is found to be Rh– she is screened at regular intervals during pregnancy for Rh antibodies. Her partner is also screened and grouped. If the father is Rh–, no further action is needed; the baby also will be Rh–. If the father is Rh+, he may be either heterozygous for the Rhesus D factor, in which case the baby has a 50% chance of being Rh+, or homozygous when the baby will certainly be Rh+.
- A sample of cord blood is taken at birth to confirm the baby's blood group. The mother is given a standard injection of anti-D immunoglobulin which destroys circulating Rh+ antigens, preventing them from activating the immune system. Timing is critical and anti-D must be given within 72 hours of birth, or following abortion.
- In subsequent pregnancies, as well as routine maternal and paternal blood tests, the antibody levels (*titres*) in the blood are regularly monitored. Amniotic fluid many also be tested for antibodies through a procedure known as *amniocentesis*.

As a result of routine antenatal screening and prompt administration of anti-D immunoglobulin, erythroblastosis fetalis is now uncommon in the West.

Table 4.4 Bloods grouped according to the ABO system that can (√) and cannot (x) be safely transferred						
Donor's blood			*Recipient's blood group*			
Group	Antigens present	Antibodies present	A	AB	B	O
A	A	Anti-B	√	?	x	x
AB	A,B	—	x	√	x	x
B	B	Anti-A	x	?	√	x
O	—	Anti-A, Anti-B	?	?	?	√

? These bloods can be mixed, if used with care. Antibodies in the donor blood will attack some of the recipient's cells, but if the volume of donor blood is small compared with the volume of the recipient's blood the effects are relatively minor.

③

What precautions do you take before administering each new bag of blood or blood component to avoid adverse reactions from the recipient?

④

What routine observations do you make on a patient who is undergoing blood transfusion and why?

Iso-antibodies

Antibodies to the A and B antigens of the ABO system develop in the blood in many people very soon after birth. The origin of these so-called *iso-antibodies* was a mystery for many years.

It is now known that substances that act like A and B antigens are quite common in nature. B antigens for example are present in bacteria like *Escherichia coli* (*Esch. coli*). The new-born baby absorbs small amounts of intact proteins through its digestive tract for a short while after birth. A and B antigens, picked up orally, can therefore slip into the bloodstream and trigger the production of anti-A and anti-B antibodies.

It is the natural presence of the anti-A and anti-B antibodies in the blood that makes blood transfusion a hazardous procedure for many people unless blood has been previously typed and matched (Table 4.4).

Transfusion reactions

If red cell antigens encounter their corresponding antibodies, they bind to one another. This coating of antibody has several effects. It:

- makes the cells adhere to one another (*agglutinate*)
- activates the *complement system*, which breaks open (*lyses*) the cell (see Ch. 15)
- singles out the cells for attack by macrophages.

The consequences of these reactions can be life-threatening if a large number of red cells are affected. In particular the sudden rupture of cells (*haemolysis*) by the complement system releases intracellular constituents,

such as haemoglobin and potassium, into the plasma. The haemoglobin released passes through the urinary filter (see Ch. 8) into the urine and together with other released constituents can cause renal failure. Potassium affects the functioning of nerve and muscle cells (see Ch. 13). In addition, products of digestion released by activated macrophages reduce blood pressure and add to the overall shock to body systems. ③④

LEUCOCYTES

Significance

The leucocytes (*white blood cells*) form a tiny part (5%) of the nomadic population of defence cells scattered throughout the tissues of the body.

Defence cells are divided into two groups:

- lymphocytes
- phagocytic cells (granulocytes and macrophages).

Both groups work together to protect the body against invasion by foreign cells and molecules. Lymphocytes identify the invaders and phagocytic cells engulf and dispose of them (see Ch. 15 for details).

Origins

Defence cells develop from stem cells in the bone marrow. Once they have left the marrow they may (Fig. 4.11):

- circulate in the blood (then known as *leucocytes*)
- lodge in the walls of blood vessels in some organs (macrophages lodged in the liver are *Kupffer cells*; see Ch. 9)
- enter the interstitial space
- pass into the lymph
- accumulate in some organs and tissues (lymphocytes in lymphoid tissue).

The cells present in blood (leucocytes: $4–11 \times 10^9$/l) thus include some defence cells newly formed by the bone marrow as well as others that have spent time in tissues and organs before returning to the blood.

Before a patient receives a transfusion of blood products that contain red or white cells, a sample of blood is drawn for cross-matching (x-matching) with that of the donor. This is necessary in order to avoid incompatibility, and very stringent procedures are followed in identifying the patient and his blood group and ensuring that the blood to be transfused is compatible.

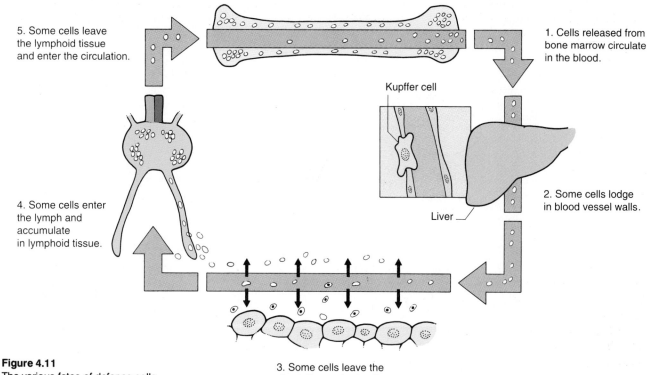

5. Some cells leave the lymphoid tissue and enter the circulation.

1. Cells released from bone marrow circulate in the blood.

Kupffer cell

4. Some cells enter the lymph and accumulate in lymphoid tissue.

Liver

2. Some cells lodge in blood vessel walls.

Figure 4.11
The various fates of defence cells released from the bone marrow.

3. Some cells leave the circulation and enter the interstitial space.

Types

Leucocytes are divided into three groups according to their appearance:

- granulocytes (42–82%)
- monocytes (2–10%)
- lymphocytes (20–45%).

Granulocytes (polymorphonuclear leucocytes) are normally in the majority (42–82%) followed by lymphocytes (20–45%) and monocytes (2–10%). Their distinctive features and development are summarised in Figure 4.12.

Granulocytes

Granulocytes have a granular appearance due to the presence of many vesicles. These vesicles contain different chemicals involved in the role of the cells in defence. Three different types of granulocyte have been distinguished on the basis of their reaction with different histochemical stains:

- neutrophils (90–95%)
- basophils (<1%).
- eosinophils (2–8%).

All are phagocytic. Neutrophils are the first phagocytic cells to be called into action in large numbers in response to injury or bacterial invasion. Their life span is relatively short, 1 to 2 days. The *pus* that collects at a wound consists mostly of dead neutrophils.

Basophils secrete *histamine* which dilates small blood vessels and *heparin* which is an anticoagulant (see below). Eosinophils inactivate histamine and leukotrienes (see Ch. 10) and kill parasitic worms.

Monocytes

Monocytes are the circulating precursors of *macrophages*. Some monocytes lodge in the walls of blood vessels and develop there into active macrophages (*fixed macrophages*, such as *Kupffer cells* of the liver, *littoral cells* of the spleen). Others are attracted into the tissues and are transformed into active cells whose characteristics vary according to the tissue in which they are found, such as:

- *alveolar macrophages* of the lungs
- *microglia* in the brain
- *histiocytes* in connective tissue
- *osteoclasts* in bone.

Macrophages are large, highly active, long-lived phagocytic cells. Because of their size they are able to engulf very large particles, and even intact cells, such as red cells.

Lymphocytes

Lymphocytes differ from most other leucocytes in that they are *not* phagocytic. Their function is the recognition and identification of foreign or abnormal material, such as bacteria and cancerous cells (see Ch. 15). Large

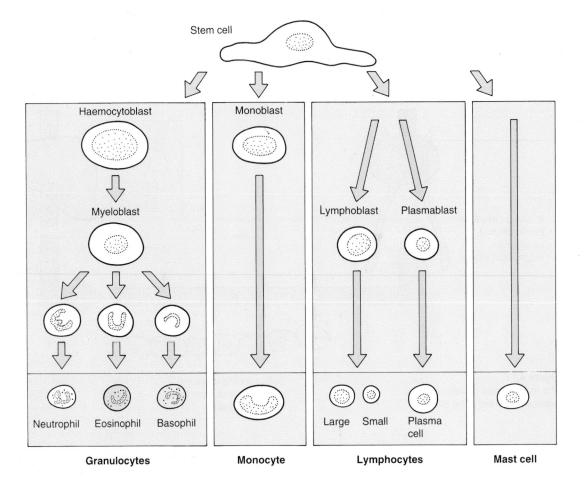

Figure 4.12
The different types of leucocyte and their development from stem cells. (Based on McDonald, Paul & Cruickshank 1988.)

numbers circulate between the blood, the tissue spaces, and the lymphatic system. Many lodge in the lymph nodes.

On encountering an antigen they recognise, they undergo transformation in structure and activity, and are stimulated to reproduce in large numbers. They manufacture and secrete substances, such as *antibodies*, which attach to the antigen and begin the process of its destruction and disposal. Their life spans vary. Some survive for many years.

PLATELETS

Platelets are tiny cellular fragments whose main function is sealing off leaks in blood vessels.

Origin and nature

Platelets are derived from the same pool, of pluripotent stem cells in the bone marrow as the other cellular constituents of blood. *Megakaryocytes* (Fig. 4.13), from which platelets are formed, develop from haemocytoblasts. Platelets consist of budded-off fragments of the megakaryocytes and contain very few cellular structures, but they secrete and produce a variety of chemicals (Table 4.5).

Circulation and fate

After leaving the bone marrow, platelets tend to lodge in the spleen for a few days before circulating freely in the bloodstream. There are normally about 150 to 400 ×

SIGNIFICANCE OF A DIFFERENTIAL WHITE BLOOD CELL COUNT

Leucocytosis – an increase in the total number of white blood cells (WBCs) – is a normal response to invading microorganisms and tissue destruction. As it is known that specific types of WBCs increase in certain disease conditions, a differential count may be ordered as an aid to diagnosis. For example:

- in acute infections, such as appendicitis and pneumonia, and following tissue destruction, as in myocardial infarction, the neutrophils increase rapidly (*neutrophil leucocytosis*)
- in chronic infections and diseases such as measles, mumps, pertussis and infectious hepatitis, lymphocytes increase (*lymphocytosis*)
- the number of monocytes is increased in protozoal infections such as malaria (*monocytosis*)
- the eosinophil count rises in allergic reactions and with parasitic invasion of the body (*eosinophilia*).

The WBC count returns to normal when the infection is controlled, or initiating factor disposed of.

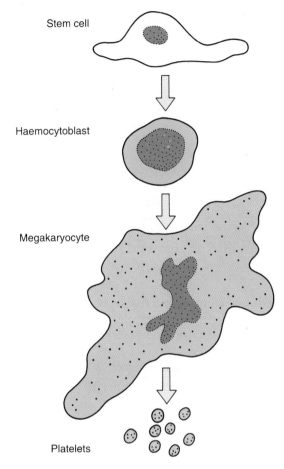

Stem cell

Haemocytoblast

Megakaryocyte

Platelets

Figure 4.13
Stages in the development of platelets. (Based on McDonald, Paul & Cruickshank 1988.)

Table 4.5 Some of the substances produced by platelets

Substance	Function
Serotonin (5-HT)	Vasoconstriction
Adenosine diphosphate (ADP)	Promotes platelet aggregation
Thromboxane	Vasoconstriction and platelet aggregation
Clotting factors	Promotes coagulation
Platelet-derived growth factor	Stimulates wound healing

10^9/litre. They are attracted to sites of blood vessel injury. Their average life span is between 9 and 12 days.

PLASMA

Blood cells and platelets are suspended in plasma (Table 4.6). Apart from the *plasma proteins* and substances which bind to them, such as calcium, the concentrations of substances present in plasma are almost the same as those in the interstitial fluid (see Ch. 2, Table 2.3).

WHITE BLOOD CELL DISORDERS

There are a number of diseases associated with disorders of the white blood cells and the following are examples.

In *leukaemia* (cancer of the blood) there is an excessive proliferation of leucocytes. Many cells remain immature (at the blast stage) and are therefore unable to perform their normal role in body defence. This renders the individual very susceptible to infection and system dysfunction as the circulating leukaemic cells infiltrate organs and tissues and impose an imbalance. The proliferation of white cells also reduces the production of red cells and platelets to the extent that patients with leukaemia are anaemic and have a tendency to bleed.

Treatment is directed towards suppressing the abnormal cell production and preventing complications. Radiation therapy or chemotherapy is often the treatment of choice followed by bone marrow transplantation.

In *leukopenia* there is a marked reduction in the number of circulating WBCs. As the most significant reduction is usually in the neutrophils, it may also be known as *neutropenia* or *agranulocytosis*.

Neutropenia is a consequence of bone marrow depression often caused by the toxic effects of drugs in people with a sensitivity or idiosyncrasy. The most frequently implicated drugs include, sulphonomides, chlorpromazine, thiouracil derivatives and gold salts. It may also be an integral part of aplastic anaemia as a consequence of radiation or anti-cancer drug therapy, or associated with typhoid fever, malaria or any overwhelming infection. It may also be due to excessive destruction of neutrophils by the spleen (*hypersplenism*).

Treatment is directed towards identifying the cause, removing or treating it and keeping the patient free from infection in a controlled environment. A gradual increase in neutrophil numbers can be expected in 2 to 3 weeks providing the bone marrow is able to perform its normal function.

Q: During the period of neutropenia patients have to be nursed in a protective environment. What basic principles of infection control would you apply in nursing such patients?

Table 4.6 Composition of plasma

	mmol/l
Sodium	145
Chloride	105
Hydrogen carbonate	25
Glucose	5
Organic anions*	5
Potassium	4
Protein	2 ≡ 60–80 g/l
Amino acids	2
Calcium	2
Magnesium	1
Phosphate	1
Sulphate	0.5

*Various substances produced by cell metabolism including: citrate, lactate, aceto-acetate, beta-hydroxybutyrate.

Table 4.7   A selection of plasma proteins

Name	Function(s)	Concentration	
		g/l	mg/l
Albumin	Transport (fatty acids, bilirubin etc.) Contributes most to oncotic pressure (see Ch. 5)	40	
Transferrin	Transports iron	2	
Transcobalamin	Transports vitamin B_{12}	—	—
Transcortin	Transports cortisol (see Ch. 10)	—	—
Fibrinogen		2–4	
Prothrombin	Coagulation		100–150
Factor V			10
Factor VIII			0.5
Angiotensinogen	Precursor of peptide hormone	—	—
Plasminogen	Precursor of enzyme	—	—

Plasma proteins

Nature and functions

The number of different proteins present in blood is very large and their functions are diverse (Table 4.7). Modern techniques such as radioimmunoassay allow individual proteins to be identified and quantified. In the past only a crude separation of the proteins was achieved, first into two fractions, *albumin* and *globulin*. Later the globulin fraction was further subdivided into alpha, beta and delta subgroups using the technique of electrophoresis. These names still persist although specific names for individual proteins are now more commonly used.

Sources

Plasma proteins come from two main sources:

- most are synthesised and secreted by the liver
- some are produced and secreted by lymphocytes (*immunoglobulins*, which are antibodies; see Ch. 15).

A small proportion of the total are proteins specifically manufactured and secreted by other cells, such as hormones secreted by endocrine cells. Others are incidental constituents of plasma released from injured or dead cells. An increased concentration of these in plasma can indicate injury to a particular tissue. For example in *myocardial infarction* the blood concentrations of the enzymes *creatine phosphokinase* and *glutamic oxaloacetic transaminase (GOT)* are usually increased.

HAEMOSTASIS

OVERVIEW

The functions of the blood in transport, communication and defence depend upon its free circulation as a liquid between different organs and tissues. Should any part of the circulatory system develop a leak through injury or weakness, the fluidity of blood becomes a grave threat to the body as a whole.

If a leak develops, several protective measures act to curb the loss of blood from the body. These include:

- constriction of the blood vessels
- formation of a platelet plug
- formation of fibrin (*coagulation*).

However, should any of these processes be triggered inappropriately, the normal circulation of blood to the tissues will be cut off. A delicate balance exists therefore between the factors that maintain the flow and fluidity of blood *within* the vessels of the circulation and the mechanisms that prevent its loss *from* the circulation (Fig. 4.14).

Sequence of events

When a leak occurs, the loss of blood is curbed first by:

- constriction of the injured blood vessels
- accumulation of platelets at the leak point.

These events narrow and plug the vessels. Simultaneously, blood at the site of injury begins to be converted from a fluid into a gel by the formation of fibrin strands (*coagulation*). As the injury is being repaired by the formation of new tissue, the gelled blood is liquefied by the breakdown of fibrin (*fibrinolysis*) and circulation is restored.

VASCULAR REACTIONS TO INJURY

If a blood vessel is cut, the immediate response is contraction of the smooth muscle in the vessel wall (see Chs 22 and 5). Contraction narrows and may even block off the vessel, reducing blood flow locally and restricting blood loss. The degree and duration of the

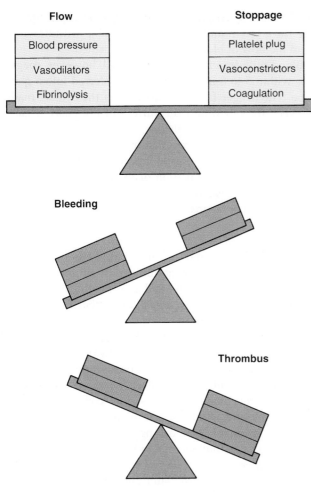

Flow   Stoppage

Blood pressure		Platelet plug
Vasodilators		Vasoconstrictors
Fibrinolysis		Coagulation

Bleeding

Thrombus

Figure 4.14
The delicate balance of factors which preserves blood flow through
the circulation whilst stopping the leakage of blood from it. Shifting
the balance results either in loss of blood from the circulation by
bleeding, or blockage of the circulation by a thrombus.

constriction is related to the extent of the injury. A clean
cut is sealed off less well by this means than one that
involves more trauma, probably because there is less
release of *vasoactive* chemicals (see Ch. 5) from the cut
tissues, and less stimulation of nerve and muscle fibres.

PLATELETS (THROMBOCYTES)

Adhesion

When injury occurs to a blood vessel, such that the
endothelial cells are traumatised or underlying tissues
consisting of collagen are exposed, platelets adhere to
the injured cells and tissues. Platelets are also good at
lodging in and sealing off any tiny gaps that may
appear in the endothelial lining of the blood vessels.
This is particularly important in the blood capillaries
(which consist entirely of endothelial cells; see Ch. 5).
Small gaps occur all the time and platelets act as the
main protection against these spontaneously occurring
leaks. ⑤

> **BLEEDING FROM INJURED VESSELS**
>
> Bleeding may be external and observable or internal and
> hidden.
>
>   The observable differences between arterial, venous and
> capillary bleeding reflect the structure and function of the
> particular vessels and the pressure within them.
>
>   In arterial bleeding, bright red oxygenated blood spurts
> out with each wave of arterial distension as the heart pumps
> blood around the body. Because of high pressure within
> arteries, blood loss may be considerable and is potentially
> fatal.
>
>   De-oxygenated venous blood, which is bluish in colour,
> flows more evenly from damaged vessels because it is not
> under pressure.
>
>   Capillary bleeding is characterised by oozing and is
> reddish in colour.
>
>   Haemostasis can be achieved by appropriate first-aid
> treatment, which facilitates the body's defence mechanisms.
> When a vessel is injured, these mechanisms are triggered to
> prevent undue blood loss and include reflex
> vasoconstriction, formation of haemostatic plug and blood
> coagulation (see main text). Initial first-aid treatment is the
> same for all types of bleeding: direct, firm pressure over the
> injury until haemostasis is achieved or, when major vessels
> are involved, surgical intervention to tie off or repair the
> injured vessels.

Release of chemicals

The adhesion of platelets to one another and to other
surfaces triggers the release of a variety of chemicals
stored within the vesicles (Table 4.5). These have a
number of different functions. Some:

● promote adhesion of platelets
● contract smooth muscle in the blood vessels
● participate in coagulation.

   Aggregation of platelets at the site of injury creates a
temporary plug. This is most effective in sealing small
vessels. Coagulation may follow, enhanced by platelet
factors, and a firmer seal is formed (see below).

Abnormalities

If the number of platelets in blood is much lower than
normal (*thrombocytopenia*) there is an increased tendency
for bleeding to occur spontaneously, particularly from
smaller blood vessels. When injury occurs haemostasis
is also less effective. Thrombocytopenia can result from:

● bone marrow deficiencies
● accumulation of platelets in the spleen in *splenomegaly*
● an *autoimmune* disorder.

COAGULATION

The blood clot

In coagulation, interlacing strands of *fibrin* are formed
when a precursor plasma protein, *fibrinogen*, is exposed

⑤
*If there are not
enough
platelets to
plug all the
gaps in the
capillary
endothelium
there will be
more
spontaneous
leaks. How
does this affect
the tendency to
bruise?*

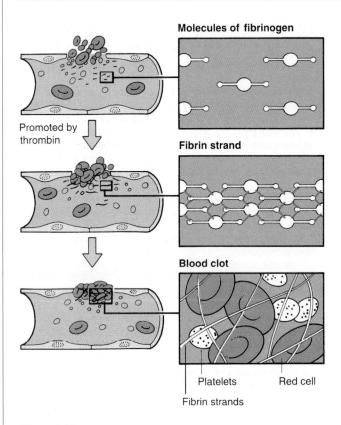

Molecules of fibrinogen

Promoted by thrombin

Fibrin strand

Blood clot

Platelets   Red cell

Fibrin strands

Figure 4.15
The process of coagulation and formation of a blood clot.

to the enzyme *thrombin* (Fig. 4.15). The meshwork of fibrin strands traps water and its dissolved constituents to form a gel, and erythrocytes, leucocytes and platelets get tangled up in it too. This is the *blood clot* or *thrombus*. It is soft at first but then further chemical changes occur which include strengthening of the fibrin strands. Later *clot retraction* occurs, caused by the platelets in the clot contracting, and some fluid (*serum*) is squeezed out in the process. Serum contains all the constituents of plasma except those, such as fibrinogen, that have been used up in coagulation.

The clot acts as a temporary seal to the damaged vessel, and also as a scaffold for the repairs made subsequently to the vessel itself. ⑥

Formation of fibrin

The formation of fibrin from fibrinogen is triggered in one of two ways by:

- chemicals released from injured tissues (*extrinsic pathway*)
- contact with an abnormal surface (*intrinsic pathway*).

When injury occurs there is usually a release of factors from the tissues (*tissue thromboplastin*) as well as a change in the surface of the vessel. If both changes are only slight, as they may be in a skillfully performed venepuncture, then coagulation will not occur very

⑥
If a wound continues to bleed profusely it is recommended that the dressing be reinforced (i.e. more dressing applied on top of it) rather than changed. What is the logic behind this?

quickly and pressure must be applied to the puncture site for a few minutes after the needle is withdrawn to stem the flow of blood until a clot is formed.

Blood withdrawn from the vein will, however, coagulate within 5 to 8 minutes if it is transferred into a glass tube. The trigger factor in this case is the contact made between the blood and the surface of the glass. If glass has been coated with silicone, which alters its surface characteristics, then coagulation does not occur as quickly. However, if tissue injury occurred in taking the blood sample, activation of the clotting factors will proceed more swiftly because of the release of more tissue thromboplastins.

Clotting factors

Both the extrinsic and intrinsic pathways involve the sequential activation of a number of different factors (Fig. 4.16 and Table 4.8) and require the presence of *calcium* and *platelet phospholipid*, and other factors facilitating the process.

Most, but not all, of the clotting factors are proteins normally present in plasma in an inactive form. Those which are earlier in the coagulation sequence are present in low concentration (Table 4.7) and have a short life span in the blood, whereas the concentrations of *prothrombin* and *fibrinogen* are relatively high and their life span is longer. This arrangement has the benefit of allowing just a small change in the concentration of one of the earlier activated factors to bring about progressively larger effects in the later ones. In other words, the effect snowballs. If the synthesis of plasma proteins is threatened, as in liver disease (see Ch. 9), deficiencies arise first in the earlier factors preventing the process of coagulation from getting underway.

FIBRINOLYSIS

While the injured blood vessel is repaired by the growth of new cells, the clot is broken down gradually by the action of the enzyme *plasmin*, which breaks down fibrin (Fig. 4.17). Plasmin is formed from the plasma protein *plasminogen* by the action of activators secreted chiefly by the endothelial cells of the blood vessel wall.

In capillaries

The concentration of activating factors is especially high in capillary blood, largely because the space into which they are secreted is small. Consequently fibrin is broken down easily in capillaries. This feature in fact makes it difficult for clots to form in the capillary circulation. Any fibrin that is formed is rapidly broken down. Thus the balance between the *fluid* and the *gel* forms of blood is tipped towards fluidity within the capillaries. This is important in preserving the flow of blood through these tiny vessels and thus in maintaining the supply of oxygen and nutrients to the tissues.

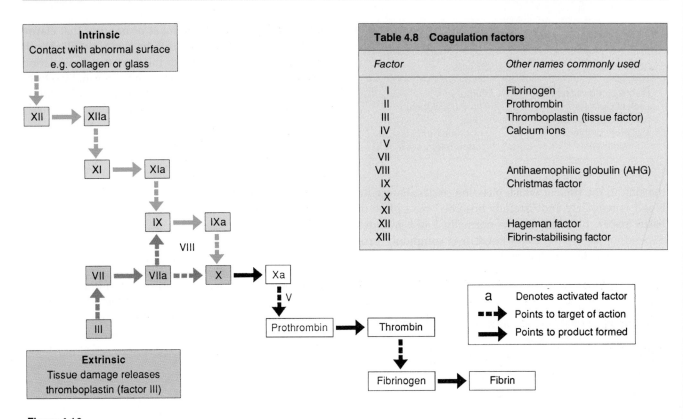

Table 4.8	Coagulation factors
Factor	*Other names commonly used*
I	Fibrinogen
II	Prothrombin
III	Thromboplastin (tissue factor)
IV	Calcium ions
V	
VII	
VIII	Antihaemophilic globulin (AHG)
IX	Christmas factor
X	
XI	
XII	Hageman factor
XIII	Fibrin-stabilising factor

Figure 4.16
Intrinsic and extrinsic pathways of coagulation. Factors are activated in turn resulting eventually in the formation of fibrin. Factors VIII and V are additional factors needed for coagulation to proceed.

In large blood vessels

In the largest blood vessels the situation is different. Here the plasminogen activating factors released from the endothelial cells are diluted in a larger volume of blood, and fibrinolysis does not occur as easily. Consequently, clots are broken down more slowly. However, the pressure of blood in the larger arterial vessels is much higher (see Ch. 5, Fig. 5.22A) and, though the chemical balance favours coagulation, the high pressures may dislodge clots forming after injury. Clots that form and then break away can form blockages (*emboli*) in other parts of the circulation.

ABNORMALITIES

The delicate balance achieved between keeping blood flowing and preventing its loss from the circulation can easily be tipped inappropriately in the direction of *bleeding* or *thrombus formation* by defects in any one of the component systems (Table 4.9). Although identification of the exact defect requires sophisticated tests, relatively simple measurements like bleeding time and clotting time allow some distinctions to be made.

The *bleeding time* is the number of minutes that elapse from the time at which a standard puncture is made of

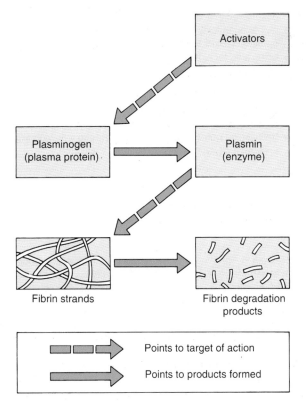

Figure 4.17
The process of fibrinolysis.

Table 4.9 Abnormalities of haemostasis

Abnormality	Disease
Fragile blood vessels	Purpura
Lack of platelets	Thrombocytopenia
Lack of clotting factors	
e.g. prothrombin	Hypoprothrombinaemia
factor VIII	Classic haemophilia

the skin to the time at which bleeding ceases. Emerging blood is regularly and carefully absorbed by a piece of tissue paper. Bleeding time is normally 2 to 9 minutes depending on the technique used. It is commonly prolonged if platelets are few or defective.

PRINCIPLES OF NURSING CARE ASSOCIATED WITH BLEEDING TENDENCIES

Failure of the coagulation process may be due to a reduction in the number of platelets (*thrombocytopenia*) or to a deficiency of any one of the blood clotting factors. For example, *haemophilia A and B* are rare, inherited coagulation disorders caused by factor VIII and factor IX deficiency respectively. Whatever the cause, it is essential for nurses caring for patients with a tendency to bleed to be aware of the origin and degree of that tendency and initiate appropriate nursing care. This would include:

- discussing the condition and the precautions to be observed in activities of daily living with the patient
- preparing quickly for prophylactic transfusions of depleted factors to cover invasive procedures or trauma
- being alert for signs of internal bleeding
- monitoring for haematuria (see Ch. 5) by regular urinalysis
- handling patients gently to avoid bruising
- avoiding intramuscular injections and other invasive procedures
- maintaining continuous pressure on the site following any invasive procedure until haemostasis is assured.

The *clotting time* is the number of minutes that elapse from the time a glass capillary tube is rapidly filled with blood, from a finger prick, to the time that coagulation occurs within the tube. Clotting time is normally 5 to 11 minutes. It is prolonged if there is deficiency of clotting factors, particularly of the intrinsic pathway. Other tests (such as the *prothrombin time*) are needed to identify which of the clotting factors is deficient.

ANTICOAGULANTS

Anticoagulants are commonly used in two ways, to:

- prevent the coagulation of a sample of blood collected for analysis
- reduce the chance of thrombus formation in a patient.

Examples of both kinds of anticoagulant and how they work are given in Table 4.10. Some of the anticoagulants used to prevent coagulation in blood samples, such as EDTA, are harmful to the body and therefore cannot be used in patients.

VENOUS THROMBOSIS

Although risk factors are known and routine precautions are taken, venous thrombosis is still relatively common in hospitalised patients and occasionally may lead to a life-threatening pulmonary embolus. This is when a clot breaks free from the site of origin, often the deep veins of the legs, and lodges in the pulmonary vessels. It usually follows a period of immobilisation during the perioperative period, or bed rest during debilitating disease or after extensive trauma. Blood flow is reduced and slowed by immobility, while surgery and trauma carry a double risk because of activation of clotting factors in response to blood vessel and tissue damage.

Prevention is through early mobilisation and physiotherapy, administration of anticoagulants and the use of anti-embolitic stockings.

Table 4.10 Anticoagulants

Name	Mode of action	Use
Heparin	Promotes action of antithrombin III*	Clinical treatment of thrombosis (by injection)
Warfarin	Reduces synthesis of factors II, VII, IX and X	Clinical prevention of thrombosis (oral)
Sodium citrate	Removes calcium from solution	Collection of blood for transfusion
EDTA	Binds calcium	Laboratory blood samples

* An inhibitor circulating in the blood that blocks the action of some clotting factors.

ANTICOAGULANT THERAPY

Anticoagulants are used to reduce the risk of thrombosis and to prevent extension of clot by disrupting the natural blood clotting mechanism. They are not fibrolytic and do not dissolve existing clots.

Heparin given by subcutaneous injection is used as a short-term anticoagulant as its action is immediate. Small doses are given to high-risk perioperative patients because it has been found to reduce the incidence of postoperative deep vein thrombosis. With these routinely small doses, there is little risk of excessive bleeding but the patient should always be carefully monitored.

Larger doses are given by continuous intravenous infusion when a thrombus has already formed, and are adjusted according to regular tests of bleeding and clotting times.

If long-term anticoagulant therapy is necessary, oral drugs such as warfarin are used. Again the dosage is calculated according to clotting times but, as the individual dose becomes established, these tests are done less frequently. It should be noted that it takes 24 to 36 hours for warfarin to influence coagulation and its effects continue for a similar period after it has been discontinued.

There is a delicate balance between clotting and increased risk of haemorrhage, and the nurse needs to be constantly alert and the patient well briefed on self-monitoring and care. It is wise for the patient to carry a Medialert card indicating the name and dose of the drug.

KEY POINTS

What you should now understand about blood and related tissues:

- what blood consists of
- how and where red cells are formed and destroyed and the factors affecting these processes
- what anaemia is and how it may be caused
- how and where white cells and platelets are formed and destroyed and factors affecting the numbers circulating
- what is meant by lymphoid tissue, where it is found and what it does
- what blood groups are and the situations in which they matter
- why blood transfusions are not given indiscriminately and why they are given with great care
- what makes blood clot and what stops it from clotting and why
- why someone may have a tendency to bleed
- what a thrombus is and conditions favouring its formation.

REFERENCES AND FURTHER READING

Bain B J 1989 Blood cells: a practical guide. J B Lippincott, Philadelphia
(Attractive specialist book giving useful information about the practicalities of taking blood and performing blood tests, as well as specific details about different blood disorders)

Contreras M 1990 ABC of transfusion. British Medical Journal, London
(Attractive collection of interesting articles from the British Medical Journal)

Dacie J V, Lewis S M (1990) Practical haematology, 7th edn. Churchill Livingstone, Edinburgh
(Explains techniques used in laboratory investigation of blood. Useful for reference)

Federation of American Societies for Experimental Biology 1971 Blood and other body fluids. FASEB

Hillman R S, Finch C A 1992 Red cell manual. F A Davis, Philadelphia
(Small paperback giving further information about red cells and their function, and the identification and management of anaemia)

Hughes-Jones N C, Wickramasinghe S N 1991 Lecture notes on haematology, 5th edn. Blackwell Scientific Publications, Oxford
(Blood diseases and their treatment. Useful for information)

Kelton J G, Heddle N M, Blajchman M A 1984 Blood transfusion: a conceptual approach. Churchill Livingstone, Edinburgh
(Unusual format of friendly diagrams and adjacent explanatory notes conveys a lot of information in a simple way)

Kendal M D 1981 The thymus gland. Academic Press, London
(Specialist book for reference)

Ludlam C (ed) 1990 Clinical haematology. Churchill Livingstone, Edinburgh
(Blood diseases and their treatment. Useful for reference)

McDonald G A, Paul J, Cruickshank B 1988 Atlas of haematology, 5th edn. Churchill Livingstone, Edinburgh

Ogston D 1983 The physiology of haemostasis. Croom Helm, London
(Specialist book, useful for reference)

Race R R, Sanger R 1971 Blood groups in man. Blackwell Scientific Publications, Oxford

Rogers A W 1992 Textbook of anatomy. Churchill Livingstone, Edinburgh

Russell N J, Powell G M, Jones J G, Winterburn P J, Basford J M 1982 Blood biochemistry. Croom Helm, London
(Concise book; useful source of further information)

Trubowitz S, Davis S 1982 The human bone marrow: anatomy, physiology and pathophysiology. CRC Press, Florida
(Specialist two volume work for reference)

Williams P L, Warwick R, Dyson M, Bannister L H 1989 Gray's Anatomy. Churchill Livingstone, Edinburgh

Chapter 5
CIRCULATION

Maintenance of an adequate blood flow is essential to cell function. If blood flow is reduced, the correct internal environment is not preserved and cell function deteriorates.

Blood is driven around the vessels of the circulation by the pressure developed by contraction of the heart. Each day the heart beats 100 000 times, its pumping action adjusted according to our needs by neural, hormonal and intrinsic regulatory mechanisms. Blood is delivered to the tissues and returned to the heart through a series of vessels that differ in structure and function:

- arteries control the distribution of blood
- capillaries allow interchange of blood constituents with the interstitial fluid
- veins act as a controllable reservoir returning blood to the heart.

PRINCIPLES

The flow of blood through the vessels of the circulation can be likened to the flow of visitors out of a ward along the corridors of a hospital at the end of visiting hours. It depends on the:

- pressure to move
- resistance encountered.

Flow is directly related to pressure (the bigger the pressure the bigger the flow), and inversely related to resistance (the greater the resistance the smaller the flow). Thus:

$$\text{Flow} = \frac{\text{Pressure}}{\text{Resistance}}$$

In the circulation, pressure is created by contraction of the heart, and resistance to flow is created by the blood vessels and by the blood itself.

RESISTANCE

If a lot of people are moving along a corridor in the same direction, the flow of people occurs most easily if the corridor is wide, and is difficult if it is narrow. If people are also chatting with one another as they walk, movement is usually slowed. Both the narrowness of the corridor and the interaction between people creates resistance to flow. The resistance to the flow of blood in the circulation is determined by similar factors:

- size of the blood vessels (particularly their *radius*)
- interactions between constituents of the blood (*viscosity*).

The ease with which flow occurs depends also upon whether it is *streamlined* or *turbulent* (Fig. 5.1). Streamlined flow is like that occurring in an orderly evacuation from a building when the fire alarm rings. All movement is in the same direction. If, however, some people choose to go back for personal belongings or there is confusion about the evacuation procedure, the flow of people is disordered (*turbulent*) and evacuation occurs more slowly.

Streamlined flow

When flow is streamlined, the factors determining resistance are related in the following way:

$$\text{Resistance is proportional to: } \frac{\text{Viscosity} \times \text{Length}}{(\text{Radius})^4}$$

'Length' and 'radius' apply to the size of the vessel; 'viscosity' applies to the fluid within it.

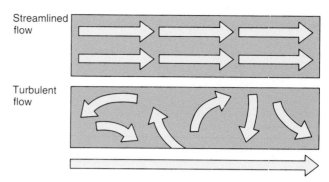

Figure 5.1
Streamlined and turbulent flow.

Of these three factors, the one having the greatest influence on blood flow is the radius of the vessel. The radius of some of the blood vessels can be altered by contraction and relaxation of muscle in their walls (see p. 92). This has an enormous influence on the ease with which blood can flow. If the muscle contracts, the vessel is constricted and flow is reduced. If the muscle relaxes, the vessel dilates and flow increases (Fig. 5.2). ①

The next most important factor in resistance is the viscosity of blood. This is chiefly affected by the proportion of red cells to plasma in blood (packed cell volume (PCV); see Ch. 4). The greater the PCV, the greater is the viscosity and the greater is the resistance to blood flow. If the proportion of red cells in blood increases, as in polycythaemia for example (see Ch. 4), blood is more viscous. The pressure required to drive blood through the circulation at the same flow rate is

① *By how much would the resistance of a vessel change if the radius doubled?*

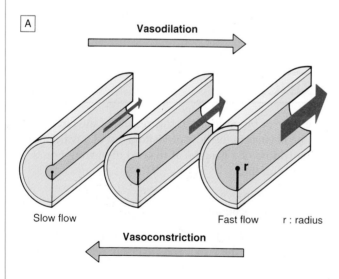

Figure 5.2
Effects of dilation and constriction on flow:
A Contraction of the muscle in the wall of blood vessels constricts the vessel and reduces flow, whereas relaxation of the muscle dilates the vessel and increases flow (radius = diameter ÷ 2)
B Altering the resistance to flow by constricting the tube.

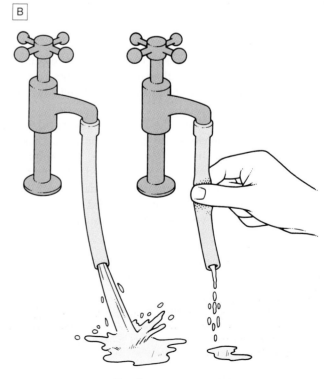

Fast flow   Slow flow

Many medical and nursing terms can be bewildering to the new student, and polycythaemia may be just such a term. If the reader does not understand these long words, before turning to the medical dictionary, try breaking them down into their component parts (e.g. *poly cyt(e) haem*) and then working out their meaning. Then check your findings with the definition in a medical or nursing dictionary.

then greater. Conversely in anaemia, blood is less viscous and flows more easily. ②

Turbulent flow

If there is turbulence, the resistance to flow is greater, and the pressure required to achieve the same blood flow is greater. Within the circulation, blood flow is mostly streamlined but turbulence can occur whenever there are obstructions to flow, as for example in the heart because of the valves, and in blood vessels if there are irregularities in the walls (*atherosclerotic plaques*).

Turbulence may also occur in the flow of blood through an unobstructed vessel if:

- the vessel is large (aorta)
- viscosity and density of blood is low (e.g. in anaemia)
- blood is moving very fast (as it does in arteries).

When turbulence occurs it usually causes vibration and this creates sound waves which can be heard through a stethoscope. Examples include the turbulence caused by closure of the valves in the heart, which gives rise to the heart sounds (see p. 88), the tapping sounds heard through a stethoscope when taking blood pressures (see p. 97), and the specific murmurs associated with diseases of the heart valves.

PRESSURE

Units

The pressure in a fluid (*hydrostatic pressure*) can be expressed in various ways:

- cm of H_2O
- mm of mercury (Hg)
- kilopascals (kPa).

cmH₂O and mmHg

The first two of these are units referring to the length of the vertical column of either water or mercury that exactly balances the pressure being measured (Fig. 5.3). In a vertical column of fluid the pressure at any level is proportional to the height of the column of fluid above it. The pressure is created by the weight of all the

② *Why is the level of red blood cells so significant? Why not the level of white blood cells, or platelets?*

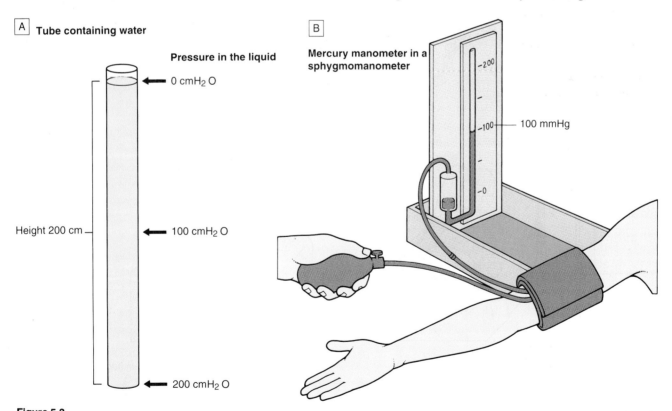

Figure 5.3

Units of hydrostatic pressure:

A cmH₂O: the molecules at the base of the tube are under pressure because of the weight of the water molecules above. The pressure is proportional to the height of the column of water. At the base this is 200 cmH₂O; half-way down it is 100 cmH₂O.

B mmHg: a column of mercury 100 mm high exerts a similar pressure to a column of water 100 cm high. A 'manometer' is an instrument for measuring pressure.

molecules of the fluid that are stacked vertically above one another. The weight is caused by gravity.

The heavier the molecules are the greater is the pressure exerted. As one atom of mercury is just over 10 times as heavy as one molecule of water, and as they each occupy about the same volume, a 1 mm column of mercury exerts nearly the same pressure as a 1 cm column of water (in fact 1.36 cm $H_2O \equiv$ 1 mm Hg).

> Until recently in clinical practice, mmHg has been the unit of choice because a column of mercury (in a sphygmomanometer) has been easy to transport and convenient to use. Imagine the difficulties you would have if you had to use a large column of water instead.

kPa

The third unit is the Système International (SI) unit for pressure (*pascal*) which gives the force per unit area expressed in newtons per square metre. One pascal (1 Pa) is an exceedingly small pressure. The smallest of pressures commonly measured in the body are about 1000 times as big. Consequently kilopascals (kPa) are

> While blood pressure is still measured in millimetres of mercury (mmHg), blood gas analysis (that is, the measurement of the pressures of important gases like oxygen and carbon dioxide in both arterial and venous blood) now uses the SI units, kilopascals (kPa). Find out what are the normal oxygen (PO_2) and carbon dioxide (PCO_2) levels in arterial blood.

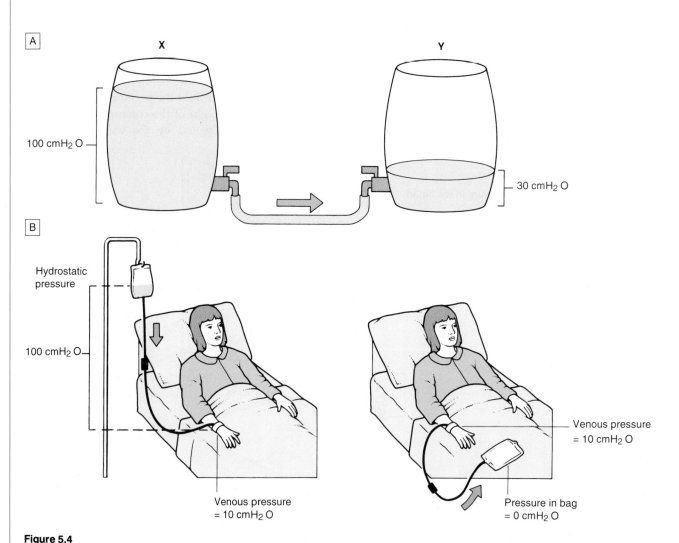

Figure 5.4

Effects of hydrostatic pressure on flow:

A Water flows from X to Y, driven by the difference in hydrostatic pressure (100 – 30 cmH$_2$O) between the two containers. When will it stop flowing?

B Fluids flow into or out of a patient, driven by the difference in hydrostatic pressure between the patient and the bag. In the first panel, fluid in the drip is flowing in (pressure difference = 90 cmH$_2$O); in the second panel, blood is flowing out of the patient into the bag (pressure difference = 10 cmH$_2$O).

used (1 kPa = 1000 Pa). 1 kPa is approximately the same as a pressure of 7.6 mmHg.

Pressure and flow

Fluids flow from one place to another if there is a difference in hydrostatic pressure between the two sites, as between the two containers X and Y in Figure 5.4A, or between a drip bottle and a patient (Fig. 5.4B). The rate of flow depends on the difference in pressure:

Flow is proportional to Pressure$_A$ – Pressure$_B$

The bigger the difference in pressure the greater is the rate of flow.

Gravitational pressure

In a column of fluid, pressure at the bottom of the column is greater than that at the top, but fluid does not flow upwards! This is because of the gravitational force which is holding it down. Similarly, when a person of average height (170 cm) is standing upright, the pressure of blood in the feet is 170 cmH$_2$O greater than at the top of the head (Fig. 5.5). This difference in pressure does not make blood flow up from the feet to the head. It is important to grasp that the actual driving force causing blood to flow in the circulation is the difference in hydrostatic pressure between two sites once the pressures due to gravity have been taken into account.

Atmospheric pressure

The atoms and molecules making up the atmosphere also exert a pressure on us due to the effects of gravity. This *atmospheric (barometric) pressure* is normally about 760 mmHg ($\approx$ 100 kPa). In the circulation, extra pressure is produced by the contraction of the heart (110 mmHg in a healthy young person at rest). Thus the actual physical pressure within the heart is 760 plus 110 mmHg (i.e. 870 mmHg). As the atmospheric pressure exerted on the body is the same all over, in practice atmospheric pressure is forgotten about and physiological pressures are quoted as net pressures *above* or *below* atmospheric. Thus pressures in the heart vary between 0 and 110 mmHg, and some venous pressures may be –10 mmHg (i.e. 10 mmHg *less* than atmospheric pressure).

Osmotic pressure

Fluids can possess osmotic pressure as well as hydrostatic pressure. Osmotic pressure is caused by dissolved solutes. Osmotic pressure does not drive the flow of fluid through vessels, but it is important in the circulatory system in affecting the movement of fluid between plasma and interstitial fluid at the capillaries.

As explained in Chapter 3, if the free diffusion of one or more solutes in a solution is restricted by a barrier permeable to water, and the solute concentration differs on either side, water moves by osmosis into the

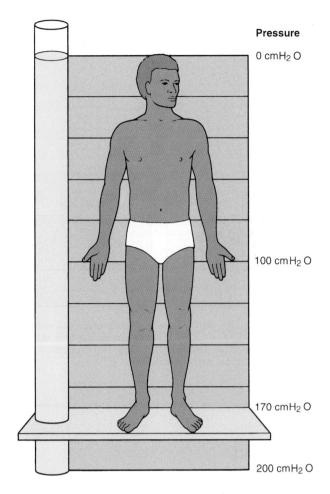

Pressure

0 cmH$_2$O

100 cmH$_2$O

170 cmH$_2$O

200 cmH$_2$O

Figure 5.5
When a person is standing, the pressure of blood in the circulation is greater in the feet than in the head because of the weight of blood created by gravity.

compartment containing more solute and makes the volume of that compartment expand (Fig. 5.6). This expansion can be counteracted by applying hydrostatic pressure to the same compartment forcing the water to flow back out again. The hydrostatic pressure needed to do this is that which balances the *osmotic pressure* drawing water in.

The osmotic potential of a solution depends on its solute concentration and this is measured as milliosmoles/litre of solution (*osmolarity*) or milliosmoles/kg of solution (*osmolality*). This osmotic potential is only translated into osmotic pressure if the solution is separated from another of lower concentration by a barrier that the solutes cannot penetrate.

As osmotic pressures can be exactly balanced by hydrostatic pressures, they are often referred to by the same units as hydrostatic pressure, namely mmHg and kPa. But a crucial fact to remember is that a fluid that has an osmotic pressure is *drawing water into itself* rather than driving it away.

Hydrostatic pressure (mmHg) needed to balance osmotic pressure
Mercury manometer
200
100
0
Solution
Water
Barrier permeable to water but not to solute
1. Water drawn into solution by osmosis. Volume of fluid in chamber expands.
2. Osmosis counteracted by applying pressure. Water movement out balances water movement in.

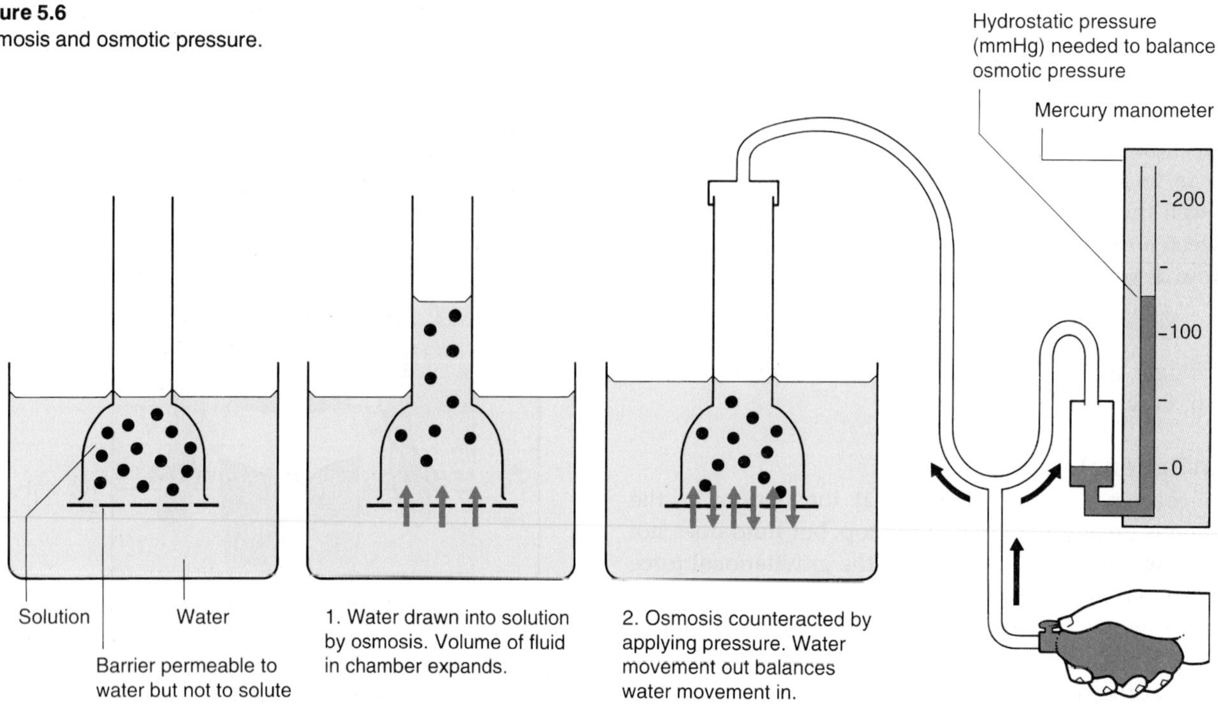

Figure 5.6
Osmosis and osmotic pressure.

HEART

STRUCTURE

The heart lies in the thorax (Fig. 5.7A & B) beneath the sternum of the rib cage. The heart consists largely of muscle tissue (*cardiac muscle*; see Ch. 22) and has four chambers (Fig. 5.8):

- two atria which receive blood from the veins
- two ventricles which pump blood out into the arteries.

The entry and exit points into the ventricles are guarded by valves.

Tissue layers

The walls of the heart consist of three layers:

- pericardium
- myocardium
- endocardium.

Pericardium

This outer part of the heart consists of a double layer of epithelium (*serous pericardium*) and some connective tissue. A tiny amount of fluid secreted by the epithelial

A
Pulmonary valve
Sternum
Right border
Tricuspid valve
Aortic valve
Left border
Rib cage
Mitral valve
B
Superior vena cava
Arch of aorta
2nd costal cartilage
Pulmonary artery
Right atrium
Ventricles
Inferior vena cava

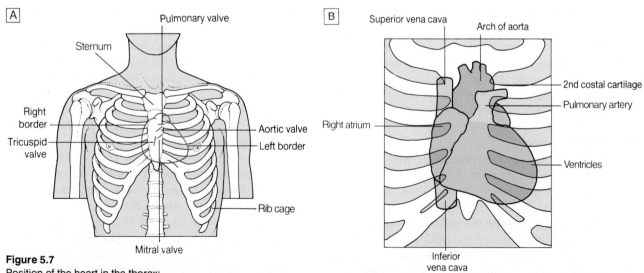

Figure 5.7
Position of the heart in the thorax:
A Heart and valves in relation to the rib cage
B Chambers and vessels in relation to the rib cage. (Reproduced from Rogers 1992 (Figs 7.7 & 38.1) by permission of the publishers.)

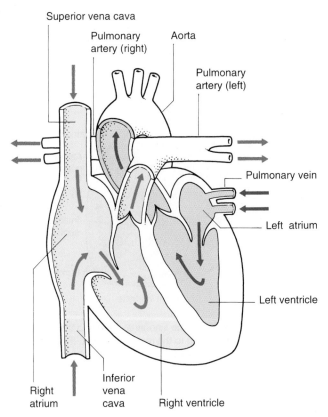

Figure 5.8
Chambers and vessels of the heart. Deoxygenated blood (blue) is pumped by the right heart to the lungs. Oxygenated blood (red) from the lungs is pumped by the left heart to the rest of the body.

cells is present between the two layers. Surrounding the heart as a whole and anchored to the diaphragm is the *fibrous pericardium* which supports the heart rather like an elastic stocking. The connective tissue between the pericardium and the myocardium contains blood vessels, nerves and autonomic ganglia.

Myocardium

The myocardium (*myo = muscle*) consists of muscle cells and forms the bulk of the wall of each of the chambers. The myocardium of the left ventricle is much thicker than that of the right. Consequently, the left ventricle can develop much greater pressures when it contracts.

Some muscle cells are specialised in a way that makes them behave more like nerves than muscle cells. They generate and transmit impulses causing the heart to contract. These cells include:

- sino-atrial node cells
- atrio-ventricular node cells
- Purkinje fibres of the *bundle of His* and the ventricles.

Endocardium

The innermost layer consists of connective tissue, blood vessels, and nerves, covered by a layer of endothelial cells continuous with the endothelial lining of the blood vessels (see p. 92). ③

Chambers

Blood enters the *right atrium* from the *venae cavae* (Fig. 5.8), is pumped from there into the *right ventricle*, and from the right ventricle into the *pulmonary circulation* (see Ch. 7). The blood picks up oxygen as it passes through the lungs and releases carbon dioxide before returning to the *left atrium* in the *pulmonary veins*. It is pumped from the left atrium to the *left ventricle* and is then ejected from the heart into the *aorta*. The wall (*septum*) separating the right and left sides of the heart normally prevents blood passing directly from one side to the other.

The atria and ventricles are separated by a dense fibrous structure, the *fibrous skeleton* of the heart, into which muscle cells are inserted. Openings in this band of tissue, between the atria and ventricles, are guarded by valves, consisting of flaps of connective tissue. There are valves also at the exit points from the ventricles into the pulmonary artery and aorta.

Valves

Atrio-ventricular (AV) valves

The valves between the atria and the ventricles on the left and right sides of the heart are the *mitral* and *tricuspid* valves respectively (Fig. 5.9). When the ventricle contracts, the flaps (*cusps*) of the valves are forced together, closing off the opening so that blood is prevented from re-entering the atria. The ends of the cusps of the valves are attached to cords, *chordae tendineae*, inserted into the wall of the ventricle. These help to prevent the flaps of the valves from being pushed right through into the atria when the ventricles contract.

③
The endocardium and the endothelial lining of blood vessels are, in health, extremely smooth. What difference might it make if they were rough?

Note how the heart is protected to some extent from trauma by the rib cage and the intercostal muscles. Where severe pressure is applied to the chest – as in a road traffic accident, or even during external cardiac massage – a sharp end of a broken rib can pierce the heart or lungs causing grave damage. In the case of cardiac massage, rib damage is less likely to occur if the resuscitator's hands are placed above the sternum and not to one side, over the ribs.

Certain disease processes can affect the flow of blood through the heart valves. The mitral valve seems to be the most commonly affected. Sometimes the valve can be *incompetent*, allowing blood to flow back through it when it should have closed. Sometimes the valve can become thickened and narrowed (*mitral stenosis*) so that the heart muscle has to pump harder to force blood through. Diseased valves can be replaced by artificial valves.

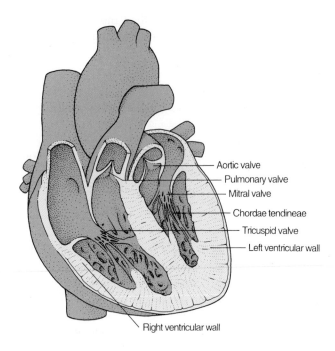

Figure 5.9
Valves of the heart. (Reproduced from Rogers 1992 (Fig. 7.3) by permission of the publishers.)

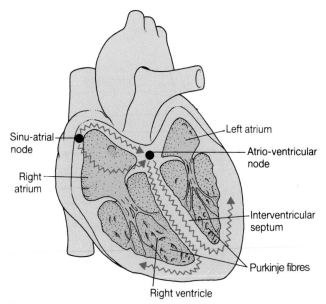

Figure 5.10
Origin of cardiac impulses in the sino-atrial node and the pathway by which they are conducted to the rest of the heart. (Reproduced from Rogers 1992 (Fig. 7.4) by permission of the publishers.)

> In certain cardiac conditions, such as sinus bradycardia, or complete heart block where no impulses from the SA node get through to the ventricles, the patient's pulse falls to as low as 40 beats per minute. If drugs fail to help, the condition can be overcome by the insertion under local anaesthetic of an artificial pacemaker, a battery driven device which stimulates the ventricles at a set rate nearer to that of a healthy heart – about 70 beats per minute. The battery will need to be changed about every 2 years. As the device is situated just under the skin, this may easily be achieved.

Arterial valves

The valves guarding the exits from the left and right ventricles (*aortic* and *pulmonary valves*) are termed *semilunar* because of their shape. Unlike the AV valves the flaps of the arterial valves are not tethered by cords of connective tissue.

Venous entrances

The openings between the veins and the atria on both sides of the heart are not guarded by valves (Fig. 5.8). Consequently some blood can be forced backwards into the veins, as well as forward into the ventricles when the atria contract.

EXCITATION

The impulses making the heart contract originate usually in the sino-atrial node (SA node) and are conducted from there to the ventricles (Fig. 5.10). The electrical activity of the heart is recorded routinely as an *electrocardiogram (ECG)*.

Pacemaker cells

All the specialised muscle cells of the heart (SA node, AV node, and Purkinje fibres) can generate impulses spontaneously, and regularly. But the cells of the SA node have the highest frequency of discharge (normally 110 impulses per minute) and therefore dominate the other cells, such as those in the ventricles which fire off more slowly (about 40 impulses per minute). The SA node acts as the *pacemaker* of the heart.

Conduction of the impulse

The impulses generated by the cells of the SA node are carried across the right atrium, to the left atrium (causing both of these to contract) and to the AV node (Fig. 5.10). The impulses travel relatively slowly through the AV node (*AV nodal delay*) and are then carried along a bundle of Purkinje fibres (*bundle of His*) running downwards in the wall between the two ventricles. These fibres transmit the impulses to the ventricles. The bundle splits into two, a *left* and *right bundle* each of which conducts the impulse to the Purkinje fibres of the ventricle. These fibres excite the cardiac muscle cells to contract.

Throughout this conducting system, and within the cardiac muscle, the impulses are carried from cell to cell via gap junctions (see Chs 2 and 22).

Because the Purkinje fibres are able to conduct the impulse rapidly (2–4 metres per second), all the muscle cells in each ventricle are excited almost simultaneously and the blood within the ventricle is compressed from all sides.

Electrocardiogram

The electrical activity generated, by the sequential activation of the conducting cells and then the muscle cells is relatively small (a few millivolts), but it can be detected by means of *electrodes* placed on the surface of the skin. The activity recorded is the *electrocardiogram* (Fig. 5.11A).

Shape and interpretation

The precise shape of the ECG depends on where the electrodes are placed (see below) but the sequence of waves is always the same. The example shown in Figure 5.11A is the ECG obtained from a recording electrode placed on the chest over the heart.

The first wave, termed *P*, is caused by electrical excitation of the atria. The complicated pattern that follows, *QRST*, is largely caused by the electrical activity of the ventricles. Most of this is due to the left ventricle as it has the larger muscle mass.

Much can be learnt from the pattern of the ECG about the heart's activity (Fig. 5.11B). If there are more P waves than QRST complexes *heart block* exists (impulses generated by the SA node are not getting through to the ventricles). If the time between the P wave and the QRST is prolonged (measured as the *PR interval*) the conduction of the impulse is delayed (*incomplete heart block*). If the QRST is abnormal in shape the activity of the ventricles is different from usual, as in *myocardial infarction*. A more detailed description of the basis of the ECG is given in Chapter 22.

Leads

In electrocardiography, recordings are made from a number of electrodes placed on different parts of the body. Each electrode system is referred to as a *lead*. Recordings may be made from electrodes sited on the arms and legs (*limb leads*) or from the chest (*chest leads*) (Fig. 5.11C and Table 5.1, p. 86). The conventional limb leads are labelled I, II, and III, and the chest leads as V$_{1-6}$. A variant of the limb leads are the *augmented limb leads*. These are labelled as 'aV' and given the subscripts 'l', 'r', and 'f' to denote left arm, right arm and foot respectively.

Conventional limb leads are *bipolar* in that electrical activity is monitored at two sites (an arm and a leg for example) and compared by the recording equipment, whereas the chest leads are *unipolar* (they monitor activity at just one site).

The exact shape of the ECG differs according to the lead which is used (Fig. 5.11C). The same components (PQRST) are there, and their timing is the same, but their shape and size differ. Just as at a football match the

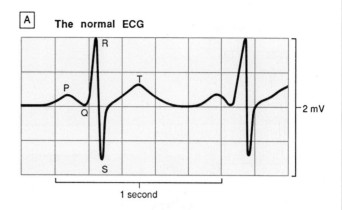

A The normal ECG

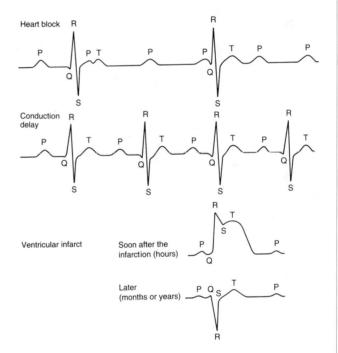

B Abnormal ECGs

Figure 5.11
The electrocardiogram.
A Normal
B Examples of abnormal ECGs. In heart block, the atria and ventricles are working independently as the impulse cannot be transmitted from one to the other. In conduction delay, the transmission of the impulse from atria to ventricles is slowed, making the PR interval longer than normal. The shape of the ECG after an infarction depends on the size and site of the damage. As the heart recovers the ECG changes shape again. Differences from normal reveal that damage remains even in a patient who in other respects appears to be 'back to normal'.

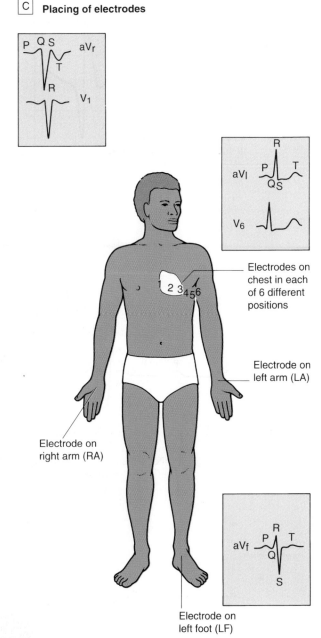

C   Placing of electrodes

Table 5.1   ECG leads

	Limb leads		Chest leads	
Name	Electrodes used*	Name	Electrodes used*
I	RA + LA	V_1	1 + reference†
II	RA + LF	V_2	2 + reference†
III	LA + LF	V_3	3 + reference†
aV_l	LA + reference‡	V_4	4 + reference†
aV_r	RA + reference‡	V_5	5 + reference†
aV_f	LF + reference‡	V_6	6 + reference†

* The 'reference electrode' provides a control against which electrical activity at the other sites is measured.
† Pooled activity recorded from RA, LA, and LF.
‡ Pooled activity recorded from the other two limbs.

Electrodes on chest in each of 6 different positions

Electrode on left arm (LA)

Electrode on right arm (RA)

Electrode on left foot (LF)

Figure 5.11 (continued)
C Placing of electrodes and typical recordings obtained from different leads.
(Based on Goldschlager & Goldman 1989.)

view of the game obtained by spectators differs according to their position on the terraces, so the wave of electrical activity sweeping around the atria and ventricles 'looks' different when 'viewed' by different leads.

CARDIAC EVENTS (MECHANICAL)

The atria and the ventricles contract in a set order in response to electrical excitation. As a result the pressure of blood in the different chambers of the heart varies in a regular pattern, and blood is moved through the heart,

from atria to ventricles, and transferred from the entry vessels (*veins*) to the exit tubes (*arteries*). The direction of flow is determined by the difference in pressure between the chambers and by the valves (Fig. 5.12).

Left ventricle

The greatest pressure changes occur in the left ventricle. When the muscle contracts, pressure increases from about zero to about 110 mmHg during a normal cardiac cycle in a young adult person. The maximum attained is termed *systolic pressure* (Fig. 5.13) and the period of contraction of the ventricle is referred to as *systole*. It is followed by a period (*diastole*) when the ventricle relaxes and remains relaxed for a short while.

THE ELECTROCARDIOGRAM

If all leads described in the text are used (a 12-lead ECG), detailed information is obtained about the spread of depolarisation and repolarisation through the heart muscle. From this, the physician is able to diagnose myocardial infarction and pinpoint the area of damage. Where needed, ECGs are usually recorded on successive days of a patient's stay in hospital in order to show changing patterns which are of significance to the physician.

Coronary care nurses also use cardiac monitors, which consist of three chest leads attached to the patient. The resultant electrical read-out is presented on a small screen by the bed or may be conveyed to a central monitor.

Cardiac monitors are used for observing the heart's *rate* and *rhythm*. While certain changes in shape of the ECG can be seen on the screen, such as a deepening Q wave or a raised ST segment, the cardiac monitor will not pinpoint areas of myocardial damage as does the 12-lead ECG.

On a coronary care unit, specially trained nurses watch the monitors for the appearance of cardiac arrhythmias, some of which may be life threatening. Courses are held that enable such nurses to identify a wide range of arrhythmias and to respond in certain emergency situations with immediate treatments. These may include giving drugs intravenously and applying a direct current shock (defibrillation) to the heart (see p. 90).

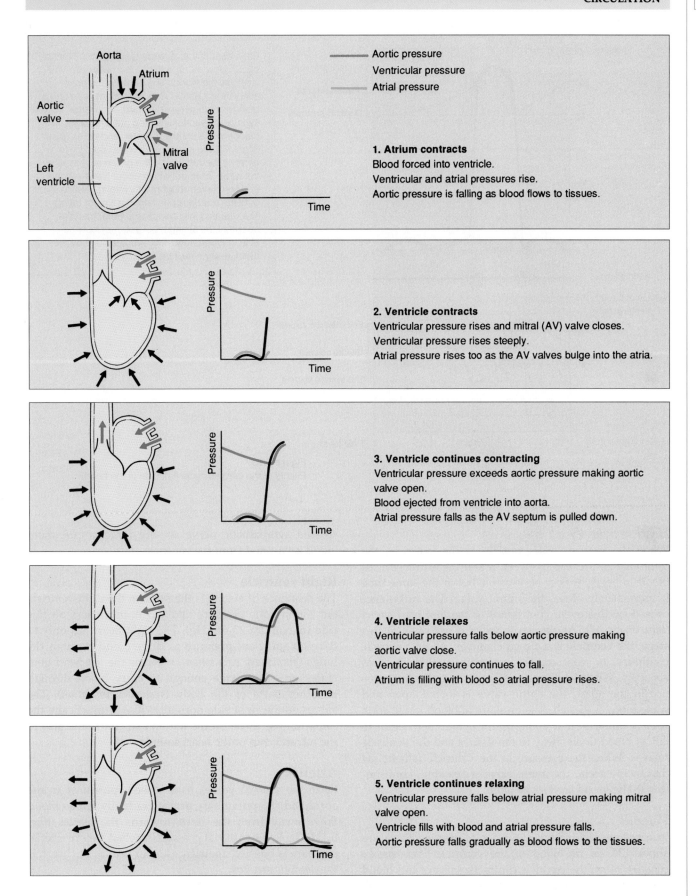

Aortic pressure
Ventricular pressure
Atrial pressure

1. Atrium contracts
Blood forced into ventricle.
Ventricular and atrial pressures rise.
Aortic pressure is falling as blood flows to tissues.

2. Ventricle contracts
Ventricular pressure rises and mitral (AV) valve closes.
Ventricular pressure rises steeply.
Atrial pressure rises too as the AV valves bulge into the atria.

3. Ventricle continues contracting
Ventricular pressure exceeds aortic pressure making aortic valve open.
Blood ejected from ventricle into aorta.
Atrial pressure falls as the AV septum is pulled down.

4. Ventricle relaxes
Ventricular pressure falls below aortic pressure making aortic valve close.
Ventricular pressure continues to fall.
Atrium is filling with blood so atrial pressure rises.

5. Ventricle continues relaxing
Ventricular pressure falls below atrial pressure making mitral valve open.
Ventricle fills with blood and atrial pressure falls.
Aortic pressure falls gradually as blood flows to the tissues.

Figure 5.12
Sequence of events in the left side of the heart.

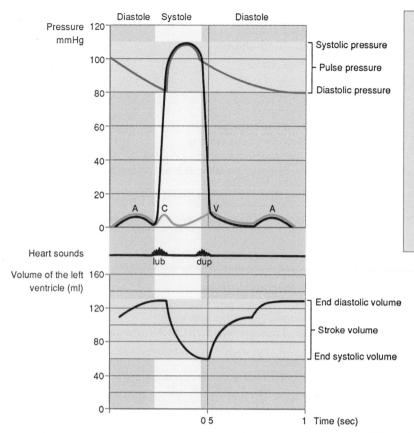

Figure 5.13
Events of the cardiac cycle (left side of the heart).

Each beat of the ventricle ejects about 70 ml of blood. How much is this? How easily can you visualise the work being done by the heart every time it beats? One way might be to find a bladder syringe on your ward – this large syringe is used for washing out a patient's bladder via a urinary catheter, and holds about 60 ml. Fill the syringe with water, then try to empty it by depressing the piston so that all of the water flows out within about half a second (the time taken roughly for systole). (Make sure the nozzle is pointing at a sink or bath!) The opening into the aorta is wider than the nozzle of the syringe, but you may now be able to judge how much work is done by the heart, every time it beats.

Heart sounds

When the pressure rises rapidly in the ventricle, the difference in pressure between it and the atrium causes blood to begin to flow backwards, but at the same time it immediately closes the mitral valve. The turbulence caused by this event contributes to the *first heart sound (lub)* (Fig. 5.13). As the aortic valve is not open at this stage, the ventricle is a closed chamber. As the ventricle continues to contract the pressure within it rises abruptly. When ventricular pressure exceeds the pressure in the aorta, the aortic valve is forced open and some blood is ejected. The pressure of blood in the aorta rises in line with that in the ventricle, and then begins to fall as blood flows away to the tissues and the ventricle relaxes. When the pressure in the ventricle falls below that in the aorta, the aortic valve snaps shut, contributing to the *second heart sound (dup)*.

Volumes

In a resting individual, just prior to ejection there are about 130 ml of blood in the ventricle (*end-diastolic volume*). When the ventricle contracts, some of this blood is ejected (*stroke volume*). About 70 ml are ejected at each beat, so that 60 ml remain (*end-systolic volume*). If the heart is stimulated to contract more forcibly, by in-creased sympathetic nerve activity for example, more blood is emptied from the ventricle.

Right ventricle

The sequence of events is the same in the right ventricle but the systolic pressure attained is much less on this side (maximum 25 mmHg). The right heart has only to develop sufficient pressure to drive blood through the lungs (*pulmonary circulation*), whereas the left heart generates pressures large enough to carry blood through all other parts of the body (*systemic circulation*). The valves on the right side normally close at practically the same time as those on the left and so contribute also to the lub and dup of the heart sounds.

Arteries

Once the arterial valves have closed, pressures in the aorta and the pulmonary artery gradually fall as blood flows away from the heart towards the tissues (Fig. 5.13). The lowest arterial pressure reached, before arterial pressure is boosted again by another beat of the heart, is the *diastolic pressure*.

Aorta

Diastolic pressure in the aorta is normally about 70 to 80

mmHg. The difference between this and the systolic pressure (about 40 to 50 mmHg) is termed the *pulse pressure*. This variation in the arterial pressure caused by the beating of the heart can be sensed in any artery as the *pulse*. ④

Pulmonary artery
Diastolic pressure is much lower in the pulmonary artery (about 8 mmHg), and the pulse pressure is also correspondingly smaller.

Atria and veins
The pressure in the atria varies during the cardiac cycle. As there are no valves between the atria and the veins, a similar variation in pressure occurs in the veins near to the heart such as the *jugular vein*. Three pulsations occur during each cycle, namely the 'a', 'c' and 'v' waves (Fig. 5.13):

- *a* is due to atrial contraction
- *c* occurs as the ventricle contracts
- *v* coincides with opening of the AV valves.

The c wave is caused by the bulging of the AV valves into the atria, which compresses the blood there. In the case of the v wave, pressure in the atria rises as blood flows into these chambers but then falls abruptly when the AV valve opens during diastole.

CARDIAC OUTPUT AND ITS REGULATION

The amount of blood ejected from the heart per minute (*cardiac output* – CO) is equal to the product of the heart rate (HR) and the stroke volume (SV):

$$CO = HR \times SV$$

In healthy individuals heart rate can range from 60 to 80 beats per minute at rest to 180 when the heart is maximally stimulated, as, for example, in physical activity. Stroke volume ranges between 70 and 120 ml. Thus cardiac output can be adjusted between 5 litres per minute at rest to a maximum of over 20 litres per minute. By physical training some people achieve higher values as a result of *hypertrophy* of the heart (growth of a larger, more muscular heart) (see Ch. 17). ⑤

Heart rate
As mentioned previously (p. 84), the heart is excited to contract by impulses generated spontaneously by cells of the SA node. The activity of these cells is influenced by neurotransmitters and hormones. The SA node is innervated by both parasympathetic and sympathetic nerves.

Parasympathetic nerves release *acetylcholine*. This makes the cells less excitable and the heart rate decreases. Sympathetic fibres release *noradrenaline* which, like adrenaline, makes the cells more excitable and

the heart rate increases. At rest, the influence of the parasympathetic fibres is dominant. Consequently the resting heart rate (70/minute) is below the natural firing rate of the SA node (110/minute). In circumstances such as emotional excitement and increased physical activity, activity in the sympathetic fibres increases and that in the parasympathetic fibres decreases so that heart rate increases (see Ch. 17). The hormone adrenaline is released too and this also increases the heart rate.

Stroke volume
The stroke volume can be varied in two ways:

- extrinsically (nerves and hormones)
- intrinsically (Starling's law of the heart).

Extrinsic control
The atria and the ventricles are richly innervated by sympathetic nerves, releasing noradrenaline. Parasympathetic innervation is sparse and largely restricted to the atria. When sympathetic activity increases, each beat of the heart is stronger and more blood is expelled per beat. In other words the stroke volume increases. This extra volume is drawn from the volume normally remaining (end-systolic volume).

The action of the sympathetic nerves is reinforced by hormones secreted by the adrenal medulla, chiefly *adrenaline*. This increases the force of contraction and the heart rate, and speeds the excitation of the cardiac tissue in general.

Noradrenaline and adrenaline act on receptors that control channels in the cell membrane which regulate the entry of calcium. This affects both the electrical excitation of the cell and the intracellular concentration of calcium which is so important for muscle contraction (see Ch. 22). Some drugs used in treating cardiac conditions, such as the calcium antagonists *nicardipine* and *verapamil*, act on these channels and thereby modify cardiac function.

Intrinsic control
Stroke volume is also affected by the degree to which the ventricles are filled during diastole (Fig. 5.14). The greater the filling, the greater the end-diastolic pressure and the greater is the degree to which the muscle fibres are stretched. Cardiac muscle, like skeletal muscle (see Ch. 22) responds to stretch by contracting more forcibly. In the heart, this property allows the force of contraction to be matched to the amount of blood returning to the heart.

The more blood delivered to the heart, the greater is the volume expelled. This relationship was first described by E. H. Starling (1915) and is popularly known as *Starling's law of the heart*. However, the work done by the heart cannot increase indefinitely. A maximum is reached, so that, although increased filling

④
Whereabouts on the body can the pulse be felt? What are each of these pulses called and what is the significance of the names?

⑤
What distinguishes the resting pulse of someone who exercises regularly? How might it differ from someone, also at rest, who hardly ever takes exercise?

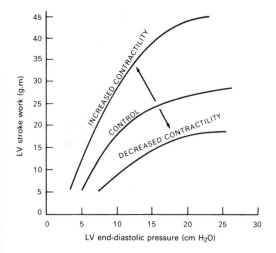

Figure 5.14
How the strength of the heart beat, and therefore the volume of blood ejected from the heart, varies with the degree to which the heart is filled. The relationship is affected by the presence of factors such as hormones and neurotransmitters which increase or decrease contractility. (From Braunwald E, Ross J, Sonnenblick E H, Mechanisms of contraction of the normal and failing heart, Figure 13. Reprinted by permission of The New England Journal of Medicine, Vol. 277, p. 911, 1967.)

produces increased contraction over the normal range of ventricular volumes, beyond this the heart becomes overdistended and less effective as a pump (Fig. 5.14), as it does in heart failure.

The property of cardiac muscle described by Starling's law is most useful in allowing adjustments to be made in response to beat to beat variations in the volume of blood returned to the heart. It cannot however fully cope with the greater challenges posed for example in exercise. Here the sympathetic nervous system is important because, by increasing the volume of blood expelled from the heart and decreasing end-systolic volume, it ensures that the volume of the heart is kept within the range over which Starling's law operates most effectively.

CORONARY BLOOD SUPPLY

The coronary arteries are the first vessels to branch from the aorta. The right coronary artery supplies the right heart and a little of the left; the left coronary artery supplies the major part of the left heart (Fig. 5.15). Cardiac muscle is very richly supplied with blood. Venous

---

EMERGENCY – CARDIAC ARREST

A nurse is returning home when a man in front of her suddenly collapses. She quickly examines him: his face is grey and pouring with sweat; he does not appear to be breathing; and there is no carotid pulse. She diagnoses that the man has suffered a cardiac arrest and proceeds with the resuscitation measures she has learned and practised in her hospital.

What has happened to the man? What does cardiac arrest mean?

The fact that the nurse cannot feel a pulse does not mean that the heart has given up completely, that there is no electrical activity. What it does mean is that the heart has ceased to pump blood around the body.

In cardiac arrest there are two basic arrhythmias that can cause death (although others may precede these or have a profound effect on cardiac output). These arrhythmias are *asystole* and *ventricular fibrillation*. The nurse in the scenario above does not know which of these has occurred; she is only aware that the victim has no effective cardiac output. By performing external cardiac massage she is attempting to provide such an output.

Within a few minutes, however, the ambulance arrives, the patient is attached to a cardiac monitor and it is possible to see what electrical activity is going on in his heart. Asystole shows as a straight line on the monitor screen, and is the result of a loss of electrical activity within the heart muscle. Ventricular fibrillation results from excessive, uncontrolled electrical activity, and shows as an irregular, bizarre tracing on the screen. Electrical activity within the myocardium is so uncoordinated that no effective pumping of the heart occurs. (During heart surgery, theatre staff can observe a heart that is in ventricular fibrillation; they describe it as quivering or trembling.)

Asystole is treated by cardiac stimulant drugs and external cardiac massage (together with the provision of air or oxygen by whatever means are available). The *sympathomimetic* drug, adrenaline (see Ch. 3), is used to counteract asystole. It increases the rate and strength of each heart contraction. Early in the resuscitation procedure, adrenaline can be injected directly into the myocardium through the chest wall. Once an intravenous line has been established, it may be given intravenously in combination with external cardiac massage, which 'flushes' the drug through the veins towards the heart.

Adrenaline may cause ventricular fibrillation and the student may wonder what advantage there is in precipitating the patient from one form of arrest into another. However, ventricular fibrillation can often be reversed with a direct current electric shock from a machine called a *defibrillator*. The monitor would show ventricular fibrillation followed by a 1 or 2 second pause immediately after shock, then, hopefully, normal rhythm resumes as the sino-atrial node takes over as pacemaker.

Calcium chloride is also a cardiac stimulant and is usually given intravenously, although it may be given directly into the myocardium. It excites the heart muscle, strengthens contractility and, like adrenaline, may enhance defibrillation by lowering the heart's defibrillation threshold. Calcium chloride is therefore used in cases of asystole with the intention of bringing about some electrical activity to the heart.

Lignocaine, unlike the previous two drugs, is given when the heart muscle is over-excitable. It has a membrane stabilising action, reducing the passage of ions through the nerve membrane, thus reducing its excitability. Lignocaine is used in cardiac arrest situations where defibrillation leads repeatedly to yet more ventricular fibrillation. By reducing the heart's excitability it is hoped that a further DC shock will convert its rhythm to normal.

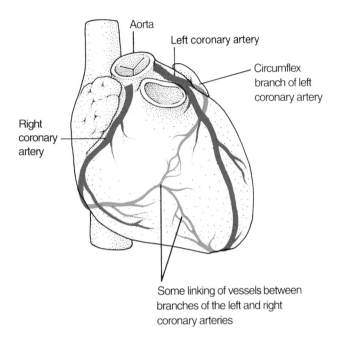

blood drains either directly into the four chambers of the heart or flows into the *coronary sinus*.

The flow of blood through the coronary circulation is pulsatile. It is reduced during systole and flows most easily during diastole. When the heart rate increases and the duration of diastole is shortened, the flow of blood to the heart per beat is reduced. This restricts the delivery of oxygen and nutrients to the cells, and may be insufficient to maintain adequate contraction. If the arterial vessels are narrowed through *atherosclerosis* the delivery of blood is then especially theatened when heart rate increases.

Local conditions around the vessels are very import-ant in determining blood flow (see p. 96). Factors increasing flow include:

- low oxygen concentrations (resulting from increased demand)
- increased concentrations of products of metabolism (such as CO_2, H^+, adenosine)
- other changes in ionic concentration (such as increased K^+).

Through these factors the flow of blood is closely matched to cardiac activity.

The coronary blood vessels are innervated by sym-pathetic nerves that exert some control over blood flow (see p. 96) but their effect is much less than that of local factors.

STRESS AND CARDIAC FUNCTION

Is a coronary care unit (CCU) necessarily beneficial to its patients? This may sound a strange question in the light of earlier acknowledgements of the advanced role of coronary care nurses and their specialised equipment. However, it has been suggested that the 'high technology' atmosphere inside such a unit could affect patients; that the sight of monitors, of resuscitation equipment, perhaps the witnessing of a cardiac arrest, could raise stress levels to such an extent that cardiac arrhythmias might occur.

Initial hopes that the use of specialised units would significantly reduce mortality in MI patients have not been realised. Some research shows that caring for the patient at home can be as effective (perhaps because it is less stressful) than admitting him to a CCU. Other research suggests that coronary care ambulances, staffed by specially trained personnel, have a greater effect on survival than CCUs.

The problem seems to centre on the patient's experience of stress. When someone is stressed, adrenaline production increases (among other physiological changes) so that peripheral vasoconstriction occurs, the pulse rate and blood pressure rise, and respirations increase. If a patient suddenly produces a dangerous cardiac arrhythmia in the period following myocardial infarction (MI), there is therefore a dilemma. On the one hand, the CCU is probably the best place for him, because the arrhythmia can be observed, identified, and treated quickly by medical and nursing staff. (Notice, incidentally, how this succession of events follows the stages of the nursing process, but in very rapid succession.) On the other hand, it may be that the atmosphere of these 'life-saving' units could raise the patient's stress level, increase the production of adrenaline and precipitate those same life-threatening arrhythmias.

Generally speaking, hospitals may have a policy whereby patients over a certain age, suffering an MI, are cared for at home, or possibly on a general medical or elderly care ward. Factors to be considered as well as age, however, are:

- the likelihood of cardiac arrhythmias (as judged by the diagnosing 12-lead ECG)
- the degree of pain and the ease with which it can be controlled at home
- the presence or absence of someone at home to care for the patient.

Within a coronary care unit, a calm, 'homely' atmosphere should exist whenever possible. Even during emergencies, staff should be aware of how they might appear to the other patients, and of the language that they use. Patients can be reassured that the nurses' attention centres on them rather than on machines; indeed, some patients report that they find the constant presence of the cardiac monitor (as well as the high staffing level) a comfort. On transferral to a general medical ward after 2 or 3 days, patients may feel extremely vulnerable – no watchful monitors and fewer nurses.

For further discussion of this topic, the reader is referred to Boore et al (1987).

ANGINA PECTORIS

Narrowing of the coronary arteries by the disease process atherosclerosis can lead to a characteristic symptom, the pain of *angina pectoris*. Here, exertion such as climbing stairs can cause severe 'crushing' central chest pain and referred pain (see Ch. 32) down the left arm. When the individual is resting, blood flow through the coronary arteries is adequate to meet the heart muscle's demands for oxygen and nutrients. During activity, however, those demands increase beyond the level that can be supplied by the narrowed coronary circulation. Pain then results, caused by substances, such as bradykinin, histamine and serotonin, produced from the ischaemic tissues.

To reduce demands on the heart, the patient is advised to restrict activity to that which does not bring on chest pain. How might stopping smoking and losing weight also help?

Glyceryl trinitrate is a drug commonly and effectively used in the treatment of angina. It is believed to bring about a generalised peripheral vasodilation by relaxing the smooth muscle of the systemic venous system (Hopkins 1992). This decreases venous return to the heart, and so reduces the output of the left ventricle (Reynolds 1993).

BLOOD VESSELS: STRUCTURE AND FUNCTION

The vessels through which blood flows from the heart to the tissues and then back to the heart (*systemic circulation*) are (Fig. 5.16):

1. arteries
2. arterioles
3. capillaries
4. venules
5. veins.

GENERAL STRUCTURE

The walls of blood vessels, capillaries excepted, consist of three layers of tissue (Fig. 5.17):

● intima   ● media   ● adventitia.

The inner layer (*intima*) consists almost entirely of a layer of *endothelial cells* in contact with the blood, to-

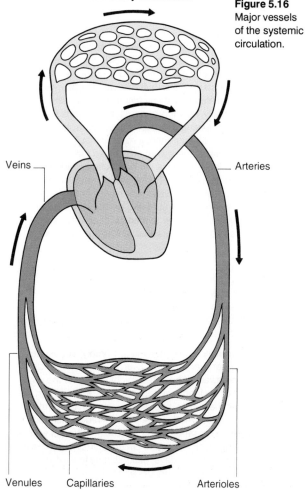

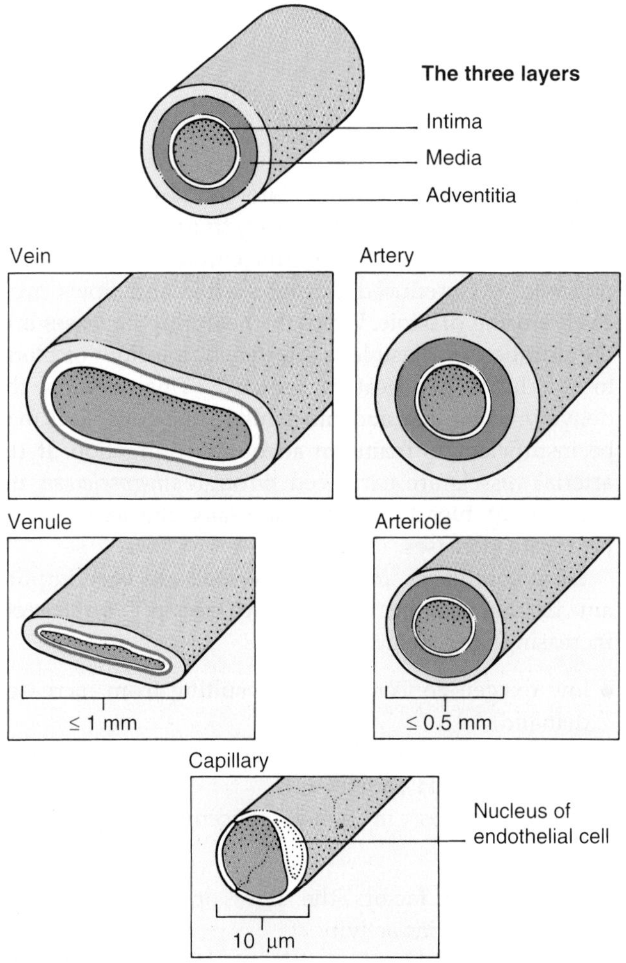

Pulmonary circulation

Figure 5.16 Major vessels of the systemic circulation.

Veins

Arteries

Venules   Capillaries   Arterioles

Systemic circulation

The three layers

Intima

Media

Adventitia

Vein

Artery

Venule

≤ 1 mm

Arteriole

≤ 0.5 mm

Capillary

Nucleus of endothelial cell

10 µm

Figure 5.17
The structure of blood vessels showing the relative proportion of each component of the wall (intima, media and adventitia) in each type of vessel.

Figure 5.18
The major arteries of the systemic circulation. (Reproduced from
Rogers 1992 (Fig. 7.9) by permission of the publishers.)

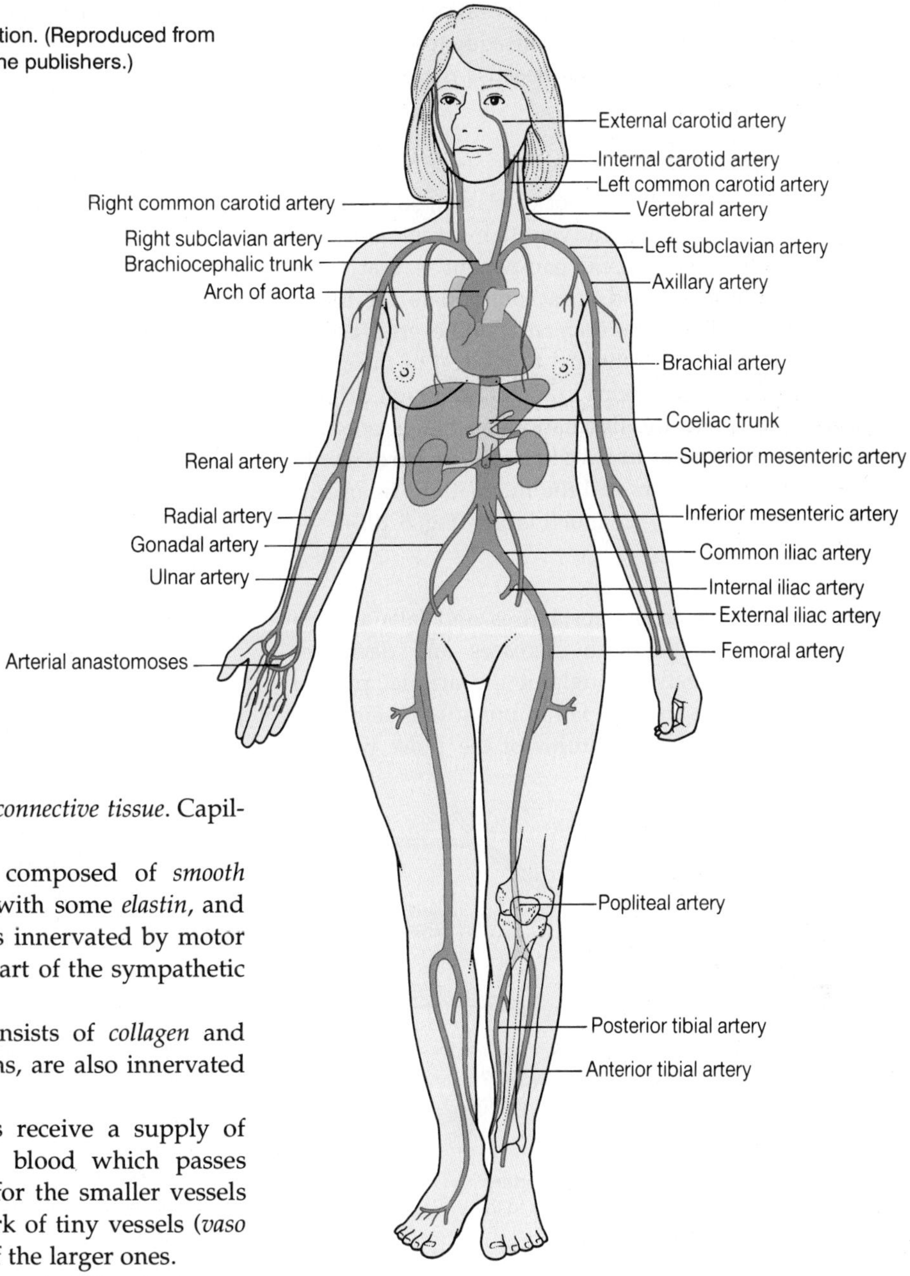

gether with a variable amount of *connective tissue*. Capillaries consist of this layer alone.

The middle layer (*media*), is composed of *smooth
muscle cells* (see Ch. 22) together with some *elastin*, and
collagen (see Ch. 2). The muscle is innervated by motor
nerve fibres, most of which are part of the sympathetic
nervous system (see Ch. 3).

The outer layer (*adventitia*) consists of *collagen* and
elastin. Some vessels, such as veins, are also innervated
by sensory neurones.

The cells of the blood vessels receive a supply of
nutrients and oxygen from the blood which passes
through them. This is sufficient for the smaller vessels
but is supplemented by a network of tiny vessels (*vaso
vasorum*) in the adventitial layer of the larger ones.

The several types of blood vessel differ from one
another in the contribution made by each of the three
constituent layers to the wall as a whole (Fig. 5.17).
These differences in structure are related to differences
in the functions of each type of vessel.

ARTERIES

The arteries (Fig. 5.18) distribute blood to the tissues.
They are elastic vessels and help to maintain the driving
pressure in the circulation. They also offer a variable
resistance to the flow of blood.

Arrangement

The arteries branch, much like a tree, and, in some
organs and tissues, *end arteries* exclusively supply dis-

crete areas of tissue (Fig. 5.19A). Should there be an
obstruction to flow then the tissue supplied by the
blocked end artery will be starved of vital supplies, and
the cells will die. Such an area is an *infarct*. This can
occur in the heart, large parts of the brain, and the
kidneys.

Anastomoses

Often, however, there are linking vessels (*anastomoses*)
between different arteries (Fig. 5.19B). In this case, a
blockage in one artery does not necessarily lead to cell
death because the anastomoses may allow the blockage
to be bypassed. Anastomoses are particularly common
in the skin, and skeletal muscle.

When arteries become narrowed with age, and by

disease, all arteries in the body are affected, but the deterioration has more serious consequences in organs such as the heart and the brain because there are fewer anastomoses.

Elastic recoil

The largest arteries contain a lot of elastin, some in the media and some in the adventitial layer. The significance of the large elastin component is that these vessels are able to distend, to accommodate the blood ejected from the heart, and then *recoil* and exert pressure on the blood as it flows onward to the rest of the circulation (Fig. 5.20A). This helps to maintain a high driving pressure and causes the fluctuations in blood pressure in these vessels to be *damped*. When arteries harden with age, less damping occurs and the fluctuations in arterial pressure (*pulse pressure*) are much larger (Fig. 5.20B).

Arterial pulse

When the pressure in the aorta rises and falls at each beat of the heart, pressure increases and decreases almost simultaneously throughout the arterial part of the circulation. This rise and fall in pressure is sensed as the *arterial pulse*. Several features of the pulse provide

⑥
If a cardiac arrest is suspected, which pulse should be felt for? If a patient has both arms and wrists in plaster, where might his pulse be taken?

important information about the circulation:

● number of pulsations per minute (heart rate)
● irregularities in rhythm (information about the pattern of electrical excitation)
● strength (clues about cardiac output)
● character or form of the pulse (may suggest leaky or narrowed valves – Fig. 5.20B).

Even the 'feel' of the arteries themselves (whether they are sinewy or soft) provides useful information. With advancing age arteries stiffen. ⑥

RECORDING THE PATIENT'S PULSE

Taking the patient's pulse is probably the most common nursing observation, but the frequency and repetitiveness of the task should not detract from the nurse's awareness of its significance. A rise in a patient's pulse rate in the first few hours following an operation may signify that there is loss of blood. A fast heart beat following a myocardial infarction may accompany a low blood pressure; the heart, because it is damaged, is a less efficient pump, and so it speeds up in order to compensate. Sometimes, after MI, damage to the heart's muscle gives rise to an irregular heart beat.

There are different forms of irregularity observable in a pulse. In one, *regularly irregular*, there is a fixed pattern to the irregularity. An example of this would be *bigeminy* or '*coupled beats*', such as may occur in digoxin overdose (see p. 392). Here, each normal beat of the heart is closely followed by a ventricular ectopic (see Fig. 162 in Schamroth 1982). The ectopic beat is felt as a somewhat weaker pulse, whereas the normal ventricular contraction, which follows it, might be felt as a particularly powerful pulse.

The ectopic beat is also referred to as a *premature* beat – it occurs sooner than anticipated if the heart beat were regular. The fact that the ectopic beat arrives prematurely explains why it is perceived as a weaker pulse; the ventricles have less time to fill with blood. Consequently, each premature contraction results in a reduced cardiac output, and a weaker pulse. Conversely, each premature beat is followed by a compensatory pause, during which the ventricles fill more than if the beat were absolutely regular. The pulse following the pause is therefore particularly strong. Bigeminy would therefore be felt thus: strong–weak . . . , strong–weak . . . , strong–weak . . .

Atrial fibrillation is an example of an *irregularly irregular* pulse. Here, no regular pattern is discernible and such a pulse should unquestionably be recorded for a full minute. Some instances of atrial fibrillation can be extremely rapid – this, and the irregularity of the beat make it difficult to count.

A patient's radial pulse may be sometimes so weak that it is difficult to feel. This is often the case where the blood pressure has fallen to a systolic of 60 or 70 mmHg. In such cases, the femoral or carotid pulse should be felt. Cardiac arrest is not diagnosed on the basis of absence of radial pulse; when cardiac arrest is suspected, the carotid pulse should be sought.

The effectiveness of resuscitation procedures may be judged by one of the team feeling for the patient's femoral pulse while cardiac massage is being performed. A palpable femoral pulse indicates the achievement of some degree of cardiac output.

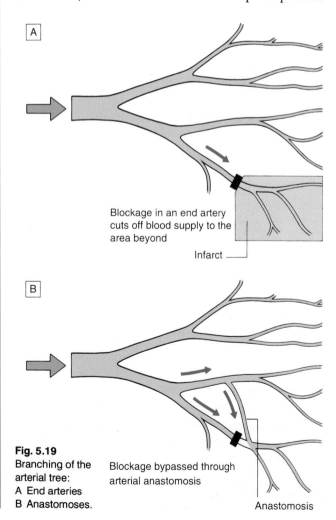

Fig. 5.19
Branching of the arterial tree:
A End arteries
B Anastomoses.

Blockage in an end artery cuts off blood supply to the area beyond

Infarct

Blockage bypassed through arterial anastomosis

Anastomosis

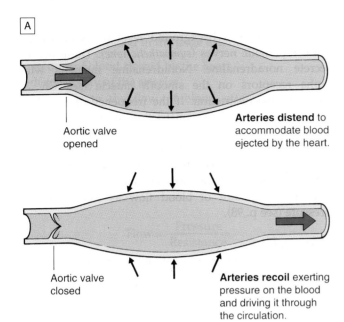

Aortic valve
opened

Arteries distend to accommodate blood ejected by the heart.

Aortic valve
closed

Arteries recoil exerting pressure on the blood and driving it through the circulation.

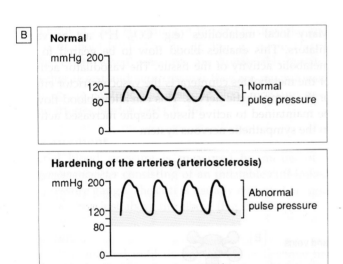

Normal

mmHg 200

120
80

} Normal pulse pressure

0

Hardening of the arteries (arteriosclerosis)

mmHg 200

120
80

] Abnormal pulse pressure

0

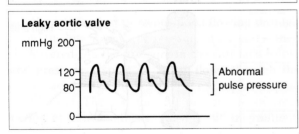

Leaky aortic valve

mmHg 200

120
80

] Abnormal pulse pressure

0

Figure 5.20
Arterial function and arterial pressure:
A How the arteries respond to the inflow of blood at each beat of the heart
B The rise and fall of arterial blood pressure at each beat of the heart and how this is altered by disease. (Adapted from Guyton 1986.)

Vasoconstriction and vasodilation

As arteries branch and become smaller in diameter further along in the circulation, the proportion of muscle to elastic tissue in their walls increases (Fig. 5.17). Contraction of the muscle reduces the internal diameter of the vessel (*vasoconstriction*). Whereas relaxation increases the internal diameter (*vasodilation*). Usually the muscle is in a state of partial contraction. The vessels are then said to possess *tone*. This tone can be either increased or decreased by the action of a wide variety of substances including neurotransmitters, hormones and local factors. Such substances are termed *vasoactive*. Examples are listed in Table 5.2.

ARTERIOLES

Resistance

In the smallest arteries, the *arterioles*, the internal diameter of the vessel is small in comparison with the thickness of the muscle layer. Consequently, small changes in muscle contraction have a large effect on the size of the vessel and thus on the flow of blood (Fig. 5.21). Contraction of the muscle can almost close the *lumen* (the space inside) and severely reduce blood flow. Conversely, relaxation dilates the vessels and increases the flow of blood.

Collectively, the arterioles offer the greatest resistance

Table 5.2 Examples of vasoactive substances		
Substance	Action*	
	Constrictor	Dilator
Neurotransmitters		
– noradrenaline	via α receptors	—
– acetylcholine	—	√
– substance P	—	√
– VIP[†]	—	√
Hormones		
– adrenaline	via α receptors	via β receptors
– angiotensin	√	—
– progesterone	—	√
Local hormones		
– serotonin (5-HT)[‡]	√	—
– bradykinin	—	√
– histamine	—	√
– prostaglandins	F series	E series
Local factors		
– carbon dioxide	—	√
– hydrogen ions	—	√
– oxygen lack	—	√
– potassium	—	√

* Action in the systemic circulation. Effects on pulmonary blood vessels may differ (see Ch. 7).
† Vasoactive intestinal polypeptide.
‡ 5-hydroxytryptamine.

It is important for the doctor to know that any change occurring in a patient's diastolic reading has been caused by altered physiology rather than varying techniques in recording it. Consequently, there needs to be uniformity of practice, so that all staff take the muffling of sounds as the diastolic pressure, or all staff note the point at which sounds disappear. Everyone involved in the recording of patients' blood pressures, needs to be aware of the local policy regarding the measurement of diastolic pressure.

However, if the upper arm is raised, for example to shoulder height, then the pressure recorded will be less because of gravity (see p. 81).

It is also important to ensure that the person is in a calm, restful state. A last minute dash to get to the surgery, or a lengthy wait, coupled with anger at the delay, is likely to raise blood pressure because of increased activity in the sympathetic nervous system. This increases cardiac output and arteriolar tone and causes more blood to be pumped into a narrowed set of vessels. Consequently arterial pressure increases. A few minutes of rest and reassurance should reduce sympathetic activity and lower pressure.

Control of blood pressure

Need for control

In order for an adequate flow of blood to be supplied to all tissues, arterial pressure has to be maintained at an adequate level. If it is not, the flow of blood to tissues such as the brain may become insufficient, and consciousness will be lost very rapidly.

Conversely, blood pressure must also not become too high. If the hydrostatic pressure in the capillaries increased greatly, more fluid would be driven from the blood into the tissue spaces, causing oedema and adversely affecting cell nutrition (see p. 101 and Ch. 3).

Baroreceptors

The pressure of blood in the circulation is sensed by *baroreceptors* located in the walls of some of the major vessels. Important locations include the *carotid sinus* at the bifurcation of the carotid arteries, and the *arch of the aorta* (Fig. 5.24). Baroreceptors consist of branching nerve endings, inserted between the tissues of the wall. They are excited by stretch. An increase in blood pressure distends the vessel, compresses the endings and excites them. Because pressure rises and falls at each beat of the heart, the frequency of nerve impulses generated by the receptors varies. Thus the receptors monitor not only the mean blood pressure but the rate of change of pressure from beat to beat.

Neural control centres

Impulses are transmitted from the receptors along

BLOOD PRESSURE

The importance of achieving an accurate measurement of a patient's blood pressure cannot be overemphasised. Many details of recording technique are contained within the main text: correct positioning of the patient's arm and of the cuff; allowing the patient to rest following exercise or relax after stress. In addition, the cuff of the sphygmomanometer should be correctly applied to the arm. The purpose of the inflated cuff is to compress the arm and its arteries. The cuff must therefore be of the correct size, be tightly wrapped around the arm – it should be firm enough to remain in position of its own accord – and not be hampered by clothing.

Not only should the sphygmomanometer be at the level of the patient's heart, but for accurate reading the mercury column needs to be at the nurse's eye level. An accurate reading will not be achieved if the nurse is looking down on to the top of the column. The student will deduce from this that the patient's heart, the mercury column, and the recorder's eye all need to be roughly at the same level. However, even when all possible care has been taken to obtain an accurate reading, a single isolated measurement of blood pressure may not be meaningful; an abnormal result should always be repeated.

Blood pressure is rarely taken in young children, since the distress caused by the procedure will alter the reading (and may make the actual recording impossible). However, children suffering from cardiac conditions may require their blood pressure to be recorded, and a small-sized cuff is used. Using an adult cuff on a young child's arm will result in an inaccurate reading.

sensory nerve fibres to the spinal cord, and from there to the *medulla* and *hypothalamus* (see Ch. 3). Within these areas of the brain are groups of nerve cells (formerly known as the *cardio-inhibitory* and the *vasomotor centres*) that are involved in the regulation of cardiac function and the control of vascular smooth muscle. These groups of cells influence the activity of sympathetic and parasympathetic nerve fibres innervating the heart and blood vessels.

Reflexes

If an increase in blood pressure is sensed by the baroreceptors, this stimulus acts reflexly through the control centres in the brain to reduce cardiac output and arterial resistance to blood flow (Fig. 5.25). The balance of parasympathetic and sympathetic activity acting on the heart shifts in favour of the parasympathetic resulting in a decrease in heart rate and stroke volume. At the same time the activity of the sympathetic nerves innervating the arterial smooth muscle decreases, the muscle relaxes and the vessels dilate. As less blood is being pumped into the arterial system, and it is able to leave more easily, the mean arterial pressure falls.

Conversely, if blood pressure falls, the balance of autonomic activity shifts in favour of the sympathetic. Consequently, heart rate and stroke volume increase,

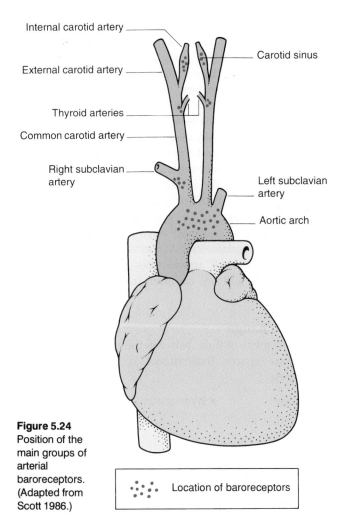

Internal carotid artery

External carotid artery

Thyroid arteries

Common carotid artery

Right subclavian artery

Carotid sinus

Left subclavian artery

Aortic arch

Figure 5.24
Position of the main groups of arterial baroreceptors. (Adapted from Scott 1986.)

Location of baroreceptors

arterial vasoconstriction occurs, and arterial blood pressure returns towards normal. ⑦

In this way, mean arterial blood pressure, and therefore an adequate flow of blood, is maintained. The particular adjustments made in response to the challenges posed by everyday activities such as eating, exercising, standing up and sitting down are described later (Chs 11 and 17).

Blood volume
Mean arterial blood pressure also depends on the volume of blood filling the circulation. If this is low then pressure is low and vice versa. Blood volume depends crucially on fluid and electrolyte balances, and their control (see Ch. 13).

CAPILLARIES

Capillaries are the simplest of the blood vessels, consisting only of a single layer of cells. They form a network of vessels between the arterioles and the venules and are the site at which exchange of substances occurs between the blood and the tissue fluid (see Ch. 3). They play an important role in determining the distribution of fluids between the blood and the interstitial fluid.

Structure and permeability
Capillary walls consist of a single layer of endothelial cells, surrounded by a basement membrane (Fig. 5.17, and Chs 2 and 3). They are the barrier between blood and tissue fluid, and determine which blood constituents are able to pass easily from the blood into the tissue fluid, and which cannot. Some capillaries (*sinusoids*) are very leaky; others, such as those in the brain (*cerebral capillaries*) are more selective. The differences in permeability are due to differences in capillary structure and activity.

Capillaries differ in:

- the nature and extent of the basement membrane
- the presence and size of 'pores' in, and between, the endothelial cells
- the degree of endocytotic and exocytotic activity.

Sinusoids
This is the name given to capillaries in the liver, spleen and bone marrow. They are very permeable to all the constituents of plasma including plasma proteins, and have very little basement membrane. Sinusoids of the

⑦
Can you explain the tachycardia and cold skin of someone who has lost blood?

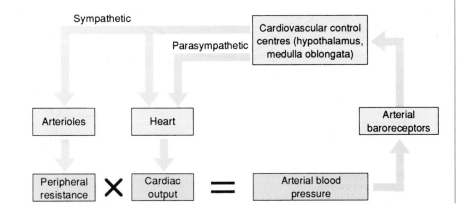

Sympathetic

Parasympathetic

Cardiovascular control centres (hypothalamus, medulla oblongata)

Arterioles

Heart

Arterial baroreceptors

Figure 5.25
The control of arterial blood pressure: cardiac output and peripheral resistance are reflexly adjusted according to the pressure monitored by the baroreceptors.

Peripheral resistance ✕ Cardiac output = Arterial blood pressure spleen and bone marrow appear to have gaps between the cells and even permit the passage of blood cells.

Cerebral capillaries

At the other extreme, capillaries in the brain only permit easy movement of very small molecules such as oxygen, water, and carbon dioxide, and restrict the passage of small ions such as K^+ and H^+. This unusual selectivity led researchers to coin the term *blood–brain barrier*, to emphasise its distinctiveness.

Cerebral capillaries have a basement membrane, lack pores and have no gaps between the cells. In addition, adjacent cells are linked very closely by tight junctions (Ch. 2).

Other capillaries

Capillaries in other tissues are intermediate in structure and permeability. Capillaries in skeletal muscle are, for example, more permeable than those in the brain but much less permeable than those in the liver.

Penicillin is one of many drugs which cross the blood–brain barrier with great difficulty. In cases of *meningitis* (inflammation of the membranes covering the brain and spinal cord) penicillin is usually given intravenously. In order to be effective, a sufficiently high dose needs to be given to permit an adequate therapeutic dose to enter the brain.

Q. How else might antibiotics be given, in the case of meningitis, in order to be certain that they reach the cerebrospinal fluid?

Arrangement

Capillaries form a network of interconnected vessels between the arterioles and the venules (Fig. 5.26A). Some of these are thoroughfare channels which allow the size of the capillary network being used to be adjusted. In skeletal muscle, for example, there is a huge difference in the metabolic needs of the tissue at rest and during activity. At rest, most blood passes through the thoroughfares, and bypasses much of the capillary bed (Fig. 5.26B). When muscles are active, however, the smooth muscle in the arterioles and at the opening of the capillaries (*pre-capillary sphincters*) relaxes and blood flows through more of the capillary bed.

Occasionally arteries and veins are linked directly by *arteriovenous anastomoses (AV anastomoses)*. They act as a capillary bypass. AV anastomoses have smooth muscle in their walls and are common in the skin circulation (see Ch. 16).

Fluid exchange

The movement of fluid between the vascular space and the tissue spaces (*interstitium*) is governed by two pressures:

- oncotic
- hydrostatic.

Inactive tissue

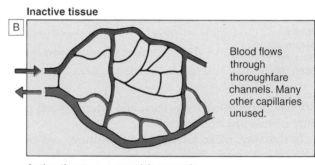

Blood flows through thoroughfare channels. Many other capillaries unused.

Active tissue e.g. exercising muscle

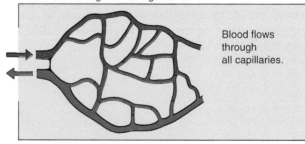

Blood flows through all capillaries.

AV anastomosis open

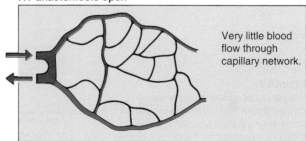

Very little blood flow through capillary network.

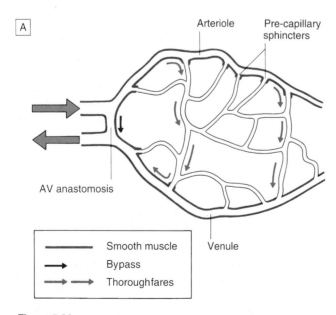

Arteriole — Pre-capillary sphincters

AV anastomosis

Venule

——	Smooth muscle
→	Bypass
⇒ →	Thoroughfares

Figure 5.26
The capillary network:
A Arrangement of vessels
B Patterns of blood flow in different circumstances.

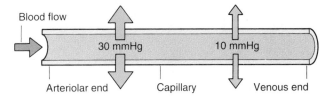

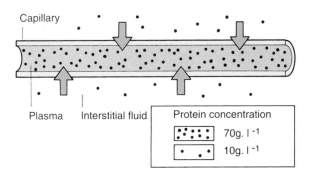

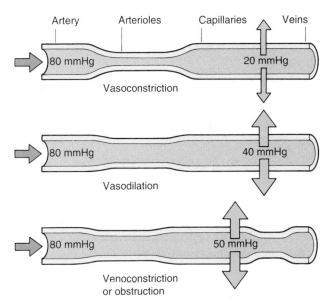

Figure 5.27
Oncotic and hydrostatic pressures:
A Oncotic pressure: osmotic pressure created by the difference in protein concentration – draws water *into* the capillary
B Hydrostatic pressure: pressure within the capillaries created by the pumping action of the heart – forces water (and dissolved solutes) *out* of the capillary. Capillary pressure is decreased by constriction of the arterioles and increased by constriction of the veins and venules.

Oncotic pressure

Most capillaries are relatively impermeable to plasma proteins. Consequently, the concentrations of plasma proteins in the plasma and in the interstitial fluid differ (Fig. 5.27A) creating a difference in osmotic pressure between the two sides. This tends to draw water *from* the interstitial fluid *into* the plasma. This osmotic force created by the plasma proteins is often referred to as *oncotic pressure* or *colloidal osmotic pressure*, meaning the osmotic pressure created by the dissolved *macro-molecules*.

Hydrostatic pressure

The oncotic force drawing fluid into the capillaries is opposed by the hydrostatic pressure of the blood within the capillaries driving fluid in the opposite direction (Fig. 5.27B). Hydrostatic pressure in the capillaries increases if the arterioles dilate, and decreases if they constrict. If there is any obstruction to the flow of blood from the capillaries into the venules and veins, capillary hydrostatic pressure also increases.

> Colloidal osmotic pressure can be reduced where there is a significant fall in plasma protein levels. This can occur with prolonged starvation, for example, or a diet with a greatly reduced protein intake. Certain kidney diseases lead to loss of proteins in the urine. In severe burns, fluid and protein are lost in the form of plasma. Intravenous replacement therapy consists of plasma or other plasma volume expanders (see Ch. 13). An infusion of normal saline, while providing fluid, would decrease rather than increase the colloidal osmotic pressure.

Balance and imbalance

It is the balance of these two forces, oncotic and hydro-static, which determines how much fluid is pushed out of the capillaries and how much is drawn back in. If hydrostatic pressure exceeds oncotic pressure, as it does at the arterial end of all capillaries, then fluid is forced out of the blood into the interstitium (Fig. 5.28A). By contrast, if oncotic pressure exceeds hydrostatic pressure, as at the venous end of the capillary bed, fluid is drawn from the interstitium into the blood. These two processes occur simultaneously so that overall the volume of fluid in the blood and in the interstitium remains constant. If one or other of the forces changes, the balance is altered and there will be a shift of fluid either out of, or into the blood.

After haemorrhage, for example, reflex arteriolar vasoconstriction occurs in response to the decreased arterial blood pressure (see p. 99) and this lowers the hydrostatic pressure of blood in the capillaries (Fig. 5.28B). Consequently, fluid is drawn into the blood and helps to make up for the volume of blood lost.

In contrast, in some forms of renal disease there are losses of plasma proteins into the urine through injured renal capillaries, and this leads to a decrease in plasma protein concentration in the blood. Consequently more

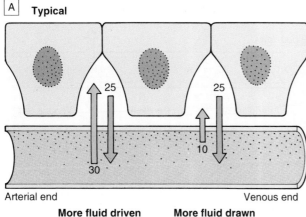

A   **Typical**

Arterial end   Venous end

More fluid driven out than drawn in   **More fluid drawn in than driven out**

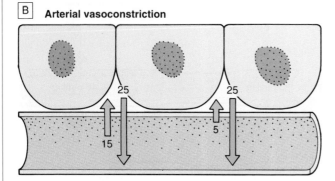

B   **Arterial vasoconstriction**

Fluid drawn into the blood from the interstitial space

C   **Plasma proteins reduced**

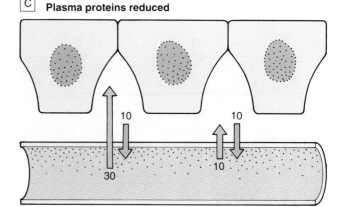

Fluid driven out into the interstitium resulting in oedema

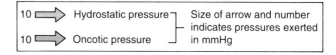

10 ⟹ Hydrostatic pressure ⎤ Size of arrow and number
                              ⎥ indicates pressures exerted
10 ⟹ Oncotic pressure   ⎦ in mmHg

Figure 5.28
Tissue fluid balance:
A Typical balance of hydrostatic and oncotic pressures
B Effects of arterial vasoconstriction
C Effects of lowered plasma protein concentration.

⑧
What happens to tissue fluid balance in heart failure and why?

⑨
What are the plasma proteins? Which of them occurs in the greatest quantity in plasma (thereby contributing most to its oncotic pull)?

fluid is pushed out of the capillaries into the interstitium and the volume of interstitial fluid expands (Fig. 5.28C). The accumulation of abnormally large amounts of fluid in the interstitium is termed *oedema*. ⑧

Lymphatic capillaries

Some fluid escapes from the interstitium through a different set of capillaries not forming part of the circulation (*lymphatic capillaries*) (Fig. 5.29). These are small blind-ending vessels consisting of a single layer of endothelial cells. They are present in most tissues, brain

excepted. Unlike blood capillaries, lymphatic capillaries are freely permeable to plasma proteins. Thus any proteins that leak from the blood into the tissues can pass into the lymphatics. These vessels join larger lymphatic vessels, similar in structure to veins (see below). The fluid within them (*lymph*) flows via lymph nodes (see Ch. 4) into the *lymphatic ducts* emptying into the subclavian veins. The composition of lymph varies according to the tissue from which it is derived. Constituents may include plasma proteins, leucocytes (Ch. 4), and chylomicrons (Ch. 6). ⑨

The lymphatic system acts as an overflow for the fluid in the tissue spaces. If lymphatics are blocked, oedema will occur.

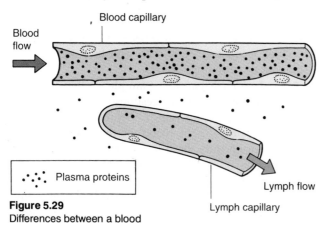

Blood capillary

Blood flow

Lymph flow

Lymph capillary

·:·: Plasma proteins

Figure 5.29
Differences between a blood capillary and a lymph capillary.

Obstruction to lymphatic drainage can lead to marked swelling of the affected part because of the accumulation of tissue fluid. Following axillary lymph node removal (usually associated with mastectomy) the patient may find that her arm on the affected side becomes heavy and swollen. It is usually rested in a raised sling to assist venous return and lymphatic drainage.

Chronic obstruction to lymphatic drainage can occur where the lymph nodes become blocked by thread-like parasites called *Wuchereria bancrofti*. This leads to severe swelling, usually of the legs and external genitalia. The parasite is carried by mosquitoes and is commonest in Central Africa. The heavy, swollen appearance of the leg has led to the condition being called elephantiasis.

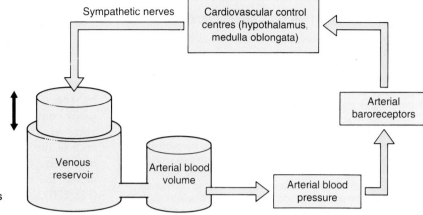

Figure 5.30
Role of the venous reservoir in the control of
blood pressure. The capacity of the reservoir is
controlled by sympathetic nerves.

VENULES AND VEINS

Venules and veins are very distensible vessels acting as
a reservoir that can expand and contract to accommodate changing volumes of blood in the circulation. The
pressure of blood in the veins, which drives the flow of
blood back to the heart (*venous return*) is very low and is
therefore easily influenced by external pressures. ⑩

Distensibility

Venules and veins are very thin walled by comparison
with the arterial vessels. Of the three layers of tissue
present in the wall, the outer adventitial layer is the
most prominent. It consists largely of collagen fibres.

These features make the veins very distensible. They
are therefore able to accommodate an increase in blood
volume without much rise in pressure. This makes it
possible for the volume of blood in the circulation to
change without seriously threatening the pressures in
the system. If blood volume increases, most of the
increase is taken up by the distensible veins. If decreases, blood can be shifted from the venous reservoir
into the arterial vessels.

Venoconstriction and venodilation

Almost all veins and venules have some smooth muscle
in their walls. Like that of the arterioles, it is innervated
by sympathetic nerve fibres, and is influenced by vasoactive substances (see p. 95). However, contraction
of the muscle has very little effect on the resistance to
the flow of blood through the veins. It does not narrow
the vessels to the same extent. Instead it stiffens them,
holding them firm and making them less distensible.
Consequently the veins cannot expand as easily in response to an increase in venous pressure and their
capacity as a venous reservoir is reduced.

If blood volume falls, as for example in haemorrhage,
reflex venoconstriction occurs. This displaces blood held
in the venous reservoir into the arterial side of the circulation and helps to maintain blood pressure (Fig. 5.30).

Valves

Many of the small and medium-sized veins, especially
those in the limbs, have valves. These consist of flaps of
the intima projecting into the lumen (Fig. 5.31). They
prevent backflow of blood towards the capillaries. ⑪

Venous return

As the resistance to blood flow through the veins is very
low (because the internal diameter is large), only a small
driving pressure is needed to return blood to the heart.
When you are lying flat venous pressures normally
range between 0 and 15 mmHg. When you stand, they

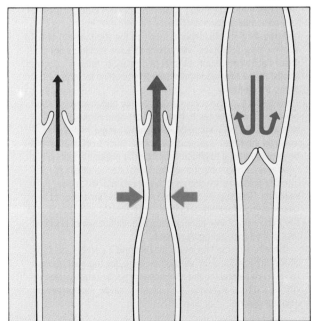

Flaps forced apart
by pressure of
blood returning to
the heart

Limb veins squeezed
when limb muscles
contract in walking

Valve prevents
backflow when limb
muscles relax

Figure 5.31
Valves in the veins and how they work.

⑩
*How would
haemorrhage
from a vein be
distinguished
in appearance
from
haemorrhage
from an artery?*

⑪
*How can you
show that there
are valves in
some of the
veins of your
hand or arm?*

DRUG ADMINISTRATION IN AN EMERGENCY

The almost instantaneous action of intravenous drugs makes this route mandatory during resuscitation. In contrast, drugs given intramuscularly or subcutaneously to a shocked patient may take a long time to work. Poor tissue perfusion in shock (see Ch. 11) means that the injected drug lingers in the muscle or fatty tissue at the injection site and is not 'flushed out' into the bloodstream. This has been seen in moutaineering casualties, where the patient may be cold as well as shocked, and an intramuscular injection of morphine appears to have little effect. Then, on evacuating the casualty from the cold mountain to a relatively warm ambulance, where an infusion may be started to counteract the shock, the patient's blood pressure rises, tissue perfusion increases, and there is a sudden release of the drug into the bloodstream. Rescuers need to be aware of this complication if they are faced with a casualty who, on reaching warmth and apparent safety, suddenly begins to lose consciousness, with decreased respiration rate and lowered blood pressure. One possible reason, though there are others, is the sudden release into the system of morphine, injected some time earlier but stored in poorly perfused tissues (Steele 1988).

Most nurses will, however, be more familiar with an emergency on a hospital ward, or in the street, rather than on a mountain. When cardiac arrest occurs, or in severe shock, thin-walled veins appear to 'collapse', so that the physician may find it difficult to insert a cannula through which to give intravenous fluid and/or drugs. Consequently, it is often the case that a patient admitted with an MI has an intravenous cannula inserted as a precautionary measure. The patient may not require intravenous fluid (in the case of MI, additional fluid may precipitate heart failure) but has the means of receiving such fluid should it be necessary. The cannula has a small amount of the anticoagulant heparin injected, to prevent it blocking with blood clot (see Ch. 4).

Why do the peripheral veins of a severely shocked patient appear to 'collapse'? One explanation is that when the individual's blood pressure falls sharply the blood supply to non-essential organs and tissues is reduced in order to maintain flow to vital organs, such as the heart and brain. To achieve this, arterioles, veins and venules serving non-essential tissues, such as skin and muscle, reflexly constrict and blood is displaced from peripheral veins to maintain pressure centrally.

Insertion of a cannula is aided by the constriction of the patient's arm *proximal* to the point of venipuncture. This congests the vein, since blood can no longer move on towards the heart, causing it to swell. Such constriction may be provided by a tourniquet or manual pressure from a colleague. The student may demonstrate the effect of manual pressure by gripping the upper arm for a few seconds. The superficial veins of the lower arm should become more visible, and thus more readily punctured. It is the thin walls of the veins, compared with those of arteries, that permit manual compression.

Once a cannula has been established it can be used for giving analgesia, such as diamorphine, for the swift pain relief so essential for the MI patient; and for emergency drugs, such as adrenaline, calcium chloride, isoprenaline and lignocaine.

increase because of the effects of gravity (see p. 81 and Ch. 17).

Muscle pump

Because venous pressures are low, and because the vessels are thin walled, local changes in pressure caused by the contraction of surrounding skeletal muscles easily compress the vessels and affect blood flow. When you walk the veins are massaged. Because of the presence of the valves, blood can be squeezed in one direction only, back towards the heart. This *muscle pump* assists the return of blood (*venous return*) to the heart (Fig. 5.31).

Respiratory pump

Venous return is also affected by breathing. This is because inspiration and expiration affect the pressure of blood in the atria and around the veins in the thorax (see Ch. 7). In inspiration, atrial pressure falls and

VARICOSE VEINS

Failure of the valves in the superficial veins of the leg results in a condition called *varicose veins*. Valves in veins assist the passage of blood towards the heart by preventing backflow. When they fail, the columns of blood within the veins are no longer supported at intervals, and the vessels become dilated and tortuous. Varicose veins may ache and are liable to haemorrhage if knocked, but the sufferer's main complaint is usually of their appearance. Increased venous pressure leads to leakage of fluid into the surrounding tissues, which therefore become oedematous. Oxygen and nutrients have greater difficulty in diffusing from the blood into tissue cells, leading to both aching in the muscles and the formation of ulcers in the skin (Guyton 1991).

There is a genetic factor in the development of varicose veins, but one important occupational factor is standing for long periods. Here, there is reduced muscular activity of the legs and, hence, less activity of the muscle pump that assists venous return from the lower limbs. Another reason for the development of varicose veins is pregnancy, women with several offspring being more liable to them. The growing fetus causes increased pressure on veins flowing through the pelvic cavity, impeding venous return (see Ch. 34).

There is no cure for this condition, but an operation can be performed that strips out the affected vein, with ligatures to supplying veins. Non-surgical relief may be had by the wearing of support tights or stockings. These are stronger than the normal type of tights and, without actually constricting vessels, assist venous return by maintaining pressure on the legs.

An effective preventive measure is sitting down at intervals throughout the day with the feet raised on a stool. Crossing the legs while sitting should be avoided, since this practice obstructs blood flow through vessels behind the knees. If long periods of standing are unavoidable, the individual could try wriggling the toes, thus increasing calf muscle compression of the veins, and therefore venous return. Venous return will also be assisted by deep breathing (see p. 105).

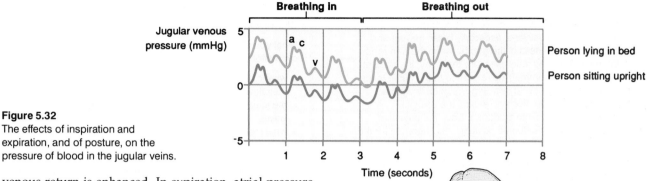

Figure 5.32
The effects of inspiration and expiration, and of posture, on the pressure of blood in the jugular veins.

venous return is enhanced. In expiration, atrial pressure rises and venous return is reduced. The pressure of blood in the veins entering the heart thus rises and falls during the breathing cycle (Fig. 5.32). These changes are superimposed on the a, c, and v waves of the jugular venous pulse (see p. 89).

When your breathing is fairly gentle the effects are relatively minor, but if you take a bigger breath, breathe out hard against a resistance (blowing up a balloon), or increase pressures in the thorax (by straining to lift something, or straining to defaecate) the resulting changes in blood pressure and the reflexly evoked changes in heart rate can be considerable.

Venous pulse

Venous pulses differ from arterial pulses in that they are very small and cannot normally be felt. Light pressure of the fingers over a vein will compress it and obstruct blood flow. However, much can be learnt from observation of the veins (Figs 5.33 and 5.34). When a person is

Normal venous pressure

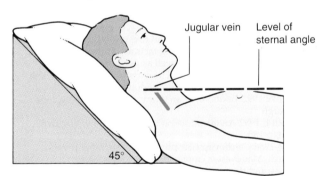

Raised venous pressure

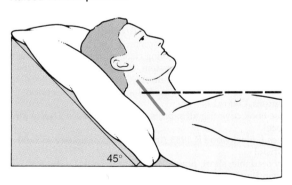

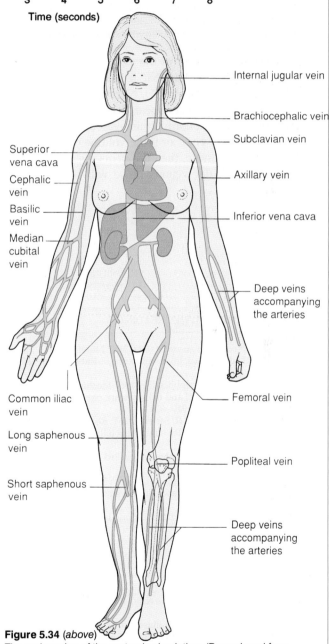

Figure 5.34 (*above*)
The major veins of the systemic circulation. (Reproduced from Rogers 1992 (Fig. 7.10) by permission of the publishers.)

Figure 5.33 (*left*)
Assessment of central venous pressure by observation of the neck veins. When pressure is high much more of the jugular vein can be seen to be filled with blood and to be pulsating.

Forced expiration is practised for prolonged periods by some orchestral musicians, especially brass players and oboists (the narrowness of the gap between the twin reeds of the oboe requiring more pressure than, say, the clarinet).

Perhaps of more immediate relevance to the nurse is the need for patients to avoid straining at stool following a myocardial infarction. For this reason, the use of a commode is preferred to a bedpan, since the patient is sitting in a more accustomed position. It is important for the nurse to prevent such a patient from becoming constipated. Suppositories, which soften stool and make defaecation less strenuous, are often used.

KEY POINTS

What you should now know and understand about the circulation:

- what makes blood and other fluids flow and what affects their flow rate
- the structure of the heart: its chambers, vessels and valves
- what makes cardiac muscle contract regularly, and how this is influenced by the autonomic nervous system and by hormones
- what an ECG is and some of the many things it reveals about cardiac functioning
- the sequence of events occurring at each beat of the heart and how these are related to the ECG, heart sounds, blood pressure and pulses
- some of the ways in which cardiac function may be disrupted and how this gives rise to signs and symptoms
- the different types of blood vessel and their distinctive structures and functions
- what arterial blood pressure is, how it is controlled, and how it is measured
- what pulses are and what they can tell you about circulatory fitness and why
- what is meant by hydrostatic and oncotic pressures, and what factors affect them
- what oedema is and how it may be caused
- what the venous system does and how its function is controlled in health, and may be altered in disease.

sitting upright, pressure in the veins of the neck, such as the jugular, is less than that at heart level because of the effect of gravity (see p. 81). Normally, therefore, the veins of the neck do not appear distended. However if venous pressure is abnormally increased, for example if cardiac function is poor, or if the volume of fluid in the circulation is excessive, then the veins distend, and the ripple of the jugular venous pulse will be seen quite clearly.

REFERENCES AND FURTHER READING

Boore J, Champion R, Ferguson M (eds) 1987 Nursing the physically ill adult. Churchill Livingstone, Edinburgh, pp 669–676

Braunwald E, Ross J, Sonnenblick E H 1967 Mechanisms of contraction of the normal and failing heart: part 3. New England Journal of Medicine 277: 910–920

Emslie-Smith D, Paterson C R, Scratcherd T, Read N W (eds) 1988 Textbook of physiology, 11th edn. Churchill Livingstone, Edinburgh

Evans D E (ed) 1992 Practical physiology, 3rd edn. University of Manchester, Manchester

Fozzard H A, Haber E, Jennings R B, Katz A M, Morgan H E (eds) 1986 The heart and cardiovascular system. Raven Press, New York
(Huge two volume work, written for and by specialists. Reference only)

Goldschlager N, Goldman M J 1989 Principles of clinical electrocardiography, 13th edn. Appleton & Lange, East Norwalk, Connecticut

Guyton A C 1991 Textbook of medical physiology, 8th edn. W B Saunders, Philadelphia, p 166–167

Hampton J R 1986 The ECG made easy, 4th edn. Churchill Livingstone, Edinburgh
(Concise little book with clear illustrations. Easy to follow. Explains why waves are as they are and gives useful clinical applications)

Hollman A 1992 Plants in cardiology. British Medical Journal, London
(Small book composed of a collection of one page articles, reproduced from the British Heart Journal. Gives fascinating snapshots of the history of how some drugs have come into use)

Hopkins S J 1992 Drugs and pharmacology for nurses, 11th edn. Churchill Livingstone, Edinburgh

Julian D, Marley C 1991 Coronary heart disease: the facts. Oxford University Press, Oxford
(Practical text for people with the disease and for those caring for them)

Levick J R 1991 An introduction to cardiovascular physiology. Butterworth-Heinemann, London
(Lucidly written advanced student text providing more detailed information. Includes interesting facts about the historical and experimental background, as well as useful further reading)

Reynolds J E F 1993 Martindale: The extra pharmacopoeia, 30th edn. The Pharmaceutical Press, London

Rogers A W 1992 Textbook of anatomy. Churchill Livingstone, Edinburgh

Schamroth L 1982 An introduction to cardiography. Blackwell, Oxford, p 185

Scott E M 1986 Cardiovascular physiology: an integrative approach. Manchester University Press, Manchester
(Short, straightforward student textbook providing more information about the system)

Steele P 1988 Medical handbook for mountaineers. Constable, London

Thomas C, Gebert G, Hombach V 1992 Textbook and colour atlas of the cardiovascular system. Chapman & Hall Medical, London
(Attractively produced book giving clear information about the structure and function of the system, clinical methods, diseases and pathology. Useful for reference)

Timmins A D 1988 Essentials of cardiology. Blackwell Scientific Publications, Oxford
(Concise book covering all aspects of cardiac disease. Useful for reference)

Vann Jones J, Blackwood R 1983 An outline of cardiology. Wright PSG, Bristol
(A very readable, short, practically oriented book. Useful for understanding the treatment and care of cardiac patients)

Chapter 6
DIGESTIVE SYSTEM

The food we eat consists of cells, tissues, and macromolecules that need to be broken down into smaller units before they can be absorbed. This breakdown is achieved by the cooperative activity of the organs of the digestive system. This system consists of the *digestive tract* (mouth, oesophagus, stomach, and intestines) plus a few additional digestive glands (salivary glands, pancreas and biliary system). The food we swallow is:

- propelled along the tract
- mixed with secretions formed by the glands
- digested.

Nutrients, water and salts are absorbed from the digested food, and products that cannot be absorbed are retained in the tract until they are evacuated.

All these processes are controlled and coordinated by the autonomic nervous system acting in concert with a variety of hormones.

Before reading this chapter it may be helpful to review the chemistry of carbohydrates, proteins and fats (see Ch. 2). The nature of food, its nutritional value, and our nutritional requirements are described in Chapter 14.

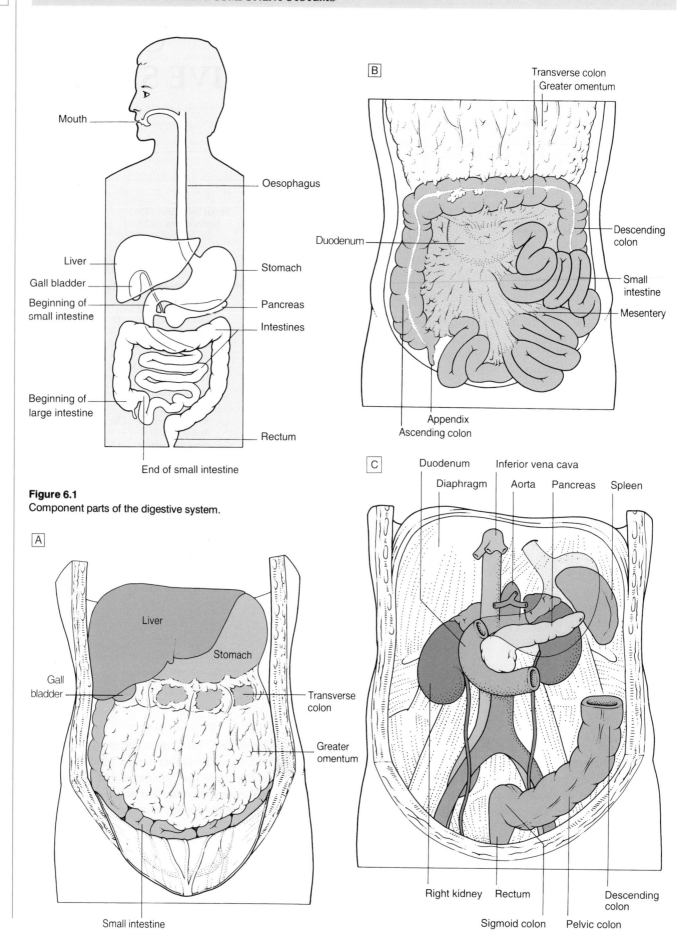

Figure 6.1
Component parts of the digestive system.

STRUCTURE

COMPONENT PARTS OF THE DIGESTIVE SYSTEM

The component parts of the digestive system are shown in Figure 6.1. Most are located within the abdominal cavity.

Organisation

Mouth, pharynx and oesophagus

The anatomy of the mouth and throat is detailed in Chapter 29, which describes the structures involved in a variety of actions, including speaking and smiling as well as eating, chewing and swallowing. Any impairment of the muscles or nerves involved in these actions, as for example in a stroke, is likely to affect a person's ability to communicate, as well as how easy it is for them to eat and to swallow. For this reason, all these activities are considered together in Chapter 29.

Stomach, intestines and accessory glands

The arrangement of these organs is illustrated in Figure 6.2A, B & C. The liver (see Ch. 9) sits snugly under the arch of the diaphragm. The stomach lies under the left lobe of the liver. The gall bladder and the first part of the small intestine (*duodenum*) lie under the right lobe. Lying close to the U-shaped duodenum and the stomach is the *pancreas*, which is a delicate structure as compared with the other organs. ①

> The pancreas may be damaged as a result of trauma caused by a seat belt injury in a road accident. This is one of the causes of pancreatitis.

Digestive secretions formed by the liver and the pancreas pass through separate ducts, eventually emptying into the duodenum through a common passage (*ampulla*) (Fig. 6.3). In some individuals an extra pancreatic duct opens separately into a different part of the duodenum.

The small intestine is divided (by convention) into

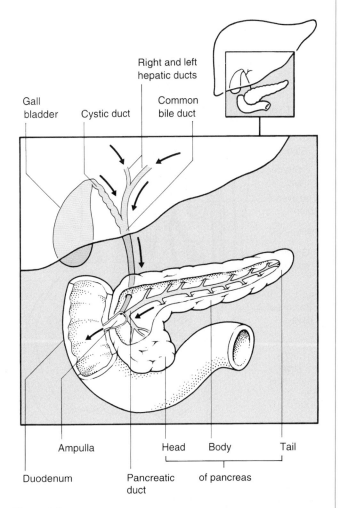

Figure 6.3
The biliary system (liver, gall bladder and bile ducts) and pancreas. Parts of the pancreas and duodenum are shown cut away to reveal the structures within.

three parts corresponding to the top, middle and bottom sections:

- duodenum (the first loop – about 30 cm)
- jejunum (the next metre)
- ileum (the last two 2 metres).

The large intestine is also subdivided into different parts:

- caecum   • colon   • rectum.

The colon is further subdivided into different sections (Fig. 6.2A, B & C):

1. ascending   4. pelvic
2. transverse   5. sigmoid.
3. descending

The last part, the *sigmoid colon*, merges into the *rectum*, the exit of which is guarded by the muscular sphincters of the *anus*.

The abdominal organs of the digestive system are enveloped by a thin epithelium, *peritoneum*, that is

Figure 6.2 (*left*)
Position of the digestive organs and associated structures within the abdominal cavity:
A Stomach, liver and greater omentum as seen beneath the anterior abdominal wall
B Greater omentum raised to show intestines lying below
C The organs lying at the back of the abdominal cavity hidden from view in A and B. The stomach is outlined to show its position in relation to the organs beneath it.
(Parts A & B reproduced from Rogers 1992 (Figs 29.2 & 29.3) by permission of the publishers.)

① *Do you understand why overeating may lead to difficulty in breathing?*

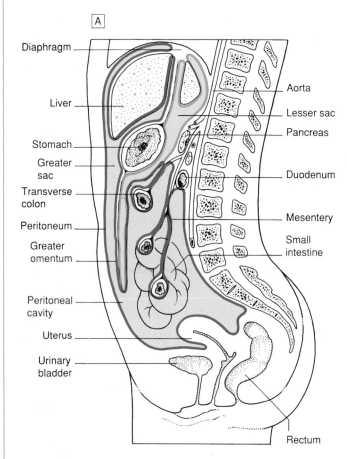

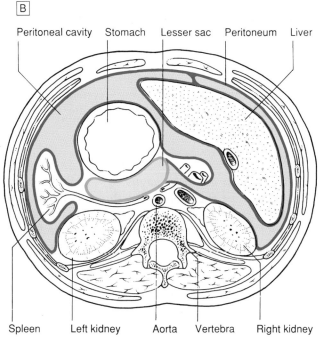

Figure 6.4

The epithelium (peritoneum) lining the anterior abdominal wall and wrapped around many of the abdominal organs. The size of the peritoneal cavity has been grossly enlarged for clarity. Normally there is very little fluid within the peritoneal cavity.

A Side view of a head to toe section through the midline of the body

B View from above of a transverse section at the level of thoracic vertebra 12.

(Reproduced from Rogers 1992. (Fig. 29.1) by permission of the publishers.)

doubled back on itself to line the anterior abdominal wall also (Fig. 6.4A & B). The small space between the two layers of peritoneum (*peritoneal cavity*) is filled with fluid. Some of the peritoneal layers become bonded together to form tissue, such as the *greater omentum* (Fig. 6.2), overlying the intestines; other peritoneal tissue forms *ligaments* attaching one organ to another. ②

Blood supply

The arteries supplying the abdominal organs of the digestive system are the *coeliac* and the *superior* and *inferior mesenteric arteries*. The coeliac artery branches to give rise to the *gastric*, *splenic*, and *hepatic arteries* that supply the stomach, pancreas, spleen and liver. The mesenteric arteries supply the intestines.

Venous blood from the stomach, pancreas, spleen and liver is collected together and routed through the liver via the *hepatic portal vein* (see Ch. 9). Blood from the remainder of the digestive tract (namely the oesophagus and above, and the rectum) escapes the hepatic filter and drains directly into the venous system. ③

Nerve supply

The digestive system is innervated almost entirely by autonomic nerves (see Ch. 3). The *vagus* (a parasympathetic nerve) innervates everything from the

oesophagus to the mid portion of the transverse colon. The remainder of the large intestine and the rectum is innervated by the *pelvic nerve*.

Sympathetic nerves innervating the system include the *splanchnic* and *mesenteric nerves*. It is important to remember that all these nerves, parasympathetic and sympathetic, contain sensory neurones as well as motoneurones. Indeed the majority of nerve fibres in the vagus nerve are sensory rather than motor.

DIGESTIVE TRACT

General structure

The digestive tract (oesophagus, stomach, and intestines) is basically a hollow muscular tube, lined on its inner surface by a layer of cells (*mucosal epithelium*) that, in the intestines, is specialised for absorption. Although the structure of the various parts of the digestive tract differs in specific details the basic form of the 'tube' is similar (Fig. 6.5).

The muscle in the wall of the tube is *smooth muscle* (see Ch. 22). It is mostly arranged in two layers, *circular* and *longitudinal*.

②
What is peritonitis?

③
How does hepatic portal blood differ in composition from other venous blood?

Figure 6.5
Basic structure of the wall of the digestive 'tube' (oesophagus, stomach and intestines).

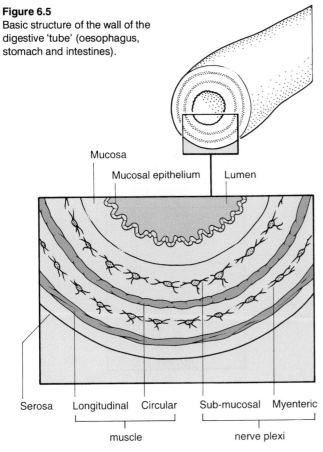

The inner lining of the tract facing the digestive contents in the lumen is the *mucosa*. The mucosa is richly supplied by blood vessels and includes nerve fibres and endocrine cells. It is covered by a layer of cells (*epithelium*) specialised for absorption or for secretion depending on their location.

The tract is covered on the outside by the *serosa*, a layer of connective tissue.

Enteric nervous system

There are two networks of nerve fibres in the wall of the gastrointestinal tract:

- submucosal plexus
- myenteric plexus.

(The plural of plexus is *plexi*.) These neural networks contain the cell bodies of *post-ganglionic parasympathetic nerve fibres* (see Ch. 3) plus the cell bodies of sensory neurones monitoring the state of the digestive tract and its contents, and many interneurones. The gastro-intestinal tract thus possesses its own nervous system (*enteric nervous system*), which is important in controlling the digestive process and can function independently of outside control. It is, however, influenced by the parasympathetic and sympathetic nerves terminating within or close to the plexi (see Ch. 3).

MOVEMENTS

The movement and mixing of food residues in the digestive tract and their eventual elimination from the body is largely brought about through the contraction of smooth muscle. Only at the top of the tract (mouth, pharynx, upper oesophagus) and at its bottom (external anal sphincter) is striated muscle involved. Smooth muscle differs in a number of ways from striated muscle (Table 6.1 and Ch. 22). These various properties enable:

- contractile tone to be maintained even in the absence of food
- activity to be increased and decreased as necessary
- the tract to distend to accommodate different volumes.

OESOPHAGUS

Structure and function

This thin-walled tube, joining the pharynx to the stomach (Fig. 6.6A & B), is composed of striated muscle at the top and smooth muscle at the bottom, with a transitional zone from one to the other in between. There are two sphincters, one at either end:

- upper oesophageal sphincter (crico-pharyngeal)
- lower oesophageal spincter (LOS or cardiac sphincter). ④

④
What is a sphincter?

Table 6.1 Differences between smooth muscle and striated muscle (see also Ch. 22)		
	Smooth muscle	*Striated muscle*
Cell structure	Small spindle shaped cells	Very long thin fibres
Excitation	Contracts spontaneously Excitation spreads from cell to cell	Contracts when excited by nerve impulses No communication between cells
Nervous control	Autonomic nerves	Somatic nerves
Hormonal control	Excites or inhibits contraction	Not involved in controlling contraction
Response to prolonged stretch	Adapts to new length	Does not adapt

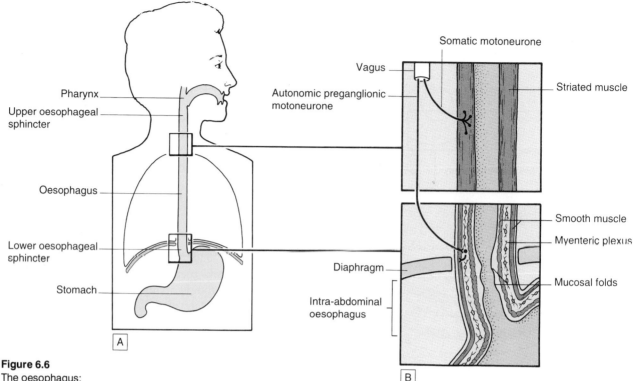

Figure 6.6
The oesophagus:
A Position in relation to other organs and structures
B Structure and innervation.

When food is swallowed, the upper oesophageal sphincter relaxes, and the food is propelled along the oesophagus by a wave of *peristalsis*. ⑤

Peristalsis

Peristalsis is a coordinated wave of contraction proceeding in an orderly direction from one part of the digestive

⑤
Which structure lying between the thorax and abdomen does the oesophagus penetrate?

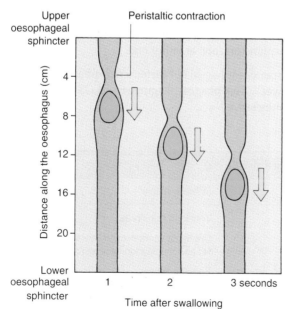

Figure 6.7
A wave of peristalsis in the oesophagus.

tract to the next (Fig. 6.7). In the oesophagus, the wave of contraction is controlled by nerve impulses in the vagus. Should any food particles remain in the oesophagus after the first wave of peristalsis, irritation of the mucosa by the particles evokes secondary waves of peristalsis that help to dislodge the food particles and sweep them into the stomach.

A wave of peristalsis is also evoked when liquids are swallowed, although, when a person is upright, gravity will carry the liquid down the oesophagus faster than the wave of contraction can. The act of swallowing (see Ch. 29) reflexly triggers the opening of the lower oesophageal sphincter so that the food propelled through the oesophagus enters the stomach.

Lower oesophageal sphincter

The lower oesophageal sphincter (Fig. 6.6B) plays an important role in resisting the regurgitation of stomach contents into the oesophagus (see Heartburn, p. 131). Several factors contribute to the action of the sphincter:

● sensitivity of the smooth muscle at the LOS
● mucosal folds
● intra-abdominal section of the oesophagus.

The bands of smooth muscle at the level of the sphincter are more sensitive to neurotransmitters and hormones than the muscle on either side. They are thus normally in a more contracted state but relax in response to specific reflexes and some hormones (see Heartburn, p. 131).

There are folds of mucosa at the site of the sphincter. These may provide some resistance to the backflow of stomach contents.

The last few centimetres of the oesophagus actually lie within the abdominal cavity. Thus, if abdominal pressure increases, as it does when you cough or lift a heavy object, this terminal section is compressed at the same time as pressure is exerted on the stomach. Consequently the stomach contents, though increased in pressure, are not forced into the oesophagus.

STOMACH

Structure and function
The stomach is divided into several parts (Fig. 6.8):

- fundus
- body
- pyloric antrum.

The fundus and body are relatively thin walled and exhibit little contractile activity. These two parts of the stomach serve as a distensible reservoir for ingested food. The muscle layers here relax when food is swallowed. This vagally mediated reflex is known as *receptive relaxation*. If this relaxation does not occur, a person feels full very quickly after just a few mouthfuls of food.

The walls of the pyloric antrum are thicker and more active. Strong waves of contraction occur here during the digestion of a meal, acting to churn and mix the food with gastric juices. Food passes from the stomach to the duodenum via the pyloric canal. The pyloric canal is encircled by a band of smooth muscle, the *pyloric sphincter*.

Mixing of food
When a meal is ingested, the sequence of events is as follows (Fig. 6.9). First the body and fundus distend as food is layered there. Then ripples of contraction, beginning at about the middle of the stomach, press the stomach contents towards the pyloric antrum and pyloric canal. These peristaltic waves of contraction, occurring about three times a minute, do not occlude

---

A patient who has had a *vagotomy* (transection of some or all vagal nerve fibres) for the treatment of gastric or duodenal ulcers may be able to cope with only small quantities of food at a time. This is because some of the nerve fibres controlling receptive relaxation may have been cut through as well as those influencing gastric secretion.

Q. How does a vagotomy help to treat gastric and duodenal ulcers?

Figure 6.8
View of the stomach, cut in half from top to bottom, showing its various regions.

Fundus

Body

Duodenum

Pyloric canal

Pyloric sphincter   **Pyloric antrum**

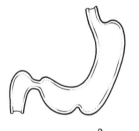

1. Empty stomach.

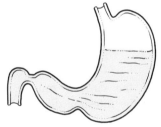

2. Distension of the body and fundus to accommodate ingested food.

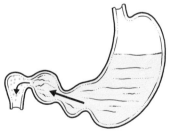

3. Peristaltic wave of contraction squeezes a little of the stomach contents towards the pyloric canal and duodenum.

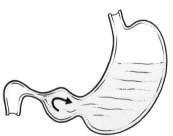

4. Pyloric sphincter and terminal antrum contracts. Stomach contents pushed back towards the body of the stomach.

5. Steps '3' and '4' repeat every 20 seconds.

Figure 6.9
How the stomach responds to the ingestion of a meal.

the stomach. As they approach the pyloric canal, they become more powerful and travel faster, and terminate in an abrupt closure of the canal itself. Thus, every 20 seconds or so, a small fraction of the stomach contents is nudged towards the pyloric canal.

Unless the mixture is very fluid, little is actually propelled into the small intestine. When the pyloric sphincter contracts abruptly, most of the mixture is turned back into the body of the stomach. Thus, solid materials are progressively reduced to a semifluid mixture known as *chyme*.

Emptying

About 6 to 10 ml of chyme are emptied into the intestine every minute. The main factor promoting strong peristaltic contractions is activity in the vagal nerve fibres supplying the antrum. If these are cut, as in a *vagotomy*, the rate of emptying of the stomach is reduced.

Under ordinary circumstances, the amount of chyme emptied per minute depends upon the nature (solid or fluid), and the quantity of the food ingested. Bigger and more fluid meals empty more quickly, whereas fatty meals empty relatively slowly (see p. 135).

SMALL INTESTINE

The pattern of contraction seen most often in the small intestine is *segmentation* rather than peristalsis. As a result chyme moves relatively slowly from one end of the intestine to the other.

Segmentation

Simultaneous contraction of the circular muscle at several discrete places along the intestine divides the intestine into a series of sacs (Fig. 6.10). A few moments later, this is followed by the simultaneous contraction of

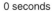
0 seconds

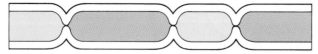

5 seconds later

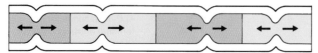

10 seconds later

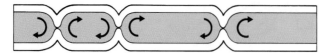

Figure 6.10
Segmentation contractions of the intestine, showing how the intestinal contents are mixed together.

muscle at a different set of places. The result is that chyme is shuttled backwards and forwards over a short distance and mixed well with the digestive secretions. The longitudinal muscle also regularly contracts and relaxes and massages the intestinal contents.

Peristalsis

Occasionally, local distension of the intestine provokes short bursts of peristalsis. The peristaltic contractions move the intestinal contents along but not very far. Their function is to even out the distribution of the contents and prevent any part of the intestines from becoming overdistended.

The rate at which chyme moves through the intestine is thus relatively slow. This is very important for the proper digestion and absorption of food substances.

Propulsion of contents

A small pressure difference exists between the upper and lower intestine caused by the slightly greater frequency of contractions in the duodenum (9/minute) as compared with those in the ileum (6/minute). It is this pressure difference that slowly moves the intestinal contents from one end of the small intestine to the other.

PARALYTIC ILEUS

The importance of peristaltic movement in the gastrointestinal tract, particularly in the small intestine, can be demonstrated by the condition of *paralytic ileus*. This condition is common after surgery where the gastrointestinal tract has been handled, and also as a result of prolonged anaesthesia for surgical procedures. It can also arise from abdominal conditions such as peritonitis. The precise cause, whether it is stimulation of the sympathetic nervous system or inhibition of the parasympathetic nervous system, is not known but the effect is the relaxation of the smooth muscle in the gastrointestinal tract.

The outcome of paralytic ileus is, in effect, the same as an intestinal obstruction. Gastrointestinal contents, either fluid or gas, cannot pass down the tract and the passage of flatus stops. If the condition is not recognised, the patient who is suffering from paralytic ileus will develop a very painful and distended abdomen, and the condition can also lead to fluid and electrolyte imbalance.

The condition usually resolves after 2 to 3 days and, during this time, it is necessary to prevent the patient from eating or drinking. This can be compensated by giving intravenous fluids and allowing the patient to have mouthwashes. Secretions will not cease during paralytic ileus and, in order to prevent gastric secretions from gathering in the small intestine, it is necessary to remove them by regular aspiration of the stomach contents. This is achieved by means of a tube (nasogastric tube) inserted via the nose into the stomach. The return of normal function in the gastrointestinal tract is indicated by the return of flatus and by an increase in bowel sounds, which can be heard by means of a stethoscope on the abdomen.

The first food residues reach the end of the ileum about 3 to 4 hours after their ingestion.

LARGE INTESTINE

Structure and function

The longitudinal muscle of the large intestine is gathered into three major strips (*taeniae coli*) (Fig. 6.11B). When they contract they gather up the wall of the intestine rather in the way that curtain-header tape gathers curtains. Because of this, and because the dominant pattern of contraction is again segmentation, the large intestine has the appearance of a series of sacs (*haustrations*) (Fig. 6.11B).

Food residues may remain in the colonic part of the large intestine for 2 to 3 days being shuttled backwards and forwards and massaged gently as water and salts are reabsorbed. When the diet is rich in fibre the

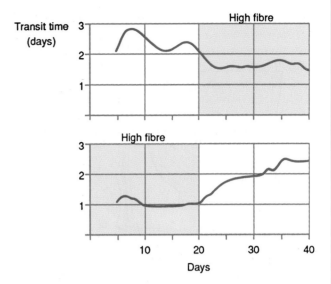

Figure 6.12
Effects of dietary fibre on transit time. (Transit time is the time taken for an ingested substance to pass right through the digestive system. Most of this time is taken up by the slow passage of material through the large intestine.) (Adapted from Cummings et al 1976.)

residues pass through the bowel much more quickly than when it is not (Fig. 6.12). The longer the residues remain in the colon the more compacted and hard they become. The *ascending colon* is the site at which most fluid absorption occurs. The *transverse* and *descending* parts of the *colon* are involved more with the storage and evacuation of faeces.

Mass peristalsis

Very occasionally, a wave of mass peristalsis propels food residues over a considerable distance. This occurs most often in the transverse and descending colon. Peristaltic waves are provoked by sudden stretch (caused by bulky food residues, for example) or reflexly in response to events elsewhere in the digestive tract. For example, the distension of the stomach by the ingestion of a meal reflexly promotes mass peristalsis (*gastrocolic reflex*; see p. 134).

Defaecation

The structures involved are illustrated in Figure 6.13. Normally the rectum is empty.

Sphincters

The exit to the rectum is guarded by two sphincters:

- the internal sphincter (smooth muscle; autonomic control – pelvic nerve)
- the external sphincter (striated muscle; somatic control – pudendal nerve).

In addition the pubo-rectalis muscle acts as a sling around the anal canal. Faeces are propelled into the rectum from the colon by a wave of mass peristalsis.

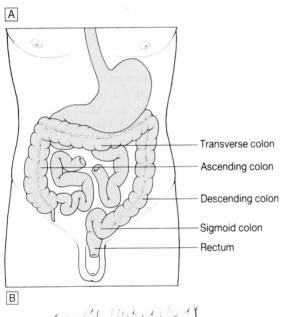

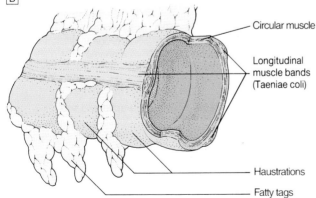

Figure 6.11
Large intestine:
A Arrangement and parts
B Structure.
(Reproduced from Rogers 1992 (Figs 5.17 & 5.18) by permission of the publishers.)

Transverse colon
Ascending colon
Descending colon
Sigmoid colon
Rectum

Circular muscle
Longitudinal muscle bands (Taeniae coli)
Haustrations
Fatty tags

⑥
Why is the urge to defaecate commonly experienced after a meal?

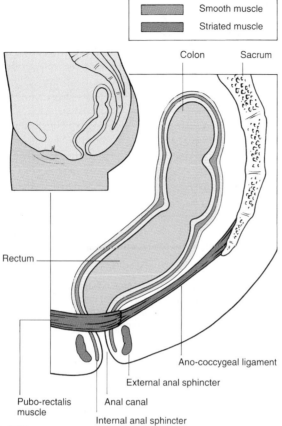

Figure 6.13
Structures involved in the storage and evacuation of faeces.

This stimulates sensory receptors in the wall of the rectum and in the anal canal that trigger a spinal reflex via the pelvic nerves, resulting in contraction of the rectum and relaxation of the internal anal sphincter. Simultaneously, the external sphincter reflexly contracts. Faeces are retained until, at an appropriate opportunity, defaecation is allowed by voluntary inhibition of contraction of the external sphincter and the pubo-rectalis muscle. ⑥

Passage of faeces through the anal canal reinforces the spinal reflex contracting the rectum and relaxing the internal sphincter. Evacuation is assisted by an increase in abdominal pressure caused by contraction of the abdominal muscle coupled with an increase in thoracic pressure (see Ch. 7). If defaecation is not permitted, the rectal receptors adapt to the continuing presence of faeces, the reflex responses abate, and the residues are returned to the colon, where more fluid is removed from them.

SECRETIONS

The secretions of the digestive system and their chief constituents are listed in Table 6.2. Altogether, 7 to 8 litres of secretion are formed per day. Most are absorbed and the constituents are recycled and re-used.

Table 6.2	Major constituents of the digestive secretions				
	Saliva	*Gastric juice*	*Pancreatic juice*	*Bile*	*Intestinal juice*
Water	√	√	√	√	√
Electrolytes (mmol/l)	Sodium (10–80) Potassium (10–40) Chloride (10–50) Hydrogen carbonate (10–40)	Hydrion (120) Chloride (140)	Sodium (150) Hydrogen carbonate (140)	Sodium (150) Chloride (100) Hydrogen carbonate (40)	Sodium Potassium Chloride Hydrogen carbonate } variable*
pH	6–8	1–2	8	7–8	7–8
Enzymes	Amylase	Pepsinogens Gastric lipase	Amylase Proteases Lipases Nucleases	None	Peptidases and disaccharidases from shed epithelial cells
Glycoproteins (mucus)	√	√	A little	A little	√
Other constituents		Intrinsic factor	Trypsin inhibitors	Bile salts	
Volume (ml/day)	1000	2500	1500	1000	1000
* Depends on specific site.					

SALIVA

Saliva is a mixture of secretions formed by three pairs of glands (*parotid, submandibular* and *sublingual*) (Fig. 6.14) together with a small number of cells scattered throughout the mouth.

Formation

The *acini* of the glands (Fig. 6.14B) consist of cells that secrete either the enzyme *amylase* or *mucus*, dissolved in a solution of salts, chiefly sodium chloride. The secretion produced by the acini (*primary secretion*) is modified in composition as it flows through the striated ducts. Sodium chloride is reabsorbed unaccompanied by water so that the fluid becomes progressively more dilute.

The concentration of sodium in saliva may be as low as 5 to 10 mmol/litre. This is much lower than plasma sodium concentration (140 mmol/litre). As flow rate increases, the concentration of sodium chloride in saliva gets closer to that in the plasma but never quite reaches it.

SALIVA AND PATIENT CARE

One of the functions of saliva is to moisten the mouth and, at the same time, to remove food particles. If food debris is allowed to accumulate in a dry mouth the decomposing food provides a good medium for the growth of organisms. The result may be painful sores and, possibly, inflammation of one or both of the parotid glands (*parotitis*). It is therefore important to ensure that the patient's mouth is kept clean and moist. This is particularly relevant for the highly dependent patient, the elderly patient and the pyrexial patient, all of whom may have a reduced flow of saliva due to some degree of dehydration.

The flow of saliva is controlled by the autonomic nervous system. The salivary glands are innervated by both parasympathetic and sympathetic nerves; impulses are received from the salivary centre in the medulla of the brain stem. Sensory messages are initiated by taste and pressure within the mouth, causing the parasympathetic nerves to stimulate the flow of saliva. The pressure can be from sources other than food, for example dental instruments (most people have experienced the need to swallow saliva as soon as the dentist starts work!) and the toddler dribbling copiously while sucking a dummy. Therefore, the action of a nurse cleaning the mouth of an unconscious patient may help to stimulate the flow of saliva as well as provide moisture in the form of a mouthwash.

Another function of saliva is to moisten food to facilitate swallowing. For some people, the smell, sight, or even thought of food can increase the flow of saliva; therefore the nurse has an important role at mealtimes in preparing patients to receive food. The present-day, plated meal system neither provides the patient with anticipatory smells nor the sight of food being served. However, the nurse should take time to make sure that the patient is comfortable and is aware that a meal is on the way, perhaps reminding him of his choice from the menu. Prompt help with eating should be offered before interest in the meal is lost.

The generalised increase in sympathetic activity associated with anxiety, fear and stress causes dryness of the mouth, often to such a degree that the person is unable to speak clearly, if at all. This has particular significance for patients who are being fasted prior to anaesthesia. The combination of fear and a certain amount of dehydration may cause a distressingly dry mouth. In addition to providing reassurance and mouthwashes the nurse should ensure that the patient is not fasted for an unnecessarily long period. When operations are postponed, the anaesthetist may agree to the patient being offered a bland drink.

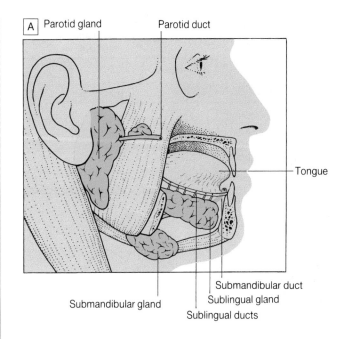

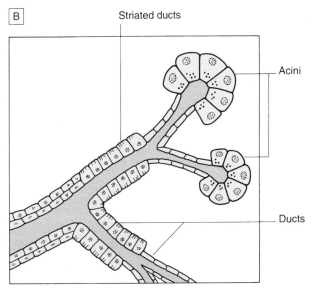

Figure 6.14
The salivary glands:
A Position
B Arrangement of cells in the parotid gland.
(Part A reproduced from Rogers 1992 (Fig. 28.10) by permission of the publishers.)

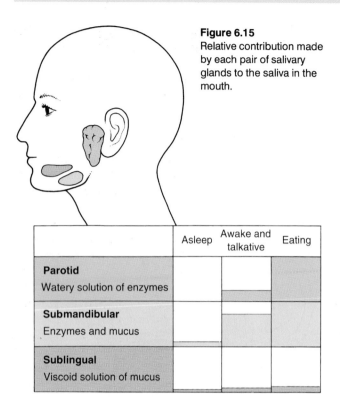

Figure 6.15
Relative contribution made by each pair of salivary glands to the saliva in the mouth.

	Asleep	Awake and talkative	Eating
Parotid Watery solution of enzymes			
Submandibular Enzymes and mucus			
Sublingual Viscoid solution of mucus			

A variety of other substances (such as plasma proteins, blood group substances and iodide) are also found in saliva in low concentration. Most diffuse into saliva from the blood.

Control

The salivary glands are innervated by parasympathetic and sympathetic nerves. The parasympathetic nerves are the most important in controlling secretion. Acetylcholine released when these nerve fibres are stimulated provokes a large increase in salivation.

The contribution made by each pair of glands to the saliva in our mouths varies during the day and night (Fig. 6.15). When we eat a meal it is the parotid glands that increase their secretion most of all.

> Drugs such as *atropine* and *hyoscine* that block the effect of acetylcholine on the salivary glands, and therefore reduce secretions, are used in premedication before intubation or inhalational anaesthesia. This reduces the danger of secretions trickling down into the trachea.

Figure 6.16
Structure of a gastric gland in the body of the stomach.

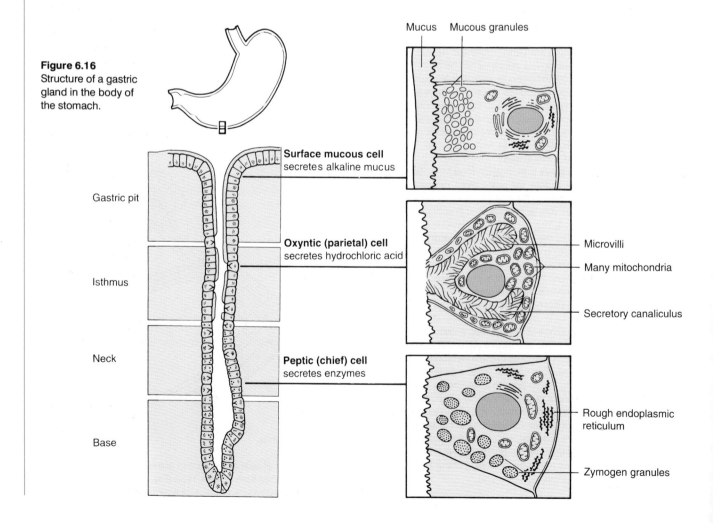

Mucus   Mucous granules

Surface mucous cell
secretes alkaline mucus

Gastric pit

Isthmus

Oxyntic (parietal) cell
secretes hydrochloric acid

Microvilli

Many mitochondria

Secretory canaliculus

Neck

Peptic (chief) cell
secretes enzymes

Rough endoplasmic reticulum

Base

Zymogen granules

GASTRIC JUICE

If the surface of the stomach is viewed through a gastro-scope it is seen to be pitted with numerous tiny openings. These are the openings of the tubular gastric glands (Fig. 6.16).

Formation

At least three different cell types can be identified in the glands, each of which produces a different secretion:

- *oxyntic (parietal) cells* (hydrochloric acid)
- *peptic (chief) cells* (digestive enzymes)
- *mucous cells* (alkaline mucus).

Oxyntic cells are found only in the glands of the body of the stomach. Peptic cells are found here in large numbers too, although some are present also in the fundus and the antrum. Thus acid secretion, and most enzyme secretion, is localised to the body of the stomach.

The alkaline mucus clings to the surface and protects the stomach itself against the potent digestive effects of acid and enzymes.

Control

The secretory activity of the cells is controlled both by the autonomic nervous system and by hormones (Table 6.3).

Enzyme secretion by the peptic cells is chiefly stimulated by vagal nerve fibres whereas acid secretion is most affected by hormonal stimulants such as *gastrin* (see p. 132) and *histamine*. The vagal nerve fibres do, however, have a small but important effect in that they sensitise the cells to the other stimulants.

Histamine is released locally from mast cells (see Ch. 4, p. 68). Its action on the stomach is blocked by a different class of *antihistamines* (H_2 receptor blockers) from those used in the relief of inflammatory responses

(see Ch. 15) such as the swelling caused by insect bites, and the symptoms of hay fever (H_1 receptor blockers).

The secretion of mucus is regulated by local hormones, such as prostaglandins (see Ch. 10), that are released in response to minor local injury of the mucosa.

PANCREATIC JUICE

The histological structure of the pancreas (Fig. 6.17) is similar in many respects to that of the salivary glands, as are some features of the secretory process.

Formation

Cells of the acini (*zymogen cells*) produce a secretion rich in enzymes (Table 6.4). All the different pancreatic enzymes are manufactured by the same cells. Like other digestive enzymes, they are secreted in an inactive form, and become activated within the digestive tract. One important activator is the protein-digesting (*proteolytic*) enzyme *trypsin*. Premature activation of pancreatic enzymes is resisted by the presence of *trypsin inhibitors* in pancreatic juice. ⑦

Centro-acinar cells and duct cells secrete an alkaline

---

⑦
Why are proteolytic enzymes stored in inactive forms?

> H_2 receptor blockers are used in the treatment of gastric and duodenal ulcers because they reduce the secretion of acid by the oxyntic cells.

Table 6.3   Factors stimulating gastric secretion

Stimulant	Site of action	
	Major	Minor
Acetylcholine (vagus)	Peptic cells	Oxyntic cells Mucous cells
Gastrin	Oxyntic cells	Peptic cells
Histamine	Oxyntic cells	—
Prostaglandins	Mucous cells	—

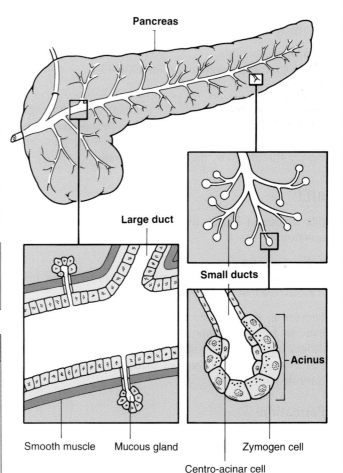

Figure 6.17
Arrangement of cells and tissues in the pancreas.

Table 6.4   Pancreatic enzymes: targets, names and activators

Targets	Enzymes	Activators
Proteins	Trypsinogen	Enteropeptidase*
	Chymotrypsinogen	
	Proelastase	
	Procarboxypeptidase A & B	Trypsin
Fats	Prophospholipase A$_2$	
	Pancreatic lipase	—
	Cholesterol ester hydrolase	—
Starch	Pancreatic amylase	Chloride
Nucleic acids	Ribonuclease	—
	Deoxyribonuclease	—

*Literally intestinal (entero) enzyme (ase) that breaks peptide bonds.

Table 6.5   Factors stimulating pancreatic secretion

Stimulant	Site of action	
	Major	Minor
Acetylcholine (vagus)	—	Zymogen cells
CCK-PZ	Zymogen cells	Ducts (small)
Secretin	Ducts (small) Centroacinar cells	—

fluid rich in sodium hydrogen carbonate but free of enzymes. This is added to the primary secretion formed by the zymogen cells.

Control

Acinar and duct cells differ in their sensitivity to the following neural and hormonal stimuli (Table 6.5):

- vagal stimulation
- cholecystokinin-pancreozymin (CCK-PZ)
- secretin.

The zymogen cells are chiefly stimulated by the vagal nerves and the hormone CCK-PZ, whereas the ducts, producing most of the fluid component of the juice, are mainly stimulated by the hormone secretin.

BILE

Bile is formed by the liver (see Ch. 9) and has a dual function. It is a:

- digestive secretion
- route of excretion for waste products (such as bilirubin; see Chs 4 and 15).

Because of its excretory function, bile is formed by the liver in large amounts all the time. In this respect it differs from other digestive secretions. Between meals, bile is diverted into the gall bladder where it is concentrated and stored.

Formation

Hepatocytes secrete the organic constituents of bile, dissolved in a solution consisting mainly of sodium chloride and sodium hydrogen carbonate (Fig. 6.18) (see Ch. 9). This primary secretion is, like pancreatic juice, added to by an alkaline secretion formed by the ducts within the liver, which are also stimulated by secretin.

Bile salts

Bile salts, sometimes referred to as *bile acids* (see Ch. 9 and Fig. 9.11), are organic molecules involved in the digestion and absorption of fat. They are manufactured in the liver from *cholesterol*. Only small amounts are synthesised each day because most of the bile salts used in digestion are absorbed from the small intestine (particularly the ileum), returned to the liver and resecreted in bile (an *enterohepatic circulation*) (Fig. 6.19).

Gall bladder

Although a little bile trickles into the duodenum all the time between meals, most of the bile formed by the liver flows into the gall bladder. When a meal is ingested the gall bladder contracts and concentrated bile is expelled into the duodenum.

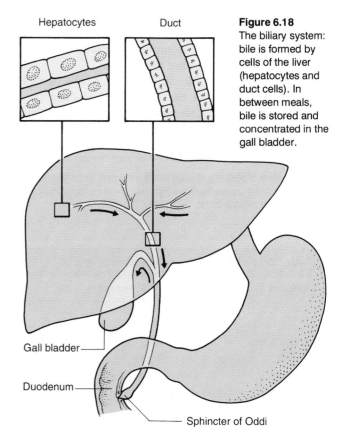

Figure 6.18
The biliary system: bile is formed by cells of the liver (hepatocytes and duct cells). In between meals, bile is stored and concentrated in the gall bladder.

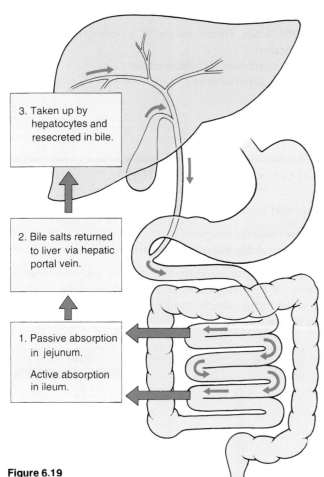

Figure 6.19
Enterohepatic circulation of bile salts.

Concentration of bile

Bile is concentrated in the gall bladder by the reabsorption of sodium chloride, sodium hydrogen carbonate and water. This may increase the concentration of the remaining constituents by about 10-fold (Table 6.6). Whereas hepatic bile is yellowish in colour due to the presence of *bilirubin*, gall bladder bile is much darker because it has been concentrated. Sometimes bile is greenish in colour because bilirubin is converted to *biliverdin*.

Table 6.6 Composition of bile (mmol/l)*		
	Hepatic	*Gall bladder*
Bile salts	20	200
Phospholipid	7	30
Cholesterol	3	7
Bilirubin glucuronide	0.4	4
Na$^+$	150	230
K$^+$	5	8
Cl$^-$	100	20
HCO$_3^-$	40	10
Ca^{2+}	1.5	3
* Average values.		

Contraction

The gall bladder distends as it fills with bile. The smooth muscle in its wall and in the ducts leading to the duodenum (*cystic duct* and *common bile duct*; Fig. 6.3) contracts rhythmically. Contractions are stimulated by the hormone CCK-PZ, which also relaxes the sphincter muscle at the end of the common bile duct (*sphincter of Oddi*; Fig. 6.18). These events are promoted by vagally mediated nervous reflexes.

INTESTINAL SECRETIONS

Intestinal secretions are not as easily measured and studied as the others because they are formed by numerous tiny glands and secretory cells throughout the intestinal tract.

Small intestine

The best characterised glands are the *glands of Brunner* in the upper duodenum (Fig. 6.20), which form a thick alkaline mucus. *Goblet cells* secreting mucus are found in

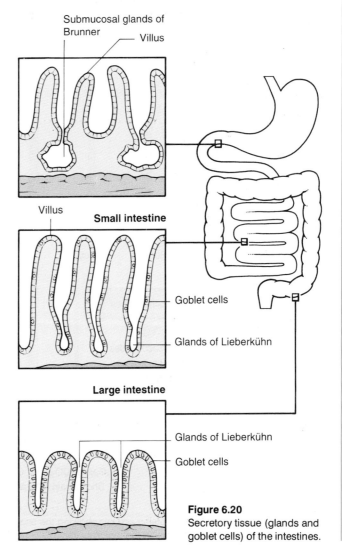

Figure 6.20
Secretory tissue (glands and goblet cells) of the intestines.

the epithelium throughout the rest of the small intestine. Cells in the *crypts (glands) of Lieberkühn* (Fig. 6.20) secrete a solution of sodium chloride, sodium hydrogen carbonate (sodium bicarbonate) and water. This secretion is stimulated by:

- bacterial toxins (such as cholera toxin)
- neurotransmitters (such as vasoactive polypeptide – VIP)
- hormones (such as prostaglandins).

Juice collected from the intestine contains some digestive enzymes, *peptidases* and *disaccharidases*, derived from the break-up of epithelial cells.

Large intestine

Glands secreting mucus, salts and water are also found in the large intestine. Potassium is secreted rather than sodium. Consequently significant losses of potassium can occur in diarrhoea. Factors stimulating colonic secretion include:

- bile acids
- fatty acids (from bacterial metabolism of carbohydrates)
- local hormones (prostaglandins)
- enteric nerve activity.

DIGESTION OF FOOD

Ingested foods are broken down by a combination of:

- mechanical disruption
- chemical digestion aided by enzymes.

The chief constituents of food, the enzymes responsible for their digestion, and the nature of the products formed in the mouth, stomach and intestines are shown in Figure 6.21.

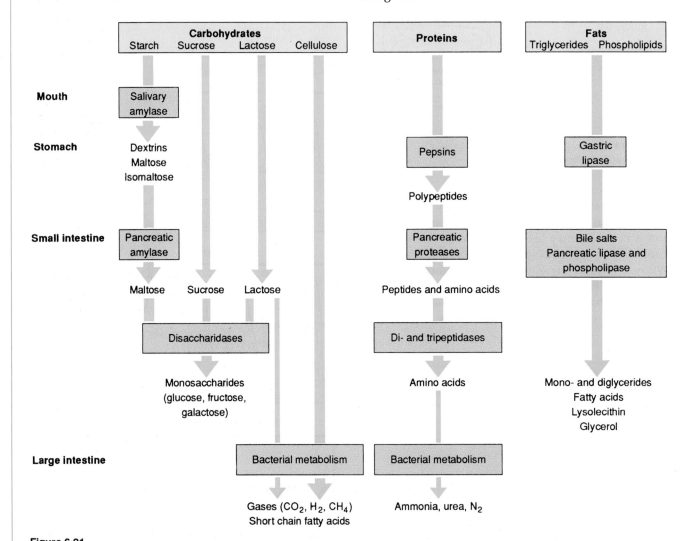

Figure 6.21
The digestion of carbohydrates, proteins and fats showing the enzymes and digestive agents involved (purple background) and the products formed at different sites within the digestive tract.

MOUTH

Disruption of food begins in the mouth. By biting and chewing, food is moulded into malleable, well lubricated portions (single portion = *bolus*), which can be swallowed. Salivary amylase is mixed into the bolus and begins the digestion of starch. ⑧

STOMACH

Amylase continues to work in the stomach despite the secretion of gastric acid which inactivates the enzyme. This is because the mixing of food with gastric juice occurs chiefly in the antrum. Most of an ingested meal collects first in the distensible body of the stomach (see Fig. 6.9) and is stored there while small amounts are steadily supplied to the antral 'mixer'. The combined action of acid, pepsins and the mixing movements gently disrupts the plant and/or animal tissues and cells in the food and creates a partially digested suspension (*chyme*) of products that is slowly fed into the duodenum.

SMALL INTESTINE

Most chemical digestion of food occurs in the small intestine. Pancreatic juice is the most important of all the digestive secretions. Its galaxy of digestive enzymes can attack carbohydrates, proteins, fats and nucleotides and reduce them to much smaller subunits. ⑨

LACTOSE INTOLERANCE

Lactose is the disaccharide (composed of glucose and galactose) that is contained in milk. Before being absorbed from the small intestine it has to be broken down into its constituent monosaccharides by the action of an enzyme called lactase. This enzyme, which is present in childhood, virtually disappears in adulthood in most of the world's population, resulting in lactose intolerance (Passmore & Eastwood 1986). (See also Ch. 14.) Consequently, if milk is drunk, the lactose is not digested and remains unabsorbed in the small intestine. The effects of this are retention of water in the small intestine due to an osmotic effect exerted by the disaccharide and, when the lactose reaches the large intestine, fermentation by commensal bacteria. The retention of water in the gastrointestinal tract causes diarrhoea – the production of watery faeces. Fermentation results in the production of abnormally high levels of gas in the large intestine, which leads to distension and pain.

The outcome of lactose intolerance for the individual can range from mild inconvenience to extreme fluid and electrolyte imbalance. Dietary modification, by either cutting down on dairy products or omitting them altogether, is the only way in which the effects of this complaint can be alleviated. In some people, the enzyme lactase persists into adulthood. These are ethnic groups, including most Caucasians (e.g. North Europeans), whose ancestors were dairy farmers.

Carbohydrates and proteins

The digestion of carbohydrates and proteins is completed on the surface of the intestinal epithelial cells where enzymes (*peptidases* and *disaccharidases*) generate monosaccharides and amino acids from the smaller peptides and sugars.

Fats

Fats present a special digestive problem because they are not very soluble in water and tend to separate out in a mixture, as oil and vinegar do when they are left to stand. This problem is solved by the bile acids. They:

* emulsify fat
* form micelles.

Emulsification

Bile acids are partly water loving (*hydrophilic*) and partly fat loving (*lipophilic*) (see Ch. 2). They can thus mix in with fat (see Ch. 2) and allow a stable suspension (*emulsion*) of tiny fat droplets to be formed. One immediate benefit of this is that it provides a larger surface area of fat that is open to attack by *pancreatic lipase* (Fig. 6.22).

Micelle formation

Bile acids also associate with the individual molecules generated by the action of lipase (mono- and diglycerides, and fatty acids) and form tiny aggregates of these products (*micelles*) (see Ch. 2 and Fig. 2.2B), which are perfectly stable in a watery environment. Other fatty molecules, such as cholesterol and the fat-soluble vitamins, are also incorporated into the micelles.

Undigested residues

Some organic dietary constituents (*dietary fibre*) are resistant to chemical digestion. This applies to a variety of non-starch polysaccharides, the chief of which is cellulose. Cellulose consists entirely of glucose subunits, but these are joined together by chemical linkages that are resistant to attack by our digestive enzymes. Undigested residues and other unabsorbed constituents pass on into the large intestine.

LARGE INTESTINE

There are no digestive enzymes in the large intestine, but there is a large population of bacteria (400–4000 different types) that can metabolise food residues and other substances in a variety of ways (Table 6.7).

Bacterial activity

The products of bacterial metabolism depend upon the types of bacteria present, which vary from one individual to another. Total numbers of bacteria vary considerably. They multiply if the supply of food residues from the small intestine increases. This happens if the amount

⑧ How do the articulations of the tempero-mandibular joint facilitate chewing?

⑨ Pancreatic juices leak out into surrounding tissues when the pancreas is injured. What do you think will be the consequence of this?

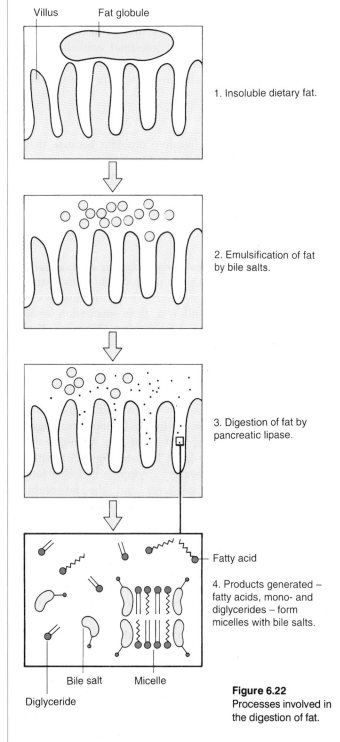

Villus   Fat globule

1. Insoluble dietary fat.

2. Emulsification of fat by bile salts.

3. Digestion of fat by pancreatic lipase.

Fatty acid

4. Products generated – fatty acids, mono- and diglycerides – form micelles with bile salts.

Bile salt   Micelle

Diglyceride

Figure 6.22
Processes involved in the digestion of fat.

Table 6.7	Metabolic activities of colonic bacteria
Target	*Products*
Proteins	Ammonia (NH_3) Urea Nitrogen (N_2)
Dietary fibre	Short chain fatty acids CO_2 Methane (CH_4) H_2
Bile salts (primary)	Secondary bile salts (see Ch. 9)
Bilirubin glucuronide	Stercobilinogen

CONSTIPATION AND LAXATIVES

Normal bowel habit is hard to define since the frequency with which people defaecate is an individual phenomenon. When defaecation takes place less frequently than an individual thinks is normal (constipation) that person will often employ laxatives in order to achieve regular defaecation. Laxatives can be bought across the counter in pharmacies or they can be prescribed by a physician. Predisposing factors to constipation can include a poor diet that is low in fibre (indigestible material largely derived from plants), low fluid intake and lack of exercise. There may also be psychological factors.

Laxatives work in several ways. Some are designed to increase the bulk of faeces (e.g. lactulose) by increasing the water that is retained in the large intestine. This also has the effect of softening the faeces. The laxative effect is brought about by the increased bulk of faeces in the large intestine stimulating defaecation, and their softer consistency making it easier to defaecate.

Other preparations directly stimulate the smooth muscle of the gastrointestinal tract, and these are called the stimulant laxatives (e.g. bisacodyl). They can be administered orally, as tablets, or rectally, in the form of a suppository. Glycerine, which softens faeces in the rectum, is also administered rectally in the form of a suppository.

Enemas are administered rectally and contain fluids that stimulate the rectum (e.g. microlette), or stimulate the rectum and also increase the water content of the faeces within it by an osmotic effect (e.g. phosphate enema).

Laxatives can become habit forming, especially if they are used indiscriminately and, for this reason, constipation is best avoided. Attention to diet and exercise, and adequate fluid intake are usually sufficient to maintain proper bowel function.

of fibre in the diet is increased, or if proteins and carbohydrates are incompletely digested in the small intestine because of an enzyme deficiency, for example lactase. Bacterial numbers are reduced by antibiotics. Antibiotic treatment consequently alters the kinds and amounts of products generated. ⑩

Faeces

Faeces consist largely of bacteria (60% of faecal solids). Only a small proportion is actually undigested food residues. The volume of faeces produced daily depends on diet, activity and bowel habits.

ABSORPTION

The epithelium lining the inside of the digestive tract separates the contents of the gut from the interstitial

⑩
Does antibiotic treatment have any effect on bowel motions? If so, what different explanations can you think of?

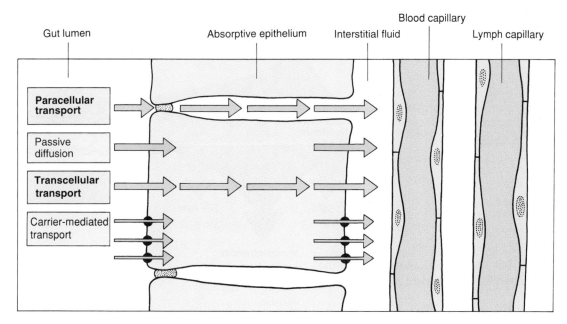

Figure 6.23
Basic structure of the absorptive epithelium and ways in which substances get across it to enter blood and lymph capillaries.

fluid that is in communication with the blood and lymph capillaries of the mucosa (Fig. 6.23). Substances cross the epithelium in a variety of ways: some pass through the cells (*transcellularly*); others pass through the junctions between the cells (*paracellularly*). Some simply diffuse across; others are transported across the epithelial cell membranes by carrier proteins.

Most absorption occurs in the small intestine (Fig. 6.24). A small quantity of fatty substances, water and salts normally pass on into the large intestine, where most of the remaining water and salts are absorbed.

HOW SUBSTANCES ARE ABSORBED

Substances cross the epithelium by:

- passive diffusion
- carrier-mediated transport
- endocytosis and exocytosis.

Passive diffusion

If the concentration of a substance is higher within the gut lumen than it is in the fluids on the other side of the epithelial barrier, absorption will occur by passive diffusion (see Ch. 3) provided the substance can get across the barrier.

However, the epithelium is normally impermeable to all molecules except those that are:

- very small and water soluble
- fat soluble.

Small water-soluble molecules pass through the junctions between cells (*paracellularly*), and through pores in

> **INFLAMMATORY BOWEL DISORDERS**
>
> *Crohn's disease* and *ulcerative colitis* are names for inflammatory bowel disorders, of which there are several. The distinction between these conditions is not entirely clear and the cause of such disorders is not known either. At the very least, there may be an element of autoimmunity (see Ch. 15), which leads to inflammation at various sites in the small and large intestines and affects the mucosa, submucosa and the muscle layers of the gastrointestinal tract. The person suffering from an inflammatory bowel disorder will experience recurrent bouts of diarrhoea and concomitant weight loss. These disorders are chronic and occur mainly in young Caucasians.
>
> Inflammatory bowel disorders cannot be cured, but treatment of symptoms is possible. Evidence of infection can be treated with antibiotics, diarrhoea can be alleviated with codeine phosphate, which reduces gastric motility, and the inflammation can be treated with steroids administered either orally or rectally. In severe cases it is necessary to hospitalise patients in order to ensure that they get adequate rest, privacy and diet. The chronic diarrhoea has consequences for the perianal region, which can become painful and excoriated. In severe cases it is necessary to intervene surgically in order to excise affected parts of bowel or to form an ileostomy. In any of the above cases, the main support required by patients with inflammatory bowel disorders is psychological – they feel embarrassed by the effects of the condition (diarrhoea) and they worry about the consequences.

the membranes of the epithelial cells, but cannot easily penetrate the lipid part of cell membranes (see Ch. 2).

However, fatty substances, such as fatty acids, pass through the lipid layers of the cell membranes with relative ease. Consequently large quantities of fat are

Figure 6.24
Major sites of absorption of different components of the diet and the digestive secretions.

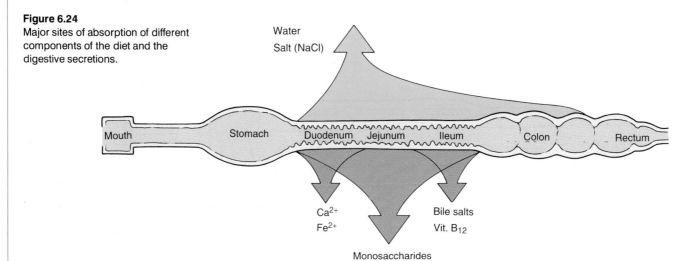

Water
Salt (NaCl)

Mouth   Stomach   Duodenum   Jejunum   Ileum   Colon   Rectum

Ca^{2+}
Fe^{2+}

Bile salts
Vit. B_{12}

Monosaccharides
Amino acids
Fats
Vitamins
K^+, HCO_3^-

absorbed passively, but only small amounts of amino acids and monosaccharides are absorbed in this way.

Carrier-mediated transport

Selected water-soluble substances, such as glucose, amino acids and calcium, that cannot cross the epithelium easily by diffusion because they are too large are assisted in their passage by *carrier proteins*.

Each carrier protein is able to link with only a limited group of molecules. For example, the carrier protein that transports glucose can transport the similar monosaccharide galactose, but cannot transport amino acids or calcium. There are several forms of carrier-mediated transport (Fig. 6.25):

- facilitated diffusion
- co-transport
- active transport.

Facilitated diffusion

When the movement of the carrier across the membrane occurs entirely passively, driven by the difference in concentration of the transported substance, such as glucose, the process is termed *facilitated diffusion*.

Co-transport

If two or more different substances bind to the same carrier, but at different sites, and are transported across the membrane together the process is termed *co-transport*. For example one of the carriers that transports glucose also carries sodium. In fact sodium influences the ability of the carrier to bind to glucose. When sodium is abundant, as it is in the intestinal contents within the gut lumen, the carrier binds glucose avidly. However, when sodium is scarce, as it is inside cells (see Ch. 2), glucose is not bound as firmly. In this way the uptake of glucose into intestinal epithelial cells is normally favoured by the composition of the intestinal contents, and the release of glucose inside the epithelial cells is favoured by the low intracellular sodium concentration. This particular form of transport is termed *sodium dependent*.

Active transport

If movement of the carrier requires the input of energy the process is termed *active transport*. ATP manufactured by cell mitochondria (see Chs 2 and 11) is usually used to power the movement of the carrier.

This form of transport moves substances 'uphill' against their natural tendency for passive diffusion. It is therefore able to create and sustain a difference in concentration, such as that of sodium, inside and outside cells.

The commonest example of this type of carrier-mediated transport is the *sodium–potassium pump*, which evicts sodium from cells, and builds up potassium inside them. This pump is present in all cells including those of the intestinal epithelium. In the intestinal epithelium it is located on the sides of the cell that face the interstitial fluid (*baso-lateral membrane*) and carries sodium from the cell into the interstitial fluid.

Endocytosis and exocytosis

In endocytosis, a small part of the cell membrane becomes invaginated, forming a vesicle that is drawn into the cytoplasm (see Fig. 2.4, Ch. 2). Fluid and/or particles can be engulfed in this way. Exocytosis is the process in reverse: an intracellular vesicle fusing with the cell membrane and releasing its contents.

SMALL INTESTINE

Several distinctive features make the small intestine the most important site of absorption:

- surface area available for absorption
- presence of many types of carrier proteins
- permeability of the epithelium to salts and water.

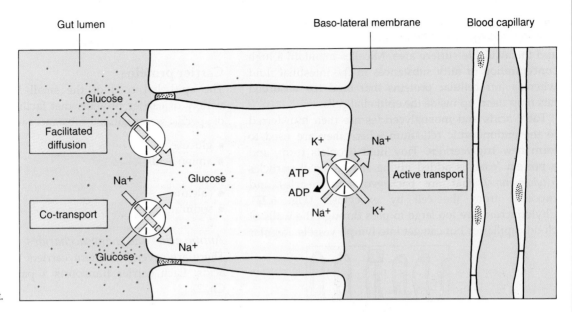

Figure 6.25
Three different forms of carrier-mediated transport.

Surface area

The surface area is very large because of numerous folds and *villi* (Fig. 6.26). This is very important for the absorption of fat. If the surface area is reduced through disease (coeliac disease), or surgery (removal of some bowel) not as much fat can be absorbed, and this results in *steatorrhoea* (fatty stools). ⑪

Concentration	Sodium	Glucose
High		
Low		

⑪
How would you recognise fatty stools?

Fat absorption

Monoglycerides, fatty acids and fat-soluble vitamins enter the epithelial cells by passive diffusion. Their rate

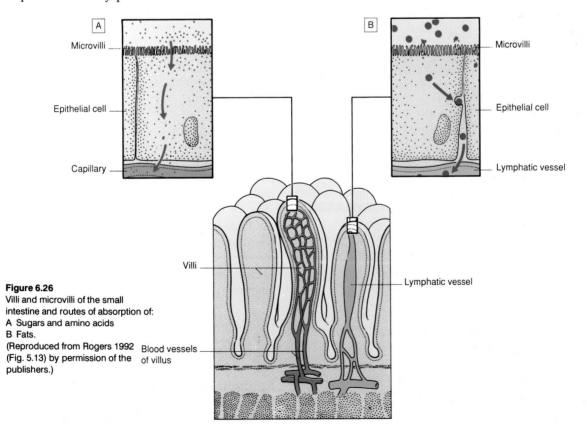

Figure 6.26
Villi and microvilli of the small intestine and routes of absorption of:
A Sugars and amino acids
B Fats.
(Reproduced from Rogers 1992 (Fig. 5.13) by permission of the publishers.)

of uptake depends on the difference in concentration of fatty substances on either side of the cell membrane and the available surface area. Micelles maintain a high concentration of fatty substances in the intestinal fluid whereas intracellular proteins that bind the absorbed fats mop them up inside the epithelial cells.

Fatty acids and monoglycerides are then transferred to the endoplasmic reticulum where they are used to form new triglycerides. Tiny lipid droplets form, and a protein 'coat' is added giving rise to small particles (*chylomicrons*) that are packaged into vesicles and exported from the cell by exocytosis (Fig. 6.27). Chylomicrons are too large to pass through the walls of blood capillaries but can get into lymph vessels. Regular

contractions of the villi help to 'milk' the lymphatics so that lymph is driven towards the larger vessels.

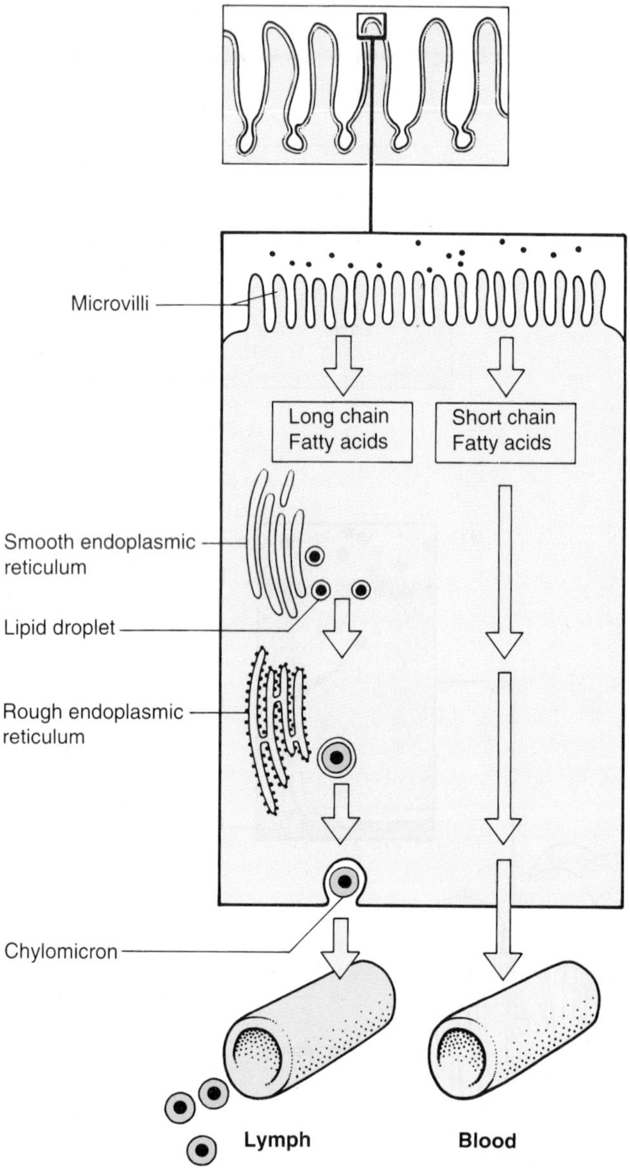

Carrier proteins

The epithelial cells of the small intestine possess a variety of carrier proteins that facilitate the absorption of specific water-soluble substances including:

- glucose
- amino acids
- iron
- calcium
- sodium.

Amino acids and monosaccharides

There are several different carriers transporting amino acids. Each carrier transports a particular group (see Ch. 2):

- acidic
- basic
- neutral.

If one of the carriers is absent, due to a genetic defect, the absorption of some but not all amino acids is therefore reduced.

Some absorption of monosaccharides and amino acids occurs by sodium dependent co-transport.

> Oral glucose is useful in the treatment of toxin-induced diarrhoea as it promotes the absorption of sodium by sodium dependent glucose transport, and the absorption of solutes like these promotes the absorption of water.

Carrier proteins for di- and tripeptides also exist. Complete digestion of proteins to amino acids is therefore not essential.

Calcium and iron

Calcium and iron are most easily absorbed in the upper small intestine. The intestinal contents are slightly more acid here than further down and this helps to dissolve the iron and calcium in the diet and make it more available for absorption. However, both of these elements can form insoluble complexes with other constituents of the diet, such as phytic acid, present in unrefined cereals, and phosphates. Both hinder the absorption of calcium and iron if they are present in the diet in large amounts. ⑫

Other substances

Carrier systems are also involved in the absorption of sodium, chloride, hydrogen carbonate, and bile salts.

Epithelial permeability

The intestinal epithelium is more permeable to the passive diffusion of water and salts than any other epithelia

⑫
What advice might you give to a patient taking iron supplements, and why?

Figure 6.27
The absorption of fat by intestinal epithelial cells. Fat is absorbed by diffusion, and most is packaged by the cells as protein-coated lipid droplets (chylomicrons). Chylomicrons are extruded from the cells by exocytosis and carried away in the lymph.

Labels on figure: Microvilli; Long chain Fatty acids; Short chain Fatty acids; Smooth endoplasmic reticulum; Lipid droplet; Rough endoplasmic reticulum; Chylomicron; Lymph; Blood

Figure 6.28
Consequences of food being broken down too rapidly in the intestine.

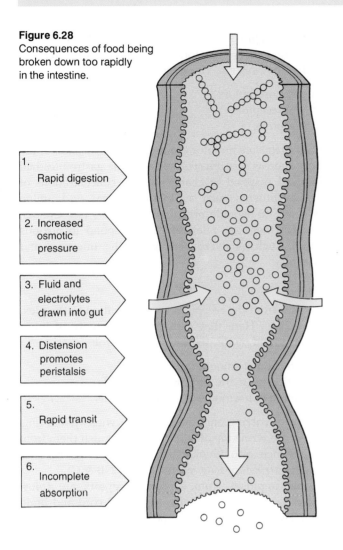

1. Rapid digestion

2. Increased osmotic pressure

3. Fluid and electrolytes drawn into gut

4. Distension promotes peristalsis

5. Rapid transit

6. Incomplete absorption

INTESTINAL STOMAS

Any artificial opening between a hollow organ and the surface of the skin is described as a *stoma*. A stoma of the small intestine is called an *ileostomy* and a stoma of the large intestine is called a *colostomy*. Intestinal stomas are necessary for several reasons, such as obstruction of the intestine (cancer), damage (gunshot wound) and in some inflammatory bowel diseases. Stomas can be either temporary or permanent but in either case it is necessary, for the duration of the stoma, to collect the contents of the intestine outside the body at the surface of the skin. For this purpose, specialised bags have been developed and specialist nursing advice is available to help people, and their families, adjust to having this kind of surgical procedure.

The intestinal stomas present their own particular complications. A colostomy is probably easier to manage than an ileostomy. A colostomy bag collects formed faecal material and it is sometimes possible for people with colostomies to exert some control over the expulsion of faeces. A major problem, however, is odour from the colostomy and people need to become proficient at fitting colostomy bags securely.

In contrast, the product of an ileostomy is much less formed because much less water has been absorbed from the contents of the small intestine than from material in the large intestine. The contents of the small intestine still contain active proteolytic enzymes and these can harm the skin if ileostomy bags are not fitted securely and proper skin hygiene is not carried out. It is also the case that a person with an ileostomy will lose a greater amount of fluid and electrolytes than normal and this needs to be compensated for in the diet.

Dietary changes may be required of people who have intestinal stomas. It is necessary to avoid food, according to individual experience, that will cause diarrhoea as this can lead to severe fluid loss and difficulty in managing the stoma.

in the digestive system, and the duodenum is the most permeable part of all. Water is absorbed always by osmosis, secondary usually to the absorption of solutes.

Duodenum

Water and salts diffuse relatively easily in either direction across the duodenal epithelium. This means that water and salts can be drawn into the digestive tract or be absorbed from it depending upon the concentration gradients.

If food is broken down too rapidly and many molecules of glucose and amino acids are suddenly generated from polysaccharides and polypeptides, the osmotic pressure of the intestinal contents may exceed that of the plasma and interstitial fluid, and water will be drawn into the digestive tract from the blood (Fig. 6.28). This can happen if the stomach empties too quickly because of disordered function after some forms of surgery. If a lot of fluid is suddenly drawn out of the body fluids into the digestive tract, blood volume and blood pressure fall and the patient feels faint (*dumping syndrome*).

Water absorption

The absorption of water is always a passive process driven by osmosis, secondary usually to the absorption of amino acids, glucose and salts. If you drink water by itself the difference in osmotic pressure between it and the interstitial fluid guarantees its absorption.

Water-soluble substances that are not absorbed can create an opposing osmotic gradient restricting water absorption. This can happen if there is a defect in digestion (such as lactase deficiency) so that digestion products (in this case the disaccharide lactose) remain unabsorbed, or if the epithelium lacks the ability or capacity to absorb all the solutes presented to it, as is the case with a large dose of magnesium sulphate (*Epsom salts*). In both cases the result is diarrhoea.

LARGE INTESTINE

Sodium is absorbed in the colon by active transport, followed by chloride and water. In this way the concentration of sodium in faecal fluid is reduced to very low amounts and losses of this important ion are minimised (see Ch. 13).

Absorption of other substances occurs simply by passive diffusion depending on how easily the substance can penetrate the epithelium. Water-soluble substances do not diffuse across at all easily, whereas those that have some lipid solubility, such as some products of bacterial metabolism (fatty acids, ammonia and secondary bile acids; Table 6.7), can do so. Usually the amounts absorbed are quite small.

> Substances administered rectally in the form of suppositories may be absorbed passively provided they have some lipid solubility.

OTHER SITES OF ABSORPTION

In the remainder of the tract, namely the mouth and stomach, there are no specialised forms of transport, but small amounts of various substances can be absorbed by passive diffusion. For example, the drug glyceryl trinitrate (used for the rapid relief of angina) is absorbed in the mouth from tablets placed under the tongue, and water and alcohol are absorbed in the stomach.

CONTROL AND COORDINATION OF ACTIVITY

For food to be efficiently digested and absorbed the activities of the several parts of the digestive system need to be controlled. Control is exercised by:

- the nervous system
- gastrointestinal hormones.

These systems regulate the digestive process and co-ordinate activity in different parts of the digestive tract. They also regulate activity between meals and influence the growth and renewal of the tract as a whole.

MECHANISMS

Nervous system
The somatic nervous system plays only a small part in control. It's activites are limited to the control of the muscles involved in chewing and swallowing (Ch. 29), and the control of the external anal sphincter. The autonomic nervous system controls salivary secretion and is involved in the control of all of the rest of the digestive system, from the smooth muscle of the oesophagus to the internal anal sphincter.

Sensory receptors
There are sensory receptors of various kinds throughout the digestive system. These include:

- mechanoreceptors
- chemoreceptors
- nociceptors.

Mechanoreceptors monitor the degree of distension of the tract, whereas *chemoreceptors* sample the gastrointestinal fluid and respond to changes in the concentrations of key constituents such as hydrogen ions and amino acids, and to osmotic pressure. *Nociceptors* (see Ch. 32), of which there are relatively few, respond to noxious stimuli, such as overdistension of the intestine, and ischaemia.

Reflexes
Impulses from the receptors are transmitted to the plexi (Fig. 6.29A). Here they influence the activity of inter-neurones, and motor neurones that control:

- contraction of smooth muscle
- secretion of gastric and intestinal glands
- secretion of hormones by endocrine cells.

Reflexes involving only the enteric nervous system (Fig. 6.29A), are termed *local reflexes* to distinguish them from those which also involve other parts of the nervous system (*extrinsic* or *long reflexes*) (Fig. 6.29B & C).

Some impulses from sensory receptors are transmitted to abdominal ganglia, the spinal cord and brain stem. These impulses are responsible for eliciting more complex reflex responses via parasympathetic and sympathetic nerve fibres (see Ch. 3). For example, distension of the stomach reflexly excites pancreatic secretion and gall bladder contraction as well as stimulating gastric activity.

Some impulses are transmitted to the cerebral cortex (see Ch. 23) and create the limited awareness we have of our internal state, such as feeling 'full up' or 'bloated'.

Neurotransmitters
Many different neurotransmitters have now been identified within the enteric nervous system. Some are listed in Table 6.8. Some of these substances, such as

Table 6.8 Neurotransmitters of the enteric nervous system
Acetylcholine
Noradrenaline
Serotonin (5-hydroxytryptamine) (5-HT)
Vasoactive intestinal polypeptide (VIP)
Substance P
Somatostatin
Enkephalins
Gastrin releasing peptide (GRP)
Neurotensin

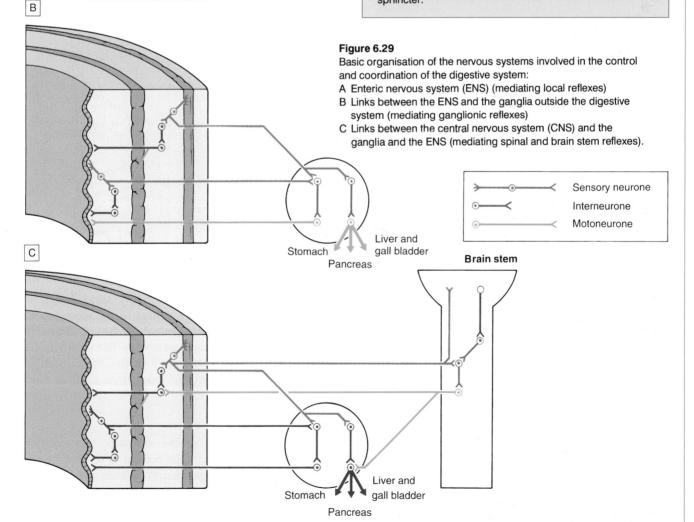

Figure 6.29
Basic organisation of the nervous systems involved in the control and coordination of the digestive system:
A Enteric nervous system (ENS) (mediating local reflexes)
B Links between the ENS and the ganglia outside the digestive system (mediating ganglionic reflexes)
C Links between the central nervous system (CNS) and the ganglia and the ENS (mediating spinal and brain stem reflexes).

Table 6.9 Gastrointestinal hormones	
Name(s)	*Major actions*
Gastrin	Stimulates gastric secretion
Cholecystokinin-pancreozymin (CCK-PZ)	Stimulates pancreatic enzyme secretion Contracts the gall bladder
Secretin	Stimulates pancreatic secretion
Gastric inhibitory polypeptide (GIP)	Inhibits gastric activity Promotes release of insulin by the pancreas
Motilin	Stimulates intestinal activity
Neurotensin	Inhibits gastrointestinal motility

Table 6.10 Chief locations of endocrine cells in the gastrointestinal tract	
Location	*Hormones secreted*
Stomach (antrum)	Gastrin
Upper small intestine	CCK-PZ Secretin GIP Motilin
Lower small intestine	Neurotensin

substance P, have also been found in endocrine cells of the digestive tract, and may in some circumstances be referred to as hormones if they are released into the bloodstream in appreciable amounts (see Chs 3 and 10).

Hormones

Many gastrointestinal hormones are also involved in the control of digestive function (Table 6.9). The chief locations of the endocrine cells that secrete them are listed in Table 6.10. Occasionally in disease, tumour cells secreting one of these hormones may be found elsewhere in the digestive system, such as a *gastrinoma* in the pancreas.

The secretion of hormones is regulated by:

- chemical conditions within the digestive tract
- nervous reflexes
- other hormones.

REGULATION OF DIGESTION

The efficient digestion of a meal depends upon:

- the readiness of the digestive system to receive food
- optimal composition of the gastric and intestinal contents for digestion and absorption
- a transit rate which maximises absorption and minimises waste.

Preliminary events

When food is smelt, ingested, chewed and swallowed, chemoreceptors (*taste buds* in the mouth and *olfactory receptors* in the nose) and mechanoreceptors are stimulated. As well as exciting salivary secretion many other parts of the digestive system are excited too via the vagus nerve (Fig. 6.30), including:

- stomach
- pancreas
- gall bladder.

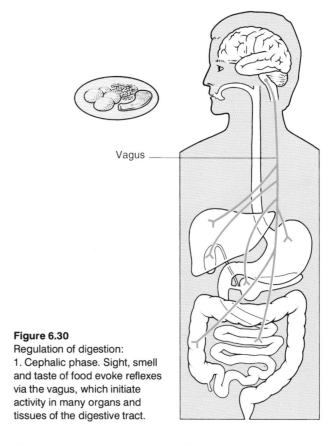

Vagus

Figure 6.30
Regulation of digestion:
1. Cephalic phase. Sight, smell and taste of food evoke reflexes via the vagus, which initiate activity in many organs and tissues of the digestive tract.

The increase in activity is relatively small but it is important in sensitising the system to the more potent stimuli that follow. This initial phase of digestive activity is termed *cephalic* because the initiating stimuli all arise from sensory receptors in the head. In some but not all people, even the thought or sight of food is an effective stimulus. ⑬

Stomach

As food accumulates in the stomach, the stomach distends and the gastric juice present is diluted by the food. These events trigger neural reflexes and hormone secretion (Fig. 6.31) which:

- promote gastric activity
- control gastric acidity (*pH*)
- alert organs downstream to the arrival of food.

⑬
How appetising is the food served to patients in your hospital? Does it matter?

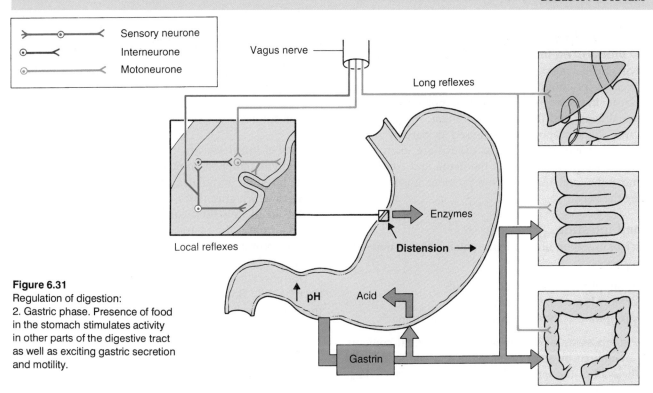

Sensory neurone	
Interneurone	
Motoneurone	

Vagus nerve

Long reflexes

Local reflexes

Enzymes

Distension →

↑ **pH**   Acid

Gastrin

Figure 6.31
Regulation of digestion:
2. Gastric phase. Presence of food
in the stomach stimulates activity
in other parts of the digestive tract
as well as exciting gastric secretion
and motility.

Gastric activity

Excitation of *stretch receptors* (a form of mechano-receptor) in the wall of the stomach evokes local and long reflexes (chiefly vagal), which stimulate gastric contractions and promote secretion of gastric enzymes (see p. 116).

Control of gastric acidity (pH)

The enzymes secreted by the stomach (*pepsinogens*) need an acid environment to work efficiently. When food enters the stomach the acid juice is diluted and the acidity decreases (pH increases; see Ch. 12). The acid is diluted even more if there is protein in the diet because the protein acts as a buffer (Ch. 12) and takes up some hydrogen ions (*hydrions*). As the pH increases, G cells in the antrum of the stomach, which are sensitive to the pH of gastric juice, increase their secretion of gastrin. Gastrin stimulates the oxyntic cells to secrete acid, which progressively lowers the pH of the gastric contents. In turn, the lowered pH inhibits the secretion of gastrin. In this way the pH of the gastric contents is brought to a suitable level for the gastric enzymes to work.

The acidity of the gastric fluid is in fact greatest when there is no food in the stomach, and least immediately after a meal (Fig. 6.32). Consequently, someone with a gastric ulcer is more likely to complain of discomfort during the night than during the daytime when regular small snacks may be eaten. ⑭

⑭
When is someone most likely to feel pain from a duodenal ulcer?

Figure 6.32
Acidity of the gastric contents over 24 hours.
Whenever food is ingested, the acid juice is
diluted and constituents of the food (such as
proteins) take up some of the hydrogen ions
(buffer action; see Ch. 12). Consequently, the
acidity of the contents falls (pH rises; see Ch. 12).
(Adapted from James & Pickering 1949.)

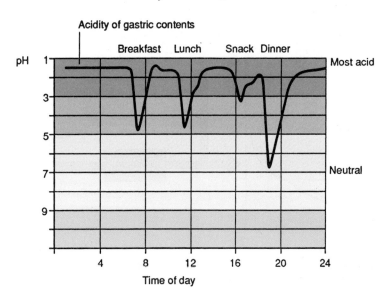

Acidity of gastric contents

Breakfast   Lunch   Snack   Dinner

pH

Most acid

Neutral

Time of day

Alerting the ileum and colon

The presence of food in the stomach also triggers activity further along the digestive tract. For example, as well as promoting secretion by the liver and the pancreas, increased peristaltic contractions occur in the terminal ileum and the colon (*gastro-ileal*, and *gastrocolic reflexes*). These responses are caused in part by neural reflexes, but hormones such as gastrin are likely to be involved too. Contractions of the ileum and colon help to move the food residues from previous meals further along the tract.

Small intestine

Efficient digestion of food in the small intestine depends on:

- the supply of enzymes and bile acids
- correct pH for enzyme activity
- appropriate delivery of chyme from the stomach.

The composition and volume of the intestinal contents are monitored by sensory receptors and endocrine cells in the wall of the intestine that respond in ways which create the right conditions (Fig. 6.33).

Supply of enzymes and bile acids

Amino acids and fatty acids in the intestinal contents stimulate the secretion of CCK-PZ, which stimulates the pancreas to secrete large amount of enzymes and the gall bladder to contract and expel bile through the relaxed sphincter of Oddi into the duodenum.

Control of intestinal pH

Acid chyme emptied from the stomach into the upper small intestine stimulates the release of the hormone secretin, which stimulates the pancreas and the liver to secrete an alkaline fluid containing hydrogen carbonate. This neutralises the gastric acid and brings the pH closer to the optimum for the pancreatic enzymes to work (about pH 7.0).

The effect of secretin on the pancreas is enhanced by CCK-PZ. Both hormones inhibit gastric emptying, thereby reducing the delivery of acid to the duodenum.

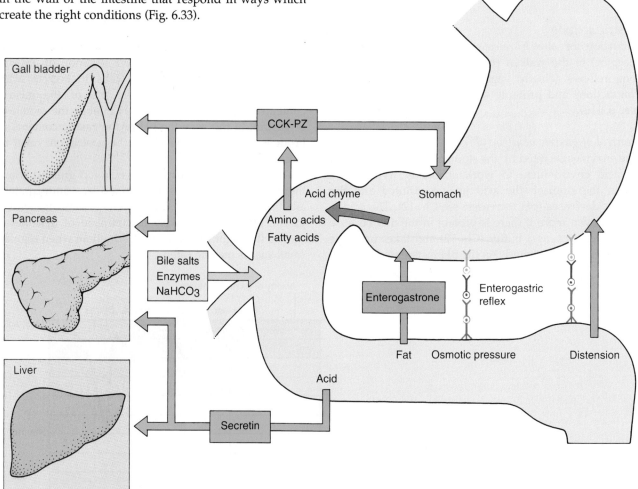

Figure 6.33
Regulation of digestion: 3. Intestinal phase. Presence of food in the intestine regulates the emptying of acid chyme from the stomach as well as the secretion of bile and pancreatic juice into the small intestine.

Feedback to the stomach

The delivery of chyme to the duodenum needs to be regulated so that the intestine is not overloaded. To do this, several characteristics of the intestinal contents, in addition to acidity, are monitored:

- fat content
- osmotic pressure
- volume.

Fat is the most difficult of the nutrients to digest and absorb properly. If too much fat enters the duodenum gastric emptying is inhibited by a hormonal mechanism. The name *enterogastrone* has been given to the hormonal factors involved, but their specific identity is still uncertain.

Osmotic pressure matters because it determines water movement into and out of the tissues. Too great a flow in either direction creates problems: water may be drawn out of the blood (see p. 129) if the osmotic pressure of the intestinal contents is greater than that of plasma; or it may flood into the blood and cause cells to swell if it is much lower than plasma. Thus if the osmotic pressure of the intestinal contents deviates a lot from that of plasma, in *either* direction, gastric emptying is inhibited by a neural reflex (*enterogastric reflex*).

Distension of the intestine also reduces gastric emptying. Distension of the ileum for example evokes the *ileogastric reflex*. It may also decrease appetite, particularly if distension is caused by unabsorbed food residues.

INTERDIGESTIVE ACTIVITY

The digestive tract is not inactive in the absence of food. About 4 to 5 hours after a meal, when the stomach is 'empty' peristaltic contractions similar to those evoked by a meal occur in the stomach. These become stronger (really strong contractions are felt as 'hunger pangs') and change in character from mixing movements to those of a propulsive kind. The duodenum in turn becomes active and a band of contractile activity slowly progresses along the intestine, with activity dying away behind it. The end of the ileum is reached in about 2 hours and, as soon as it is, another wave of contractions begins in the stomach.

This complex activity is referred to as the *interdigestive migrating contractions* or the *migrating myoelectric complex (MMC)*. It is accompanied by increased secretion from gastrointestinal glands, the pancreas and biliary system. The control of these events is not fully understood, but it is clear that the hormone *motilin* is involved in stimulating muscle contraction. The role of the complex may be to 'sweep out' the gastrointestinal tract regularly, thereby discouraging bacteria from the large intestine from colonising the small intestine as well.

KEY POINTS

What you should now know and understand about the digestive system:

- the various parts of the system, their key features and major functions
- what digestive secretions are formed, what they contain and what they do
- how the contents of the digestive tract are mixed, and moved from one end of the tract to the other
- what happens to food after it has been chewed and swallowed
- the factors promoting digestion of food and those hindering it
- where and how ingested substances (drugs as well as food and drink) are absorbed
- the factors promoting absorption and those hindering it
- what faeces consist of, why their consistency may alter, and how they are evacuated
- some of the consequences of disordered function of individual parts of the digestive system
- the basis of some common symptoms such as dry mouth, heartburn, 'wind', constipation and diarrhoea.

REFERENCES AND FURTHER READING

Cummings J H, Jenkins D J A, Wiggins H S 1976 Measurement of the mean transit time of dietary residue through the human gut. Gut 17: 210–218

Davenport H W 1982 Physiology of the digestive tract. Year Book Medical Publishers, Chicago
(Clearly presented student text explaining some experimental background and linking well with clinical applications)

Davison J S 1989 Gastrointestinal secretion. Wright, London
(Advanced student text consisting of a collection of well referenced articles by different authors)

Ferguson D B F 1988 Physiology for dental students. Butterworth, London
(Concise textbook covering all aspects of physiology but with rather more information than usual about aspects of oral physiology)

Hamilton Smith S 1972 Nil by mouth. RCN, London

Hayes P C, Gimson A E S, Westaby D 1988 Aids to gastroenterology and hepatology. Churchill Livingstone, Edinburgh
(Small book summarising useful clinical facts)

Hobsley M 1982 Disorders of the digestive system. Edward Arnold, London
(Companion to Sanford P A; concise coverage of different diseases explained in terms of disturbed structure and function)

James A H, Pickering G W 1949 The role of gastric acidity in the pathogenesis of peptic ulcer. Clinical Science 8: 181–210

Johnson L R, Christenson J, Jackson M, Jacobson E, Walsh J H (eds) 1986, 1987 Physiology of the gastrointestinal tract. Raven Press, New York
(Huge two volume work, written for and by specialists, relating physiology to pathophysiology and clinical dysfunction)

Magee D F, Dalley A F 1986 Digestion and the structure and function of the gut. Karger, Basel
(Advanced student text giving more detailed information. Includes clinical application, experimental background and references)

Passmore R, Eastwood M A 1986 Davidson's Human nutrition and dietetics, 8th edn. Churchill Livingstone, Edinburgh

Polak J M, Bloom S R, Wright N A, Butler A G 1984 Basic science in gastroenterology: physiology of the gut. Glaxo Group Research, Ware

Rogers A W 1992 Textbook of anatomy. Churchill Livingstone, Edinburgh

Sanford P A 1992 Digestive system physiology, 2nd edn. Edward Arnold, London
(Student text taking an organ by organ approach. Includes experimental basis of facts and has good bibliography)

Chapter 7
RESPIRATION

Most cells in the human body need oxygen (O_2) to survive and to carry out their functions. As cells work, they use up O_2 and produce carbon dioxide (CO_2) as a waste product that must be eliminated.

The term *respiration* refers to the processes by which O_2 is transported to and used by the cells and CO_2 is produced and eliminated (Fig. 7.1). This complicated task is achieved by the cooperative work of:

- the respiratory system
- red cells in the blood
- the circulatory system.

This chapter describes (1) the respiratory system and the respiratory process and (2) how O_2 and CO_2 are transported in the blood. The circulatory system is dealt with in detail in Chapter 5.

The oxygenation of the blood and the elimination of carbon dioxide from the body is termed *external respiration*. The use of O_2 by cells and their production of CO_2, sometimes described as *internal* or *cellular respiration*, is covered in Chapter 11.

The respiratory process and respiratory system

The main components of the respiratory *system* (Fig. 7.2) are:

- airways
- lungs
- thoracic cage and respiratory muscles
- pulmonary circulation.

These structures cooperate in the respiratory *process*, which can be subdivided into three parts (Fig. 7.3):

- *ventilation* of the lungs with air
- *gas exchange* between air and blood
- *perfusion* of the lungs with blood.

Each of these is vital for the efficient uptake of O_2 into the body and for the elimination of CO_2. Each will be described in turn together with the relevant structure of the parts of the respiratory system.

VENTILATION

The first step in the respiratory process is ventilation – that is, getting air into and out of the lungs. When we breathe, air is alternately sucked into and blown out of the lungs. This process is powered by the respiratory muscles, which are stimulated by nervous signals generated in the brain. Ventilation can feel effortless or laboured depending on the stiffness of the respiratory system and on the narrowness of the airways.

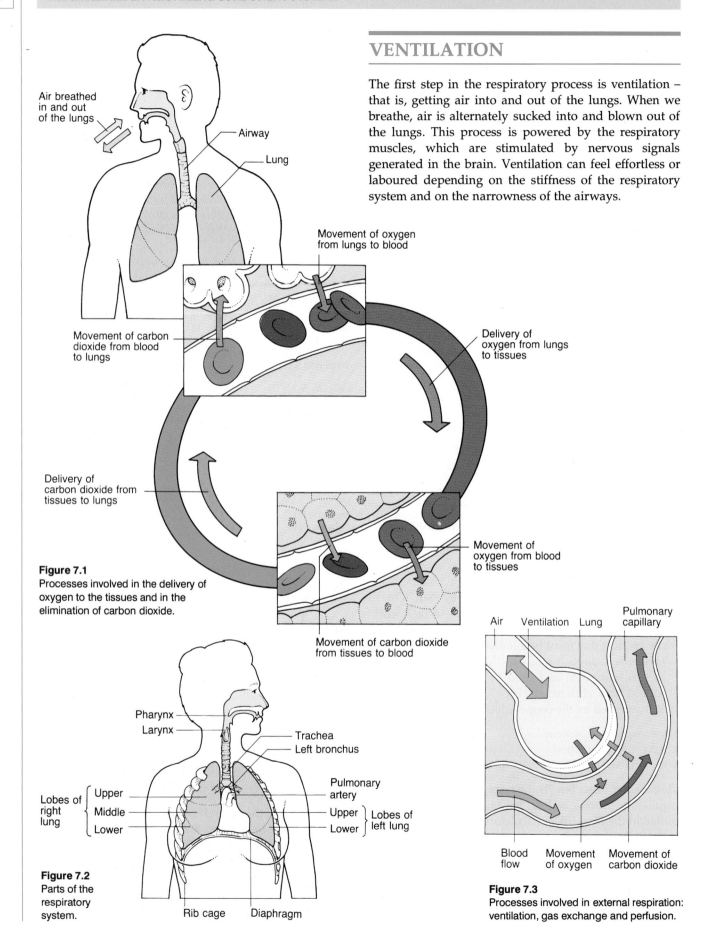

Air breathed in and out of the lungs

Airway

Lung

Movement of oxygen from lungs to blood

Movement of carbon dioxide from blood to lungs

Delivery of oxygen from lungs to tissues

Delivery of carbon dioxide from tissues to lungs

Movement of oxygen from blood to tissues

Movement of carbon dioxide from tissues to blood

Figure 7.1
Processes involved in the delivery of oxygen to the tissues and in the elimination of carbon dioxide.

Pharynx
Larynx
Trachea
Left bronchus
Pulmonary artery

Lobes of right lung { Upper, Middle, Lower }

Upper, Lower } Lobes of left lung

Rib cage   Diaphragm

Figure 7.2
Parts of the respiratory system.

Air   Ventilation   Lung   Pulmonary capillary

Blood flow   Movement of oxygen   Movement of carbon dioxide

Figure 7.3
Processes involved in external respiration: ventilation, gas exchange and perfusion.

AIRWAYS

Air breathed in through the mouth and nose reaches the lungs via the *pharynx* and *larynx* and then a branching system of tubes beginning with the *trachea* (Fig. 7.4A). The trachea divides into the *left bronchus* and *right bronchus* (plural = bronchi), which divide in turn into *lobar* and then *segmental bronchi* (Fig. 7.4B). Branching continues, with the airways becoming progressively smaller at each branch point. These smaller airways (Fig. 7.4B & C), listed in order of decreasing size, are:

1. *bronchioles*   3. *respiratory bronchioles*
2. *terminal bronchioles* 4. *alveolar ducts*.

The airways lead to the *alveoli*, which are tiny distensible sacs where gas exchange occurs between air and blood.

The trachea and the large bronchi are supported by rings of cartilage that normally prevent their compression. The smaller airways have progressively less cartilage in their walls, while the smallest have none at all and so can be compressed and closed in some circumstances. ①

Respiratory epithelium

The airways are lined internally by a ciliated layer of cells, the *respiratory epithelium* (Fig. 7.4D). Glands and goblet cells of the epithelium secrete *mucus*, a sticky substance that coats the inner surface of the airways and traps inhaled particles. The cilia drive these secretions away from the alveoli, up and out of the airways into the throat, or pharynx, where they are swallowed. Each day, about 100 ml of mucus are secreted and moved

CHOKING

Normally, only air is drawn into the respiratory system, as the entrance to the airways is protected during the act of swallowing by the epiglottis, which closes off the larynx (see Ch. 29). However, we have all choked on something that has suddenly 'gone down the wrong way'. The offending item is usually coughed up and then swallowed as it should have been in the first place.

Occasionally, an object that is accidentally inhaled is large enough to obstruct the airway and completely cut off air supply. If it is not removed, the person will become unconscious, collapse and may die from asphyxiation in a few minutes. Emergency action must be taken immediately.

A sharp below on the victim's back may loosen the object by force. Small children can be turned upside down first as gravity may help to remove the obstruction. An alternative and increasingly recommended method is to use the *Heimlich manoeuvre* (or *Heimlich abdominal thrust*), which uses the person's own lungs as an air pump to propel the object out with the force from a sudden increase in air pressure.

To perform the Heimlich manoeuvre, the first-aider stands behind with arms high around the victim's waist, making a fist against the upper abdomen and quickly and firmly thrusting the fist upwards towards the diaphragm. The compression causes a sudden rise in air pressure within the lungs, which, if sufficient, may dislodge the obstructing object upwards and out of the windpipe.

To help you picture what's happening, imagine a cork in a plastic bottle that can be squeezed – the increased pressure caused by a sudden and firm squeeze will pop the cork out.

① *Where can you feel the rings of cartilage through the skin just by pressing (lightly!) with your fingers?*

upwards at a rate of 1 to 2 cm/hour.

Lower down in the respiratory tract, closer to the alveoli, *Clara cells* are found in the epithelium. They

Tobacco smoke not only stimulates more mucus secretion but can destroy the ciliary epithelium. This means that smokers have more mucus to clear from their airways but have a reduced mechanism for doing so. They – and the people around them – are very conscious of the smokers' productive cough.

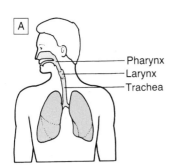

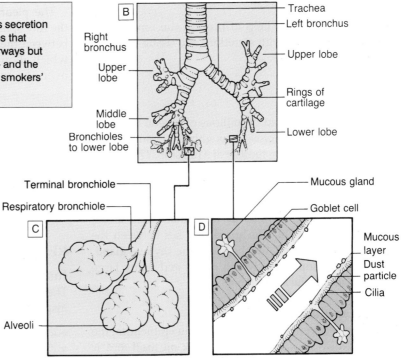

Figure 7.4
Structure of the airways and lungs:
A Upper airways
B Bronchial tree
C Terminal airways and alveoli
D Lining of the airways.

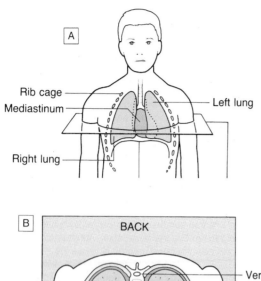

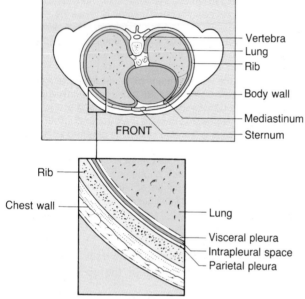

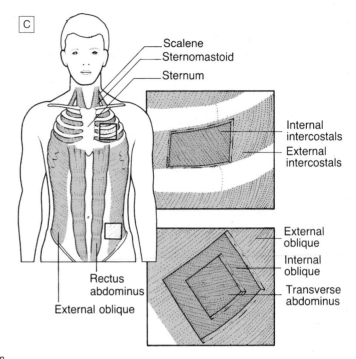

Figure 7.5
The thorax and associated structures:
A Structures within the thoracic cavity
B Cross-section of the thorax showing the pleurae
C Rib cage and muscles. The enlarged insets show the different layers of muscle.

absorb fluid and may help to prevent the tiny alveoli from becoming filled with secretions and tissue fluid.

LUNGS

Alveoli

The lungs are composed of millions of alveoli (singular = alveolus). Each alveolus is roughly 1/3 mm in diameter, which is less than the size of a full stop. The alveoli are bounded by elastic connective tissue and are covered on their outer surface by pulmonary capillaries.

The lungs are located in the *thoracic cavity* (Fig. 7.5A). They are held in place only by their attachment to the left and right bronchi. The space that lies between the two lungs, which contains the heart, the thymus gland, most of the oesophagus, lymph nodes and many large blood vessels, is the *mediastinum*. ②

Pleural epithelium

Each lung is covered externally by a thin epithelium, the *visceral pleura*. This layer doubles back on itself and is continued over the structures surrounding the lungs

(chest wall, diaphragm and organs of the mediastinum) to form the *parietal pleura*. Thus, each lung is enveloped separately by a double layer of pleural epithelium (Fig. 7.5B).

The pleural cells secrete a watery (*serous*) fluid into the tiny space (*intrapleural space* or *pleural cavity*) existing between them. The intrapleural fluid acts as a lubricant which allows the lungs and adjacent structures to slide over one another while remaining firmly together.

> *Pleurisy* is an inflammation of a part of the pleural epithelium. In 'dry' pleurisy, every breath can be quite painful as the inflamed layers rub against rather than glide over the opposing surfaces. People with painful pleurisy try to reduce their pain by taking small shallow breaths and may also restrict chest movement by holding, or splinting, the painful area with their hands.

RESPIRATORY MUSCLES

Inspiratory muscles

The respiratory muscles (Fig. 7.5C) used chiefly for inspiration include:

- *diaphragm*
- *external intercostals*
- *scalene* and *sternomastoid muscles* (*accessory muscles*).

② One lung is slightly larger than the other. Which one and why?

Diaphragm

The most important of these is the diaphragm, a sheet of muscle separating the thoracic cavity from the abdominal cavity. The edge of this sheet is anchored to the lower ribs (Fig. 7.6). When the diaphragm contracts, it pushes the abdominal organs down and increases the distance between the top and bottom of the thorax. At the same time, the lower ribs are swung outwards a little, so that the width of the thorax also increases (Fig. 7.6). ③

Intercostals

The intercostals link adjacent ribs (Fig. 7.5C). Their contraction in inspiration raises the rib cage, so that the front-to-back dimension of the thorax increases as well.

Accessory muscles

The accessory muscles are used in inspiration only when breathing is vigorous. The scalene muscle elevates the first two ribs and the sternomastoids raise the sternum.

Expiratory muscles

When the thoracic cavity is expanded by contraction of the muscles of inspiration, the lungs also expand. The size of the alveoli and of the smaller airways increases, and the elastic tissue in the lung and in the airways stretches. When the muscles relax, this elastic tissue recoils, in much the same way as a stretched elastic band does, and air is forced out of the lungs. Thus, expiration is normally an entirely passive process – no extra muscular effort is needed.

However, when expiration needs to be more forcible (blowing up a balloon) or more controlled (playing a wind instrument or speaking), muscular effort is required. The most powerful of the muscles used are in the abdominal wall:

- *rectus abdominus*
- *internal* and *external oblique muscles*
- *transverse abdominus.*

Contraction of these muscles increases abdominal pressure and drives the diaphragm upwards. In addition, contraction of the internal intercostals assists by pulling the ribs in and stiffening the rib cage.

NEURAL CONTROL OF THE RESPIRATORY MUSCLES

The respiratory muscles are innervated by somatic motoneurones (see Chs 3 and 20), which are controlled by two different systems (Figs 7.7 and 7.8): ④

- *involuntary* – to control ventilation
- *voluntary* – for speech, singing etc.

The involuntary system includes the respiratory centres

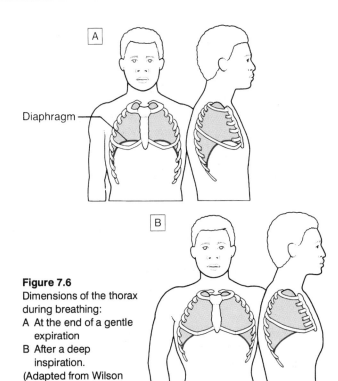

Figure 7.6
Dimensions of the thorax during breathing:
A At the end of a gentle expiration
B After a deep inspiration.
(Adapted from Wilson 1987.)

OUT OF BREATH

Normally, we are not conscious of the work that our respiratory muscles do except when we are 'out of breath' after exercise, when the natural tendency is to remain still so that no further demands for O_2 are made and we can concentrate on 'getting our breath back'. The work of the respiratory muscles becomes obvious when we are 'breathing hard' (for example, the sternomastoid muscles may be seen contracted in the neck), and we instinctively want to loosen any tight clothing so that respiratory muscle movement is not restricted.

Patients who are very breathless because of a respiratory problem react in exactly the same way. They don't want to be moved unnecessarily and they need to have the freedom to use their muscles to capacity.

Because so many muscles, thoracic as well as abdominal, are involved in the work of respiration, any local injury can disrupt the normal smooth pattern of breathing because of the associated pain.

Following thoracic or upper abdominal surgery where the surgical incision is in or very close to respiratory muscles, patients naturally attempt to control pain and discomfort by minimising respiratory muscle movement. The very shallow respirations that result, along with their natural reluctance to cough, are counterproductive – mucous secretions remain in the lungs and form a potential site for infection.

Various strategies are sometimes used to help patients contract their muscles properly in order to breathe deeply and cough effectively. For example, analgesics given before breathing exercises work by reducing pain perception. The nurse can use her hands to support the patient's wound on either side or she may use a pillow to control tension on the wound edges. Only the wounded area is splinted so that the healthy surrounding muscle can contract and move normally.

③ *Hiccups are caused by sudden involuntary spasmodic contractions of one of the respiratory muscles. Which muscle do you think is affected?*

④ *What are some differences between the autonomic and somatic nervous systems?*

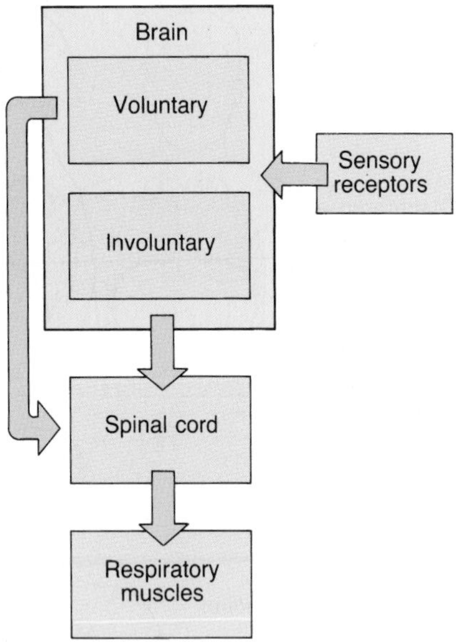

Figure 7.7
Control of the
respiratory muscles.

The phrenic nerve includes nerve axons that leave the spinal cord in cervical nerves 3 to 5 (Fig. 7.8). Damage to the spinal cord at or above this level paralyses all the respiratory muscles. If spinal injury occurs below cervical nerve 5, the diaphragm will function normally but control of the intercostal and abdominal muscles will be disordered.

in the brain stem and many different sensory receptors. The voluntary system, which involves other brain areas, is dealt with in detail later (Chs 27 and 29).

Nerve supply

The cell bodies of the neurones that innervate the respiratory muscles are in the ventral horn of the spinal cord (see Ch. 20) and their axons are found within:

- the *phrenic nerve* (for the diaphragm)
- the *intercostal nerves* (for most other muscles).

Involuntary and voluntary control

Impulses from the involuntary and voluntary systems converge on the motoneurones in the spinal cord. Most of the time, the motoneurones are driven by the involuntary system to give the regular inspiration/expiration breathing cycle, which we normally don't notice. But when we choose to speak or play a musical instrument, the voluntary system interrupts this cycle.

The voluntary system cannot, however, overrule the involuntary one completely. When the signals from the two systems conflict, the involuntary system usually wins, although attention-seeking children have been known to hold their breath long enough to go blue in the face and even faint before the involuntary system triumphs! ⑤

Respiratory centres

The clusters of cells in the brain that control the automatic breathing cycle are in the *medulla* and the *pons* of the brain stem (Fig. 7.8; see also Ch. 3). Regular bursts of activity in the cluster termed the *inspiratory centre* set the basic rhythm of breathing. Other clusters of cells, such as the pneumotaxic centre (also shown in Fig. 7.8), regulate the size and duration of each breath.

Sensory receptors

The respiratory centres receive a multitude of information from a variety of sensory receptors located

⑤
Why do you count a patient's respiratory rate without his knowledge?

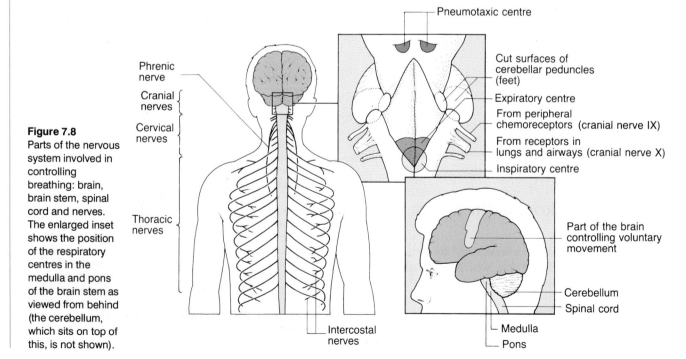

Figure 7.8
Parts of the nervous system involved in controlling breathing: brain, brain stem, spinal cord and nerves. The enlarged inset shows the position of the respiratory centres in the medulla and pons of the brain stem as viewed from behind (the cerebellum, which sits on top of this, is not shown).

Table 7.1   Sensory receptors involved in the control of breathing

Type	Location	Stimulus	Effect on breathing
(A) Within the respiratory system			
	Nose		Sneeze
Irritant receptor	Airway epithelium — Trachea and bronchi	Inhaled particles and vapours	Cough
	Bronchioles		Increased rate and depth
Stretch receptors	Airway smooth muscle	Inflation	Slowed down
J receptors	Alveolar wall	Interstitial oedema Pulmonary emboli	Rapid and shallow
Muscle spindles (see Ch. 24)	Respiratory muscles (e.g. diaphragm, intercostals)	Elongation of the muscles	Made smoother and more efficient
(B) Elsewhere Chemoreceptors (see Chs 11 and 12)	Carotid artery Aorta	↑ CO_2 ↓ O_2 } in blood ↑ H^+	
	Brain (medulla)	↑ H^+ in CSF }	Increased rate and depth

throughout the respiratory system (Table 7.1). These receptors monitor the state of expansion of the lungs and other local conditions (such as inhaled dust) and bring about reflex changes in the pattern of breathing.

Other sensory receptors located elsewhere in the body also provide information to the respiratory centres. These include *chemoreceptors* that monitor the amounts of O_2 and CO_2 in the blood and reflexly alter the ventilation of the lungs to stabilise the concentrations of these two gases in the blood. Their function is described in detail later (Chs 11 and 12). ⑥

> The cough reflex is triggered by stimulation of sensory receptors in the lining of the airways. A cough is not always a symptom of disorder – most of us cough several times every day. A cough is a natural defence mechanism designed to clear the airways of irritants such as dust and excess mucus.

LUNG VOLUMES

The volume of air breathed in and out and the number of breaths taken per minute vary between people according to age, sex, build and activity. At rest, about 500 ml of air are inspired and expired with each breath (*tidal volume*) and the frequency of breathing is about 10 to 15 breaths per minute. This pattern of gentle breathing is shown in the recording obtained from a *spirometer* (literally breath-meter) in Figure 7.9. ⑦⑧

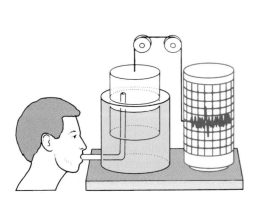
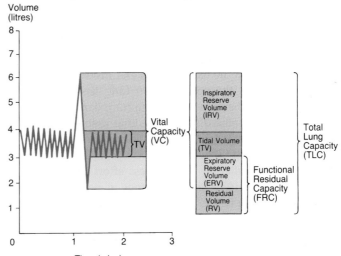

Figure 7.9
Measurement of lung volumes by spirometry. The spirometer consists of a cylinder filled with air which is inverted into a container of water. As air is breathed in and out, the cylinder rises and falls. This movements is inscribed on the chart fixed to a slowly revolving drum. (Note: the valves in the system, and the CO_2 absorbant within the spirometer, are not shown.)

⑥
What changes occur in the pattern of breathing when the level of CO_2 in the body goes up?

⑦
The tidal volume in the record is larger than 500 ml. Why might this be?

⑧
You can easily count the number of breaths you take per minute. How does your respiratory rate compare with that of your friends?

With maximum effort, the lungs can be expanded to hold between 4 and 6 litres of air (*total lung capacity*). Most, but not all, of this can be expelled. The maximum volume expelled (*vital capacity*) is one of several measurements used to assess respiratory function. Any respiratory disorder, such as pulmonary fibrosis, that reduces the ability of the lungs to expand also reduces vital capacity.

In ordinary gentle breathing, about 2 litres of air remain in the lungs at the end of expiration (*functional residual capacity*). Some of this can be breathed out forcibly, but even after a maximum expiration, about 1 litre of air still remains trapped in the lungs (*residual volume*).

Factors that may affect vital capacity include:

- age, sex and build
- position of person during measurement
- strength of respiratory muscles
- distensibility of lungs and chest cage.

EASE OF LUNG EXPANSION AND RECOIL

When we breathe, expansion of the lungs requires effort. The amount needed depends on the *compliance* of the respiratory system. Expiration may require effort but can occur without it powered by the *elastic recoil* of the lungs.

Compliance

In health, the effort required to expand the lungs in gentle breathing is very small. The lungs and associated structures easily yield to (or comply with) the forces acting on them – that is, their compliance (volume change per unit of effort) is high.

If the respiratory system becomes stiffer, as it does in old age, compliance is reduced. A bigger force is then required to expand the lungs to the same extent. Compliance is also reduced in some respiratory disorders, such as pulmonary oedema. In this condition, the fluid present in the tissue spaces and inside some of the alveoli causes the normally soft lung tissue to be much firmer and therefore reduced in compliance.

Conversely, in some diseases, the lung tissue is more rather than less compliant. In emphysema, for example, there is loss of lung tissue. As there is less tissue present to be stretched, inflation requires less effort. However, the power of elastic recoil of the lungs is also reduced by the loss of lung tissue. Consequently, expiration may require muscle power even when breathing at rest. ⑨

Surfactant

One of the natural factors that makes the lungs compliant is *surfactant* in the fluid lining the inner surface of the alveoli. Surfactant is a mixture of substances

---

THE FIRST BREATH

At the moment of birth, we all wait expectantly for the baby to take his first breath (perhaps holding our own breath in anticipation). This is not just a special moment emotionally but a crucial one physiologically. In going from the mother's womb to the outside world, the baby's respiratory system must undergo a tremendous adaptation to make the transition from the fluid intrauterine environment to the air outside (see Ch. 35).

Even in a healthy, full-term baby, that first breath is not an easy one. Before birth, fluid fills the respiratory passageways and the alveoli are collapsed, like empty balloons. At birth, air must replace this fluid and the alveoli must expand to be able to take part in gas exchange. The baby must make a tremendous effort to replace the fluid with air and to inflate the alveoli. Surfactant plays a vital role in the success of this transition and, most importantly, helps to make each subsequent breath a bit easier.

Because surfactant is not formed by the growing fetus until the last few weeks before birth, infants who are born prematurely often develop breathing problems. The lack of surfactant means that some of the little alveolar sacs remain collapsed (*atelectasis*), as they were in fetal life, and others open stiffly and only with some difficulty (reduced compliance) when the baby first tries to breathe as well as with each subsequent breath.

Because fluid passes easily into the alveoli from the capillaries (*transudation* of fluid) when the level of surfactant is low, alveolar space within the baby's lungs is also reduced. These clinical problems, when present, form the *infant respiratory distress syndrome*.

Respiratory difficulty increases with the degree of prematurity. Often some assistance with ventilation is necessary until the baby reaches the normal gestational age at which surfactant is produced. Once this is present, the lungs easily expand with each breath and ventilation becomes normal.

ADULT RESPIRATORY DISTRESS SYNDROME

Surfactant deficiency can also occur in adults when changes develop inside the lungs similar to those in infants with low surfactant. *Adult respiratory distress syndrome* can occur following severe shock, trauma or massive blood transfusion. These patients, who are very ill, develop increasing respiratory distress with rapid, shallow, ineffectual breathing, and many, like the infants, require some assistance with ventilation.

Q: What would you expect a spirometer trace to look like in these patients? In particular, what would happen to tidal volume?

(chiefly lipids) secreted by cells of the alveolar epithelium. It lowers the *surface tension* of the fluid lining the alveoli, making the alveoli easier to expand.

Surface tension is caused by strong forces of attraction between molecules in a liquid, which make the surface molecules hold tightly together and resist being spread out. An analogy might be the way that a clique of people tend to stay together at a party and resist being drawn into other conversations. At a party, cliques can be dispersed if other people with wider associations can break in and form new points of contact.

Surfactant plays a similar role. For alveoli to expand, the fluid lining their interior has to spread out over a larger area. Surfactant allows this to happen by associating with the water molecules in the fluid layer and weakening the attraction between them.

By reducing surface tension, surfactant also helps to prevent fluid being sucked into the alveoli from the interstitial space.

Recoil forces

The lungs have a natural tendency to recoil caused by:

● stretched elastic fibres in the lung tissue
● surface tension of the fluid lining the alveoli.

Despite this, the lungs do not fully empty at the end of expiration in gentle breathing. The reason for this is that, at the end of a gentle expiration, the recoil of the lungs is exactly counterbalanced by the recoil of the chest wall and diaphragm, which are being pulled away from their natural rest-point by the lungs (Fig. 7.10A). These structures are held together by the intrapleural fluid and, while they are, neither the lungs nor the chest wall and diaphragm are free to recoil completely to their non-stretched state.

Intrapleural pressure

Because the intrapleural fluid is pulled in opposite directions, its pressure is less than atmospheric (Fig. 7.10B). If the atmospheric pressure is 100 kPa, the intrapleural pressure will be around 99.6 kPa. As the atmospheric pressure varies slightly from day to day, sometimes being 'high' and sometimes 'low', it is simpler to describe intrapleural pressure as 0.4 kPa less than atmospheric, in other words, as –0.4 kPa.

Intrapleural pressure changes during the breathing cycle, becoming even more sub-atmospheric as we breathe in. The bigger the breath, the more sub-atmospheric the pressure becomes. Conversely, after a forcible expiration, when air is trapped in the lungs, the space may be compressed and then the pressure rises above atmospheric (see Ch. 5, Respiratory pump).

Most of the time though, the pressure is sub-atmospheric. This is possible because the space is sealed off both from the atmosphere outside the body and from the air in the alveoli. If, however, the chest wall is stabbed or, more likely, if the lung tissue is torn, the intrapleural space may then be opened to air from the lungs or the atmosphere.

As air will always flow from an area of higher pressure to an area of lower pressure, the difference in pressure between the air outside and the fluid inside causes air to be sucked in, forming a *pneumothorax*. At that site the lung is no longer held to the adjacent structures. The

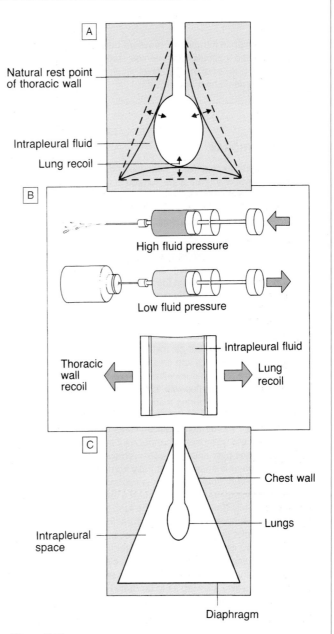

Figure 7.10
Recoil tendencies of the lungs and thoracic wall:
A Act against one another so long as pleural fluid holds the two together; consequently the lungs cannot collapse, and the chest wall and diaphragm are pulled away from their natural rest points
B Create a sub-atmospheric intrapleural pressure
C Cause lung collapse and thoracic expansion if a large amount of air enters the intrapleural space (pneumothorax).

tendency of the lungs to recoil is no longer restrained by the opposing tendencies of the chest wall and the lung gradually collapses as air is drawn in (Fig. 7.10C). Fortunately, as the intrapleural space of the left lung is not continuous with that of the right lung (see Fig. 7.5B), only one lung may be affected at a time.

The fluctuation in intrapleural pressure between each expiration and inspiration can be seen reflected in the steady rise and fall of the fluid level within the tube of an underwater seal chest drainage set.

PNEUMOTHORAX

A pneumothorax may occur because of damage either to the chest wall or to part of the surface of the lung. The degree of breathlessness depends upon the suddenness of onset and the size of the pneumothorax.

The consequences of a pneumothorax depend upon the type:

- In an *open pneumothorax*, air is drawn into the pleural space through the area of damage, such as a wound in the chest wall or a tear in the visceral pleura. In other words, air is 'breathed' in via the abnormal opening with each inspiration and, once the pneumothorax is established, blown out again with each expiration. The air that occupies the pleural space obviously contributes nothing to gas exchange. Instead, it interferes with inflation of the lungs and creates breathing problems.

  Because the pressure within the pleural space eventually equilibrates with atmospheric pressure (with small fluctuations during respiration), there is nothing to hold the lung in its normal position tightly against the chest wall. The stretched elastic fibres recoil and the lung deflates and collapses. It cannot reinflate until the injured area closes over and air is either removed by pleural aspiration or is absorbed naturally from the pleural cavity.
- In a *closed pneumothorax*, air is sucked out of the lung into the intrapleural space through a tear in the lung tissue, which then seals over, the lung collapses with the loss of the normal negative pressure. In time, as the air in the intrapleural space is gradually absorbed, the lung will reinflate to its normal shape and size.
- In a *valvular pneumothorax*, a type of closed pneumothorax, the small injury in the pleura acts as a one-way valve allowing air to be drawn into the intrapleural space but with no way of escape during expiration. If the air tries to escape, the increased intrapleural pressure forces the edges of the damaged area to collapse together and block the flow of air (like the valve on a bicycle tyre). The result is that each breath adds to the air volume and pressure within the intrapleural space. The increase in volume and pressure not only causes the affected lung to collapse but also pushes the mediastinal structures towards the opposite chest wall (*mediastinal shift*), compressing the other lung as well. The consequences of this type of pneumothorax are very grave and, unless treated, the patient may suffocate.

⑩
Which of the other lung volumes would be affected and how?

AIRFLOW THROUGH THE AIRWAYS

The forces that we have looked at so far are those that affect the volume of the lungs. The changes in lung volume that occur when we breathe alter the pressure of air inside the alveoli, and this in turn drives the flow of air into and out of the lungs. The ease with which air flows depends largely on the size of the airways.

Pressure

The pressure of any gas changes when the volume that it occupies is altered. This is Boyle's law, which states that the product of pressure (P) and volume (V) of a fixed amount of gas does not change:

$$P \times V = a \text{ constant}$$

If the volume is doubled, the pressure is halved, and so on.

In principle, this is what happens to the air in the alveoli when the lungs expand (Fig. 7.11A). During a gentle inspiration, the pressure of the air in the alveoli drops below atmospheric by about 0.1 to 0.2 kPa. This small pressure difference between the air in the lungs and the air outside the body is sufficient to drive air into the expanding lungs. The flow of air continues until the pressures inside the alveoli and outside the body are the same – that is, atmospheric.

When the lungs recoil, their volume decreases and the air within them is compressed. The pressure rises above atmospheric, again by about 0.1 to 0.2 kPa. The pressure difference is now in the opposite direction and air is forced out of the lungs.

Size of airways

The size of the airways is very important in determining how easily air flows into and out of the lungs. The wider the airways are, the easier it is for air to flow (Fig. 7.11B). If they are narrowed (for example through inflammation or the accumulation of secretions), then air flow is more difficult.

The size of all but the larger airways (those stiffened by cartilage) changes appreciably during the breathing cycle. When we breathe in, the airways as well as the alveoli expand. This makes airflow progressively easier. When we breathe out, however, the airways get narrower and narrower and the resistance to the flow of air increases. In a forced expiration, the smallest airways close completely and trap air in the alveoli. If the airways are already narrowed because of disease, such as bronchitis, closure occurs sooner and more air is trapped (that is, the residual volume increases; see p. 144). ⑩

The diameter of the airways is also affected by contraction and relaxation of the smooth muscle in their walls. Bronchodilators relax the smooth muscle while bronchoconstrictors contract it.

Bronchodilators	*Bronchoconstrictors*
sympathetic nerves	parasympathetic nerves
adrenaline	histamine
CO_2	

As the smallest airways are very tiny, it might be assumed that these create the most difficulty for airflow. However, what they lack in size they make up for

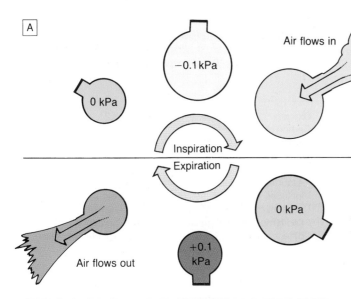

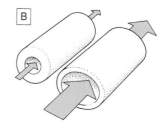

Figure 7.11
Airflow through the airways:
A Depends on the change in alveolar air pressure caused by the expansion and compression of the alveoli during the breathing cycle
B Is affected by airway size.

> Airways close prematurely in emphysema, a condition where there is loss of lung tissue. Patients often find it easier to exhale through pursed lips. This prolongs expiratory time and maintains pressure in the airways, which helps to keep the small airways open.

in numbers. The tiniest branches can probably be numbered in millions, and this increase in numbers outweighs the decrease in size. Collectively, they offer less resistance to flow than the trachea and bronchi (Fig. 7.12). At least 50% of the total resistance to airflow

is normally contributed by the upper airways – mouth, nose and pharynx.

Assessment of airflow

The maximum rate of airflow that we can achieve when we breathe out as hard and quickly as possible, starting from full lungs, is the *peak expiratory flow rate (PEFR)*. It is measured using a simple instrument (peak flow meter) that registers the maximum airflow achieved during a breath. In health, PEFR ranges from 400 to 600 litres/minute.

Airway function can also be assessed by determining the proportion of the vital capacity that can be expelled from the lungs in 1 and then 3 seconds, again while breathing out as quickly as possible. In health, at least

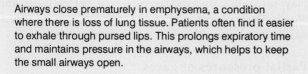

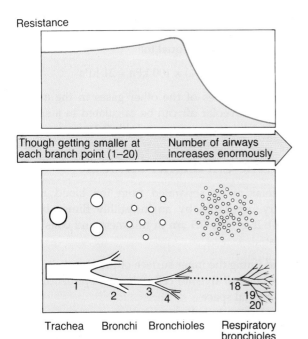

Figure 7.12
The resistance to airflow offered by different sections of the airways. (Adapted from West 1990, based on Pedley et al 1970 and Weibel 1963.)

PEAK FLOW

In conditions such as asthma where the bronchioles are narrowed (that is, in *bronchospasm*), measurements of peak expiratory flow rate (PEFR) can provide an objective measurement of the severity of bronchiole constriction.

Many asthma sufferers are now taught to take and record their peak flow rates at regular intervals throughout the day. In this way they know what is normal for them. They usually take the recordings in the morning and in the evening. When they are well, these recordings should be no different from those of someone without asthma; that is, their peak flow rate should be within normal limits for their age, size and sex, with evening recording slightly higher than the morning recording.

When mild bronchospasm occurs, a fall in the PEFR occurs even before breathlessness becomes evident, so it is a helpful early warning measure and can alert someone in good time to the need to take prescribed bronchodilators or to seek medical help before the bronchospasm gets worse.

Peak flow measurements are also used to assess the effect and, therefore, the effectiveness of a particular type of bronchodilator or a particular course of bronchodilator drugs. To do this, PEFR is measured before and after the drug is administered.

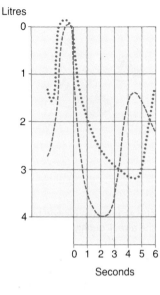

Figure 7.13
Forced expiratory volume (FEV) measured by spirometry in two adult men, one of whom has asthma. Each man filled his lungs to capacity and then at 0 seconds breathed out as hard and fast as he could. (Data courtesy of D. E. Evans.)

Table 7.2 Composition of air				
	Dry atmosphere		Alveolar air (37°C)	
	%	kPa*	%	kPa*
Oxygen	21	21	13.2	13.2
Carbon dioxide	0.04	0.04	5.3	5.3
Nitrogen†	79	79	75.2	75.2
Water vapour	‡	‡	6.3	6.3

* Assuming barometric pressure is 100 kPa.
† Includes <1% rare gases (argon, helium etc.).
‡ Amount of moisture in atmosphere depends on humidity and temperature. If moisture is present, percentage of other constituents will then be correspondingly decreased.

80% can be expelled in the 1st second and about 100% by the 3rd. This measurement is the *forced expiratory volume* and is abbreviated to FEV_1 and FEV_3 for 1 and 3 seconds, respectively. If the airways are narrowed, as in asthma, both PEFR and FEV will be lower than normal (Fig. 7.13).

GAS EXCHANGE

After the alveoli are ventilated with fresh air, the next step in the respiratory process is the transfer of gases between the air in the alveoli (alveolar air) and the pulmonary blood.

COMPOSITION OF AIR

Alveolar air
The air inside the alveoli is not the same as that in the atmosphere (Table 7.2). It is different because it gains water from the moist epithelia lining the respiratory tract and picks up CO_2 and loses O_2 within the alveoli. The composition changes during the breathing cycle as fresh air is drawn into the lungs and some alveolar air is expelled. In gentle breathing these changes are not dramatic because the volume of fresh air added at each breath (tidal volume – about 500 ml) is small compared with the volume of air already in the lungs (functional residual capacity – about 2 litres).

Deadspace air
Some of the air in each breath does not reach the alveoli but merely fills the airways and is breathed out, unaltered in composition. Only very tiny amounts of O_2

and CO_2 move across the walls of the airways, which play no useful role in gas exchange between air and blood. The volume within the airways acts as deadspace. On average, this volume is about 150 ml.

Partial pressures of gases
The composition of air containing a mixture of gases can be described in several ways:

- per cent composition
- partial pressures of the constituent gases (kPa).

Suppose, for example, that the atmospheric pressure is 100 kPa. From the per cent composition of the atmosphere (Table 7.2) we know that O_2 forms 21% of the air. Therefore, 21% of the total pressure of the atmosphere is due to O_2. So the *part* of the *pressure* due to O_2 (*partial pressure* of O_2, or PO_2) is equal to:

$$21/100 \ (21\%) \times 100 \text{ kPa} = 21 \text{ kPa}$$

The partial pressures of the other gases in the atmosphere and in alveolar air can be calculated in a similar way. Typical values are given in Table 7.2. ⑪

ALVEOLAR–CAPILLARY BARRIER

The alveolar air is separated from the blood in the pulmonary capillaries by an incredibly flimsy barrier (Fig. 7.14). It is only 0.5 μm in thickness and consists of four parts:

- the fluid lining the inner surface of the alveoli
- a single layer of alveolar cells (alveolar epithelium)
- the interstitial space
- the capillary endothelium.

The alveolar epithelium is remarkable for its extensiveness – if the 300 million alveoli were spread out to form a single sheet it would have a total surface area of about 85 square metres. Blood capillaries cover about 60% of this surface. ⑫

⑪ What is the highest percentage of O_2 you have seen prescribed? What would the PO_2 be? Do you know why the patient required that amount?

⑫ What size of hospital ward would have a similar sized area?

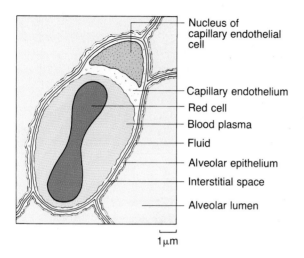

Nucleus of capillary endothelial cell
Capillary endothelium
Red cell
Blood plasma
Fluid
Alveolar epithelium
Interstitial space
Alveolar lumen

1 μm

Figure 7.14
Cross-section of a piece of lung tissue showing alveoli, a single pulmonary capillary and the alveolar–capillary barrier.

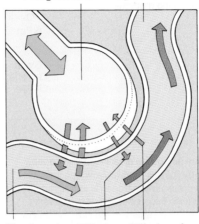

Alveolar air
PO_2 13.2 kPa
PCO_2 5.3 kPa

Blood leaving lungs
PO_2 13.2 kPa
PCO_2 5.3 kPa

Blood coming   Diffusion   Diffusion of
to lungs   of oxygen   carbon dioxide
PO_2 5.3 kPa
PCO_2 6 kPa

Figure 7.16
Gas transfer between alveolar air and blood. The gases in the blood leaving the lungs are in equilibrium with air in the alveoli.

GAS TRANSFER

Diffusion of gas molecules into liquid

By nature, gas molecules move randomly in all directions powered by their own internal energy. When they meet a liquid, they penetrate it and move around within the liquid in the same random way (Fig. 7.15). At first, there will be more gas molecules entering the liquid than leaving it. In other words, the gas is *diffusing* into the liquid.

The concentration of gas molecules dissolved in the liquid will increase until the numbers leaving the liquid equal those entering it. The gas outside the liquid and that inside it are then in *equilibrium*. We can describe the gas in the liquid as then having the same pressure as the gas outside, that is, the same partial pressure.

Diffusion of oxygen and carbon dioxide

O_2 moves from the alveolar air into the blood by diffusion (Fig. 7.16). Although the blood coming to the lungs already has some O_2 in it, the partial pressure of

O_2 in this blood (5.3 kPa) is less than that in the alveolar air (13.2 kPa). Consequently, more molecules of O_2 move into the blood than out of it. In time, equilibrium is reached and the partial pressure of O_2 in the blood becomes the same as that in the alveolar air.

CO_2 leaves the blood in the same way. Its partial pressure in the blood (6 kPa) is greater than that in the alveolar air (5.3 kPa) and so diffusion occurs from the blood to the air.

Equilibration of alveolar air with blood occurs very quickly. It takes less than a second for blood to pass through the capillary network and only 0.25 second to reach equilibrium. ⑬

Rates of transfer of oxygen and carbon dioxide

The rate at which the gases are transferred between alveolar air and blood depends upon:

- the difference in partial pressures
- the distance between the alveolar air and the blood
- the total surface area available for gas exchange.

Anything that increases the distance that the gases have to move will slow down the rate of transfer because the gradient for movement is made less steep (Fig. 7.17). In pulmonary oedema, for example, the interstitial space becomes congested with fluid and some may even accumulate in the alveoli. The distance that the gases have to diffuse is increased, transfer is slowed, and equilibrium may not be achieved before the blood leaves the lungs. Consequently, the blood does not become fully oxygenated.

An increase in the diffusion distance is more of a problem for O_2 than for CO_2 since CO_2 moves much more quickly and easily because of its chemical nature.

⑬
What might be the significance of the speed of equilibration? When would it be important?

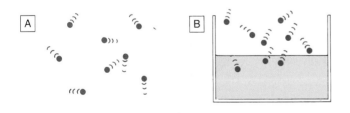
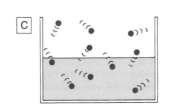

Figure 7.15
Equilibration of gas molecules between air and liquid. At equilibrium the number of molecules entering the liquid equals the number leaving.

A   B   C

Figure 7.17
The rate at which oxygen travels between the alveolar air and the blood depends on the gradient.

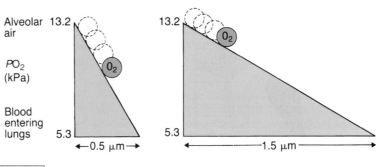

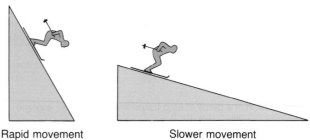

Rapid movement   Slower movement

THE BENDS

Although the most abundant gas in alveolar air is nitrogen, its concentration in body fluids is relatively low because it is not very soluble. If the pressure of nitrogen is increased, however, more of the gas is forced into solution. In divers working a long way below the surface of the sea, the weight of the water increases the pressures of the gases breathed and nitrogen dissolves in larger amounts in body fluids and body fat (nitrogen is especially soluble in fatty substances).

If a diver ascends from the depths very quickly, nitrogen is released so rapidly from the fat stores into the blood that bubbles of gas form in the body fluids, similar to the effect of opening a bottle of fizzy drink. Bubbles in drink are fine, but bubbles in blood vessels may obstruct blood flow causing ischaemia damage, pain, perhaps death.

Q: Why do you think a hyperbaric O_2 chamber is used for some divers after their return to the surface?

The area available for gas exchange will also limit the total amounts of O_2 and CO_2 that can be transferred per minute. Any pulmonary disease, such as emphysema, which severely reduces this area may result in inadequate oxygenation of the blood and retention of CO_2. ⑭

⑭
What other conditions may decrease surface area?

PERFUSION

The amounts of O_2 taken up into the body and the amounts of CO_2 that can be eliminated from it depend on the quantity of blood passing through the lungs (*perfusion*) as well as the ventilation of the lungs and the efficiency of gas exchange.

PULMONARY CIRCULATION

Blood is pumped from the right side of the heart via the *pulmonary artery* through the arteries, capillaries and veins of the *pulmonary circulation*. It is returned to the left side of the heart via the *pulmonary veins* (Fig. 7.18).

Flow

The pulmonary circulation has a very large blood flow. The entire output of the right side of the heart passes through the lungs. As the output of the right and left side of the heart is the same, the blood flow through the lungs is the same as the cardiac output (see Ch. 5), ranging between 5 litres/minute in a resting person to 25 litres/minute at the limits of physical exertion (see Ch. 17).

Pressures

Blood pressures in the pulmonary circulation are characteristically low. Pulmonary arterial pressure is only 24/8 mmHg as compared with 120/80 mmHg in the systemic circulation (see Ch. 5). This pressure is sufficient, however, to take the blood to all parts of the lungs.

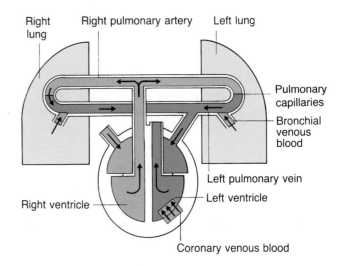

Figure 7.18
The heart and the pulmonary circulation. Oxygenated blood is delivered to the left heart via the pulmonary veins. Note that the airways receive their own blood supply (bronchial circulation) and that a little deoxygenated blood from the bronchial and coronary veins mixes with the oxygenated blood. Note also that only one pulmonary vein is shown entering the left atrium. In fact there are four.

The pressure of blood in the pulmonary capillaries (10 mmHg) is lower than in most other circulations. Consequently, the amount of tissue fluid formed is relatively small (see Ch. 3) and does not much distend the interstitial space. About 20 ml of excess tissue fluid spill over into the lymph vessels each hour.

However, if the hydrostatic pressure of the blood in the pulmonary capillaries increases acutely, as it may do in failure of the left side of the heart, the amount of tissue fluid formed increases greatly. Although the flow of lymph also increases, fluid accumulates in the interstitial space and eventually is forced into the alveoli. This accumulation of fluid, or pulmonary oedema, restricts ventilation of the lungs and impairs gas exchange. ⑮

Reservoir function

The pulmonary arterial vessels are unusually thin walled, making them much more distensible than other arteries. If pulmonary arterial pressure increases, the vessels distend (rather like veins do in the systemic circulation) and the volume of blood contained in the vessels increases. The pulmonary circulation thus acts as a blood reservoir and normally contains about 1 litre of blood.

The small amount of smooth muscle in the walls of the pulmonary vessels is innervated by sympathetic nerves. These nerves do not regulate the flow of blood through the lungs as they do in other parts of the circulatory system. Their function appears to be to stiffen the vessels, which changes the capacity of the vessels to hold blood and alters the size of the pulmonary reservoir.

Vasodilator effect of oxygen

The pulmonary circulation is the only place in the body where arteriolar smooth muscle dilates if there is an abundance of O_2 close by and constricts if there is a deficiency. In all other circulations, a lack of O_2 in the tissues promotes vasodilation, which increases the amount of O_2 to those tissues (see Ch. 5).

The distinctive response of the pulmonary arterioles is useful. If the concentration of O_2 in some alveoli is lower than average because of poor ventilation, the pulmonary arterioles supplying that part of the lung tissue constrict. This reduces the blood supply to that area and allows more blood to flow through other parts of the lung that have a higher O_2 concentration. ⑯

VENTILATION–PERFUSION BALANCE

It is important that well ventilated parts of the lung receive an adequate blood supply and that blood passing through the lungs does not escape oxygenation. In other words, for optimal gas exchange between alveoli and blood, perfusion should match ventilation in all parts of the lungs. If it does not, there may be surplus ventilation or perfusion.

Alveoli that are ventilated but not perfused with blood cannot participate in gas exchange (Fig. 7.19A). They add to the deadspace of the respiratory system. The volume of air in the respiratory system that does not participate in gas exchange is termed *physiological deadspace*. In health, this is nearly the same as the volume of air in the airways (*anatomical deadspace*; see p.

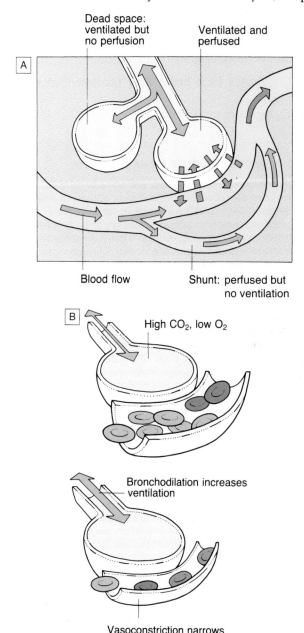

Figure 7.19

Matching ventilation and perfusion:
A How gross imbalances create deadspace and shunts
B The unit above is underventilated and overperfused, but the effects of low O_2 and high CO_2 on the blood vessels and bronchioles bring about a better match between ventilation and perfusion (unit below).

⑮
Can you explain how left heart failure results in increased pulmonary capillary pressure?

⑯
How many differences between the pulmonary and systemic circulations have you identified so far?

⑰
Can you think of an example of when this might occur?

⑱
What effect on ventilation would a chest infection have? Would a chest infection have any effect on perfusion?

148). But in disease, the physiological deadspace may be greater if there are underperfused alveoli. ⑰

If blood passes from the right heart to the left heart without coming into contact with ventilated alveoli, it also cannot pick up O_2 or off-load CO_2. A bypass route of this kind is termed a *shunt* (Fig. 7.19A). Shunts can occur in pneumonia because areas of consolidation in the lung may be perfused but not ventilated. ⑱

These situations represent extremes. Regional differences in ventilation and perfusion do exist even in health (see Ch. 17). At least two mechanisms help to match up ventilation and perfusion locally so that gas transfer occurs efficiently (Fig. 7.19B):

- O_2 regulates local blood flow (as described earlier, p. 151)
- CO_2 regulates local ventilation.

CHRONIC OBSTRUCTIVE AIRWAYS DISEASE

Chronic bronchitis, emphysema and some forms of asthma can all be described as types of *chronic obstructive airways disease* (COAD). COAD is a permanent and incurable condition in which the primary respiratory difficulty is with exhalation of air. Although asthma is generally characterised by intermittent and reversible episodes of bronchospasm, it may eventually develop into chronic bronchitis, emphysema, or both. Although the pathology of chronic bronchitis and emphysema is quite distinct, the two conditions are often found together with different degrees of severity.

The major feature of chronic bronchitis is excess mucus production from enlarged mucous glands in the bronchioles and bronchi. The mucus clogs up and partially blocks the already oedematous airways, increasing airway resistance and the work of breathing. This is often especially noticeable during expiration as the small soft airways become occluded more easily then, trapping air behind them. The reduction in ventilation with the retention of alveolar air produces a low alveolar PO_2 which is reflected in a low plasma PO_2. Again, because of the retention of air, the PCO_2 is often increased in both alveoli and plasma.

In emphysema (from the Greek, meaning bodily inflation), the walls of many of the alveoli have been destroyed and the remaining alveoli are abnormally large. This reduces not only the alveolar surface but also the pulmonary capillary bed. Because the total area over which gas exchange takes place is much reduced, breathlessness is one of the main features of emphysema.

As the tissue destruction also involves the elastic tissue in the lungs, the elastic recoil that assists in making normal expiration a passive rather than active process is lost also and expiration becomes more difficult. Again, air is trapped in the distorted, distended alveoli with a resultant increase in the amount of air left in the lungs after expiration (residual volume).

The priority for the nurse is to help these patients to breathe more easily, perhaps by finding the most comfortable position and teaching breathing techniques. Difficulty with breathing often causes anxiety and, here again, the nurse may help by teaching the patient to relax tense muscles to allow easier breathing.

The smooth muscle of the bronchioles relaxes in response to a build-up of CO_2. If ventilation of some alveoli is poor, the concentration of CO_2 increases locally and causes bronchodilation. This eases the flow of air into those alveoli and improves ventilation.

Transport of oxygen and carbon dioxide in the blood

Very large quantities of O_2 and CO_2 are carried safely and efficiently in the blood because of the presence of red cells (Fig. 7.20). Their single most important constituent is *haemoglobin*. This intricate molecule plays a vital role in the transport of both O_2 and CO_2.

OXYGEN TRANSPORT

O_2 is transported two ways:

- dissolved (1.5%)
- linked with haemoglobin (*oxyhaemoglobin*; 95%).

The amounts present in arterial and venous blood are shown in Table 7.3.

DISSOLVED OXYGEN

The solubility of a gas in a liquid depends on the chemical properties of both the gas and the liquid. O_2 is not very soluble in water and so only a little is carried dissolved in blood. The amount of O_2 dissolved is proportional to the partial pressure of the O_2 (PO_2) in the liquid. If the pressure is doubled, for example if the pressure of O_2 is increased from 13.2 kPa to 26.4 kPa by breathing in 40% O_2 instead of air, then the concentration of the dissolved gas is also doubled.

HAEMOGLOBIN

Haemoglobin is a complex molecule made up of several parts (Fig. 7.21) – two pairs of protein molecules (two *alpha* and two *beta chains*) each of which is wrapped around a *haem unit*. In the centre of each haem unit is one atom of iron to which O_2 binds.

The four protein chains (or subunits) are held together by weak chemical attractions between their constituent amino acids. The position and shape of the subunits can change according to the surrounding conditions (pH, CO_2, temperature). These changes alter the ability of the molecule to associate with O_2. One type of structure

Each gram of haemoglobin should, when fully saturated, carry 1.39 ml of O_2. If someone has a blood haemoglobin concentration of 15 g/100 ml, the maximum amount of O_2 that could be carried in blood (discounting the tiny amount in solution) is 20.8 ml per 100 ml.

Q: How would anaemia (see Ch. 4) affect the amount of O_2 carried?

Table 7.3 Oxygen and carbon dioxide in blood* (ml/litre)

	Arterial blood	Venous blood[†]
Oxygen		
– dissolved	3	1.2
– oxyhaemoglobin	195	150
Carbon dioxide		
– dissolved	26	30
– carbonic acid	[‡]	[‡]
– carbamino compounds	26	34
– hydrogen carbonate	438	463

* Assuming a haemoglobin concentration of 150 grams/litre.
[†] Composition of the mixture of venous blood entering the heart (mixed venous blood).
[‡] Very tiny amount.

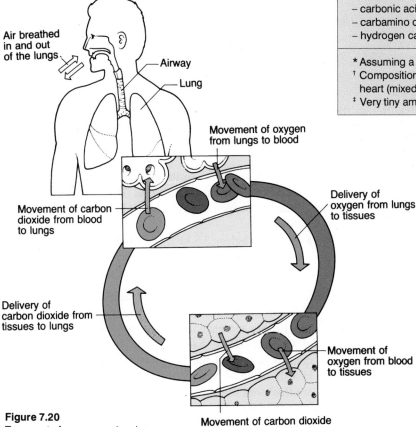

Figure 7.20
Transport of oxygen and carbon dioxide between the lungs and the tissues.

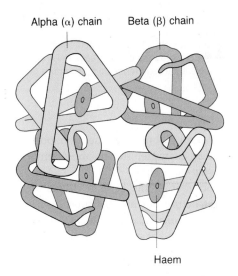

Figure 7.21
Component parts of a single molecule of haemoglobin.

makes binding easier whereas another makes it more difficult.

As each molecule of haemoglobin contains four atoms of iron, and each iron atom can link with one molecule of O_2, each molecule of haemoglobin can carry at most four molecules of O_2. When all four O_2 binding sites are occupied, haemoglobin is said to be *saturated* with O_2. The compound then formed is oxyhaemoglobin, which is bright red in colour, in contrast to deoxygenated haemoglobin, which is purplish. It is the change from *oxy*haemoglobin to *deoxy*haemoglobin that makes blood change colour between the arteries and the veins.

Different forms of haemoglobin

The site to which O_2 binds can be made unavailable to O_2 either because another substance has bound to it or because it has been altered chemically.

- Carbon monoxide binds very strongly to the O_2 binding site and forms *carboxyhaemoglobin*, which is bright red.
- Some drugs (such as sulphonamides) and chemicals (such as nitrites) can convert the iron into a form that can no longer bind O_2, thus forming *methaemoglobin*, which is very dark in colour. Small amounts exist in blood normally. [19]
- The protein components of haemoglobin may be abnormal. Sometimes an inherited mutant gene causes abnormal protein chains to be synthesised. Many such abnormal haemoglobins may be totally harmless but others are so different in properties from normal

[19]
How do we come in contact with nitrites? How common are they?

CARBON MONOXIDE POISONING

Carbon monoxide (CO) binds to haemoglobin in the same way that O_2 does, except that haemoglobin holds on to CO much more strongly – the affinity of haemoglobin for CO is about 250 times as great as for O_2. This means that when CO is inhaled, some haemoglobin that should combine with O_2 combines instead with CO. Only a relatively small concentration of the gas needs to be breathed for appreciable amounts of carboxyhaemoglobin to be formed in the blood.

CO may be formed by an ordinary gas fire that is not burning correctly or is inadequately ventilated. It is also present in car exhaust fumes and cigarette smoke – as much as 16% of the total haemoglobin of smokers can be bound to CO.

CO poisoning is particularly dangerous because it can go unnoticed, both externally and internally. If sufficient amounts of CO are breathed for a prolonged time, the person concerned will suffer progressive O_2 deficiency while maintaining apparently rosy features (carboxyhaemoglobin is bright red). The situation may not be identified clinically, either, because routine blood gases tests measure only dissolved O_2 and not that bound to haemoglobin. Similarly, the lack of O_2 bound to haemoglobin is not detected by receptors in the body, breathing is not stimulated, and the individual experiences no discomfort (see also Ch. 11).

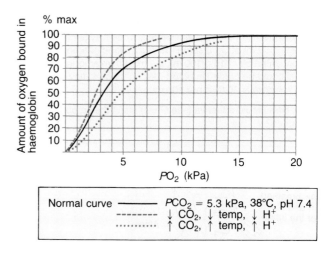

Figure 7.22
Amount of oxygen carried by haemoglobin at different pressures of oxygen and under different conditions (oxygen–haemoglobin dissociation curves).

- The PO_2 has to fall quite a bit before the amount of O_2 transported is much reduced. This ensures that very little O_2 escapes from the blood between the lungs and the tissues.
- At a PO_2 below 5.3 kPa, O_2 is released very easily. As tissue PO_2 may be only 1.5 to 2.5 kPa, a lot of O_2 will be off-loaded just where it is needed.

One further point should be noted. Because haemoglobin is fully saturated with O_2 at a PO_2 of 13.2 kPa, any further increase in PO_2 cannot increase the amount of O_2 carried by haemoglobin. It is full up. Consequently, a part of the lung having a high PO_2 (say 18.2 kPa) because of over-ventilation cannot compensate for another area that is badly ventilated and has a low PO_2 (say 8.2 kPa). In respiratory disease, patches of badly ventilated lung will always cause incomplete oxygenation of the blood.

haemoglobin that the transport of O_2 is impaired (for example, the haemoglobin present in *sickle cell anaemia* – HbS).

- Sometimes the protein chains are entirely normal in structure but are not produced in the right amounts. Occasionally, either the alpha or the beta chain is not produced at all. This group of disorders is termed the *thalassaemias*.

OXYGEN–HAEMOGLOBIN DISSOCIATION CURVE

The shape of the curve and its significance

The amount of O_2 bound to haemoglobin depends on the PO_2 of the blood (Fig. 7.22). When the PO_2 is low, most of the O_2 binding sites are empty. At higher pressures, more of the vacant sites become filled until eventually all are occupied with O_2.

The relationship between the amount of O_2 bound to haemoglobin and the PO_2 is *sigmoid* in shape (looks like a lazy 'S') because of the way that the protein subunits interact with one another and the effect this has on the affinity of O_2 for the binding site.

The shape of the curve is important for the uptake of O_2 in the lungs and its delivery to the tissues:

- First, at a PO_2 of 13.2 kPa (similar to that of the blood leaving the lungs), haemoglobin is completely saturated with O_2. Therefore, blood leaving the lungs is normally fully oxygenated.

Influential factors

Several factors influence the way that O_2 binds to haemoglobin, making it either easier or more difficult for O_2 to bind at any given PO_2. These include:

- CO_2
- H^+
- temperature
- 2,3-biphosphoglycerate (2,3-BPG for short).

An increase in any of these causes O_2 to be unloaded more easily, whereas a decrease enhances O_2 binding (Fig. 7.22). CO_2, H^+ and temperature are all slightly

The amount of 2,3-BPG decreases gradually in blood stored for transfusion. Older blood may therefore not be as good at releasing O_2 as fresh blood.

higher in the tissues than in the lungs. Therefore, these factors promote the off-loading of O_2 in the tissues and facilitate the uptake of O_2 in the lungs.

2,3-BPG is formed inside the red cell as a by-product of metabolism. Its production is increased in situations of chronic O_2 deficiency, such as anaemia.

CARBON DIOXIDE TRANSPORT

CO_2 reacts chemically with several constituents of blood and is thus carried in several forms:

- dissolved as CO_2 (5–6%)
- as carbonic acid (H_2CO_3)
- as hydrogen carbonate ion (HCO_3^-)
- linked with proteins (*carbamino compounds*, such as carbaminohaemoglobin).

The amounts present in arterial and venous blood are shown in Table 7.3.

CHEMICAL REACTIONS

CO_2 reacts with water to form carbonic acid:

$$CO_2 + H_2O \rightarrow H_2CO_3$$

The carbonic acid splits up (*dissociates*) to form H^+ and HCO_3^-. These reactions occur throughout the body, not just in the blood. However, the process occurs very efficiently in the red cells for several reasons (Fig. 7.23):

- Red cells contain the enzyme *carbonic anhydrase*, which facilitates (*catalyses*) the reaction between CO_2 and H_2O.
- Deoxyhaemoglobin, formed when O_2 is released to the tissues, acts as a buffer (see Ch. 12) and picks up much of the H^+ formed. This encourages more carbonic acid to split up and more to be formed from

CO_2 and H_2O. The result is that a lot of CO_2 is converted into HCO_3^-.

- HCO_3^- does not accumulate in the red cell but passes out into the plasma in exchange for chloride.

All these processes are reversible. In the tissues, where the concentration of CO_2 is high, the bias is towards the formation of HCO_3^-.

In the lungs, HCO_3^- is converted back into CO_2. Oxygenation of haemoglobin in the lungs causes the H^+ ions that had been bound to it in the tissues to be released. These combine with HCO_3^- to form carbonic acid again, and this in turn yields CO_2 and H_2O.

CARBON DIOXIDE DISSOCIATION CURVE

The amount of CO_2 carried in blood increases almost in proportion to the PCO_2. It does not saturate. If the PCO_2 is high, more CO_2 is carried, almost without limit (Fig. 7.24). One consequence of this is that over-ventilated

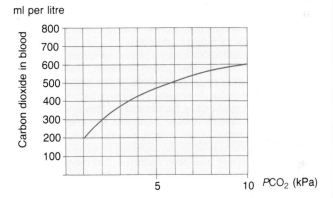

Figure 7.24
Amount of carbon dioxide carried in blood at different pressures of CO_2 (CO_2 dissociation curve).

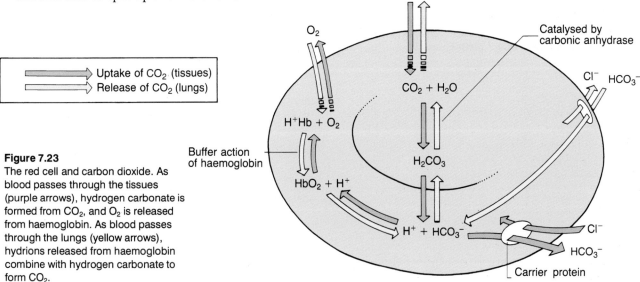

Figure 7.23
The red cell and carbon dioxide. As blood passes through the tissues (purple arrows), hydrogen carbonate is formed from CO_2, and O_2 is released from haemoglobin. As blood passes through the lungs (yellow arrows), hydrions released from haemoglobin combine with hydrogen carbonate to form CO_2.

and under-ventilated alveoli may compensate for one another in a way that is not possible for O_2. Thus, an imbalance of ventilation and perfusion does not necessarily cause retention of CO_2 in the blood.

RESPIRATORY DISEASE AND THE ENVIRONMENT

With every breath, we inhale not only air but also dust and other pollutants, such as car exhaust fumes, which may cause or contribute to respiratory disease. In addition, some people increase their exposure to lung irritants by smoking, while others may work in environments with particularly high levels of irritant substances (such as dust from coke, iron foundry pollutants and asbestos). Both smoking and occupational exposure to dust and pollution have been linked to increased risk for chronic obstructive airways disease (COAD; see p. 152). The home as well as the work environment may affect respiratory health, with old, poorly maintained housing, which is often damp and cold, identified as particularly unhealthy.

Dust or smoke that gets into the lungs stimulates mucus secretion, which is normally cleared by the action of the cilia. However, the irritants coat the cilia so that they can no longer beat normally, and the cells eventually die. The presence of the irritants and the excess mucus causes inflammation and narrowing of the airways and also provides a site for potential infection.

Cigarette smoke also contains carbon monoxide, which binds to haemoglobin (see Carbon Monoxide Poisoning, p. 154) as well as other chemicals that cause further bronchoconstriction. Eventually, the airways become permanently narrowed by the formation of fibrous tissue as inflammation persists (*chronic bronchitis*). Moreover, the prolonged irritation slowly destroys alveolar tissue, thus reducing the lung area for gas exchange (*emphysema*).

Once the alveoli have been destroyed, they cannot be repaired, but removing the source of irritation (by stopping smoking or even changing jobs) can at least prevent further damage. Giving up smoking is not so easy, though, and requires an understanding attitude. In many cases, smoking can be considered a true addiction and withdrawal symptoms can be quite distressing. Success depends on a number of factors, including the will and determination of the smoker and the availability of social and family support.

The best strategy, of course, is to decrease the risk of lung disease as much as possible by avoiding exposure to environmental irritants in the first place: use protective equipment at work and DON'T SMOKE.

KEY POINTS

What you should now understand about respiration:

- how we breathe and what we breathe
- factors that make breathing easy or difficult
- why a person's pattern of breathing may change in disease
- how respiratory function can be assessed
- the basis of some forms of respiratory disorder and their treatment
- what is meant by blood gases and the factors that affect them
- how respiration is affected by cardiac malfunction
- how gas transport in blood is affected by the environment and by disease.

REFERENCES AND FURTHER READING

Boore J R P, Champion R, Ferguson M C (eds) 1987 Nursing the physically ill adult. Churchill Livingstone, Edinburgh

Pedley T J, Schroter R C, Sudlow M F 1970 The prediction of pressure drop and variation of resistance within the human bronchial airways. Respiratory Physiology 9: 387–405

Staub N C 1991 Basic respiratory physiology. Churchill Livingstone, Edinburgh
(Very useful textbook for further study of human respiration. Includes questions and answers and provides lists of further reading)

Watson J E, Royle J R 1987 Watson's Medical–surgical nursing and related physiology, 3rd edn. Baillière Tindall, London, ch 16.

Weibel E R 1963 Morphometry of the human lung. Springer Verlag, Berlin, p 111

West J B 1990 Respiratory physiology – the essentials, 4th edn. Williams & Wilkins, Baltimore
(Concise textbook, explaining respiratory function in more detail. Includes questions and answers and further reading)

West J B 1992 Pulmonary pathophysiology – the essentials, 4th edn. Williams & Wilkins, Baltimore
(Companion to West 1990. Describes lung function tests, what happens to respiratory function in respiratory diseases, and the principles involved in oxygen therapy and mechanical ventilation)

Whipp B J (ed) 1987 The control of breathing in man. Manchester University Press, Manchester

Wilson K J W 1987 Ross & Wilson Anatomy and physiology in health and illness, 6th edn. Churchill Livingstone, Edinburgh, p 119

Chapter 8
URINARY SYSTEM

The main function of the urinary system is the elimination of water-soluble substances. Each day your kidneys filter over 150 litres of fluid from the blood plasma (about the same volume as would fill a bath). Most of this fluid, containing vital constituents such as electrolytes, nutrients and water, is recovered by the kidneys and returned to the blood, leaving only 1 to 2 litres of fluid containing water-soluble waste products to be excreted as urine. The amounts of water and electrolytes excreted by the kidneys are regulated by a variety of mechanisms.

The urine formed continually by the kidneys collects in the distensible urinary bladder. This is emptied periodically under the control of the autonomic and somatic nervous systems.

STRUCTURE

There are two kidneys, each weighing about 140 g, situated at the back of the abdomen (Fig. 8.1). Urine passes from the kidneys, through the ureters, to the urinary bladder. Each kidney is made up of about 1 million tiny tubes (*nephrons*), which are richly supplied with blood, and which empty into a smaller number of collecting ducts. ①

NEPHRONS

Each nephron consists of a long tube, closed at one end and open at the other, made up of four sections (Fig. 8.2A):

- Bowman's capsule
- proximal convoluted tubule
- loop of Henle
- distal convoluted tubule.

Arrangement
The tubule is twisted into a characteristic shape crucial to its function (Fig. 8.2A). Part of the distal convoluted tubule, the *macula densa*, lies near to Bowman's capsule of the same tubule (Fig. 8.2B). The macula densa,

① *Where are the kidneys situated in relation to the peritoneum? What is the significance of this position when surgery of the kidney is carried out?*

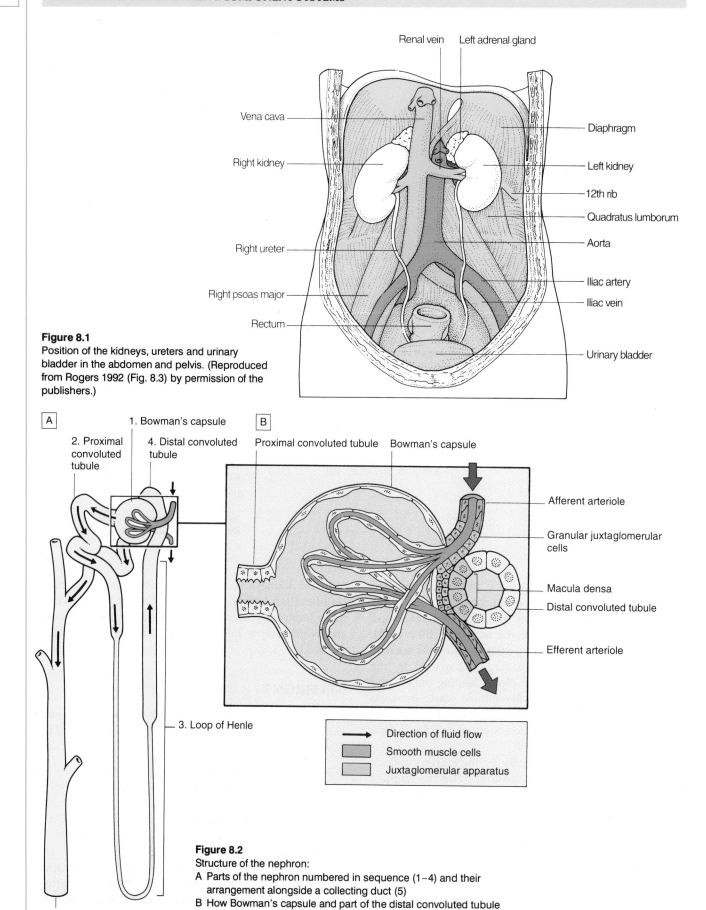

Figure 8.1
Position of the kidneys, ureters and urinary bladder in the abdomen and pelvis. (Reproduced from Rogers 1992 (Fig. 8.3) by permission of the publishers.)

Figure 8.2
Structure of the nephron:
A Parts of the nephron numbered in sequence (1–4) and their arrangement alongside a collecting duct (5)
B How Bowman's capsule and part of the distal convoluted tubule are arranged to form the juxtaglomerular apparatus.

This 'kidney slice' is sometimes called a *coronal section*. You may be able to suggest other organs where a coronal section is useful for anatomical study.

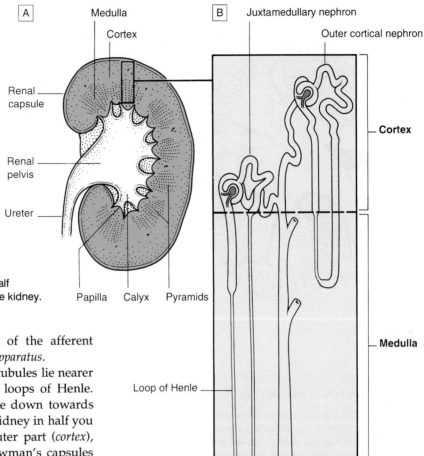

Figure 8.3
Structure of the kidney:
A Structures visible when the kidney is cut in half
B Types of nephron and their position within the kidney.

together with adjacent granular cells of the afferent arteriole, is termed the *juxtaglomerular apparatus*.

Bowman's capsules and convoluted tubules lie nearer to the surface of the kidney than the loops of Henle. These loops dip inwards and converge down towards the centre of the kidney. If you slice a kidney in half you will see that the appearance of the outer part (*cortex*), where the convoluted tubules and Bowman's capsules arc, differs from the inner section (*medulla*), occupied by the loops of Henle (Fig. 8.3A).

Types

All the nephrons have the same constituent parts but they do differ. Those with Bowman's capsules in the outer cortex have very short loops of Henle which do not extend very far into the medulla. Others, with Bowman's capsules sited close to the medulla, *juxtamedullary* nephrons, have long loops (Fig. 8.3B).

COLLECTING DUCTS, PELVIS AND URETERS

Fluid from several nephrons flows into the *collecting ducts*. These empty into large drainage vessels (*calyces*) at the *papillae* of the *medullary pyramids*. Urine flows from the calyces via the *pelvis* of the kidney into the *ureter*. The whole of each kidney is enclosed by a capsule of connective tissue (*renal capsule*).

RENAL BLOOD VESSELS

Arteries

Within each kidney the renal artery branches to form several *interlobar arteries*, which divide the medulla into sections (*medullary pyramids*) and carry the blood to the

boundary between the medulla and the cortex (Fig. 8.4). At this point each interlobar artery gives rise to *arcuate arteries* that run along the border between the medulla and the cortex. From these, small *interlobular arteries* carry the blood up into the cortex. Branching off the interlobular arteries at multiple points are tiny vessels the *afferent arterioles* ('afferent' means 'carrying to') each of which supplies blood to a tuft of capillaries (*glomerular capillaries*) lodged within the expanded end of the nephron (*Bowman's capsule*). ②

Capillaries

Glomerular capillaries

The glomerular capillaries fit into Bowman's capsule rather like a hand inserted into an incubator, or isolation chamber, through a glove. The indented part of Bowman's capsule (the glove of the incubator in the analogy) is wrapped around the glomerular capillaries (the hand). The two together form the *glomerulus* (Fig. 8.5A). The indented layer of Bowman's capsule consists of distinctive cells (*podocytes*). These have many 'feet' (*pous* in Greek means foot) that make contact with the basement membrane of the endothelial cells of the

② *What percentage of the cardiac output supplies the kidneys in a resting person?*

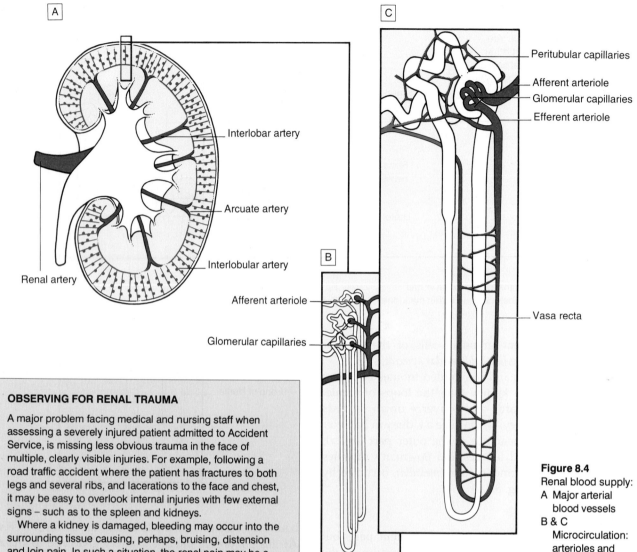

Figure 8.4
Renal blood supply:
A Major arterial
   blood vessels
B & C
   Microcirculation:
   arterioles and
   capillaries.

OBSERVING FOR RENAL TRAUMA

A major problem facing medical and nursing staff when assessing a severely injured patient admitted to Accident Service, is missing less obvious trauma in the face of multiple, clearly visible injuries. For example, following a road traffic accident where the patient has fractures to both legs and several ribs, and lacerations to the face and chest, it may be easy to overlook internal injuries with few external signs – such as to the spleen and kidneys.

Where a kidney is damaged, bleeding may occur into the surrounding tissue causing, perhaps, bruising, distension and loin pain. In such a situation, the renal pain may be a dull ache, and overlooked by the patient (and carers) in the face of much more acute pain from, say, broken bones. Severe trauma may cause the kidney to tear away from its major blood vessels so that haemorrhage is massive, and death can swiftly ensue. (Recollect what proportion of the cardiac output goes to the kidneys.)

Damage within the renal capsule may lead to visible *haematuria* (blood in the urine) and the Accident Service nurse may be asked to collect serial specimens of urine. (If the patient does not, or cannot, pass urine he may be catheterised in order to obtain a specimen for examination. Catheterisation is not carried out if damage to the urethra is suspected. Why not?)

The reason for obtaining serial specimens of urine where kidney damage is suspected is as follows. The first specimen obtained may be negative to blood, either from naked eye inspection or on testing using reagent strips. However, that first specimen consists of urine that may have been present in the bladder for some time. Damage to one of the kidneys may result in a small flow of blood which, at first, occupies the kidney pelvis and ureter. A second specimen of urine may subsequently reveal visible haematuria, as bleeding from the kidney reaches the bladder and is drained by the urinary catheter.

capillary wall (Fig. 8.5B). Fluid filtered from the capillaries passes across the endothelial cell layer, then the basement membrane and finally through gaps between the 'feet' of the podocytes, into the space inside Bowman's capsule itself (equivalent to the interior of the incubator in the analogy).

Peritubular capillaries
Blood leaves the glomerulus through a vessel which has the structure of an arteriole and is termed the *efferent arteriole* ('efferent' means 'carrying away from'). This gives rise to another set of capillaries, *peritubular capillaries*, which surround the convoluted tubules (Fig. 8.4C).

The juxtamedullary nephrons, which have long loops of Henle, have a specialised arrangement of peritubular vessels known as the *vasa recta* (Fig. 8.4C). These vessels do not branch very much. Instead they extend straight down into the medulla, following the line of the loop of

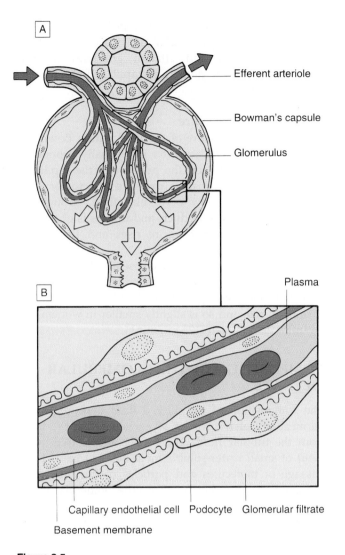

Figure 8.5
The glomerulus:
A Structure
B Microstructure of the glomerular filter.

Henle. Near the tip of the loop they double back towards the cortex, again following the route taken by the tubule.

Veins

From the peritubular capillaries, *interlobular veins* carry the blood back to *arcuate veins*, *interlobar veins*, and then the *renal vein*, along the same route, in reverse, as the arteries.

HOW FLUID IS FILTERED

The first step in the formation of urine is *glomerular filtration*, the formation of a filtrate of plasma. This filtrate contains all the constituents of plasma except the plasma proteins. The processes involved are the same as those involved in the formation of tissue fluid elsewhere in the body (see Ch. 5). However, the barrier consists of the capillary wall and basement membrane plus the podocytes (Fig. 8.5B). It is practically impermeable to plasma proteins. The blood flow to the kidneys is considerable (1200 ml/min) and capillary pressures are high. Consequently, the volume of fluid filtered is large (120 ml/min).

In some renal diseases, such as *nephrotic syndrome*, there is severe loss of protein in the urine. This is because of damage to the glomerular capillaries. Loss of protein leads to a low serum albumin level.

Q: What effect will a low serum albumin have on the formation of interstitial fluid?

HYDROSTATIC AND ONCOTIC PRESSURES

The forces that are involved in the filtration of fluid by the kidneys (Fig. 8.6) are:

- the difference in hydrostatic pressure between the fluid in the glomerular capillary and that within Bowman's capsule
- the oncotic pressure of the plasma, created by plasma proteins and the glomerular barrier.

The distinctive feature about the balance of forces in the kidney is the high hydrostatic pressure within the glomerular capillaries (45–50 mmHg).

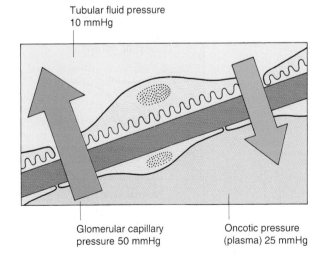

Tubular fluid pressure
10 mmHg

Glomerular capillary
pressure 50 mmHg

Oncotic pressure
(plasma) 25 mmHg

Hydrostatic pressure driving fluid out	= 50 - 10 mmHg	= 40 mmHg
Oncotic pressure drawing fluid in		= 25 mmHg
Net pressure driving filtration	= 40 - 25 mmHg	= 15 mmHg

Figure 8.6
The balance of forces determining glomerular filtration.

Glomerular capillary pressure

The glomerular capillary pressure is the highest normally present in any capillary bed in the body. As such, it normally exceeds the oncotic pressure of the plasma at *all points* of the glomerular capillaries, not just at the 'arterial' end as in other capillaries (see Ch. 5). Consequently, under normal circumstances, some fluid is driven out of the plasma across the glomerular wall and none is drawn back in.

The uniquely high capillary pressure is caused by the resistance offered by the efferent arterioles. The driving pressure for filtration is affected by constriction and dilation of the efferent arterioles as well as the afferent arterioles. Both sets of vessels are innervated by sympathetic nerves and are influenced by hormones such as angiotensin and adrenaline.

Afferent arteriole

If the afferent arteriole constricts, the hydrostatic pressure in the capillaries decreases and the rate of fluid filtration decreases also. This happens if there is a reflex increase in the activity of the sympathetic nerves innervating the vessels, as in haemorrhage (see Chs 5 and 13, Fig. 13.8).

Control of efferent arteriole

The driving pressure is also affected by the ease with which blood is able to leave the glomerulus, which depends on the degree of dilation or constriction of the efferent arteriole. If this vessel constricts, the pressure of blood upstream in the glomerulus increases, and *glomerular filtration rate* (GFR) will also increase.

If both afferent and efferent arterioles constrict simultaneously then glomerular capillary pressure, and GFR, may not change.

Tubular fluid pressure

The hydrostatic pressure of the fluid within Bowman's capsule (*tubular fluid pressure*) is normally around 10 mmHg. This counteracts the pressure in the capillaries so that the net hydrostatic pressure is actually 35 to 40 mmHg. If the flow of tubular fluid through the nephrons, the collecting ducts and ureters is obstructed in any way, tubular pressure rises and the rate of filtration decreases.

Factors which increase or decrease filtration across the glomerulus are summarised in Figure 8.7. On average, GFR (both kidneys together) is 120 ml/minute. It varies with body size and so is slightly smaller in women (110 ml/min) than in men (125 ml/min).

COMPOSITION OF THE GLOMERULAR FILTRATE

The composition of the filtered fluid depends on the permeability of the barrier layers separating the blood from the tubular fluid. The barrier allows free movement of small water-soluble molecules but restricts the passage of molecules and particles of the size of the plasma proteins and bigger. Thus the glomerular filtrate

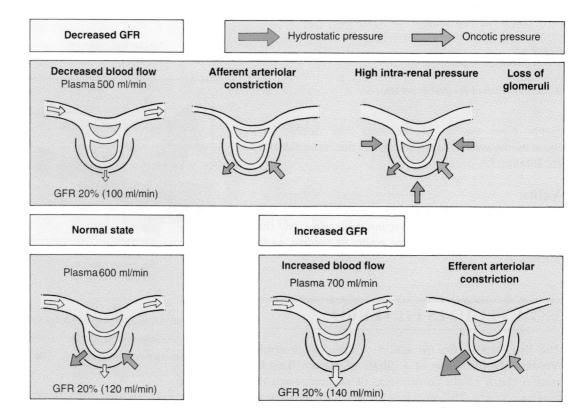

Figure 8.7
The factors decreasing and increasing glomerular filtration rate (GFR).

OBSERVING FOR RENAL FAILURE

Urine production relies on an adequate pressure of blood within the renal arteries. A fall in blood pressure, if severe or sufficiently prolonged, may cause damage to renal tissue, and the patient suffers *acute renal failure*. This condition can be fatal but, if treated swiftly, is reversible. Swift treatment relies on nursing observations of blood pressure and urine output, which can inform medical staff that renal failure is likely. Steps are then taken to prevent it.

Patients following major surgery, myocardial infarction or severe burns, for example, have frequent observations made of their pulse and blood pressure. A prolonged systolic pressure below about 60 to 70 mmHg would be regarded as possibly heralding acute renal failure. In such cases, urine output would be measured hourly; daily totals of fluid balance are insufficient. Such a severely ill patient will probably be catheterised, perhaps for the sole reason of assessing urine formation. Special collecting chambers are available, which attach to the catheter tubing and measure small amounts of urine.

Swift treatment to improve a patient's blood pressure should result in an improvement in urine output. Such treatment might include a blood transfusion to restore blood volume following severe haemorrhage. In some cases of heart failure, drugs such as dobutamine may be given intravenously to improve cardiac performance and therefore renal blood flow.

Following surgery, a brief period of *oliguria* (reduced urine output) is to be expected. (Why?) Where blood pressure is maintained, and blood volume restored, this period of oliguria should not exceed 2 to 3 hours.

Q: What are the reflex effects on the circulation of a low blood pressure and how might this affect renal blood flow and GFR?

HOW VITAL CONSTITUENTS OF THE FILTRATE ARE RECOVERED

The second step in the formation of urine is the recovery of constituents of the filtrate that must be retained within the body. These are:

- nutrients (glucose and amino acids)
- electrolytes (sodium, potassium, chloride, etc.)
- hydrogen carbonate
- water.

These constituents are returned to the blood in the peritubular capillaries from the tubular fluid in the convoluted tubules, loop of Henle and collecting ducts. ③

③
What foodstuffs are a good source of potassium and sodium? What might be the effects on the body of a significant loss of these electrolytes?

NUTRIENTS: GLUCOSE AND AMINO ACIDS

If the composition of the glomerular filtrate is compared with the composition of fluid at the end of the proximal convoluted tubule (PCT) (Table 8.1) it can be seen that almost all of the glucose and the amino acids filtered at the glomerulus have been removed by the time the fluid reaches the end of the PCT. Normally, only minute quantities of these substances, undetectable by routine clinical methods, are lost in the urine. They are recovered by carrier-mediated transport. The transport mechanisms are very similar to those described for the absorption of glucose and amino acids in the small intestine (see Ch. 6).

There is an upper limit to the amounts that can be transported by the cells. If they are presented with too much glucose or amino acids, some is not recovered, and substantial losses of these substances occur in the urine (*glycosuria* and *amino-aciduria*). The amount of glucose lost (excreted) in the urine at different plasma concentrations of glucose is shown in Figure 8.8. At normal fasting concentrations of plasma glucose (3.5–5.5 mmol/l), urinary glucose is virtually undetectable. Above

contains all the constituents of plasma with the exception of most plasma proteins. A little protein does get through, just as some escapes into the tissue space in other capillary beds, but the amounts are not large. If the permeability of the barrier increases, as in the *nephrotic syndrome*, the glomerular filtrate contains appreciable amounts of protein which then appears in the urine (*proteinuria*).

Table 8.1 Approximate composition of the tubular fluid at different sites along the nephron		Glomerular filtrate	End of proximal convoluted tubule	End of distal convoluted tubule
Albumin	g/l	0.2	0.0	0.0
Glucose		5	0.5	0.0
Amino acids		2	0.2	0.0
Sodium (Na)	mmol/l	135	135	40–135
Potassium (K)		4	4	4–40
Chloride (Cl)		115	135	35–135
Hydrogen carbonate (HCO$_3$)		25	6	1–10
Osmotic pressure	mosm/kgH$_2$O	300	300	80–300
Fluid flow rate	ml/min	120	40	5–10

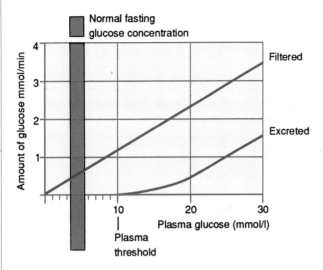

Figure 8.8
Urinary losses of glucose in humans at different plasma glucose concentrations. At high glucose concentrations (>20 mmol/l) the difference between the amount of glucose filtered and that excreted is the maximum the tubules can absorb (Tm). (Adapted from Emslie-Smith et al 1988.)

THE DIABETIC PATIENT

Glycosuria is one of the signs of *diabetes mellitus*. Lack of effective insulin production by the pancreas (see Ch. 10) means that glucose in the blood cannot be utilised by all tissues. Blood glucose levels consequently rise until the renal threshold is reached and exceeded – glycosuria then occurs. This can happen suddenly in youngsters (mostly boys) or occur more gradually in, principally, middle-aged or elderly, overweight women. (This is an extremely simplified summary of events. You may wish to read a more detailed medical–nursing text such as Boore et al 1987, pp. 492–511.)

The osmotic force of high levels of glucose excreted in urine leads to *polyuria* – excessive urine volumes. Reabsorption of water from the tubules is diminished because of the osmotic pull of glucose in the glomerular filtrate. Increased water, as well as glucose, enters the collecting tubules and is eventually excreted as urine. This loss of water from the body leads to dehydration. Reduced blood volume is balanced by withdrawal of fluid from the interstitial compartment into the blood, which in turn leads to movement of water from body cells into the interstitial compartment. In other words, there is a shift of water out of the cells into the bloodstream and then into the urine.

One of the first signs of diabetes mellitus in a young child might be excessive drinking to counteract an intense thirst (the osmoreceptors in the thirst centre being stimulated by an increase in the osmolarity of blood passing through it). Parents may then notice increased visits to the toilet. A child may even start bedwetting at night, having previously outgrown this, because of the increased urine production.

Urine is tested for glucose by reagent strips that change colour according to the level of glucose present. Incidentally, one of the earliest tests for diabetes was tasting a sufferer's urine for sugar, or leaving a container of the urine outside, where it attracted bees because of its sweetness. Present-day nurses may prefer modern scientific methods.

---

10 mmol/l appreciable amounts of glucose begin to appear, and the urinary output increases in proportion to the increase in plasma glucose concentration.

The plasma concentration of glucose at which the increase in output begins (Fig. 8.8) is the *plasma threshold*. As nephrons, like people, are not identical, some reach their maximum absorptive capacity for glucose before others. So, at first, just a trickle of glucose appears in the urine before most nephrons are overloaded.

ELECTROLYTES (SODIUM, POTASSIUM, CHLORIDE, CALCIUM)

About 70% of the electrolytes filtered at the glomerulus are returned to the blood in the peritubular capillaries surrounding the proximal convoluted tubule. Most of the remainder is recovered into the blood by distal parts of the nephron and peritubular capillaries. The amounts of electrolytes recovered and excreted are adjusted according to need.

Proximal convoluted tubule

From Table 8.1, it can be seen that the concentrations of sodium, potassium and chloride are almost the same at the end of the proximal convoluted tubule (PCT) as they were in the glomerular filtrate. However, the volume of fluid emerging from the proximal convoluted tubules (~40 ml/min) is much less than the volume entering them at the glomerulus (~120 ml/min). Thus about 70% of the electrolytes that were filtered at the glomerulus have in fact been removed from the tubular fluid by the end of the PCT.

Mechanisms
Some of the ways in which the electrolytes are returned to the blood include (Fig. 8.9):

- passive transport (either by diffusion or swept along with the water absorbed by osmosis)
- carrier-mediated transport.

Control
Most of this absorption is not under hormonal control. In that sense it is unregulated and is therefore often referred to as *obligatory*. However, the recovery of calcium is influenced by a variety of factors including the hormones *parathyrin* and *calcitonin* (see Ch. 10) and the concentration of phosphate in the tubular fluid.

Distal convoluted tubule

In Table 8.1, it can be seen that the composition of the tubular fluid at the end of the distal convoluted tubule (DCT) varies. The fluid here may be *hypotonic* (osmotic pressure less than plasma) or *isotonic* (osmotic pressure equal to plasma) (see Ch. 5). This part of the nephron

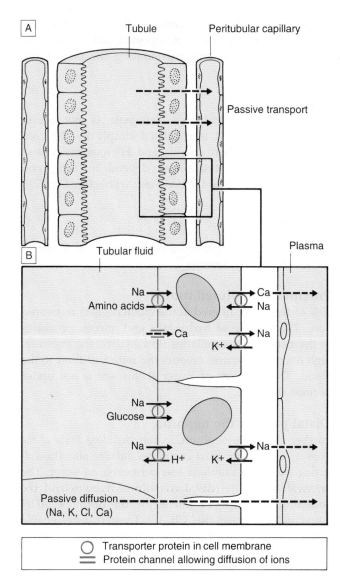

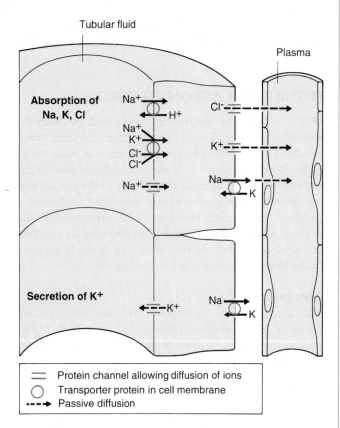

Figure 8.9
Ways in which electrolytes are absorbed into the blood from the tubular fluid by cells of the proximal convoluted tubule.

Figure 8.10
Absorption and secretion of electrolytes by cells of the distal convoluted tubule.

adjusts the amounts of sodium, potassium, water, and acid and alkali that are recovered or excreted, and so helps to maintain normal water, electrolyte and acid–base balance within the body (see Chs 12 and 13). Some of the processes involved in electrolyte transport here are summarised in Figure 8.10.

Control

The absorption of sodium by the distal convoluted tubule is increased by the steroid hormone *aldosterone* (see Chs 10 and 13). Aldosterone stimulates the synthesis of some of the transporter proteins that carry sodium. If aldosterone secretion increases, the recovery of sodium chloride is gradually enhanced over several hours. This allows the excretion of these electrolytes to be adjusted, for example, according to long-term variations in the dietary intake of sodium (see Ch. 13). Aldosterone also increases the urinary excretion of potassium.

Other parts of the nephron

Substantial amounts of sodium, potassium and chloride (25% of that filtered) are absorbed into the blood from the loop of Henle. Small amounts of electrolytes are also recovered by the collecting ducts (Table 8.2). Potassium differs from sodium in that some is added to the tubular fluid by cells of the distal convoluted tubules. Thus the amount of potassium excreted per day (150 mmol) is as large as the amount of sodium excreted (also about 150 mmol) even though there is much more sodium than potassium in the glomerular filtrate (see Table 8.1). This

Table 8.2 Amounts of sodium recovered by different parts of the nephron (as % filtered load)	
	%
Proximal convoluted tubule	66
Loop of Henle	25
Distal convoluted tubule	4
Collecting duct	4
Total	>99%

high urinary excretion of potassium is needed to balance the high dietary intake of potassium (see Ch. 13).

HYDROGEN CARBONATE (HCO₃⁻)

HCO_3^- is, like the electrolytes, recovered by both the proximal and distal convoluted tubules, but the extent to which it is recovered depends on the acid–base status of the body (see Ch. 12). If the extracellular fluid (ECF) is more acid than normal, then all the hydrogen carbonate filtered at the glomerulus is recovered, and none is excreted in the urine. However, if the extracellular fluid is more alkaline than normal then the tubular recovery of hydrogen carbonate decreases and some is excreted in the urine, making the urine alkaline. ④

④
Under what conditions might a person's extracellular fluid become more acid than normal? Think about both diet and medical conditions.

Mechanism

The absorption of hydrogen carbonate relies on the presence of the enzyme *carbonic anhydrase* both within and on the luminal surface of the tubular cells. As in red blood cells (see Ch. 7), it catalyses the reversible conversion of CO_2 and H_2O into carbonic acid. Hydrogen carbonate in the tubular fluid combines with H^+ ions, which are transported into the tubular fluid in exchange for sodium, to form carbonic acid (Fig. 8.11). Carbonic acid is rapidly converted into CO_2 and H_2O. CO_2

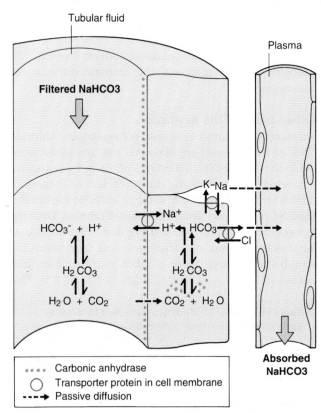

Figure 8.11
Absorption of sodium hydrogen carbonate from the tubular fluid into the blood.

diffuses easily into the tubular cells and is used to re-form HCO_3^-, which is transported out of the cells into the interstitial fluid surrounding the peritubular capillaries.

Control

The recovery of hydrogen carbonate is not under hormonal control. It is regulated simply by the concentrations of carbon dioxide and H^+ ions inside and outside the kidney cells. These depend, in turn, upon the acid–base status of the body as a whole (see Ch. 12).

WATER

Throughout the nephron, the absorption of water is driven entirely by osmosis.

Proximal convoluted tubule

70% of the water filtered at the glomerulus is recovered here. The balance of hydrostatic and oncotic pressures in the peritubular capillaries (low hydrostatic pressure, high oncotic pressure) favours the return of fluid to the blood. The recovery of water at this site is not under hormonal control.

Distal parts of the nephron

Further along the nephron, in the *ascending limbs of the loops of Henle*, the *distal convoluted tubules* and the *collecting ducts*, the tubule is less permeable to water. The permeability of the distal convoluted tubules and the collecting ducts can be altered by the hormone ADH (*antidiuretic hormone*) (see Ch. 10). These features enable water to be eliminated or conserved according to need.

Control: eliminating water

As the tubular fluid passes up the ascending limb of the loop of Henle, which is relatively impermeable to water, sodium chloride is removed and the fluid becomes dilute (Fig. 8.12). It becomes hypotonic (see p. 000). When the distal convoluted tubules and the collecting ducts are impermeable to water, water is not absorbed here even though a substantial difference of osmotic pressure exists between the tubular fluid and the blood plasma. Under these conditions, large amounts of dilute urine are formed (900 to 1500 ml/h). Massive urinary flows of this kind occur in disease in the condition known as *diabetes insipidus* in which the hormone ADH is either absent or ineffective.

Control: conserving water

ADH increases the permeability of the distal convoluted tubules and the collecting ducts to water, and thus allows water to be conserved. The volume of urine excreted can be reduced to a minimum of 18 ml/hour by concentrating the fluid. As a result it becomes *hypertonic* (meaning that it has a greater osmotic pressure

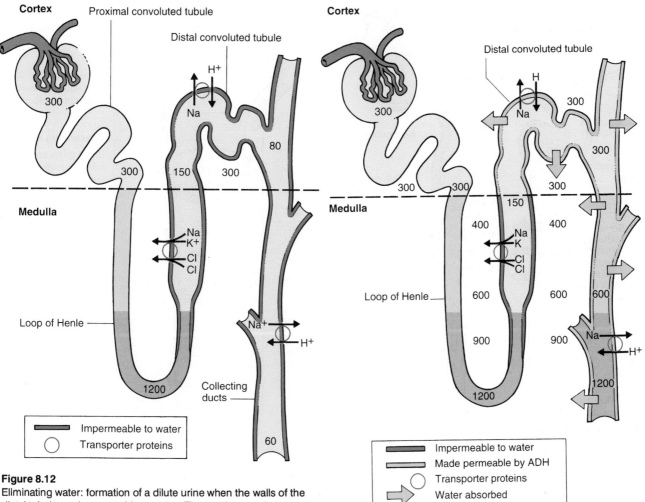

Figure 8.12
Eliminating water: formation of a dilute urine when the walls of the distal tubule are impermeable to water. The numbers and orange shading indicate how the osmotic pressure of the tubular fluid changes along the nephron and collecting duct.

Figure 8.13
Conserving water: formation of a concentrated urine when the walls of the distal tubule are made permeable to water by the action of the hormone ADH. The numbers and orange shading indicate how the osmotic pressure of the tubular fluid changes as it passes along the nephron and collecting duct.

than plasma). The power of the kidneys to achieve this is due to the distinctive arrangement and characteristics of the loop of Henle. It creates a difference in osmotic pressure between the interstitial fluid of the cortex and that of the medulla. Whereas the osmotic pressure of the cortex is similar to that of the plasma, at the tip of the medulla it may be four to five times as great (Fig. 8.13). The way in which this difference in osmotic pressure is developed is explained later.

The collecting ducts through which the tubular fluid passes are thus surrounded by an environment which becomes increasingly more concentrated as the papillae are approached. If the walls of the collecting duct are impermeable to water the tubular fluid tracking through the collecting duct remains the same as when it left the distal convoluted tubule (Fig. 8.12). However, if the walls are permeable, then water in the tubular fluid is drawn by osmosis into the hypertonic environment of the medullary interstitium, and the tubular fluid is gradually concentrated. A maximally concentrated urine

will have an osmotic pressure similar to that of the interstitial fluid at the tips of the loops of Henle (1200 mosmoles/kgH$_2$O – about four times that of blood plasma).

Loop of Henle

This consists of two limbs, descending and ascending (Fig. 8.14A). Fluid leaving the proximal convoluted tubule enters the descending limb and flows down and then up into the ascending limb. The flow of fluid in the two limbs of the loop of Henle is thus in opposite directions (*countercurrent*).

Creating hypertonicity

Cells of the ascending loop of Henle actively transport sodium chloride from the tubular fluid out into the interstitium, unaccompanied by water. The sodium

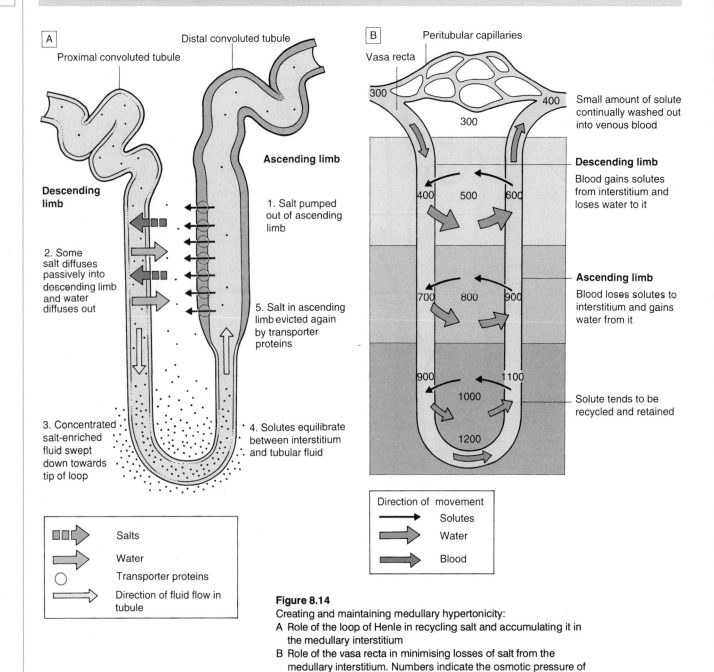

Figure 8.14
Creating and maintaining medullary hypertonicity:
A Role of the loop of Henle in recycling salt and accumulating it in the medullary interstitium
B Role of the vasa recta in minimising losses of salt from the medullary interstitium. Numbers indicate the osmotic pressure of the interstitial fluid and the blood plasma at different levels.

chloride diffuses through the interstitium. Some of it enters the fluid in the descending limb of the loop. The direction of fluid flow sweeps the sodium chloride down towards the tip of the loop. When the tubular fluid rounds the bend and flows back towards the cortex some of the sodium chloride in it is picked up again by the transporter proteins in the cells of the ascending limb and ejected once more into the interstitium. Thus, sodium chloride gets recycled and trapped in the loop and the medullary interstitium. In this way the concentration of sodium chloride builds up towards the tip and it is this which chiefly creates the difference in osmotic pressure between the cortex and the medulla.

Role of the vasa recta

If the blood capillaries supplying the loop of Henle formed a network similar to that around the convoluted tubules, then much of the sodium chloride transported out of the ascending limb would simply diffuse into the capillaries and be swept away in the bloodstream. Consequently, little salt would be trapped in the medulla and the difference in osmotic pressure between the cortex and medulla would be much less.

However, the capillaries follow the loop around. Consequently, although the blood flowing in the descending limbs of the vasa recta gains salt from the interstitium (Fig. 8.14B), that passing up the ascending limbs loses most of it again back into the medullary interstitium. Hence sodium chloride and other solutes tend to be retained in the medulla rather than washed away.

The amount of sodium chloride and other solutes retained in the medulla depends on the rate of flow of blood through the vasa recta. If flow increases, more is lost and the difference in concentration between the cortex and the medulla decreases. Consequently tubular fluid passing through the collecting ducts cannot be concentrated to the same extent and a less concentrated urine is formed. Conversely, if blood flow decreases, as it does under the action of ADH, which causes vaso-constriction of the vasa recta, the concentrating power of the kidney increases.

HOW WASTE SUBSTANCES ARE ELIMINATED

The waste substances that the kidneys eliminate are water soluble. Most get into the tubular fluid simply by being filtered at the glomerulus (Fig. 8.15). In addition to this a few substances are transported from the blood into the tubular fluid (*secreted*) by carrier proteins in the tubular cells.

FILTRATION

Any substance dissolved in plasma, which is smaller in size than the plasma proteins and which does not bind to them, will pass through the glomerular filter into the tubular fluid. Its fate thereafter depends on the tubular epithelium and the characteristics of the substance concerned, such as its:

- ability to bind to carrier proteins in the membrane of the tubular cells
- molecular size and liposolubility.

Tubular cell selectivity

The carrier proteins transporting substances across cell membranes are usually highly selective for specific molecules. The carrier that transports glucose for example does not transport mannitol, a carbohydrate molecule of similar size but differing in structure. In this way the tubular cells are able to selectively recover key molecules whilst rejecting others.

Molecular size and liposolubility

The permeability of the tubular epithelium to water-soluble molecules is much less than that of the glomerular filter. Thus some molecules, such as *creatinine* (a breakdown product of muscle metabolism), get trapped in the tubular fluid because their molecular size stops

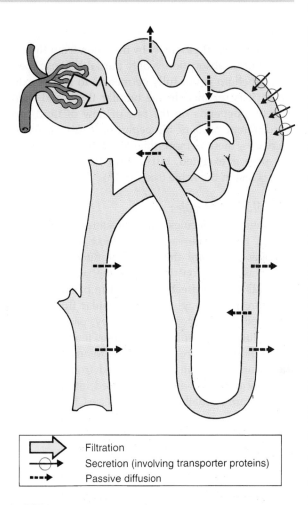

Figure 8.15
Elimination of waste materials by filtration and secretion. The amount finally excreted depends on the extent to which waste substances are absorbed by passive diffusion through the walls of the tubules.

⬜ Filtration
⊘→ Secretion (involving transporter proteins)
---▶ Passive diffusion

them from passing easily through the epithelium. They stay in the tubular fluid and their concentration increases progressively as water and other constituents of the glomerular filtrate are gradually absorbed.

Water-soluble molecules which *can* leak out of the tubular fluid back into the blood are either tiny enough to pass through the water-filled channels that do exist in the cell membranes and at the junctions between cells, or they are soluble to some extent in lipids and can simply diffuse across the cell membrane. In both cases, the driving force for absorption is the difference in concentration of the substance between the tubular fluid and the blood plasma.

Concentration differences develop as fluid is absorbed by the mechanisms described previously (see p. 166). Consequently, if a molecule can get through the epithelium it will be absorbed passively. A good example of this is *urea*, a waste product of protein metabolism (see Chs 9 and 14).

Urea

Urea is absorbed passively by diffusion from the tubular fluid, but its absorption is only partial because the tubular epithelium is not fully permeable to it. The extent to which it is retained in the tubular fluid, and therefore excreted, depends on the rate of flow of fluid through the different parts of the nephron. If tubular fluid flow decreases, there is more time for diffusion to occur and less urea is excreted, but if fluid flow increases, more urea is lost in the urine (see Ch. 15).

Liposoluble molecules

Liposoluble molecules, such as steroid hormones (see Ch. 3), tend to be carried in blood, bound to plasma proteins. They are therefore not filtered to the same extent as other constituents of the plasma. The small amounts that are freely dissolved in plasma, and which therefore get through into the tubular fluid are largely absorbed back into the blood by passive diffusion. Consequently liposoluble molecules tend to be retained in the blood and are not excreted to any great extent in the urine. They can be eliminated from the body but only once they have been converted into a more water-soluble form, usually by the liver (see Chs 9 and 15).

SECRETION

In addition to the nonspecific ways of eliminating waste materials just described, cells at the end of the proximal convoluted tubule are able to transfer some selected compounds *from* the peritubular blood into the tubular fluid. This involves transporter proteins in the membranes of the tubular cells carrying the molecules

---

DIURETICS

Any substance which increases urine flow rate is termed a *diuretic*. Alcohol is a diuretic. It inhibits the secretion of ADH and thus promotes the loss of water. Alcohol is thus not the most effective drink to have to quench a genuine thirst. Caffeine is a diuretic too, albeit a very weak one. There is evidence that it increases GFR.

Drugs that are given to increase the loss of fluid from the body work by inhibiting the recovery of one or more electrolytes, usually sodium, chloride or hydrogen carbonate. Different drugs affect different processes: some act on the transport of salt in the loop of Henle (*loop diuretics*); some inhibit the action of aldosterone; some inhibit the enzyme carbonic anhydrase and reduce the recovery of hydrogen carbonate (Table 8.3).

RENAL DIALYSIS

When renal failure occurs, whether in its acute or chronic form, and for whatever reason, the normal functions of the kidney diminish or disappear. Substances, such as urea, potassium and water, that are usually excreted are retained in the circulation. Some of these can be especially dangerous; excessive potassium, for example, will lead to cardiac arrhythmias.

Renal dialysis replaces normal kidney function by ridding the body of excess water, electrolytes and waste products. Dialysis may be a temporary measure, maintaining the person's blood chemistry within acceptable limits until kidney function returns, or it may be permanent (or at least long term, until a renal transplant is available).

There are two main types of dialysis:

- haemodialysis
- peritoneal dialysis.

The physiological principles are the same for each.

Haemodialysis is perhaps most familiar to the general public for its use of kidney machines. Blood flows along a cannula in a vein in the patient's arm, passes through the kidney machine where it is filtered of its harmful contents, and returns to the patient via a second vein. Inside the machine, the blood passes along one side of a sterile, semipermeable membrane (that is, a membrane that permits the passage of certain substances only). On the other side of this membrane flows the dialysate. This is a sterile fluid containing carefully controlled levels of electrolytes. For example, it contains very little, if any, potassium. Potassium therefore diffuses across the membrane from the patient's blood where its level is high. Other substances that can cross the membrane, such as urea and creatinine, do the same.

You may wonder what effect the blood's osmotic pull has. Since plasma proteins cannot cross the membrane, why doesn't water flow from the dialysate into the blood? To counteract this osmotic attraction, the dialysate is made hypertonic by the addition of extra glucose. Water flow is therefore usually from the patient to the dialysate. The patient's blood chemistry is carefully monitored, and frequency and length of haemodialysis (and sometimes constituency of dialysate) will be calculated from the results.

Haemodialysis is expensive, not just in equipment but in its need for specially trained nurses. Peritoneal dialysis avoids the need for expensive equipment, though it too demands careful nursing care. Here, dialysing fluid is run into the peritoneal cavity through a sterile catheter, the peritoneum acting as a semipermeable membrane. Unwanted substances diffuse across the peritoneum from the patient's blood until, after the required time, the dialysate is run out again.

Some patients with long-term renal failure can use dialysis within a comparatively normal lifestyle by the use of continuous ambulatory peritoneal dialysis (CAPD). The dialysate is contained within a sterile 2-litre plastic bag, which, for the first part of the procedure, is elevated (either hanging from a drip stand or worn around the upper part of the body) so that the fluid runs in under gravity. After approximately 4 hours, the now empty bag is lowered to below the level of the abdomen. It can be strapped to the side of the bed or to the patient's leg if he wishes to be active. The fluid can now flow out without the sterile circuit being broken, and with as little disturbance to the patient's life as possible.

This is a very brief introduction to a complex subject. You may wish to read more detailed texts, for example Boore et al 1987, pp. 851–870, and to update your knowledge from nursing journals.

Table 8.3 Diuretics and their actions

Type	Example	Trade name	Action
Loop diuretics*	Frusemide	Lasix	Inhibits transporter proteins in thick ascending limb of loop of Henle
Potassium-sparing diuretics	Spironolactone Amiloride	Aldactone Midamor	Inhibits action of aldosterone Blocks sodium channels in distal tubule
Carbonic anhydrase inhibitors	Acetazolamide	Diamox	Inhibits absorption of hydrogen carbonate
Thiazide diuretics*	Chlorothiazide	Saluric	Inhibits absorption of NaCl in first part of distal convoluted tubule
Osmotic diuretics	Mannitol		Counteracts absorption of water by exerting osmotic pressure within the tubular fluid

* These diuretics also increase the urinary loss of potassium. To avoid hypokalaemia they may be combined with a potassium supplement or a potassium-sparing diuretic.

across the cell membranes. These transporter proteins can handle a variety of different molecules including endogenous substances like some *organic acids* and drugs such as *penicillin* (see Ch. 15).

STORAGE AND EVACUATION OF URINE

Urine is formed continuously by the kidneys and passes through the ureters to the urinary bladder, where it is stored. Evacuation of the bladder via the urethra is controlled by the autonomic and somatic nervous systems.

URETERS

Urine passes to the pelvis of each kidney and is then carried via the two ureters to the bladder (Fig. 8.16). Both the ureter and the bladder are lined by an epithelium which is highly impermeable to water. Thus the osmotic pressure of urine remains the same within the ureters and the bladder even if it is different from that of the blood. The ureters, like the bladder, possess smooth muscle (see Ch. 22) in their walls. Regular

Where a small stone (*calculus*) is produced in the renal system, and then passes down the ureter, extreme pain is caused when the sharp edges of the stone scratch the smooth lining of the ureter, and its muscle wall goes into spasm. Passage of the stone is aided by the patient drinking copious amounts of fluid and by the prescription of effective analgesia, such as pethidine, or the anti-inflammatory drug diclofenac. Larger stones formed in the renal pelvis curiously cause far less pain, because they are much too big to move.

Q: Why is it important for a stone that is eventually passed from the urethra to be sent to the pathology department for analysis?

contractions of this muscle move the urine along the ureters into the bladder in spurts.

The ureters enter the bladder at an oblique angle. When the bladder contracts and the pressure of fluid inside it increases, the openings of the ureters are compressed by the bladder wall and backflow of the urine is prevented.

BLADDER

Filling

The bladder distends as urine flows into it, but the pressure inside it does not increase very much at first (Fig. 8.17). The maximum volume of fluid that a normal bladder can hold when fully distended varies between people. One student taking part in an experimental project produced almost a litre of urine at one sitting, but this is rather unusual except in cases of chronic urinary retention. Usually, the maximum volume that can be held in the bladder without too much discomfort is about 0.5 litres.

Sphincters

The neck of the bladder, which is connected to the urethra, has three distinct layers of smooth muscle. The first of these, which is really an extension of the muscle of the bladder, acts as the *internal sphincter* (Fig. 8.16C). The muscle of the bladder and the sphincter is innervated by autonomic nerves, both sympathetic and parasympathetic. The urethra (longer in men than in women) (see Ch. 34) passes through the *urogenital diaphragm* in the pelvic floor. Muscle associated with the diaphragm acts as a sphincter (the *external sphincter*). This muscle is striated (see Ch. 22) and is innervated by somatic nerves (pudendal). ⑤

Control

The passage of urine (*micturition*) is controlled both by involuntary and voluntary mechanisms (Fig. 8.18).

⑤
Where else in the body is this arrangement of sphincters, with voluntary and autonomic nerve supplies, to be found?

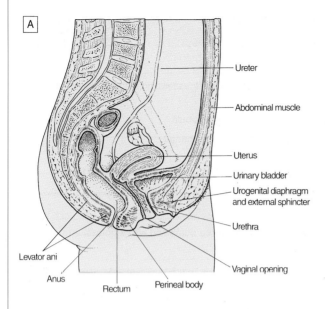

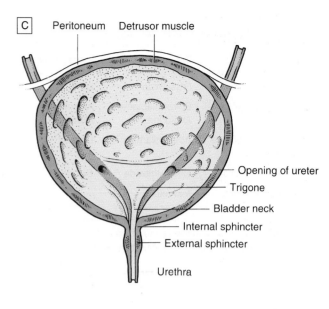

Female

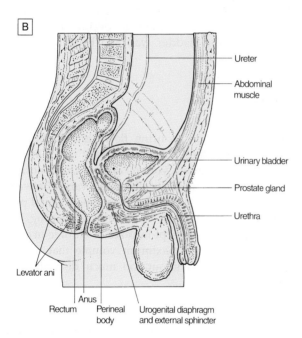

Figure 8.16 (*above and top right*)
Position and structure of the bladder, ureters, and urethra in men and women:
A Arrangement of pelvic structures in women
B Arrangement of pelvic structures in men
C Structure of the bladder.
(Parts A & B reproduced from Rogers 1992 (Figs 8.7 & 8.8) by permission of the publishers.)

Figure 8.17 (*right*)
Pressure inside the bladder as it fills. The dotted lines represent the temporary increases in pressure caused by reflex contraction of the muscle of the bladder in response to stretch caused by filling. If micturition does not occur the bladder accommodates to the new volume, adaptation occurs and the intra-vesical pressure falls. (Reproduced from Emslie-Smith et al 1988 (Fig. 12.26) by permission of the publishers.)

Involuntary control

Stretch receptors in the wall of the bladder are stimulated as the bladder distends. Via a spinal reflex they cause the smooth muscle of the bladder to contract. This increases the pressure within the bladder and opens the internal sphincter. As urine passes into the urethra, sensory receptors there sense the flow of urine and add to the reflex excitation of the bladder.

Voluntary control

If it is not possible to get to a toilet, bladder emptying is prevented by voluntary contraction of the external sphincter. If this is maintained for long enough the reflex contraction of the bladder muscles wanes. More urine flows into the bladder, which distends further, until impulses from sensory receptors reflexly stimulate the smooth muscle again (Fig. 8.17). This cycle may be repeated several times before micturition occurs. When it does happen, the flow of urine through the urethra

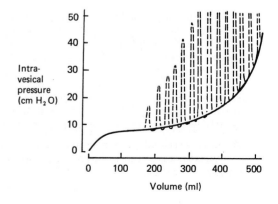

URINARY RETENTION

Hyperplasia of the prostate gland occurs in many men in middle and old age. The prostate gland (see Ch. 34) surrounds the urethra as it leaves the bladder neck (Fig. 8.17B) and, as glandular tissue increases, compresses and 'kinks' the urethra. At first, micturition is more hesitant, the individual observing a poor stream and 'end dribbling'. Frequency of micturition, even at night (*nocturia*), follows and the person may experience incontinence. Eventually, if the condition is not treated, retention will occur. This may be acute, with severe pain, or chronic, with overflow.

Even when retention has occurred, the bladder will continue to fill as the kidneys manufacture urine, and the normal bladder capacity will be exceeded. Prolonged obstruction will eventually lead to kidney damage, since urine is unable to pass down the ureters, yet is still being produced. This will lead to 'back pressure' on the kidneys. It is important, therefore, to treat urinary retention swiftly.

Catheterisation is performed aseptically, so as to avoid introducing microorganisms, and the urine drains into a sterile collecting bag. Some urologists believe that urine should be allowed to drain continuously so as to reduce 'back pressure' on the kidneys as quickly as possible. The nurse observes and records the amount drained in order to assist the urologist to assess the potential for kidney damage. Others believe that urinary drainage should be interrupted to avoid the sudden release of pressure in the abdomen, which, it is claimed, may induce shock and haemorrhage (Watson & Royle 1987). After an initial 500 ml is drained, the catheter is clamped for 15 minutes before a further 500 ml is allowed to drain. This process is repeated until the bladder is empty.

considerably strengthens the reflex contraction of the bladder by exciting sensory receptors there. In this way contraction is maintained until the bladder is emptied.

Abdominal pressure

Emptying of the bladder is also assisted by the pressure exerted by simultaneous contraction of the abdominal muscles. Sometimes an increase in abdominal pressure when coughing or lifting provokes a transient loss of urine (*stress incontinence*). This is more common in

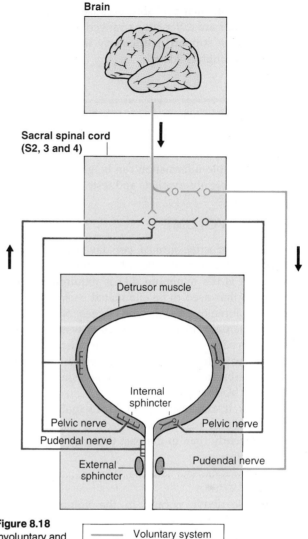

Figure 8.18
Involuntary and voluntary systems controlling the evacuation of urine from the urinary bladder.

	Voluntary system
	Involuntary system
	Sensory receptor
	Synapse

CAUSES OF URINARY INCONTINENCE

Stress incontinence can sometimes occur when childbirth has damaged the pelvic floor muscles and the external urinary sphincter. Control is maintained unless intra-abdominal pressure suddenly increases, as occurs with coughing, sneezing or even laughter. (It is well known that prolonged, helpless laughter may lead to 'accidents' even in those with an undamaged urinary system. Stress incontinence, however, occurs with ordinary, everyday laughter. Its effect on a person's social life and self-esteem may well be imagined.)

Incontinence may occur as a result of bladder inflammation, such as cystitis, or irritation, as in tuberculosis of the bladder and bladder tumours. Here the sensory nerve endings within the bladder wall are stimulated so that

frequency of micturition occurs. In the case of urinary tract infection, micturition is not only frequent but painful. Cystitis is often caused by infection with *Escherichia coli*, and is particularly prevalent in women who have commenced sexual activity.

Interestingly, certain forms of urinary retention can also cause incontinence. Prostatic hyperplasia can interfere with outflow of urine through the internal and external sphincters. Sometimes the bladder fills so as to cause great pain, and the patient is unable to pass any urine. Sometimes, however, small amounts of urine escape causing incontinence and adding to his misery. This is called retention with overflow.

Q: Why is cystitis a common problem in sexually active women? Why is a copious fluid intake recommended?

women than in men probably because the muscles of the pelvic floor are differently arranged and do not offer quite the same support, particularly if they have been weakened through childbirth.

TESTS AND MEASUREMENTS OF RENAL FUNCTION

A lot of valuable information can be gained from some relatively simple observations and tests.

URINARY VOLUME

The volume of urine formed per day normally ranges between a minimum of 500 ml to about 3 litres. The lower limit is the minimum that is required to excrete the solutes that need to be eliminated each day. Above that, the volume of urine depends largely on the balance between the daily intake and losses of water. Someone who drinks a lot, whether tea or some other beverage, is bound to have to pay rather more visits to the toilet. Frequent trips to the toilet do not necessarily indicate diabetes or bladder dysfunction. ⑥

However, if someone begins to drink more than usual for no apparent reason, and needs to visit the toilet more frequently than in the past this may indeed point to dysfunction.

Polyuria

An increase above normal in the volume of urine formed is referred to as *polyuria*. If the urine formed is very dilute this suggests a defect in water conservation. In the past, a simple way of finding out how dilute or concentrated the urine was, was to measure its specific gravity with a hydrometer. Values lower than 1.010 indicated a dilute urine. Nowadays it is preferable to use an osmometer, which, by measuring the osmolality, shows whether the urine is hypo-, iso- or hypertonic.

⑥
Have you noticed that you tend to pass urine more often in cold weather? There are several reasons why this might be. What are they?

Urinary flow rate may also increase above normal if there is an increase in solute excretion. If some glucose for example remains unabsorbed, as it does in *diabetes mellitus*, it acts as an osmotic force counteracting the forces promoting water recovery and more water will be excreted. This in turn upsets the recovery of electrolytes and more of these are excreted also. The presence of glucose in urine can be detected by using *dipsticks*. These are impregnated with chemicals that react with glucose to form a coloured compound. The depth of colour gives a rough measure of glucose concentration.

SMELL AND APPEARANCE OF URINE

Other observations that may provide clues as to renal function and the presence of abnormalities in other body systems include the smell and appearance of urine.

An offensive smell suggests infection. A sweetish smell may indicate the excretion of increased amounts of keto-acids as in diabetes mellitus (see Chs 14 and 19).

Urine is normally yellowish in colour. A very dark colour may indicate the presence of large amounts of the waste product bilirubin glucuronide formed by the liver from haemoglobin (see Chs 9 and 15). A frothy urine may suggest the presence of protein.

RENAL FUNCTION TESTS

More specialised measurements may sometimes be made to assess particular features of renal function, such as glomerular filtration rate by means of creatinine. Creatinine, a product of muscle metabolism, is freely filtered at the glomerulus, and then remains completely unabsorbed. The glomerular filtration rate is calculated

---

ACCURATE READING OF DIPSTICKS

It is important to cap the dipstick container tightly following each use, as the chemicals impregnating the sticks can deteriorate and give inaccurate readings. Similarly, the expiry date on the container should be noted.

Certain dipsticks are designed to detect substances other than glucose in the urine – for example ketones, blood and albumin. Each coloured strip on the dipstick must be read at the exact time recommended on the container's label. The timing for each strip to be read may vary: 30 seconds, 60 seconds, and so on. Each time must be measured using a watch with a second hand; a rough guess is inaccurate and unprofessional.

COLLECTING SPECIMENS OF URINE

Nursing staff may be requested to collect different types of urine specimens for different investigations. Where a urine infection is suspected, or the physician wishes to exclude this possibility, a *mid-stream* specimen of urine will be collected. The techniques of this procedure are beyond the scope of this book, but the principle behind it is to avoid contaminating the specimen with microorganisms from the skin around the urethral opening, or from the nurse's hands. An *early morning* specimen of urine is usually requested when it is to be examined for constituents such as urea, sodium and potassium (biochemical tests). An early morning specimen demonstrates better the kidney's ability to concentrate substances, before the day's normal fluid intake brings about dilution. (The individual may notice that the first urine passed in the morning is darker in colour than that later in the day.) Specimens should be sent to the pathology laboratory within 2 hours. Ideally, ward tests of urine using dipsticks should be carried out immediately, or readings may alter.

CREATININE CLEARANCE TEST

Estimation of creatinine clearance requires the collection of all urine produced by the patient over 24 hours (*a 24-hour collection of urine*). A specimen of venous blood will also be taken to estimate plasma creatinine levels.

Creatinine is formed in the muscle and passes via the blood into the urine. It is valuable in the estimation of renal function, in particular the glomerular filtration rate, because blood levels of creatinine remain fairly constant. In this respect it differs from urea, another end-product of metabolism, whose blood levels vary with protein intake and metabolic state.

Creatinine is filtered by the glomerulus and remains within the kidney tubules until excreted in the urine. It is not reabsorbed into the blood. Consequently, the amount of creatinine filtered per minute by the glomeruli is equal to the amount of creatinine excreted per minute in the urine. A 24-hour specimen of urine is collected so that the total daily amount of creatinine excreted may be measured and the excretion rate per minute calculated.

In some cases of renal disease, where there is disordered glomerular filtration, the amount of creatinine excreted in the urine will fall. This will be accompanied by an elevated plasma creatinine level, because the creatinine is not being excreted via the kidneys.

If any of the urine is accidentally discarded during the collection period, the test must recommence. Failure to do so would give a reduced total creatinine value, a reduced amount of creatinine clearance per minute, and hence an inaccurate glomerular filtration rate. Strict maintenance of the 24-hour collection is therefore an important nursing responsibility.

from the amount of creatinine excreted in the urine and its concentration in the plasma. This is known as the *creatinine clearance.*

KEY POINTS

What you should now understand about the formation and elimination of urine:

- how much urine is formed and what it normally contains and does not contain
- how urine is formed by filtration of the plasma and by tubular processing of the filtrate, and the factors influencing these processes
- how the conservation and excretion of water and electrolytes by the kidney is regulated
- what diuresis is and how it may be caused
- what can go wrong with renal function and the consequences of this
- what abnormal changes in urine flow rate and urinary composition reveal about renal and body function
- how urine is stored and evacuated by the bladder
- how urinary retention and urinary incontinence may arise.

REFERENCES AND FURTHER READING

Boore J, Champion R, Ferguson M (eds) 1987 Nursing the physically ill adult. Churchill Livingstone, Edinburgh
De Wardener H E 1985 The kidney, 5th edn. Churchill Livingstone, Edinburgh
(Comprehensive account of all aspects of the kidney in health and disease. Useful for reference and for information about clinical aspects of renal function)
Emslie-Smith D, Paterson C R, Scratcherd T, Read N W (eds) 1988 Textbook of physiology, 11th edn. Churchill Livingstone, Edinburgh, p 203
Lote C 1987 Principles of renal physiology, 2nd edn. Croom Helm, London
(An excellent, lucidly written, concise text explaining what the kidney does as well as how it does it. Includes plenty of suggestions for further reading and some problems and answers)
Rogers A W 1992 Textbook of anatomy. Churchill Livingstone, Edinburgh, p 107, 110
Seldin D W, Giebisch G (eds) 1985 The kidney: physiology and pathophysiology. Raven Press, New York
(Comprehensive, weighty, two volume coverage of the physiology and pathophysiology of renal function and electrolyte metabolism, written for and by specialists)
Tanagho E A, McAninch J W 1991 Smith's General urology, 13th edn. Appleton & Lange, East Norwalk, Connecticut
(Clinical text covering all aspects of disease of the genitourinary tract in depth. Useful for reference and for further information about the bladder and ureters)
Torrens M J, Morrison J F (eds) 1987 The physiology of the lower urinary tract. Springer Verlag, Berlin–Heidelberg
(Specialist book, reviewing current knowledge)
Valtin H 1983 Renal function mechanisms preserving fluid and solute balance in health, 2nd edn. Little Brown, Boston & Toronto
(Very well referenced, student text explaining renal mechanisms in detail and giving the experimental basis of current theory. Includes questions to think about, and answers)
Watson J, Royle J 1987 Watson's Medical–surgical nursing and related physiology, 3rd edn. Baillière Tindall, London, p 926

Chapter 9
LIVER

Whereas adjustments to plasma water and electrolytes are made mainly by the kidneys, and the supply and removal of oxygen and carbon dioxide is achieved by the lungs, the liver is concerned primarily with the provision and elimination of a wide variety of organic molecules such as glucose, amino acids, fatty acids, steroids, and plasma protcins, together with many waste products.

The liver is often likened to a chemical factory in that it is involved in the manufacture and processing of a wide range of substances. It cooperates with the digestive system in the supply of nutrients to the body, and complements the activity of other excretory systems in the processing and elimination of unwanted materials from the body.

Central to the function of the liver is its blood supply which supports the many different activities of the liver cells. These activities include the metabolism of carbohydrates, amino acids, fats and vitamins, and the formation of bile.

STRUCTURE AND BLOOD SUPPLY

GENERAL FEATURES

Anatomy

The liver is the largest soft organ in the body. In an adult person it weighs about 1.5 kg. It is located high in the abdomen, bounded above by the dome of the diaphragm (Fig. 9.1A & B). There are several lobes, the one on the right being the largest. The normal dark purplish-brown colour of the liver is evidence both of the richness of its circulation and of the fact that a sizeable fraction of the blood supply (70–80%) is already partially deoxygenated.

Histology

The liver is composed chiefly of one cell type (Fig. 9.2), the *hepatocyte* or *parenchymal cell* which is responsible for many of the functions of the liver (see p. 185). In addition to these cells, which form the major part of the liver tissue (80% by volume), there are a few other cell types present in smaller numbers. These include Kupffer cells, Ito cells and pit cells (see later Fig. 9.5).

Kupffer cells are macrophages that engulf and dispose of bacteria, cell debris and viruses. *Ito cells* (also known as fat-storing cells) contain a high concentration of vitamin A and are believed to be involved in the formation of hepatic connective tissue. The function of *pit cells* is unclear. They may have a neuroendocrine function. ①

Replacement of hepatocytes by connective tissue in disordered liver function is termed *fibrosis*.

BLOOD SUPPLY

The liver has an ample blood supply (1.25–1.5 litres/min; approximately one fifth of the cardiac output at rest) which is derived from two sources (Fig. 9.3):

- the hepatic artery
- the hepatic portal vein.

① *Can you name and describe the process whereby macrophages engulf foreign material?*

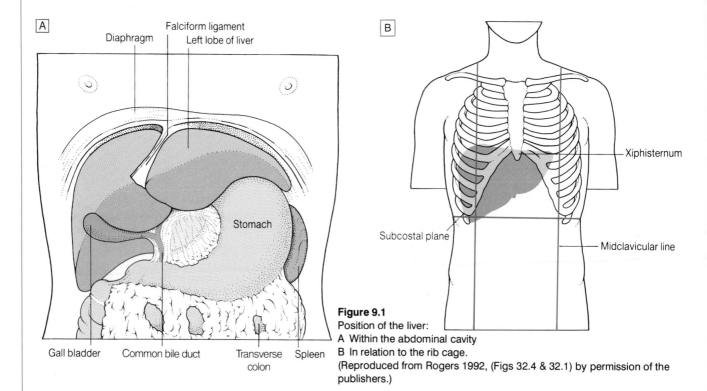

Figure 9.1
Position of the liver:
A Within the abdominal cavity
B In relation to the rib cage.
(Reproduced from Rogers 1992, (Figs 32.4 & 32.1) by permission of the publishers.)

② *Why is the blood in the portal circulation partially deoxygenated?*

The hepatic artery contributes only one fifth to one third of the supply. This blood is delivered at normal arterial pressures and is fully oxygenated. The majority of the blood supply, delivered via the portal vein, comes from the venous drainage of most of the gastrointestinal tract and is partially deoxygenated. ②

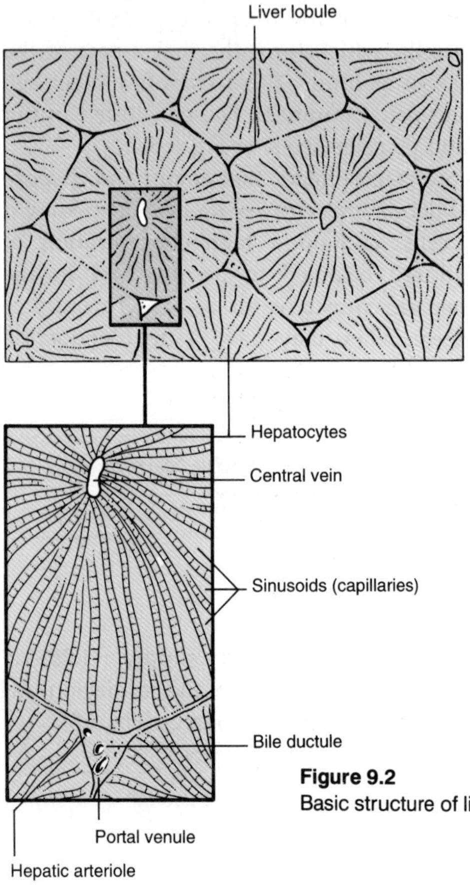

Portal blood supply

The portal supply includes *all* the venous drainage of the gastrointestinal tract from the lower part of the oesophagus through to the end of the large intestine. Only the venous blood from the mouth, most of the oesophagus and parts of the rectum escapes the hepatic 'filter' (Fig. 9.3). There are a few linking vessels (*anastomoses*) between the oesophageal veins and the portal vein. If blood flow through the liver is restricted these may open up giving rise to *oesophageal varices*.

Normal pressures in the hepatic portal vein are quite low (5–10 mmHg). If there is obstruction to flow through the liver, as for example in advanced *cirrhosis*, portal pressure rises, (*portal hypertension*). This affects tissue fluid balance in the capillaries upstream (*splanchnic capillaries*) and may lead to the accumulation of large amounts of tissue fluid in the peritoneal cavity (*ascites*; see p. 179).

Microcirculation

Both the hepatic artery and the hepatic portal vein divide into branches which carry blood to the several lobes of the liver. Thereafter these vessels divide many times again to form arterioles and venules which supply blood to a group of liver cells, which together with the terminal blood vessels is known as an *acinus* (Fig. 9.4).

Figure 9.2
Basic structure of liver tissue.

ASCITES

Ascites is both disfiguring and distressing, leading to a grossly swollen abdomen which makes movement difficult and clothing very tight, or even impossible, to wear.

Patients with ascites feel very uncomfortable. They are, quite literally, heavier than normal due to the fluid accumulation in the abdomen. One of the main nursing observations in this condition is to establish whether or not ascites is improving or deteriorating. Since ascites represents a build-up of fluid, and that fluid is mainly water, the most accurate way of establishing whether the accumulation has increased or decreased is to weigh the patient. This may not always be possible, however, and an alternative method is to measure abdominal girth. This must be done with the patient in exactly the same position each time, using a mark somewhere on the abdomen to position the tape measure. It is useful if several measurements can be made at one time in order to obtain an average and an accurate record kept.

Another aspect of ascites follows from the anatomy of the abdomen and thorax. The increasing size of the abdomen, and this is particularly true when the patient is lying down, restricts movement in the thorax by putting pressure on the diaphragm. Consequently, the patient with ascites has difficulty breathing and is prone to develop chest infections due to the fact that the lungs are not being properly ventilated.

Ascites is indicative of underlying disease which must be treated medically. Nursing actions revolve around caring for the distressed patient and keeping a record of fluid intake and output in addition to direct observation and reporting on the ascites.

OESOPHAGEAL VARICES

A varicosity is simply a part of a vein which has become dilated (stretched) and oesophageal varices are usually a sign of advanced cirrhosis of the liver. They are common in people whose livers have become severely damaged through excessive alcohol intake.

Cirrhosis is described as widespread fibrosis of the liver where functional hepatocytes are replaced by non-functional fibrous tissue. In this condition blood flow through the liver is restricted and this, in turn, increases the blood pressure within the portal circulation, which carries blood from the digestive organs to the liver. As a result of this restricted blood flow a collateral circulation, which is an alternative to the normal circulation, takes place via blood vessels in the stomach and at the lower oesophagus. The collateral circulation has a higher blood pressure than normal, causing varicosities to form in the oesophagus.

A steady small loss of blood into the oesophagus can ensue, leading to anaemia, or the loss of blood can be acute and spectacular, leading to death since the varicosities can rupture, resulting in massive loss of blood and shock.

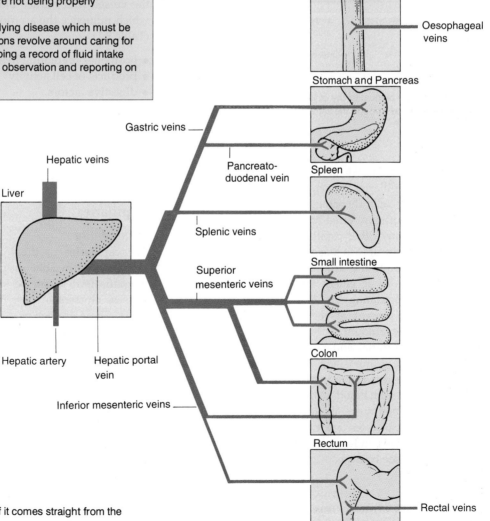

Figure 9.3
The hepatic blood supply: most of it comes straight from the digestive tract.

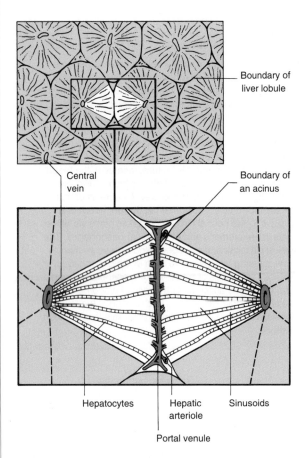

Central
vein

Boundary of
liver lobule

Boundary of
an acinus

Hepatocytes   Hepatic   Sinusoids
arteriole

Portal venule

Figure 9.4
Structure of a liver acinus: all the cells within an acinus are
supplied with blood through the same hepatic arteriole and hepatic
portal venule.

The terminal arterioles and terminal portal venules
empty into capillaries, which form 'tunnels' between
'walls' of liver cells (hepatocytes) one cell thick. Liver
capillaries are often referred to as *sinusoids* because they
differ from many other capillaries in being larger and
much more permeable to plasma proteins.

The blood from the arterioles and from the portal
venules mixes as it enters the sinusoids. Sphincters
involved in regulating the delivery of blood to the
sinusoids are present at the ends of the arterioles.
By varying the amount of arterial blood the relative
proportion of arterial and portal-venous blood can be
altered. As the composition of the blood from these
two sources differs (arterial blood is fully oxygenated,
whereas portal vein blood is partially deoxygenated and
contains absorbed nutrients, for example), the blood to
which the hepatocytes are exposed can be varied in
composition. This influences the metabolic activity of
the liver cells (see below). ③

Veins

Sinusoids from adjacent areas of liver tissue empty into
a *central hepatic vein* (Fig. 9.4). This in turn joins other

veins to form larger and larger vessels, which ultimately
form the short *hepatic veins* which drain blood into the
inferior vena cava in the abdomen.

Control of blood flow

Portal circulation
Blood flow through the portal vein normally depends
almost solely on the factors which control the blood
supply to the digestive system. When a meal is being
digested, the increased flow of blood to the digestive
system increases the flow of blood through the hepatic
portal vein to the liver. The veins entering the portal
vein, and the portal vein itself, contain some smooth
muscle innervated by sympathetic nerves. Contraction
of this muscle stiffens the veins and alters their capacity,
as it does in veins elsewhere, but has relatively little
effect on the rate of blood flow (see p. 103; Ch. 5). ④

Arterial circulation
The hepatic arterial supply is regulated independently.
The arterioles are innervated by sympathetic nerves
which when excited cause vasoconstriction, narrow
the vessels and reduce blood flow. Blood-borne factors
which influence the arterioles and regulate flow include
(Table 9.1):

- hormones regulating liver metabolism
- products of cell activity
- digestive factors.

The arterial supply is vital. Without it the liver
becomes susceptible to bacterial colonisation. In the
absence of the arterial supply, the low oxygen concentrations to which the liver is exposed favour the growth
of some types of bacteria.

Capillaries

Permeability
The capillaries of the liver are unusual in that they
are very permeable to plasma proteins. Under high
magnification it can be seen that the endothelial cells
possess clusters of pore-like structures known as *sieve
plates*. These are believed to be the route through which
plasma proteins get across the capillary wall and enter
the *space of Disse* between the capillary and the
hepatocytes (Fig. 9.5).

Table 9.1   Factors causing vasodilation of the hepatic arterioles

Hormones	Products of cell activity	Digestive factors
Adrenaline Glucagon	Adenosine CO_2 K^+	Secretin Bile salts

③
*What kind of
muscles are
sphincters
composed of?*

④
*Which
neurotransmitter
is released
by most
sympathetic
nerve fibres?*

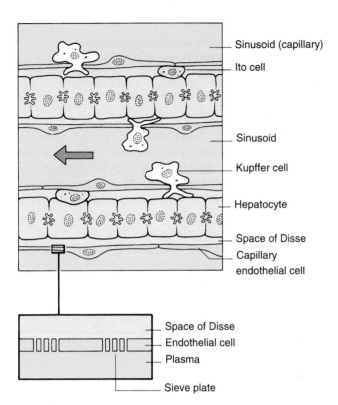

Figure 9.5
Liver capillaries and their relation to hepatocytes and other cells.

Table 9.2 Some plasma proteins manufactured by the liver
Albumin
Angiotensinogen
Factor VII
Factor IX
Factor X
Fibrinogen
Prothrombin
Transcobalamin
Transcortin
Transferrin

phages found scattered throughout the body which engulf and degrade cellular debris, bacteria and viruses (see Chs 4 and 15). Kupffer cells are estimated to make up 60% of all the cells in the macrophage system. They are strategically sited as the venous blood from the digestive system, which may be carrying bacteria, viruses, and foreign proteins absorbed through the digestive epithelium, must first pass through the liver before entering the rest of the circulation.

> Because of its siting, the liver itself is at risk of infection from viruses which enter the body via the digestive system. The most common virus is hepatitis A (*infectious hepatitis*). It can be spread by poor personal hygiene from hands to food. Care is needed in the disposal of urine and faeces from infected patients.

Substances such as bilirubin (see Ch. 4), fatty acids and heavy metals (lead, copper) which are largely transported in blood bound to plasma proteins have very easy access to the hepatocytes. This differs from other tissues and contrasts with the capillaries of the brain (see Ch. 20). The liver 'welcomes all comers'. This enables it to fulfil its major role in the processing and disposal of waste materials (see Ch. 15). Likewise, other constituents of blood that are generally too large to cross capillary walls (such as chylomicrons; see Ch. 6) have easy access to the hepatocytes.

The traffic of proteins across the capillary wall occurs in both directions as the liver is the site of manufacture of many of the plasma proteins including albumin and a variety of the clotting factors (Table 9.2 and Ch. 4).

Activity
Endothelial cells are not simply a passive, very leaky barrier. They also play an active role in the uptake, processing and degradation of macromolecules such as proteins in the blood. They engulf these molecules by *endocytosis* (see Ch. 2).

Lodged at various points in the capillary wall are larger, plumper cells (*Kupffer cells*; Fig. 9.5). Extensions of these cells protrude both into the blood on the one side and the space of Disse on the other. The cells are phagocytic and belong to the diffuse system of macro-

HEPATIC INNERVATION

Efferent nerves
The liver like other viscera is innervated by para-sympathetic and sympathetic nerves. Nerve endings have been identified in most parts of the liver, although the density of innervation differs between one part and another.

In general sympathetic nerves are most abundant. Adrenergic terminals are found in association with the smooth muscle of the blood vessels as well as with hepatocytes and other cells. The cholinergic innervation, by contrast, appears to be more limited.

Major functions of the efferent nerves includes regulation of the hepatic circulation and the regulation of glucose metabolism. ⑤

Afferent nerves
In addition to these efferent fibres, sensory fibres have also been identified. Sensory receptors, such as baroreceptors and osmoreceptors, monitor conditions within the liver, and this information is used in the overall regulation of visceral function.

⑤
During the so-called 'fight or flight' reaction do you think that blood flow to the liver will be increased or decreased?

LIVER FUNCTIONS

METABOLIC ACTIVITY OF THE HEPATOCYTES

Most of the important functions of the liver are carried out by the hepatocytes. The chief histological features of these cells are shown in Figure 9.6. Liver cells are often cited as useful examples of a typical cell because they contain a balanced range of cellular organelles. This reveals the diversity of metabolic activity of these cells, which includes:

- processing of substances in the smooth endoplasmic reticulum (steroid hormones, drugs)
- synthesis of proteins for export in the rough endoplasmic reticulum (plasma proteins)
- packaging of various secretory products by the Golgi apparatus (proteins, bile salts, drugs)
- storage of substances in vesicles (glycogen, iron, vitamins).

Much of this activity is powered by the energy generated by the mitochondria. ⑥

Regional differences in metabolic bias

All the hepatocytes carry out the same range of activities. However, they differ in the bias of their activity because the cells are not all exposed to exactly the same environment (Fig. 9.7). The cells in zone 1, close to

⑥
In what chemical form is energy produced by mitochondria? Are mitochondria involved in aerobic or anaerobic metabolism?

Liver function tests probe different aspects of metabolic activity. For example serum albumin is lowered when the liver is not synthesising as much protein, and the blood level of the enzyme alkaline phosphatase is raised when the secretion of this enzyme in bile in blocked.

the supply vessels (arterioles and portal venules), are exposed to higher concentrations of oxygen and absorbed nutrients than the hepatocytes downstream closer to the central veins (zone 3). Consequently the metabolic activities of the cells upstream in the *periportal* regions (zone 1) differ in degree from those in the *perivenous* (or *centrilobular*) regions (zone 3).

The activity of the cells closest to the supply vessels is biased towards the uptake, processing and metabolism of a variety of substances including monosaccharides

If the liver is injured by an overdose of the drug paracetamol, it is the perivenous cells that suffer most damage.

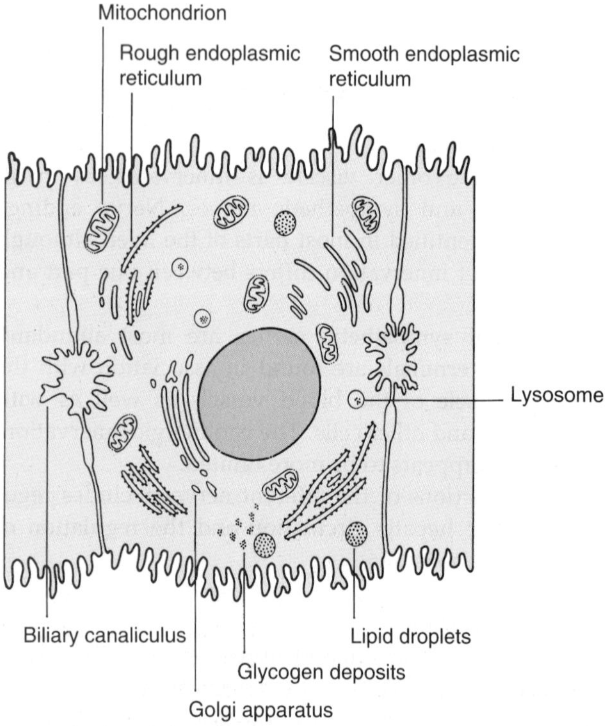

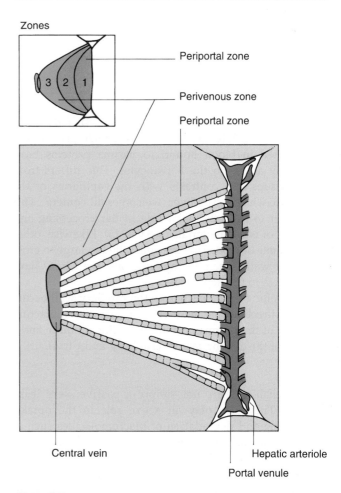

Figure 9.7
How the environment of the hepatocytes changes from one end of the sinusoid (periportal) to the other (perivenous) dividing the acinus into zones of differing metabolic activity.

Mitochondrion
Rough endoplasmic reticulum   Smooth endoplasmic reticulum

Lysosome

Biliary canaliculus
Lipid droplets
Glycogen deposits
Golgi apparatus

Figure 9.6
Chief structural features of the hepatocyte.

Table 9.3 Metabolic bias of different hepatocytes*	
Periportal (zone 1)	*Perivenous (zone 3)*
Uptake of – bilirubin – bile salts – glucose	Drug metabolism
Formation of – glycogen – glucose	Fat synthesis
ATP formed oxidatively[†]	ATP formed by glycolysis[†]

* All hepatocytes do the same things, but some are more active in some processes than others. This table shows what periportal and perivenous hepatocytes specialise in.
[†] See Chapter 11.

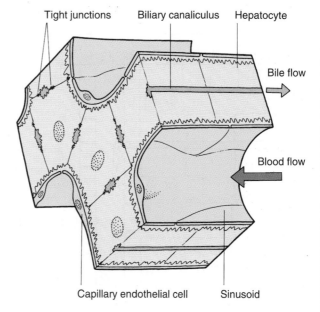

Figure 9.8
The biliary canaliculi: tiny channels running between adjacent hepatocytes.

In *cholestasis* (reduced flow of bile) substances normally excreted in bile accumulate in the body and give rise to such clinical features as itching (*pruritus*), caused probably by bile salts, and yellowing of the skin (*jaundice*), caused by bile pigments such as bilirubin.

and amino acids. Further along the sinusoid, the bias of cell activity shifts towards fat synthesis and drug metabolism (Table 9.3).

The metabolic activity of the cells is not fixed but changes with nutritional status, blood supply and hormonal balance.

BILE SECRETION

The hepatocytes are linked together by specialised junctions, including tight junctions and gap junctions (see Ch. 2), to form sheets of cells, which in cross-section look like cords radiating from the central veins (Fig. 9.2). Running between adjacent cells and sealed off on either side from the interstitial space of Disse by tight junctions are tiny (1 μ in diameter) fluid filled channels, the *biliary canaliculi* (little canals) (Fig. 9.8). The secretion of bile is one of the many functions of the hepatocytes. A variety of substances including bile salts (see Ch. 6) are excreted in bile. A few examples are listed in Table 9.4.

Bile formed by the hepatocytes flows in the opposite direction to the blood, from the canaliculi nearest the

central veins to the canaliculi nearest to the terminal arterioles and portal venules. From there it flows into the ducts of the biliary system. The biliary ducts lie alongside the blood vessels supplying blood to the liver sinusoids (Figs 9.2 and 9.9). ⑦

The primary bile formed by the hepatocytes (*canalicular bile*) is modified as it flows through the ducts. An alkaline secretion of sodium hydrogen carbonate is added here and a few selected substances such as glucose are absorbed.

LIVER FUNCTIONS IN CONTEXT

Many of the general functions of the liver (Table 9.5) are shared with other parts of the body. For example the liver has an important role in the metabolism of carbohydrates, proteins and fats but it shares this role with other tissues, particularly skeletal muscle and adipose tissue (see Ch. 14). Similarly, the liver participates in the defence of the body against invasion by bacteria and other foreign matter through the phagocytic activity of the Kupffer cells but again it is only part of the body-wide system of macrophages (see Ch. 15). As regards specific functions, however, there are certain

Table 9.4 Some substances excreted in bile	
Type	*Examples*
Bile salts	Sodium glycocholate Sodium glycochenodeoxycholate
Endogenous waste products	Bilirubin glucuronide Steroid hormones
Drugs	Erythromycin Barbiturates Digitalis glycosides
Heavy metals	Lead Copper

⑦
With reference to the biliary tree, what happens to bile once it has left the liver?

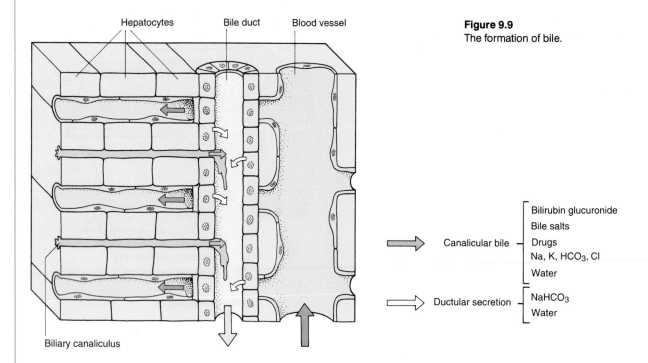

Figure 9.9
The formation of bile.

activities, such as the formation of urea, that are almost exclusively performed by the liver.

The several functions of the liver can for simplicity be divided into two groups:

- nutrient homeostasis
- elimination of waste and unwanted materials.

In nutrient homeostasis the liver cooperates with the digestive system, skeletal muscle, adipose tissue and the kidneys in controlling the circulating levels of nutrients such as glucose, amino acids and lipids. In the removal

of waste or unwanted materials, the liver cooperates with the lungs, the kidneys and phagocytic cells throughout the body to provide a comprehensive waste disposal service. How these different tissues and organs interact will be described in two later chapters (Chs 14 and 15), but a brief mention will be made here of the major activities of the liver, in order to make clear the kind of disturbances that arise if the liver is damaged or diseased.

Nutrient homeostasis

Storage

The liver acts as a storage site for some nutrients when these are surplus to immediate requirements. Examples are listed in Table 9.6. The synthesis of glycogen from glucose is called *glycogenesis*. ⑧

Amino acids are used in the body to form proteins, purines and pyrimidines. Amino acids that are surplus to requirements are not stored in a separate protein depot but are degraded instead (*deaminated*) by the liver to form *urea* as a waste product (Fig. 9.10).

⑧
Glycogen is stored in large amounts in another tissue too. Which one?

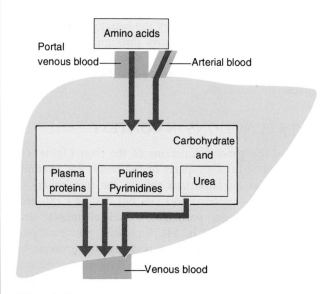

Figure 9.10
Products formed from amino acids by the liver.

> In renal disease the excretion of urea may be inadequate because of defective kidney function (see Ch. 8). In this circumstance the danger of *uraemia* (raised blood urea concentration) can be avoided by reducing the amount of protein in the diet, and thus the amount of urea manufactured by the liver.

Table 9.5 Functions of the liver

General	Specific examples
Carbohydrate metabolism	Synthesises glucose Stores glucose as glycogen Converts galactose to glucose*
Protein and amino acid metabolism	Synthesises and degrades many plasma proteins Synthesises and degrades purines and pyrimidines Forms and degrades amino acids Forms urea and uric acid*
Fat metabolism	Synthesises fatty acids Forms and secretes VLDL (very low density lipoproteins)* Forms ketone bodies* Forms bile salts from cholesterol*
Metabolism of endogenous waste	Bilirubin* Steroid hormones
Metabolism of xenobiotics	Alcohol Drugs
Phagocytosis	Bacteria, red cells
Bile secretion*	

* Functions that may be considered as exclusive to the liver as other tissues contribute so little (if at all).

Synthesis

The liver manufactures a wide variety of substances that are used by the body. Key substances are listed in Table 9.7.

Plasma proteins including some of the clotting factors (see Ch. 4 and Table 9.2) are synthesised from amino acids. In liver disease it is the shortfall in the supply of some of the earlier factors in the clotting sequence that leads to bleeding disorders.

Table 9.6 Some nutrients stored by the liver

Vitamin A	Iron
Vitamin B – riboflavin – niacin – B_6 – folic acid – B_{12}	Glucose as glycogen

Table 9.7 Some substances produced by the liver

Type	Function	Chapter reference
Plasma proteins	Coagulation Transport	4
	Prohormones	10
Glucose	Fuel	11, 14
Lipoproteins (chiefly VLDL)*	Lipid transport and metabolism	14
Ketone bodies	Fuel	14
Bile salts (acids)	Digestive agent	6
Creatine	Precursor of creatine phosphate in muscle	11, 17
Urea	Waste product (affects renal function)	8
Purines Pyrimidines	Components of DNA, RNA	2

* Very low density lipoproteins.

BLEEDING DISORDERS

The liver is responsible for the synthesis of nine of the blood clotting factors and any impairment in liver function will reduce its capacity to synthesise any of these factors. Additionally, three of the factors require the presence of vitamin K in order to be synthesised. Vitamin K, which is fat soluble, requires the presence of bile salts in the small intestine in order for it to be absorbed. Bile salts emulsify fats and form micelles which aid in the digestion and absorption of fat. In *cholestasis* there is a lack of bile in the intestine thus decreasing the absorption of vitamin K and consequent synthesis of some of the clotting factors.

An individual who has a tendency to excessive and prolonged bleeding due to liver disease will have to take precautions and be made aware of the possible signs. The kind of precautions that can be taken are common sense such as, in men, shaving with an electric rather than a wet razor. Additional care has to be taken, for example, when brushing teeth to avoid bleeding gums. A sign of internal bleeding may be the passing of blood in the urine (*haematuria*). Haematuria results from bleeding into any part of the urinary system and minor damage in a patient who has reduced blood clotting ability will lead to prolonged bleeding. This is very distressing for the patient.

A feature of the medical care of such patients will be the regular taking of blood samples for analysis of 'clotting times' (see Ch. 4). What is being sought is a reduction in clotting time to normal, which will happen when normal liver function is restored. Where there is cholestasis, vitamin K can also be administered by injection to help in the synthesis of clotting factors by the liver.

Q: What may be done to minimise the risk of blood loss when taking blood samples?

Large amounts of *glucose* (up to 250 g/day) can be formed by the liver from a variety of precursors including alanine, glycerol and lactic acid. This process is called *gluconeogenesis*.

Triglycerides are synthesised in the liver from fatty acids and glycerol. The fat formed is normally packaged together with other lipids, such as phospholipids and cholesterol, and 'coated' with protein to form lipid-rich complexes (*lipoproteins*) which are secreted into the blood (see Ch. 14). The main class of plasma lipoproteins formed by the liver is VLDL (very low density lipoprotein). If the formation and secretion of VLDL does not keep pace with the hepatic synthesis of triglycerides, the triglycerides accumulate giving rise to a fatty liver, as for example in liver disease in alcoholism.

Ketone bodies (*aceto-acetate, beta-hydroxybutyrate*) are formed from acetyl CoA which is derived from the mitochondrial oxidation of fatty acids. In starvation (see Ch. 14) large amounts of ketone bodies are formed from fat and used as an energy source.

Bile acids are synthesised in the liver from cholesterol. In humans the two major bile acids synthesised are *cholic acid* (pronounced 'ko-lic') and *chenodeoxycholic acid* (Fig. 9.11). The sodium salts of these acids are sodium cholate and sodium chenodeoxycholate. These are linked (*conjugated*) with the amino acids glycine or taurine to give *conjugated bile salts*:

- sodium glycocholate
- sodium glycochenodeoxycholate
- sodium taurocholate
- sodium taurochenodeoxycholate.

The glycine conjugated sodium salts constitute the larger proportion. All these bile salts are secreted in large amounts in bile and are necessary for the digestion and absorption of fats (see Ch. 6). They are referred to as *primary* bile salts to distinguish them from *secondary* bile salts that are formed from them by the bacteria in the large intestine (Fig. 9.11).

Elimination of waste and unwanted materials

The liver has a major role in the processing and elimination of many endogenous and exogenous substances (Table 9.8). Some of these substances are converted into products that are secreted into the blood and then excreted in body fluids such as urine and sweat, or in expired air. Ammonia for example is converted into urea and excreted in the urine whereas alcohol is converted into acetaldehyde, some of which is exhaled in expired air.

Other substances, such as bilirubin (derived from the breakdown of haemoglobin; see Ch. 4) are secreted into the bile and eliminated in the faeces. If the secretion of bile by the liver is impaired or if its delivery to the gall bladder or intestine is blocked (see Ch. 6), as for example by a gall-stone, then some waste products, such as bilirubin, will be dammed back into the liver and spill back into the blood giving rise to various clinical features including *jaundice* (yellowing of the skin and mucous membranes).

LIVER FAILURE

If liver function is inadequate the consequences will include:

- a decrease in the plasma levels of manufactured products (plasma proteins, urea, glucose)
- a build-up of waste products that are normally removed (bilirubin, ammonia and steroid hormones).

If a patient with liver failure is on any medication this has to be given with great caution since the liver is the means whereby many drugs are processed and eliminated. The effect on the patient will be that drugs will cause increased side effects and their therapeutic effects will last longer. This is often taken into account by administering smaller doses.

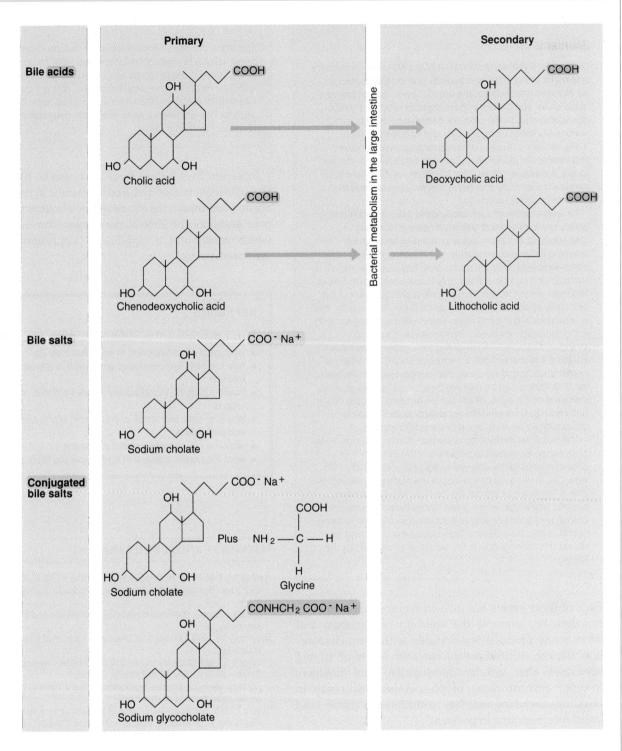

Figure 9.11
Structure of some bile acids and bile salts.

Table 9.8 Substances whose elimination from the body is assisted by the liver	
Endogenous	*Exogenous*
Ammonia	Dietary constituents e.g. alkaloids
Bilirubin	Drugs e.g. antibiotics
Steroid hormones	Heavy metals e.g. copper, lead

JAUNDICE

Defined as a yellow discoloration of the skin and conjunctiva (the moist lining of the eye socket), jaundice is caused by an increase in bilirubin in the blood. The source of bilirubin is the haem component of haemoglobin which is broken down when red blood cells are destroyed. The bilirubin is normally taken up by the liver and excreted in bile. If this excretory route is impaired through liver disease (*hepatocellular jaundice*) or failure of bile flow from the liver to the duodenum (*obstructive jaundice*), or if the liver is overloaded with bilirubin (as in *haemolytic jaundice*) then the skin becomes yellowed.

In severe cases of such disease the yellow discoloration is very obvious, even to the untrained eye. It is very distressing to the individual with jaundice and can be alarming for friends and family. On the other hand, it takes considerable experience to observe mild jaundice and sometimes it can be noticed only in the conjunctiva. This is fortunate since the definition of 'yellow discoloration of the skin' only applies to those with white skins. Incidentally, this is worth bearing in mind by nurses when assessing for any condition which involves skin discoloration such as cyanosis and pallor. When caring for a patient with severe jaundice it is prudent not to express alarm at the person's appearance and to be aware that symptoms of cholestasis such as itching can be relieved by appropriate drugs. Also, yellowing of the eyes, which can be extreme in some cases and can make the patient very self-conscious, can be concealed by wearing tinted or darkened glasses.

It is possible, through an understanding of the underlying physiology, for nurses to be aware of the different characteristics of the different types of jaundice. For example, in cholestasis the faeces are normally pale yellow due to the fact that stercobilin (see Ch. 15), an excretory product of bilirubin which gives faeces their characteristic colour, is reduced or absent because less bilirubin is being secreted into the intestine. Conversely, the urine may be darker than normal due to the excretion of bilirubin by the kidneys.

Each of these events has its own repercussions on body function. For example the build-up of ammonia and other waste products is associated with brain dysfunction (*hepatic encephalopathy*); elevated levels of steroid hormones alter cellular development and function; lowered concentrations of plasma proteins result in bleeding disorders and may contribute to tissue fluid imbalance, resulting in oedema.

The signs of hepatic encephalopathy include changes in personality and intellect and also confusion, restlessness and, in severe cases, coma and convulsions. In people with liver disease, for example cirrhosis, this will be an intermittent feature of life which is precipitated by factors such as binge drinking, drug overdose, dehydration and excessive protein intake.

In severe liver failure there may also be hypothermia as a consequence of reduced metabolic activity. Under normal conditions the extensive metabolic activity of the liver accounts for 20% of the oxygen consumed at rest which contributes a significant proportion of resting heat production.

KEY POINTS

What you should now understand about the liver:

- what cells it is composed of and what they do
- how the cells are organised and how this affects their function
- how the hepatic blood supply differs from that of other organs
- why liver cells are at risk of injury from blood-borne toxins, and pathogens
- what the major functions of the liver are
- what the consequences of liver failure are likely to be.

REFERENCES AND FURTHER READING

Arias I M, Jakoby W B, Popper H, Schachter D, Shafritz D A 1988 The liver: biology and pathobiology, 2nd edn. Raven Press, New York
(Thick volume of detailed reviews written for and by hepatologists)
Rogers A W 1992 Textbook of anatomy. Churchill Livingstone, Edinburgh
Sherlock S 1989 Diseases of the liver and biliary system, 8th edn. Blackwell Scientific Publications, Oxford
(A very useful reference book combining authority and clarity on all aspects of liver disorder)
Storer J 1988 The liver. In: Hinchliff S, Montague S (eds) Physiology for nursing practice. Baillière Tindall, London

Chapter 10
ENDOCRINE TISSUE AND HORMONES

Hormones form part of the control systems that regulate cell activity and maintain homeostasis (see Ch. 3). They complement neural control mechanisms and are integrated with them through the neural and endocrine functions of the hypothalamus. ①

Most hormones are secreted by endocrine cells, but some are secreted by nerves and others are formed in plasma and interstitial fluid from products released by cells.

Hormone-secreting tissue takes many forms. It includes:

● the neuroendocrine tissue of the hypothalamus
● discrete endocrine glands (anterior pituitary, adrenals, thyroid)
● endocrine cells lodged in other organs (pancreas, digestive system, heart and kidneys).

This chapter outlines the structure of the main types of hormone-secreting tissue, and the nature, regulation and actions of the hormones secreted. The specific roles played by different hormones in homeostasis are described later in relevant chapters (Chs 11–16). The gonads (ovaries and testes) and their role in repro-duction and development are described in Chapters 34 and 35.

NAMING OF HORMONES

The current list of recognised hormones is very long and grows longer by the year, as more are identified by experiment and analysis (Table 10.1). Each time a hormone is discovered a name has to be found for it. This is almost as problematic as finding a suitable name for a new baby. Usually, the investigators who first demonstrate the existence of a hormone give it a name that describes an aspect of its character that they have identified. Thus, some hormones have been named after the tissue from which they were first isolated, e.g. adrenaline (from the adrenal medulla); insulin (from the islets of Langerhans – *insula* means island). Sometimes the name describes the first known action of the hormone, e.g. glucagon (which increases blood glucose concentration); calcitonin (which decreases blood calcium concentration). Occasionally hormones have been renamed or possess two names when a further important action has been identified. This applies to vasopressin which is also known as antidiuretic hormone (ADH). It has two major actions. It increases blood pressure by contracting blood vessels (*vasopressor*) and it decreases urine output (*antidiuretic*).

① *What does endocrine mean?*

NEUROENDOCRINE FUNCTION OF THE HYPOTHALAMUS

The hypothalamus acts as an interface between the nervous system and the endocrine system. It receives information about the internal state of the body from many sensory receptors, and coordinates the activity of different tissues and organs through the secretion of hormones and the autonomic nervous system. Several hypothalamic hormones control the activity of the *anterior pituitary gland* which in turn secretes hormones that control selected endocrine cells including those of the adrenals, thyroid and gonads (ovaries and testes) (Fig. 10.1).

NEURAL CONNECTIONS

The hypothalamus receives information from many parts of the nervous system. These include receptor cells which monitor many aspects of the body's state:

- composition of the body fluids (such as osmotic pressure, glucose, fatty acids)
- body temperature
- pressures in the circulation
- pressures in the gastrointestinal tract.

Information is also relayed to the hypothalamus from the *limbic system*, part of the brain which is concerned with our appetites, desires and emotions (see Ch. 31).

The hypothalamus controls body systems (circulatory, digestive, respiratory, urinary) and influences many endocrine cells through the autonomic nervous system. It is also involved in the control of activities such as drinking, eating, and sexual activity, through the somatic nervous system (Ch. 31).

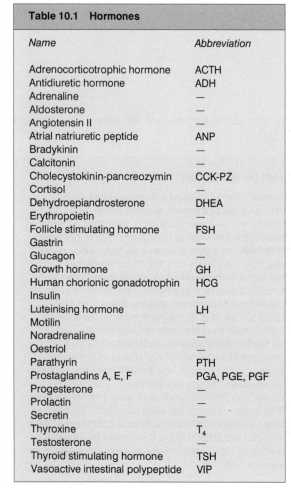

Table 10.1	Hormones
Name	*Abbreviation*
Adrenocorticotrophic hormone	ACTH
Antidiuretic hormone	ADH
Adrenaline	—
Aldosterone	—
Angiotensin II	—
Atrial natriuretic peptide	ANP
Bradykinin	—
Calcitonin	—
Cholecystokinin-pancreozymin	CCK-PZ
Cortisol	—
Dehydroepiandrosterone	DHEA
Erythropoietin	—
Follicle stimulating hormone	FSH
Gastrin	—
Glucagon	—
Growth hormone	GH
Human chorionic gonadotrophin	HCG
Insulin	—
Luteinising hormone	LH
Motilin	—
Noradrenaline	—
Oestriol	—
Parathyrin	PTH
Prostaglandins A, E, F	PGA, PGE, PGF
Progesterone	—
Prolactin	—
Secretin	—
Thyroxine	T_4
Testosterone	—
Thyroid stimulating hormone	TSH
Vasoactive intestinal polypeptide	VIP

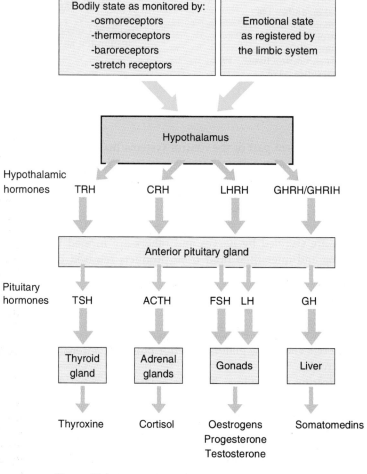

Figure 10.1
Central role of the hypothalamus in the regulation of hormone secretion by endocrine tissue (see Table 10.2, p. 192).

ENDOCRINE FUNCTION

Some neurones of the hypothalamus secrete regulatory substances into the blood. These substances are properly termed hormones even though they are manufactured and secreted by nerves.

The cell bodies of these *neuroendocrine cells* are, like other cells in the brain, grouped into clusters known as *nuclei* (see Ch. 20). Axons extend from these neuroendocrine cells to two areas adjacent to the hypothalamus (Fig. 10.2):

- median eminence
- posterior pituitary.

The nerve endings in the median eminence release hormones (*hypophysiotrophic hormones*) which control the anterior pituitary gland (or *adenohypophysis*), a small clump of endocrine cells located immediately below the hypothalamus. The nerve endings within the posterior pituitary (*neurohypophysis*) release two hormones, *ADH* and *oxytocin*, into the bloodstream.

Relation to the pituitary gland

The anterior and posterior pituitary are joined together forming a small pea-sized structure (the *pituitary gland*) which hangs below the hypothalamus. Though they are linked together to form a single anatomical structure, and though they both secrete hormones, the two parts of the pituitary differ from one another.

The anterior pituitary develops in the embryo from cells associated with structures in the mouth and consists of endocrine cells, whereas the posterior pituitary develops as part of the nervous system and consists mainly of nerve axons and nerve endings.

THE PINEAL BODY (GLAND)

The pineal body is tiny; it weighs a little more than 0.1 g and lies deep within the brain, attached to the roof of the third ventricle (Fig. 10.2.). It is believed to be an endocrine gland and the hormone of interest here is melatonin.

Melatonin, which was discovered in 1958 by Aaron B Lerner and research workers at Yale University, is present in our bodies in very small amounts depending on age. The hormone was previously known to cause the skin of amphibians to blanch but its function in mammals remained uncertain until research in the 1970s and 80s suggested that it regulates sleeping cycles and the hormonal changes that usher in sexual maturity. The pineal gland's production of melatonin varies with both time of day and age: production is dramatically increased during the night and falls off during the day; levels are much higher in children under 7 years of age than in adolescents, and lower still in adults. Melatonin is thought to act by keeping a child's body from undergoing sexual maturation, since sex hormones such as prolactin, which play a part in the development of sexual organs, emerge only after melatonin levels have declined. It has been suggested that children with germ cell tumours of the pineal body (germinomas and teratomas) often reach sexual maturity unusually early in life because the pineal gland's production of melatonin has been hampered. These tumours, albeit rare and occurring mostly in children, are malignant, invasive and may be life threatening. For instance, they may give rise to increased intracranial pressure resulting in headaches, vomiting and epileptic seizures, the care principles of which require to be known by nurses and other health workers.

Melatonin has also been observed to play an important role in regulating sleep cycles. Test subjects injected with the hormone become sleepy, suggesting that the increased production of melatonin coincident with nightfall acts as a fundamental mechanism for inducing sleep. With dawn, the pineal gland stops producing melatonin and wakefulness and alertness ensue. The high level of melatonin production in young children may explain their tendency to sleep longer than adults. The functions of the pineal body are beginning to unfold but it still remains a somewhat mysterious bit of tissue. The functions discussed are speculative; ideas may change as more information becomes available.

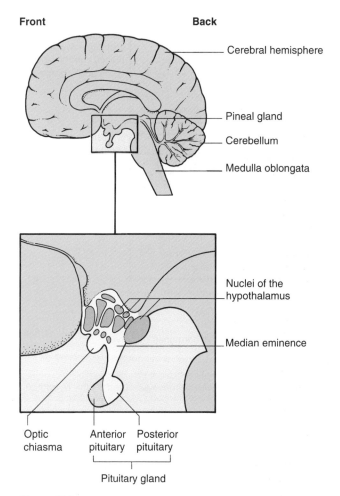

Figure 10.2
Position and structure of the hypothalamus and the pituitary gland in the brain. The diagram shows the view of the brain that you would see if you cut the brain in two, separating the left and right cerebral hemispheres, and looked at one half (in this case the right half).

Neurosecretion

Hormones are manufactured in the cell bodies of the neurones in the form of large precursor polypeptides

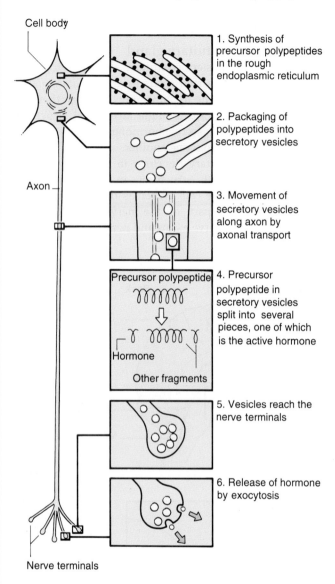

Cell body

1. Synthesis of precursor polypeptides in the rough endoplasmic reticulum

2. Packaging of polypeptides into secretory vesicles

Axon

3. Movement of secretory vesicles along axon by axonal transport

Precursor polypeptide

4. Precursor polypeptide in secretory vesicles split into several pieces, one of which is the active hormone

Hormone

Other fragments

5. Vesicles reach the nerve terminals

6. Release of hormone by exocytosis

Nerve terminals

Figure 10.3
Formation and secretion of hormones by nerves.

② *Can you think of a few examples of psychological stress?*

(*prohormones*) and are packaged into small secretory granules. The granules move down the axons of the nerve cells to the nerve endings by *axonal transport* (Fig. 10.3). During transport the precursor polypeptides in the secretory granules are split enzymically into fragments giving rise to hormones and other peptides such as *neurophysins*.

The contents of the secretory granules (hormones and other products) are released by exocytosis at the nerve endings. Secretion is evoked by nerve impulses just like the secretion of neurotransmitters (see Chs 3 and 21).

Control of secretion

The secretion of hypothalamic hormones is mainly controlled by nervous activity. Hormones are released reflexly in response to excitation of sensory receptors. For example ADH is secreted when osmoreceptors are stimulated, and oxytocin is released when touch receptors around the nipple of a woman's breast are excited during suckling by a baby (Fig. 10.4).

Because of the links between the hypothalamus and other parts of the nervous system the secretion of hormones is also affected by our emotional state and by psychological stress. ②

Hypophysiotrophic hormones

The nerve endings in the median eminence lie close to a set of blood vessels (*hypothalamo-hypophyseal portal vessels*) linking this part of the hypothalamus to the anterior pituitary (Fig. 10.5). These vessels are distinctive in that they link two networks of capillaries, those in the median eminence, and those in the anterior pituitary. They form a *portal* circulation similar in principle to the hepatic portal vein which links the digestive system to the liver (see Ch. 9). The hormones released from the nerve endings in the median eminence (*hypophysiotrophic hormones*) are thus carried directly to the cells of the anterior pituitary and regulate their secretion of hormones (Table 10.2).

Table 10.2 Effects of hormones secreted by the hypothalamus on the anterior pituitary gland		
Hypophysiotrophic hormones		*Effect on secretion of anterior pituitary hormones*
Name	Abbreviation	
Corticotrophin releasing hormone	CRH	↑ ACTH (corticotrophin)
Growth hormone releasing hormone	GHRH	↑ growth hormone (somatotrophin)
Growth hormone release inhibiting hormone (somatostatin)	GHRIH	↓ growth hormone (somatotrophin)
Luteinising hormone releasing hormone	LHRH	↑ FSH ↑ LH
Prolactin inhibiting hormone	PIH	↓ prolactin (luteotrophin)
Prolactin releasing hormone	PRH	↑ prolactin (luteotrophin)
Thyrotrophin releasing hormone	TRH	↑ TSH (thyrotrophin)

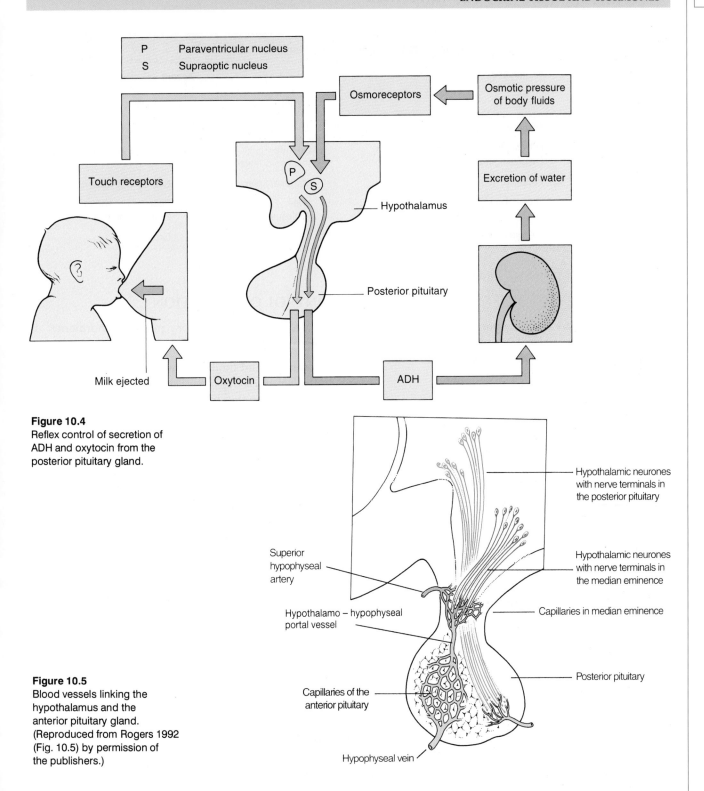

| P | Paraventricular nucleus |
| S | Supraoptic nucleus |

Figure 10.4
Reflex control of secretion of
ADH and oxytocin from the
posterior pituitary gland.

Figure 10.5
Blood vessels linking the
hypothalamus and the
anterior pituitary gland.
(Reproduced from Rogers 1992
(Fig. 10.5) by permission of
the publishers.)

ADH and oxytocin

ADH (vasopressin) and oxytocin are manufactured by
the cell bodies forming the *supraoptic* and *paraventricular
nuclei* and secreted from the nerve endings in the
posterior pituitary. ADH has a major role in the regulation of fluid balance (see Ch. 13), whereas oxytocin
is concerned chiefly with reproductive function (see
Ch. 34).

ANTERIOR PITUITARY GLAND

This collection of endocrine cells consists of a number of
cell types, distinguishable by labelling with antibodies
specific to the hormones secreted (*immunocytochemistry*).
Each cell secretes at lease one hormone (Table 10.3).

Table 10.3 Hormones of the anterior pituitary gland: their origin and actions				
Cell of origin	Pituitary hormone		Actions	
		Target	Stimulatory effect
Corticotroph	Adrenocorticotrophic hormone (ACTH)	Adrenal cortex	Secretion of hormones
Gonadotroph	Follicle stimulating hormone (FSH) Luteinising hormone (LH)	Gonads (ovaries & testes)	(See Chs 34 and 35)
Lactotroph	Prolactin	Mammary glands	Secretion of milk
Somatotroph	Growth hormone (GH)	Liver All tissues	Secretion of somatomedins Protein synthesis
Thyrotroph	Thyroid stimulating hormone (TSH)	Thyroid gland	Growth

HORMONES

All the hormones are basically polypeptides (see Ch. 3). The largest is *thyrotrophin* (*TSH*) (mol. wt. 28 000) and the smallest is *adrenocorticotrophic hormone* (*ACTH*) (mol. wt. 4500).

Trophic actions

The hormones regulate the growth and development of one or more tissues in the body, several of which are other endocrine glands (Table 10.3).

When pituitary hormones are secreted in excess the tissues and glands influenced by them enlarge (*hypertrophy*). Endocrine glands increase their secretion of hormones and this in turn stimulates their target cells. Conversely, if the secretion of anterior pituitary hormones is deficient, the target endocrine glands shrink in size (*atrophy*), and their secretion of hormones decreases.

The effects of over- and underproduction of growth hormone and prolactin depend on someone's stage of development. Growth hormone for example is necessary for the normal development of stature in a young person, but, once full height has been achieved, a deficiency of this hormone does not cause someone to shrink! Overproduction of prolactin stimulates the secretion of milk in women but not in men of reproductive age (see Chs 34 and 35).

Somatomedins

The growth promoting effects of growth hormone are not caused by the hormone itself but by the action of intermediary factors (*somatomedins*). Somatomedins are manufactured by the liver (and kidneys) and their secretion is stimulated by growth hormone. They are structurally and functionally similar to the hormone insulin and have been termed '*insulin-like growth factors*'.

CONTROL OF SECRETION

The secretion of anterior pituitary hormones is influenced by:

- stimulating and inhibiting factors from the hypothalamus (*hypophysiotrophic hormones*)
- hormones secreted by the target endocrine cells (*negative feedback*).

Hypophysiotrophic hormones

Secretion of each of the anterior pituitary hormones is influenced by at least one of the hypophysiotrophic hormones (Table 10.2). The secretion of growth hormone and of prolactin differs from the other hormones listed in that they are regulated by two hypophysiotrophic hormones, one which stimulates and one which inhibits secretion.

As the secretion of hypophysiotrophic hormones is controlled by the nervous system, the pattern of secretion of the pituitary hormones has several distinctive features. It is:

- pulsatile
- influenced by stress
- varies with the sleep/wake cycle.

Pulsatile release

Hypophysiotrophic hormones are secreted by exocytosis provoked by action potentials arriving at the nerve endings in the median eminence. Consequently, secretion of the hormones occurs in bursts, in a *pulsatile* way, as the frequency of impulses in the hypothalamic neurones changes quickly. As hypophysiotrophic hormones cause rapid changes in the secretion of pituitary hormones, these too are secreted in a pulsatile fashion.

LH, for example, is released in pulses (Fig. 10.6) from puberty onwards. Similarly bursts of secretion of growth hormone, prolactin and ACTH also occur. As pituitary hormones are cleared from the circulation

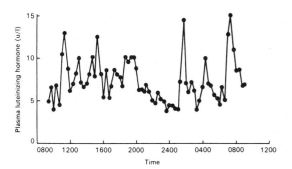

Figure 10.6
Pulsatile secretion of luteinising hormone (LH) in man.
(Reproduced from Emslie-Smith et al 1988 (Fig. 24.18, based on
Boyar et al 1972) by permission of the publishers.)

quite quickly their concentration in the blood rises and
falls rapidly.

> The rate of disposal of a hormone from the blood is
> measured as its half life. The half life is the time it takes for
> the concentration of an injected, labelled hormone in the
> blood to he halved. Half lives of the anterior pituitary
> hormones are about 30 minutes or less.

Effects of stress
Stress of various kinds, such as fear, injury, acute cold,
exercise, and low blood sugar, can affect the secretion
of the pituitary hormones through the effects of these
challenges on the nervous system. In general, secretion
of pituitary hormones is increased, but the proportion of
the different hormones secreted differs according to the
specific nature of the stress experienced.

> An example of the effects of stress is where the
> gonadotrophic hormone balance may be altered resulting in
> disturbances in the menstrual cycle that are frequently seen
> in young women when they first move away from home.

Sleep/wake cycle
The regular alternation between being awake and being
asleep is caused by periodic changes in nervous activity
(see Ch. 31). These changes affect the hypothalamus as
well and, through it, the pituitary. Secretion of growth
hormone and of prolactin, for example, is highest
during the night, whereas the secretion of ACTH is
lowest during the very 'early hours' of the morning and
peaks around the time of waking (see Ch. 18). ③

Negative feedback from target glands
The secretion of the pituitary hormones that regulate
other endocrine glands (TSH, ACTH, FSH and LH) is

OVERGROWING
Growth hormone is of major importance in controlling
growth from birth to adolescence. In certain circumstances,
because of disorders due to tumour of the pituitary gland,
there is an uncontrolled and excessive secretion of growth
hormone. If this happens in childhood it leads to
exaggerated growth known as *gigantism*.

In gigantism, growth is gradual but continuous and
consistent; the affected person, with bones in normal
proportion, may attain a height of 8 feet. Muscles may
be well developed but later undergo some atrophy and
weakening. The life span is shorter than normal because of
a greater susceptibility to infection and metabolic disorders.
The susceptibility arises because an untreated pituitary
gland tumour grows until the gland is destroyed and ceases
control of all endocrine glands. One of the glands affected
is the thyroid, leading to inadequate production of the
hormones responsible for regulating metabolism and hence
to metabolic disorders. Among such disorders is nutritional
deficiency in which body-building and energy-yielding
foods are not utilised (caloric failure). The consequence is
progressive weight loss and weakness. Opportunistic
organisms, which are normally harmless, take advantage
and invade the body giving rise to gastrointestinal or
parasitic disorders. It is thus the general deficiency of other
pituitary hormones that usually causes death in early
adulthood.

An excessive production of growth hormone in an adult
results in enlargement of skeletal extremities, a condition
known as *acromegaly*. For instance, the bones and soft
tissues of the hands, feet, face and lower jaw become
enlarged and the skin becomes coarse.

Growth hormone can also stimulate the growth of
connective tissue such as ligaments, capsules and synovial
membranes. A combination of connective tissue growth and
hypertrophied bones compresses the local nerves causing
pain, burning sensation in the joints, stiffness in the limbs,
and tingling and numbness in the hands. Another condition
commonly associated with acromegaly is diabetes mellitus
described later in this chapter. It affects approximately 20 to
40% of acromegalic individuals because the growth
hormone blocks the action of insulin.

In both gigantism and acromegaly, apart from the
physiological traumas that result from the excessive
production of growth hormone, there are also problems in
adapting to an altered body image that can cause great
embarrassment. The role of the nurse is to utilise the
principles of care that apply to difficulty in adapting to
altered body image, susceptibility to infection, injury and
pain. Examples of these principles would be rest, clean and
safe nursing environment, interaction and reassurance,
unhurried approach, respect for the expression of feelings
of clients and reduction of pain by drugs prescribed by
physicians.

also controlled by hormones released by these glands.
Thus *thyroxine* from the thyroid gland, *oestrogens* and
testosterone from the gonads (ovaries and testes) and
cortisol from the adrenal glands inhibit secretion of their
respective pituitary hormones (Fig. 10.7). This is an
example of negative feedback control (see Ch. 3). It

③
*Is the secretion
of growth
hormone and
prolactin
affected if a
person
changes
his/her pattern
of sleep, e.g.
sleeping
during the day
and staying
awake at
night?*

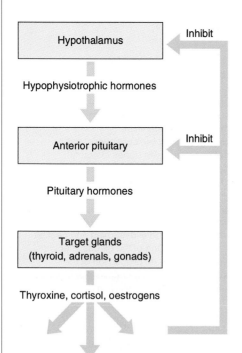

Figure 10.7
Stabilising the concentration of thyroxine, cortisol and oestrogen in the blood by negative feedback.

maintains the plasma concentrations of thyroxine, cortisol, oestrogens and testosterone at an appropriate level.

Oestrogens are unusual in that they can also have a positive feedback effect but only at a specific time during a woman's menstrual cycle (see Ch. 34).

Hormones secreted by the target endocrine glands may also influence the secretion of hypophysiotophic hormones by the hypothalamus. For example cortisol inhibits the release of CRH.

ADRENAL GLANDS

There are two adrenal glands, one on each side of the body. They are sited, as their name implies, right next to the kidneys, at their top end (Fig. 10.8A).

Like the pituitary, each adrenal gland is composed of two parts, one of which, the *medulla*, is derived embryologically from neural tissue. Enveloping the medulla are the cells of the *cortex* (Fig. 10.8B).

ADRENAL MEDULLA

The adrenal medulla consists of *chromaffin cells* (so-called because of their colour in histological sections). Embryologically they originate from the same neural tissue that forms neurones of the sympathetic ganglia

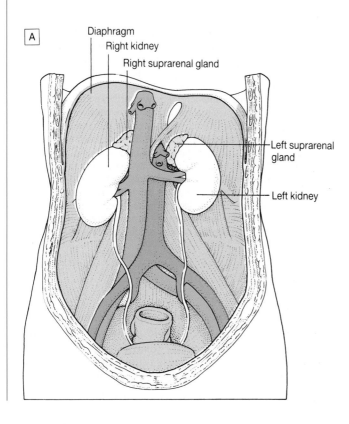

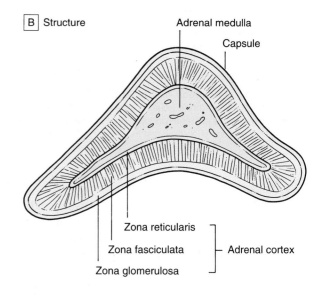

Figure 10.8
The adrenal glands:
A Position
B Structure.
(Part A reproduced from Rogers 1992 (Fig. 10.8) by permission of the publishers.)

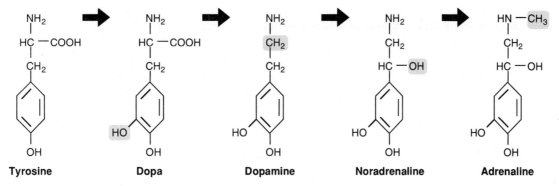

Figure 10.9
Steps in the synthesis of catecholamines from the amino acid tyrosine.

(see Ch. 3). As such, they are closely related to neurones even though they do not posses dendrites or axons.

The cells are packed full of granules (vesicles) containing storage forms of the two hormones secreted by the medulla:

- adrenaline
- noradrenaline.

Hormone synthesis
Noradrenaline and adrenaline are both synthesised from the amino acid tyrosine (Fig. 10.9). Noradrenaline is synthesised in the same way in nerve terminals. The difference, here in the adrenal medulla, is that the process is extended to the formation of adrenaline. Thus adrenaline, and not noradrenaline, is the major product secreted (80%). Adrenaline, noradrenaline, and their precursor, dopamine, are classed chemically as *catecholamines*.

Control of secretion
The secretion of medullary hormones into the bloodstream is affected by nerves and hormones that affect the chromaffin cells directly, and by factors that regulate blood flow through the gland.

Sympathetic nerves
Chromaffin cells are innervated by sympathetic nerves (Ch. 3). These nerves release the neurotransmitter acetylcholine which stimulates the cells to secrete the hormones by exocytosis. When activity in the sympathetic nervous system increases, the secretion of the medullary catecholamines increases too.

Adrenal blood flow
The adrenal medulla receives blood from two sources:

- arterial blood
- portal blood from the adrenal cortex.

Thus chromaffin cells are exposed to blood that has a high concentration of steroid hormones secreted by the cortex. Blood drains from the adrenal gland through the *central vein*. Venoconstriction can cause secreted hormones to be dammed up within the gland or to be released from it when the venules dilate.

Actions
Adrenaline and noradrenaline have widespread effects on cells and tissues (Table 10.4). They affect contraction of smooth muscle and cardiac muscle and regulate

---

As a means of protecting ourselves from harm, each one of us has an 'alarm reaction' mechanism – also frequently called the 'fight or flight reaction'. The reaction is reinforced by physiological changes in the bloodstream. Alarm causes secretion of the hormones, adrenaline and noradrenaline, which speed the heart, increase blood sugar and generally prepare the body for fight or flight.

Table 10.4 Some actions of adrenaline and noradrenaline

Cardiovascular	Metabolic	Other
Increase cardiac contraction	Increase metabolic rate	Stimulate the nervous system
Increase cardiac exitability	Increase breakdown of glycogen	Increase alertness
Increase heart rate	Increase supply of fatty acids	
Vasoconstriction (noradrenaline)	Increase plasma lactate	
Vasodilation (adrenaline)		
Increase blood pressure		

Table 10.5   Some effects of activating different adrenoreceptors

Alpha receptor	Beta₁ receptor	Beta₂ receptor
Pupil of the eye dilates	Heart rate increases	Blood vessels relax
Blood vessels constrict	Cardiac contraction increases	Bronchial smooth muscle relaxes
Gut muscle relaxes	Fat breakdown stimulated	Gut muscle relaxes

several aspects of carbohydrate and fat metabolism. They exert their effects by binding to *adrenoreceptors* on their target cells.

Adrenoreceptors

Several different adrenoreceptors (alpha and beta; see Ch. 3) have been identified. They have different affinities for adrenaline and noradrenaline and different effects (Table 10.5).

The exact effect of the medullary hormones depends on the relative numbers of the different receptors present on the target cells, as well as on the concentrations of the adrenaline and noradrenaline in the fluid surrounding them. This depends on the noradrenaline released from nerve terminals locally as well as the hormones secreted by the adrenal medulla.

For example, alpha and beta receptors are present on the smooth muscle cells of the coronary blood vessels. Activation of alpha receptors by noradrenaline, released from sympathetic nerves, causes vasoconstriction, as in most other circulations (see Ch. 5). However, in exercise, adrenaline from the adrenal medulla helps to over-rule this effect by activating beta receptors which cause vasodilation.

Other chromaffin tissue

Small clumps of cells like those in the adrenal medulla are also found associated with other parts of the autonomic nervous system. Their role and significance is not yet clear. Occasionally tumours of the chromaffin cells may develop at these sites (*phaeochromocytoma*). These secrete catecholamines.

ADRENAL CORTEX

The cortex consists of three different zones (Fig. 10.8B), named according to their histological appearance. From the outer to the inner zone these are:

Phaeochromocytoma (the only known disorder that gives rise to the excessive production of catecholamines) results in hypertension, hyperglycaemia and high metabolic rate. A patient with phaeochromocytoma is treated by surgical removal of the tumour, which is usually unilateral and benign.

- zona glomerulosa
- zona fasciculata
- zona reticularis.

The middle zone is the largest of the three, occupying about 75% of the cortex.

Hormones

The cortical cells synthesise a variety of *steroid hormones* (see Ch. 3 and Table 10.6) of which two are most important:

- cortisol   • aldosterone.

Cells of the zona fasciculata and zona reticularis produce cortisol whereas cells of the zona glomerulosa specialise in the synthesis of aldosterone.

Synthesis

The steroids are synthesised from cholesterol by inter-related metabolic pathways (Fig. 10.10). The significance of this possibly daunting picture is that, should one step be impaired, there will be 'knock-on' effects on other steroids that are part of the same integrated scheme. A build-up of earlier precursors occurs and these overflow into alternative pathways. As a result, the production of one or more of the steroids is deficient and others are produced in excess.

Transport in blood

About 80% of cortisol in plasma is bound to a specific plasma protein (*transcortin*) and 15% is bound to albumin. Only 5% therefore is free to influence cell activity. The majority of the aldosterone in plasma is unbound.

Actions

Steroid hormones influence cell activity by controlling the synthesis of specific proteins (see Ch. 2). The proteins include those involved in the transport of sodium and potassium across cell membranes (*mineralocorticoid* effect of steroids), and those which influence the metabolism of carbohydrates, amino

In *Addison's disease* there is insufficent production of steroids. It may be due to an autoimmune disorder causing atrophy of the adrenal cortex.

Table 10.6 Steroid hormones secreted by the adrenal cortex

Name	Also known as
Cortisol	Hydrocortisone
Corticosterone	—
Aldosterone	—
Deoxycorticosterone	DOC
Dehydroepiandrosterone	DHEA
Androstenedione	—

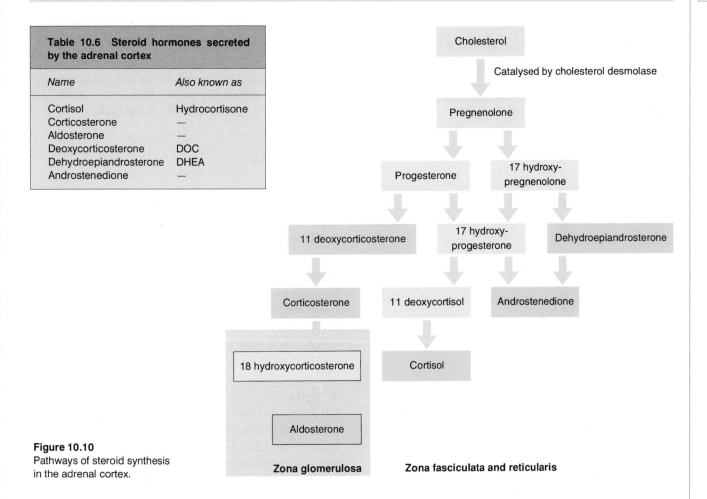

Figure 10.10
Pathways of steroid synthesis in the adrenal cortex.

acids and fats, and raise blood glucose concentration (*glucocorticoid* effect).

Mineralocorticoid activity

Aldosterone is a potent mineralocorticoid. It is important in the regulation of sodium and potassium balance (see Ch. 13). Cortisol is not as potent but, because of its structural similarities with aldosterone, it does influence sodium and potassium balance, albeit to a small extent (20% of the contribution made by aldosterone).

Glucocorticoid activity

Cortisol is much more potent as a glucocorticoid. It increases blood glucose concentration by affecting the metabolism of many tissues including muscle, adipose tissue and liver (Table 10.7). It is involved in regulating blood glucose concentration in response to starvation (see Ch. 14) and in adjusting metabolism in response to stress (see Ch. 19).

Table 10.7 Effects of cortisol on the metabolism of carbohydrates, proteins and fats

Tissue	Carbohydrates	Proteins	Fats
Muscle	Decreases glucose uptake	Increases protein breakdown	—
Adipose tissue	Decreases glucose uptake	—	Increases fat breakdown
Blood	Glucose concentration ↑	Amino acid concentration ↑	Fatty acid concentration ↑
Liver	Promotes glycogenesis (conversion of glucose to glycogen)	Promotes gluconeogenesis (conversion of amino acids and fatty acids to glucose)	

Steroids such as prednisolone (an anti-inflammatory and anti-allergic glucocorticoid) are used in the treatment of certain inflammatory diseases including dermatitis. However, their use may slow down wound healing, as inflammation promoted by the immune system is an essential stage in the process of healing.

④
Why does the thyroid gland become enlarged to form a lump in some individuals?

Other effects of steroids
The presence of cortisol is also required to maintain normal function of:

● the cardiovascular system
● the central nervous system.

At higher concentrations it also:

● decreases the effectiveness of the immune system
● increases the sensitivity of many tissues to nor-adrenaline.

Control of secretion

Aldosterone
Secretion of aldosterone by the cells of the zona glomerulosa is affected by:

● angiotensin II (see p. 207)
● ACTH from the anterior pituitary
● plasma potassium concentration.

Of these, angiotensin II is the most potent stimulus for secretion. ACTH stimulates secretion but its effects are relatively small. Secretion of aldosterone increases when plasma potassium is raised and decreases when it falls (see Ch. 13).

Cortisol
The secretion of cortisol by the adrenals is controlled by ACTH. Steroid hormones, unlike peptides and proteins, are not stored to any great extent. Thus secretion can only be increased by actually stimulating the manufacture of the hormone. The interaction of ACTH with receptors on cells of the two inner zones (fasciculata and reticularis) increases the activity of the enzyme cholesterol desmolase (see Fig. 10.10). Cortisol production increases within a few minutes. The secretion of cortisol thus closely follows changes in the plasma concentration of ACTH. The bursts of secretion of ACTH from the pituitary, and the regular 24-hourly rise and fall in its concentration, are reflected in a similar pattern of plasma cortisol concentration (see Ch. 18).

In the long term, continued stimulation of the gland by ACTH provokes an increase in the size of the two inner zones, whereas in the absence of ACTH these two zones atrophy and cortisol secretion virtually ceases.

THYROID GLAND

The thyroid gland is situated just below the larynx and lies over the front of the trachea (Fig. 10.11A & B). If it enlarges a lump (*goitre*) is visible in the neck. ④

STRUCTURE

The appearance of thyroid tissue is unmistakable (Fig. 10.11C). The tissue is made up of many *follicles* (sometimes termed *acini*) interspersed by blood and lymph capillaries, nerve fibres and 'C' cells.

Follicles
The follicles consist of a layer of *follicular cells* enclosing a non-cellular area (*follicular lumen*). The lumen stains bright pink with the chemical reagent used in histology, and is filled with *colloid*. The chief constituent of the colloid is the glycoprotein *thyroglobulin*.

'C' cells
'C' cells secrete the peptide hormone, *calcitonin*. Calcitonin is involved in the maintenance of calcium balance (see Ch. 13). Its secretion increases in response to a rise in calcium concentration in the interstitial fluid. Calcitonin increases the secretion of calcium by the kidneys and thereby lowers calcium concentration in the extracellular fluid.

HORMONES

The two major hormones secreted by the thyroid gland are:

● thyroxine
● tri-iodothyronine.

Synthesis
Thyroxine and tri-iodothyronine are iodine-containing hormones formed from tyrosine (Fig. 10.12) one of the amino acids present in the protein thyroglobulin.

Iodine
Tri-iodothyronine contains three iodine atoms, whereas thyroxine (also known as tetra-iodothyronine) contains four. For simplicity these hormones are sometimes referred to as T_3 and T_4 respectively.

An adequate dietary intake of iodine is vital for the hormones to be manufactured. Follicular cells actively extract iodine from the blood and concentrate it within the cells.

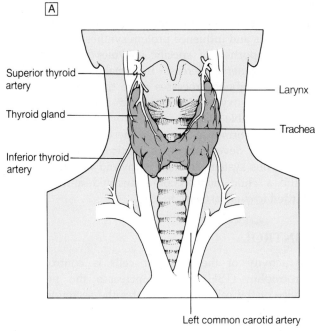

A

Superior thyroid artery

Thyroid gland

Inferior thyroid artery

Larynx

Trachea

Left common carotid artery

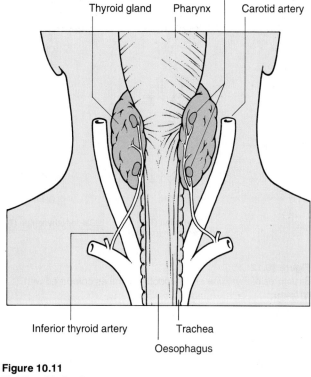

B

Thyroid gland Pharynx

Parathyroid glands

Carotid artery

Inferior thyroid artery Trachea

Oesophagus

Figure 10.11
The thyroid gland:
A Position in the neck as viewed from the front
B Position in the neck as viewed from behind, showing the parathyroid glands
C Tissue structure.
(Part A reproduced from Rogers 1992 (Fig. 10.6) by permission of the publishers.)

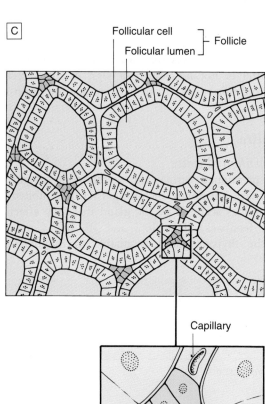

C

Follicular cell

Folicular lumen

Follicle

Capillary

Parafollicular cells ('C' cells)

Thyroglobulin

The first step in the synthesis of the thyroid hormones is the synthesis of thyroglobulin by the follicular cells (Fig. 10.13). The protein is packaged into vesicles, probably together with enzymes needed for the later stages of the manufacturing process, and is secreted into the follicular lumen by exocytosis. Further processing of the thyroglobulin molecule occurs in the follicular lumen:

- iodine combines with tyrosine residues
- two iodinated tyrosine residues become linked.

As a result molecules of T_3 and T_4 are formed attached to the main thyroglobulin molecule (Fig. 10.13).

Secretion

Secretion of thyroid hormones involves the uptake of chunks of colloid by the follicular cells by endocytosis.

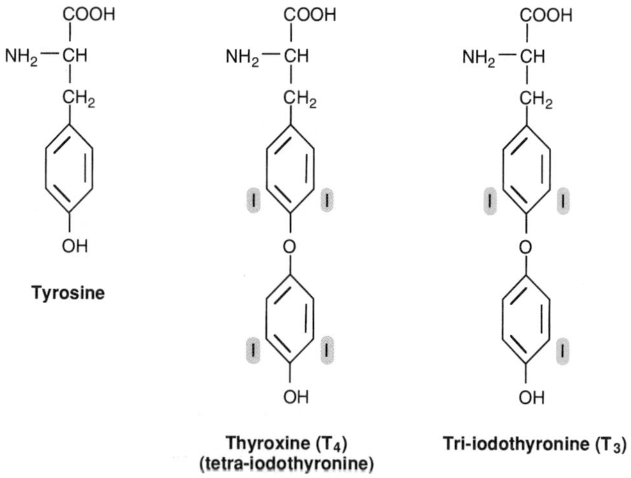

Figure 10.12
Structures of thyroxine and tri-iodothyronine as compared with tyrosine.

Large vesicles are formed which fuse with lysosomes containing enzymes that degrade thyroglobulin to liberate the free thyroid hormones. Other products of this breakdown, such as iodine, amino acids and sugars, are recycled and re-used by the follicular cells. The thyroid hormones are secreted into the bloodstream.

Transport in blood

Less than 1% of the thyroid hormones present in blood is free in plasma and able to diffuse into the interstitial spaces to influence cell activity. The vast majority is bound to plasma proteins (two specific binding proteins and albumin).

Actions

Thyroid hormones diffuse into cells, bind to receptors in the nucleus and influence protein synthesis. The change in the proportion of specific enzymes within the cell causes a general increase in metabolic activity but increases catabolic processes more than anabolic ones. Much more oxygen is consumed and more heat is generated (Table 10.8).

Thyroid hormones are also necessary for normal growth and development, in particular maturation of the nervous system. If there is thyroid deficiency early in life a child may become dwarfed and mentally retarded (*cretinism*) (see Ch. 35).

CONTROL

The activity of the follicular cells is controlled by thyrotrophin (TSH), which increases the metabolic activity of the cells and stimulates the secretion of the thyroid hormones as well as the manufacture of thyroglobulin. The cells grow in size, which adds to their overall productivity.

TSH stimulates the growth of the cells even if the manufacture of the thyroid hormones is blocked in some way. For this reason enlargement of the thyroid (*goitre*) is not necessarily a sign of oversecretion of thyroid hormones. It can indicate just the opposite (see below).

Goitre

Hypothyroid goitre

As mentioned earlier, the secretion of several of the pituitary hormones, including TSH, is inhibited by the hormones secreted by the gland that they affect (negative feedback) (Figs 10.7 and 10.14A). Consequently if the thyroid gland is unable to manufacture the

Table 10.8 Consequences of the cellular actions of thyroid hormones		
Cellular action	Consequences	
	Primary	Secondary
Increased oxygen consumption (calorigenic effect)	Increased heat production	Vasodilation
Increased protein breakdown (catabolism)	Loss of muscle mass	Muscle weakness
Increased formation of beta receptors in the heart	Promotes action of adrenaline and noradrenaline	Increased cardiac output
?	Increased intestinal absorption of glucose	Increased blood glucose after a meal
Increased formation of LDL receptors*	Increased cellular uptake of LDL*	Decreased plasma cholesterol
* LDL: low density lipoprotein (see Ch. 14).		

hormones (for example if there is a lack of iodine in the diet) then this inhibition is lacking and the secretion of TSH increases. Under the action of TSH the thyroid gland grows in size, but growth does not go hand in hand with an increase in the secretion of thyroid hormones. Thus there continues to be a deficiency of

thyroid hormones (*hypothyroidism*) despite the fact that the thyroid gland is enlarged (Fig. 10.14B).

Hyperthyroid goitre

A goitre may also develop in *hyperthyroidism* (*Graves' disease*). In this case the follicular cells are driven by abnormal stimulants present in the blood, and not by TSH. These stimulants have been identified as antibodies that bind specifically to the follicular cells and, in binding, activate the cells in a similar way to TSH. Large amounts of thyroid hormones are secreted. The raised plasma concentration of thyroid hormones suppresses

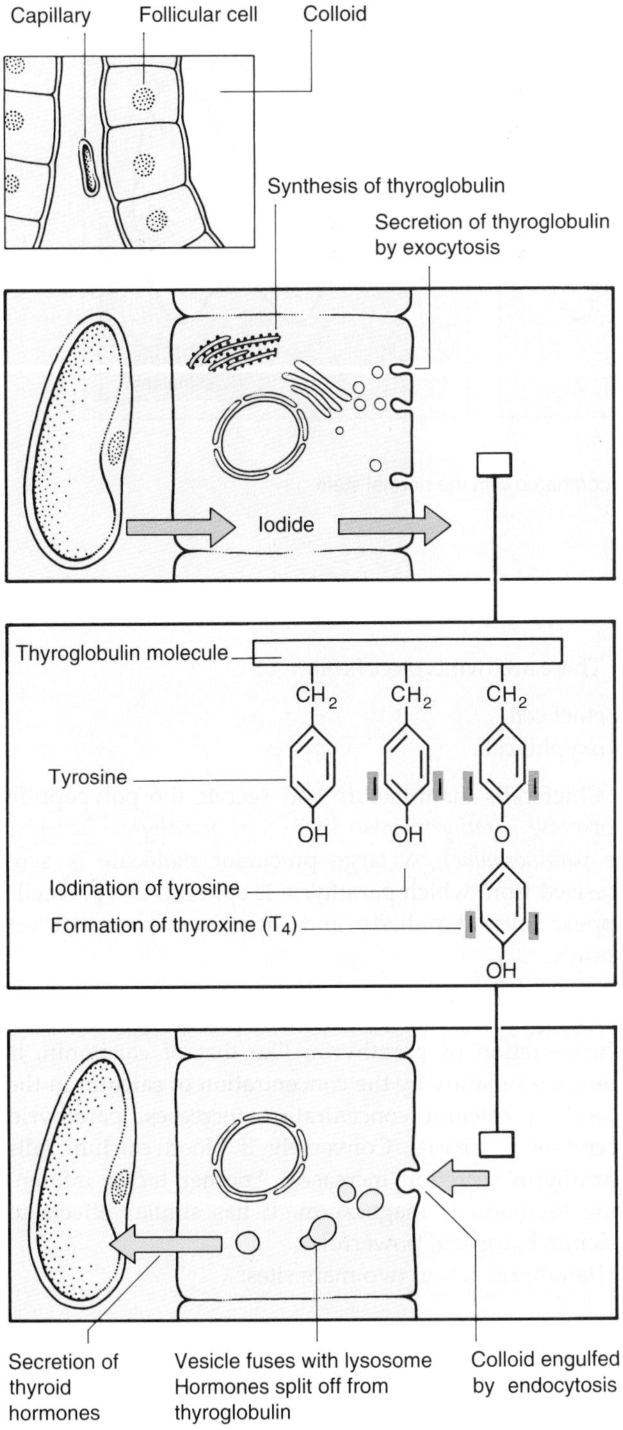

Figure 10.13
Steps in the formation of thyroid hormones.

APPETITE AND WEIGHT LOSS IN HYPERTHYROIDISM

Thyroxine is essential for normal growth. In excess, however, it results in the condition known as *hyperthyroidism*. This does not produce overgrowth as with the growth hormone but causes an increase in the catabolism of protein and other nutrients. The increased blood level of thyroid hormone accelerates the metabolic rate. In the process, the person's appetite increases and unless the food intake keeps pace with the metabolic rate, there is a marked loss of weight. The rapid metabolic rate is caused by the increased catabolism in which the additional energy produced is released in the form of heat rather than stored in adenosine triphosphate (ATP; see Ch. 11). The sufferer feels warm even in cold conditions and the body temperature may be raised, with excessive sweating.

Nervousness, apprehension, emotional instability and restlessness are evident and the hands are warm and moist in contrast to the cold moist extremities associated with anxiety. Shortness of breath on exertion and palpitation are experienced as a result of the increased metabolic rate. Although the patient tends to eat more, he complains of weakness and fatigue due to loss of weight. Also observed in the thyrotoxic patient is a fine rapid tremor of the hands, which is accentuated when they are outstretched.
Diarrhoea, resulting from increased gastrointestinal activity, may be troublesome.

Nursing principles aimed at helping the thyrotoxic client include:

- creating an environment that reduces nervousness
- encouraging him to eat a high protein, high carbohydrate diet
- encouraging him to drink extra fluids to replenish the increased fluid loss resulting from excessive heat production and perspiration
- encouraging decreased activity
- keeping him comfortably cool
- helping him to achieve self-management of the therapeutic regime.

Cretinism is a congenital disorder in which the deficiency of thyroid hormone may be primary, due to a disorder of the thyroid itself, or may be secondary as a result of pituitary or hypothalamic disturbance.

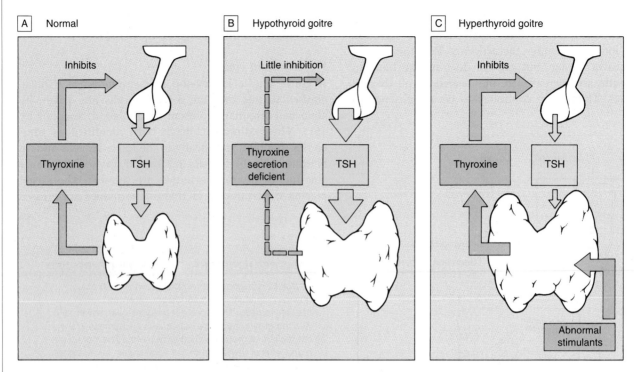

A   Normal
Inhibits
Thyroxine   TSH

B   Hypothyroid goitre
Little inhibition
Thyroxine secretion deficient   TSH

C   Hyperthyroid goitre
Inhibits
Thyroxine   TSH
Abnormal stimulants

Figure 10.14
Differences in the secretion of thyroxine and TSH in two forms of goitre as compared with the normal state.

the secretion of TSH, but as this was not the primary activator of the gland the secretion of the hormones continues unabated (Fig. 10.14C).

ENDOCRINE TISSUE LODGED IN OTHER ORGANS

THYROID

Parathyroid glands
As their name suggests, the parathyroids are found right next to the thyroid gland. They are very small glands, each weighing only about 50 mg (roughly the weight of a small postage stamp). In humans there are usually four of them situated at the back of the thyroid gland (Fig. 10.11B). Not infrequently there may be one or two more. Sometimes they are found deep in the thyroid itself or at other places, such as within the mediastinum, the space between the lungs, or in the thorax (see Ch. 7).

The parathyroid glands are supplied with blood from branches of the arteries supplying the thyroid gland. Similarly, the venous blood drains into the veins of the thyroid which then empty into the jugular veins of the neck, and the superior vena cava.

There are two types of cell:

● chief cell
● oxyphil cell.

Chief cells manufacture and secrete the polypeptide hormone *parathyrin* (also known as *parathyroid hormone* or *parathormone*). A large precursor molecule is synthesised from which parathyrin is split off. Oxyphil cells appear only at puberty and their function is not yet known.

Parathyrin
The secretion of parathyrin, like that of calcitonin, is controlled mainly by the concentration of calcium in the blood. If calcium concentration increases, parathyrin secretion decreases. Conversely if blood calcium falls parathyrin secretion increases. Another factor influencing secretion is magnesium. It has similar effects to calcium but is less powerful.

Parathyrin acts at two main sites:

● bone
● kidneys.

It stimulates osteoclasts to digest bone tissue (*resorption of bone*) and release the products, including calcium, into the blood. In the kidneys it stimulates the reabsorption of calcium by the renal tubules and the excretion of phosphate in the urine. The result is an increase in plasma calcium concentration (see Ch. 13). ⑤

PANCREAS

The pancreas consists mainly of secretory cells and ducts that form pancreatic juice (see Ch. 6). However, interspersed between this *exocrine* tissue are small islands of endocrine tissue, the *islets of Langerhans* (Fig. 10.15), named after the histologist who first described them.

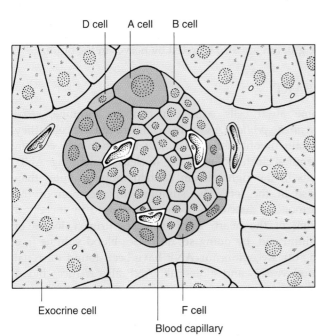

Figure 10.15
Structure of a single islet of Langerhans embedded within the exocrine tissue of the pancreas.

Islets of Langerhans

Four different types of cell have been identified in the islet tissue. All four manufacture and secrete regulatory polypeptides:

- A cells – glucagon
- B cells – insulin
- D cells – somatostatin
- F cells – pancreatic polypeptide.

Glucagon and insulin are the two major hormones secreted into the blood. Somatostatin and pancreatic polypeptide act chiefly as local hormones regulating the activity of other pancreatic cells. Somatostatin inhibits the cells which secrete insulin and glucagon, whereas pancreatic polypeptide inhibits exocrine pancreatic secretion.

Insulin and glucagon

Actions

Insulin and glucagon are involved in the regulation of nutrient metabolism (see Ch. 14). Their effects are summarised in Table 10.9. The ratio of glucagon to insulin in the blood determines the bias of cell metabolism. If insulin dominates, metabolism is directed towards the uptake of nutrients such as glucose, amino acids and fatty acids into cells, and their incorporation into glycogen, proteins and fats respectively. If glucagon dominates, metabolism shifts in favour of the breakdown of stored macromolecules particularly glycogen and triglycerides.

The cells of most tissues, including muscle and adipose tissue, need the presence of insulin to be able to take up glucose. These are *insulin-dependent tissues*. However, some cells do not require insulin for glucose

⑤
Parathyroid hormone works in association with other substances to maintain normal calcium concentration. What are they?

Table 10.9   Metabolic effects of insulin and glucagon

	Insulin	Glucagon
Blood glucose concentration	Decreased	Increased
Glucose metabolism	Promotes cellular uptake	Promotes cellular release
Amino acid metabolism	Promotes cellular uptake	—
Fatty acid metabolism	Promotes cellular uptake	—
Glycogen stores	Increased	Decreased (liver only)
Fat stores (adipose tissue)	Increased	Decreased
Protein	Promotes synthesis	—

Table 10.10   Factors affecting the secretion of insulin and glucagon

Category	Factor	Insulin	Glucagon
Nutrient concentrations in blood	↑ glucose	↑	↓
	↑ amino acids	↑	↑
Gastrointestinal hormones	GIP	↑	—
	Gastrin, CCK-PZ	↑	↑
	Somatostatin	↓	↓
Autonomic nervous system	Acetylcholine (parasympathetic nerves)	↑	↑
	Noradrenaline (sympathetic nerves)	↓	↑

uptake. These include cells of the lens, liver, kidneys and brain. These tissues are termed *insulin-independent*. This is a little misleading in that insulin influences other aspects of metabolism in these cells, such as the proportion of different enzymes within the cells. However, the term makes it clear that glucose can get into insulin-independent cells easily, which is not the case for insulin-dependent tissues. ⑥

Control of secretion

The chief factor controlling the secretion of glucagon and insulin is the concentration of glucose in the interstitial fluid surrounding the A and B cells. If glucose concentration increases above 4.5 mmol/l, insulin secretion increases and glucagon secretion is suppressed. Conversely, if glucose concentration falls, the secretion of insulin decreases and that of glucagon increases.

The secretion of insulin and glucagon is also influenced by:

- plasma amino acid concentration
- gastrointestinal hormones
- the autonomic nervous system.

The effects of these factors are detailed in Table 10.10.

DIGESTIVE SYSTEM

Many endocrine cells are scattered throughout the length of the gastrointestinal tract, usually in the mucosa. They are involved in the regulation of digestion (see Ch. 6).

Peptide hormones include *gastrin, secretin, CCK-PZ, GIP, enteroglucagon, neurotensin* and *motilin*. There are other peptides, secreted chiefly by nerves, which act as local regulators of activity. These include *gastrin-releasing peptide (GRP), VIP, substance P, endorphins* and *enkephalins*. Some gastrointestinal peptides may be classified as hormones in one situation and as neurotransmitters in another depending on where they come from and what they do. For example neurotensin and the shortened form of CCK-PZ (CCK-octapeptide) are secreted into the bloodstream by endocrine cells of the gut, but are also secreted by nerves in the brain.

HEART

Some atrial cells secrete a peptide hormone, *atrial natriuretic peptide (ANP)*. The cells are muscle cells (they contain myofibrils; see Ch. 22) but they also contain granules clustered near the nucleus, containing ANP. Cells in the right atrium contain more granules than those in the left. The stimulus for secretion of the hormone is distension of the atria caused by increased filling of the heart. ANP increases urinary losses of sodium and, by doing so, decreases blood volume (see Ch. 13). Receptors for ANP have been found on renal blood vessels and glomeruli. ANP also reduces blood pressure by causing vasodilation. ⑦

KIDNEY

Some cells of the kidney (probably the epithelial cells of the glomeruli) secrete *erythropoietin* in response to a

⑥
If the pancreas fails to produce insulin, it has to be given by injection. Why can it not be given orally?

⑦
Can you suggest a reason why cells in the right atrium contain more granules than cells in the left?

decrease in the delivery of oxygen. Erythropoietin is a peptide hormone which stimulates the development of red cells from stem cells in the bone marrow (see Chs 4 and 11).

FORMATION OF HORMONES IN THE PLASMA AND THE TISSUES

Some hormones are formed in the body fluids. Some, such as *angiotensin II* and *bradykinin* are derived from precursor proteins. Others, such as the *prostaglandins* are formed from the fatty acid arachidonic acid.

RENIN–ANGIOTENSIN SYSTEM

The hormone *angiotensin II* is formed from the plasma protein angiotensinogen, secreted by the liver, through the action of *renin* and a converting enzyme (ACE) (Fig. 10.16).

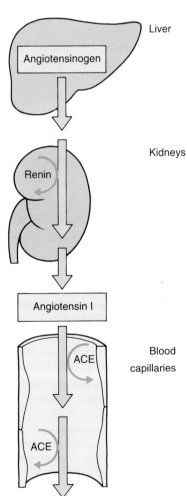

Figure 10.16
The production of angiotensin from angiotensinogen.

Renin

Renin is an enzyme formed and secreted into the blood by cells of the afferent arterioles of the kidney (see Ch. 8). Its secretion is affected by:

- sodium delivery to the distal tubule
- pressure in the afferent arteriole
- activity in the sympathetic nerves.

Renin splits off a 10 amino acid unit (a *decapeptide*), angiotensin I from angiotensinogen.

Converting enzyme

Angiotensin I is then converted into angiotensin II by an enzyme secreted by endothelial cells of the circulation, *angiotensin converting enzyme (ACE)*. Much conversion occurs in the lung capillaries.

Angiotensin II

Angiotensin II has two major effects. It:

- is a potent constrictor of arterioles
- stimulates the secretion of aldosterone.

It is rapidly broken down in the circulation having a half life of roughly 1 minute.

KININS

Kinins are peptides formed from proteins (*kininogens*), by the action of enzymes (*kallikreins*) produced in the blood and in the tissues (Fig. 10.17). There are two different kinins:

- bradykinin
- lysylbradykinin (kallidin).

Bradykinin is formed in the plasma and lysylbradykinin is formed in the tissues.

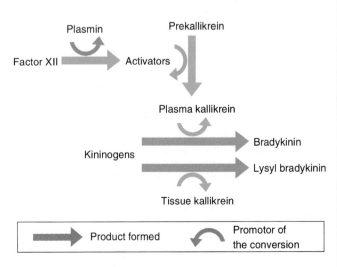

Figure 10.17
The production of kinins from kininogens.

DIABETES MELLITUS

A relative, or complete, lack of insulin secretion by the beta cells of the pancreas or defects of the insulin receptors result in a complex disorder of carbohydrate, fat and protein metabolism known as *diabetes mellitus*. The disorder, which is often familial, has been divided into a series of categories by the National Diabetes Data Group of the National Institute of Health.

Type I diabetes is characterised by a complete lack of secretion of insulin by the pancreas and occurs commonly in young people. Normally, insulin acts to lower the blood glucose level by allowing glucose to enter cells to be metabolised. It does so by binding itself firmly to a receptor site on a cell membrane. Insulin's major metabolic effects are in muscle and adipose tissue. In a diabetic person, the lack of insulin results in starvation of these tissues and this explains why the patient becomes tired and loses weight.

Since glucose is not utilised, it accumulates in the blood of the diabetic person and spills over into the urine causing thirst and passage of large amounts of urine. Unless a replacement of insulin is given, these problems would result in further physiological complications. Thus, the person suffering from type I diabetes requires regular injections of insulin for life to prevent ketosis – a complication arising from disturbed fat metabolism (see Ch. 14). For this reason type I diabetes is also known as insulin-dependent diabetes mellitus (IDDM).

Type II diabetes results from the insensitivity of the insulin receptors to the readily available insulin. In this group, special diet is prescribed to reduce weight and tablets are given to stimulate the pancreas to secrete more insulin. Since no insulin is required, type II diabetes is also known an non-insulin-dependent diabetes mellitus (NIDDM).

Those people with gestational diabetes (GDM), usually identified as type III, are women who develop glucose intolerance during pregnancy. Type IV identifies other types of diabetes including patients whose condition is associated with pancreatic disease, hormonal change, adverse effects of drugs, or genetic or other abnormalities.

Nursing consideration is directed mainly at extensive education and the giving of emotional support. The nurse may help the person to accept the diagnosis and to understand the disorder and the need for continued nursing supervision and dietary restriction. The person is also taught how to:

- administer his own medication
- test his urine and blood for sugar and interpret the results
- recognise the signs of hyperglycaemia (excessive glucose in the blood) leading to coma
- recognise the signs of hypoglycaemia (lack of glucose in the blood for the insulin to act on) leading to insulin shock.

Safety precautions, such as avoiding infection, carrying a supply of glucose at all times for emergency use, carrying an identity health alert card and the use of sterile technique in giving self-medication are all emphasised.

Kallikreins

Plasma kallikrein is activated by fragments of the activated form of Factor XII, one of the clotting factors (see Ch. 4). Tissue kallikreins are produced by many of the glands of the digestive system and by the kidneys.

Action of kinins

Kinins are involved in inflammation (see Ch. 15). They:

- cause vasodilation
- increase capillary permeability
- attract leucocytes
- stimulate cutaneous pain receptors.

Within the digestive system they also increase blood flow to secretory glands and stimulate smooth muscle.

DERIVATIVES OF ARACHIDONIC ACID

Arachidonic acid (Fig. 10.18) is one of the essential fatty acids (see Ch. 14). An enormous variety of different regulatory substances are formed from it including:

- prostaglandins
- thromboxanes
- leukotrienes.

These are all local regulators of cell activity formed in tissues throughout the body.

Prostaglandins

There are a variety of different prostaglandins, which are divided into several groups, such as *PGA, PGE, PGF*, on the basis of their chemical structure. They have many different effects in different tissues (Table 10.11).

ENDOCRINOLOGICAL DISORDERS: A SUMMARY

These may arise in one of two general ways:

- abnormal endocrine tissue
- abnormal sensitivity of the target tissues.

Abnormal endocrine tissue. Production of the hormone can be affected in several ways. It may be reduced through:

- deficiency of constituents necessary for synthesis (e.g. lack of iodine for thyroxine)
- destruction of the cells by autoimmune antibodies (e.g. idiopathic adrenal insufficiency).

Conversely, hormones may be secreted in excess when a tumour develops (e.g. phaeochromocytoma – tumour of the adrenal medulla).

Abnormal target. Where there is altered sensitivity of the target cells the secretion of hormone by the endocrine cells may be normal. One example of this is maturity-onset diabetes; another is nephrogenic diabetes insipidus. In both cases the secretion of the hormones (insulin and ADH respectively) is essentially normal but the target cells are relatively insensitive to the hormones.

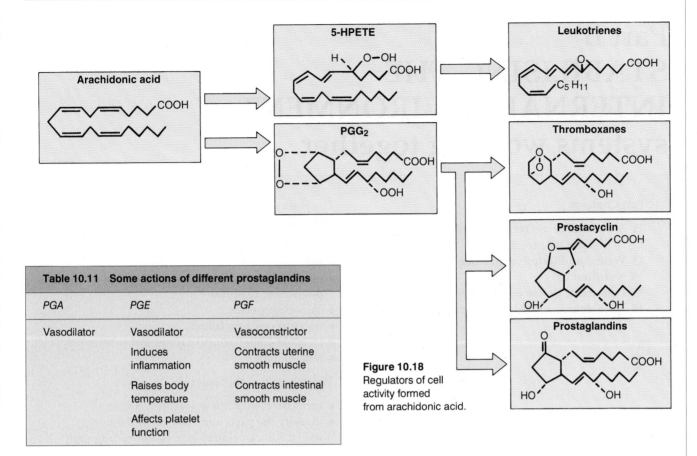

Figure 10.18
Regulators of cell activity formed from arachidonic acid.

Table 10.11   Some actions of different prostaglandins

PGA	PGE	PGF
Vasodilator	Vasodilator	Vasoconstrictor
	Induces inflammation	Contracts uterine smooth muscle
	Raises body temperature	Contracts intestinal smooth muscle
	Affects platelet function	

Thromboxanes

Thromboxane and *prostacyclin* affect blood platelets and vascular smooth muscle and thus play a role in haemostasis (see Ch. 4).

Leukotrienes

Leukotrienes are involved in inflammation and some allergic responses (see Ch. 15). They:

- cause contraction of bronchiolar and arteriolar smooth muscle
- increase capillary permeability
- attract neutrophils and basophils.

KEY POINTS

What you should now know about endocrine tissue and hormones:

- the basic structure of the pituitary, adrenal, thyroid and parathyroid glands
- the hormones produced by these glands, how they are formed and secreted, what they do and how their secretion is controlled
- the structure and function of the hypothalamus as it relates to the pituitary gland and the significance of this arrangement
- the location and structure of the islets of Langerhans and the secretion and actions of their hormones
- the endocrine function of cells within the heart, digestive system and kidney
- the origin and functions of hormones, such as angiotensin, kinins and prostaglandins, which are manufactured in body fluids and tissues
- some of the ways in which endocrine abnormalities arise
- some of the consequences of endocrine abnormality.

REFERENCES AND FURTHER READING

Boyar R, Perlow M, Hellman L, Kapen S, Weitzman E 1972 Twenty four hour patterns of luteinizing hormone secretion in normal men with sleep stage recording. Journal of Clinical Endocrinology and Metabolism 35: 73–81
Campbell C 1978 Nursing diagnosis and intervention in nursing practice. John Wiley & Sons, New York
Crapo L 1985 Hormones: messengers of life. W H Freeman, New York
(Opens windows into how endocrinological facts have been discovered. Engaging account of how hormones regulate life processes)
Emslie-Smith D, Paterson C R, Scratcherd T, Read N W (eds) Textbook of physiology, 11th edn. Churchill Livingstone, Edinburgh
Greenspan F S 1990 Basic and clinical endocrinology, 3rd edn. Appleton & Lange, Norwalk, Connecticut
(Well signposted book for finding more information. Well referenced resource)
Gupta D, Reiter R J 1986 The pineal gland during development: from fetus to adult. Croom Helm, London
Hinchliff S, Montague S 1988 Physiology for nursing practice. Baillière Tindall, London
Martini F 1989 Fundamentals of anatomy and physiology. Prentice Hall International, UK
Rogers A W 1992 Textbook of anatomy. Churchill Livingstone, Edinburgh
Watson J E, Royle J A 1991 Watson's Medical–surgical nursing and related physiology, 3rd edn. Baillière Tindall, London

Part B
STABILISING THE INTERNAL ENVIRONMENT:
systems working together

The features of the internal environment that matter for the survival of our cells are:

- oxygen concentration
- pH
- electrolyte concentrations (e.g. sodium, potassium, calcium)
- osmotic pressure
- nutrient concentrations
- freedom from harmful agents and substances
- temperature.

The chapters in this part:

- focus on each of these features in turn
- identify the parts and systems of the body which have a primary role in controlling each feature
- show how the stability of each feature is maintained by the cooperative activity of several control systems.

Chapter 11
MAINTENANCE OF OXYGEN SUPPLIES

Oxygen (O_2) is vital for life. If someone is acutely deprived of O_2, unconsciousness may occur within less than a minute followed by irreversible brain damage if deprivation continues for only a little longer.

The supply of O_2 to the tissues is normally protected by several homeostatic control mechanisms that regulate the uptake of O_2 by the lungs, the amount of O_2 carried in the blood and the delivery of O_2 to the tissues.

In health, the demand for O_2 may sometimes exceed the supplies available. In disease, the processes that normally guarantee O_2 supplies may be defective. In either case, O_2 deficiency (*hypoxia*) arises, with widespread effects on body systems.

Major life-threatening emergencies – cardiac arrest, respiratory arrest, haemorrhage and fire – all relate to sudden and severe O_2 deprivation, and the response time in restoring an adequate O_2 supply is critical. This is why it is essential for all health personnel to be familiar with the emergency procedures they may need to implement, i.e. cardiopulmonary resuscitation (CPR), first aid for massive haemorrhage, and fire drill.

Nurses and doctors in particular have a responsibility to maintain functional equipment, to practice their skills and to respond to an emergency immediately, as irreversible brain damage and death can occur within a matter of minutes.

Q: What is the critical response time in which to establish effective CPR?

THE NEED FOR OXYGEN

ATP FORMATION

The cells of the body need O_2 to form large amounts of ATP (*adenosine triphosphate*; Fig. 11.1). ATP is a high energy compound used to power many energy-requiring processes in the body. A few examples are given in Table 11.1. When ATP is broken down to form ADP (*adenosine diphosphate*) and then AMP (*adenosine monophosphate*), energy is liberated. Other high energy compounds include creatine phosphate, acetyl Co-A and compounds that are similar in nature to ATP, such as guanosine triphosphate (GTP). ATP, however, is quantitatively the most important.

ATP is formed in two main ways (Fig. 11.2):

• oxidative phosphorylation
• anaerobic glycolysis.

Oxidative phosphorylation

The overwhelming majority of ATP is produced by oxidative phosphorylation. This process is linked with a complex series of chemical reactions called the *flavoprotein cytochrome system* through which hydrogen is linked to O_2 to form water. The hydrogen atoms that are fed into this system are derived chiefly from another sequence of chemical reactions called the *citric acid cycle* or *Krebs cycle* (after the biochemist Hans Krebs). The citric acid cycle uses fragments of carbohydrates, fats

Table 11.1 Some of the processes powered by ATP	
Muscle contraction	Synthesis of DNA and RNA
Movement of cilia	Protein synthesis
Active transport of ions across cell membranes (e.g. Na$^+$, K$^+$, Ca^{2+}, H$^+$)	Gluconeogenesis

and proteins as its raw material and generates carbon dioxide (CO_2) as a waste product.

The components of these systems are located within the mitochondria (see Ch. 2). Although forming ATP in this way is complicated, it is very efficient – 34 molecules of ATP are generated by the breakdown (*catabolism*) of one molecule of glucose. The critical point to remember is that this system cannot work without O_2. It is *aerobic*, meaning 'requiring air'.

Anaerobic glycolysis

Some ATP can be formed without O_2 (*anaerobically*) by a different and much simpler process, *glycolysis*. Glucose is simply split up (that is, glyco–lysis) to yield *pyruvic acid*. In the absence of O_2, pyruvic acid is converted into *lactic acid*. Only two molecules of ATP are generated per molecule of glucose. They are, however, formed very quickly. ATP can be formed in this way only as long as stocks of glucose last because no other foodstuff

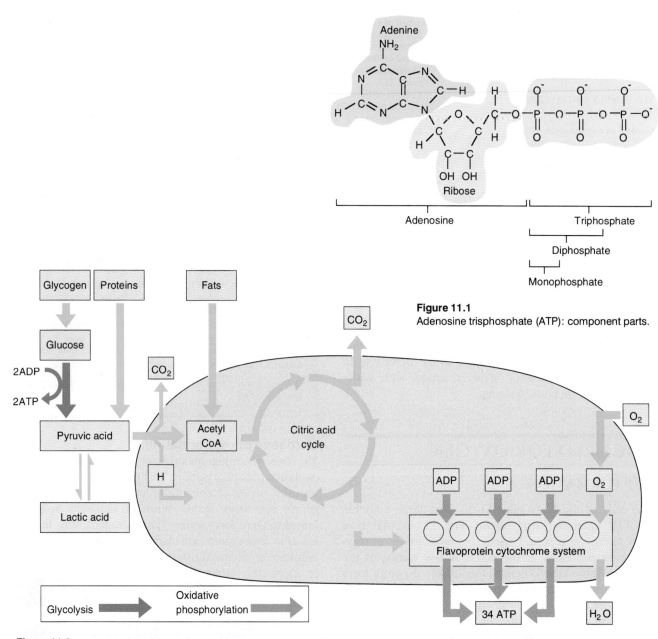

Figure 11.1
Adenosine trisphosphate (ATP): component parts.

Figure 11.2
How ATP is formed: aerobic and anaerobic processes. (Note: the number of molecules of ATP formed by the mitochondrial metabolism of glucose can appear to be contradictory in different textbooks. This is because mitochondrial metabolism is more complicated than shown here. Between 32 and 34 ATPs are formed by oxidative phosphorylation depending

on the exact metabolic pathways, and 2 extra ATPs are formed by an entirely different mitochondrial pathway. The exact numbers are not that important. The crucial point is that many more ATPs are generated by mitochondrial metabolism than by glycolysis (see Stryer 1988).)

can be used directly instead. This system of ATP production is an emergency mechanism for most tissues. It protects cells temporarily against periods of O_2 deficiency. Cells that are likely to experience O_2 deficiency on a regular basis, such as muscle, usually store their own stocks of glucose in the form of *glycogen*. ①

When the supply of O_2 is restored, ATP is formed again aerobically. Some of this energy is used to replenish the stocks of glycogen and other compounds such as creatine phosphate (see also Ch. 17) that were run down during the time of O_2 deprivation. O_2 is needed for this restocking. In other words, when ATP is being produced anaerobically, an O_2 debt is incurred, which has to be 'paid back' when O_2 supplies are restored. ②

OXYGEN REQUIREMENTS

Tissues differ in their O_2 requirements (Table 11.2). The three parts off the body that account for the majority (about 60%) of the O_2 consumed at rest are:

- brain
- liver
- skeletal muscle.

The brain needs a large amount of oxygen to generate enough ATP to power the active transport of sodium and potassium across nerve cell membranes (*sodium–potassium pump*). This pump maintains the correct intracellular concentrations of sodium and potassium which are crucial to the generation and transmission of nerve impulses (see Ch. 21).

The liver is a very active chemical factory (see Ch. 9). About 40% of its requirement for oxygen is associated with the usage of ATP in the synthesis of plasma proteins.

Although individual muscle cells at rest don't use very much O_2, the total O_2 requirement of the body's skeletal muscle, which accounts for almost half of body weight, is quite substantial.

Tissues of the body also differ in the degree to which their O_2 requirement may change. A resting person who has not eaten for a couple of hours uses about 250 ml of O_2 per minute. During intense physical activity, this can increase to 5 litres per minute. Skeletal muscle, when maximally active, may increase its O_2 requirements by 100-fold (see Ch. 17). More modest demands are made by the heart when cardiac output increases and by the digestive system during the digestion and absorption of a meal.

In contrast, the total O_2 consumption of the brain changes very little in health even with the most concentrated mental activity. Although metabolic activity in specific parts of the brain may increase during different mental tasks (see Fig. 20.14), an increased requirement for O_2 in one part of the brain is usually accompanied by a decreased requirement somewhere else. Total O_2 consumption therefore remains unchanged.

Two other regions of the body that also have relatively constant requirements for O_2 are the kidneys and the skin. The amount of fluid filtered and recovered by the kidneys each day (about 180 litres; see Ch. 8) changes very little. Thus, the kidney's energy requirements also change very little. The skin needs energy for repair and renewal, which, except in cases of extensive injury, remains fairly constant.

A general increase in tissue oxygen consumption occurs, however, if metabolism is stimulated by an increase in:

- body temperature
- thyroid hormone
- adrenaline and noradrenaline.

In a fever, oxygen consumption increases by about 14% for each degree Celsius that body temperature rises. The hormones thyroxine, tri-iodothyronine, adrenaline and noradrenaline, stimulate metabolism in many different tissues (see Ch. 10).

① *In what form and by what method can glucose be given to increase the back-up stocks of glycogen?*

② *It is preferable to use O_2 rather than air in CPR. What reasons may there be?*

Table 11.2   Oxygen consumption and blood flow of different organs and tissues (at rest)*

	Oxygen consumption			Blood flow		
	ml.100 g^{-1}.min	ml.min^{-1}	% total	ml.100 g^{-1}.min	ml.min^{-1}	% total
Heart muscle	10	30	12	80	250	5
Kidneys	6	20	8	400	1250	23
Brain	3	50	20	50	750	14
Liver	2	50	20	60	1500	28
Skin	0.3	10	4	15	500	9
Skeletal muscle	0.2	50	20	3	800	16
Other tissues	0.2	40	16	1	300	5

* Compiled from Bard 1961. Figures have been rounded for easier comparison.

THE SUPPLY OF OXYGEN TO TISSUES

Maintenance of O_2 supplies to all tissues according to need is crucial. The supply of O_2 relies basically on three things:

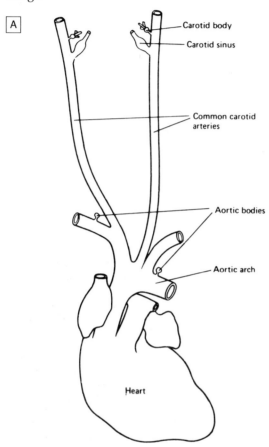

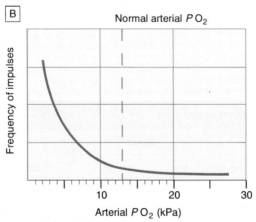

Figure 11.3
The peripheral chemoreceptors, aortic and carotid bodies:
A Location close to the heart and brain
B Sensitivity to decreasing oxygen pressures.
(Part A reproduced from Ganong 1991 Review of medical physiology, 15th edn, Figure 36.3, by permission of Appleton & Lange.)

- adequate oxygenation of the blood by the lungs
- sufficient numbers of circulating red cells
- adequate cardiac output and its appropriate distribution amongst the tissues.

Each of these is regulated by control systems that monitor the state of the body and bring about corrective adjustments should the supply of O_2 be inadequate or under threat.

CONTROL OF OXYGENATION

The oxygenation of the blood in the lungs (see Ch. 7) is controlled through feedback mechanisms that monitor O_2 and CO_2 and reflexly change the pattern of breathing to stabilise the partial pressure of these two gases in the blood. Normally, the partial pressure of O_2 (PO_2) in the arterial blood, pumped from the lungs to the rest of the body by the heart, is about 12.7 kPa in a young adult, though it can range from 11.3 to 13.3 kPa. Arterial blood PO_2 is monitored continously by specialised *chemoreceptors* located very close to the major arteries that carry blood away from the heart (Fig. 11.3A).

The chemoreceptors are found within small clumps of tissue, each of which is simply described as a body. There is one *carotid body* on each carotid artery and two or more *aortic bodies* close to the arch of the aorta.

Stimulation of chemoreceptors

When blood PO_2 decreases, the concentration of O_2 dissolved in the interstitial fluid around the receptors decreases also (see Ch. 7) and the chemoreceptors are stimulated. The receptors are also influenced by the local concentration of CO_2 and hydrogen ions (see Ch. 12).

The chemoreceptors are not stimulated much until the PO_2 in the blood falls below 8 kPa (Fig. 11.3B). Consequently, under ordinary conditions, when the PO_2 is around 13 kPa, the concentration of O_2 in blood is not an important factor in the control of breathing. It becomes important below 8 kPa. It is significant that it is at a PO_2 of about 8 to 9 kPa that oxyhaemoglobin begins

Sports medicine research supports the common-sense observation that active people who take regular aerobic exercise stay fit and healthy longer than those who are sedentary and take little or no exercise.

Benefits of physical training, providing there is an intact cardiopulmonary system and normal oxygen transport in the blood, come from both peripheral adaptation and improved cardiac function (see Ch. 17).

The functional basis of degenerative cardiovascular disease is an imbalance between O_2 requirements and available O_2, and physical training programmes counteract this by developing the essential systems (Dirix et al 1988).

Q: What do you understand by aerobic exercise?

Chemoreceptors are the body's blood gas monitoring system. In the clinical situation, arterial blood gas levels (ABGs) can be monitored by laboratory blood gas analysis.

Blood is drawn from the radial or femoral artery, or from an established arterial line, using a heparinised syringe. Air bubbles are carefully excluded from the syringe, which is capped and sent for immediate analysis.

If the patient is on O_2 therapy it is important to ensure that he has been receiving the prescribed amount for at least 15 minutes before the blood is drawn and to wait for 20 minutes following intermittent positive pressure breathing (IPPB). The prescribed amount should be indicated on the laboratory request form. Following the procedure, firm pressure must be applied to the puncture site for at least 5 minutes.

Q: Why must air be excluded from the blood sample for ABG analysis?

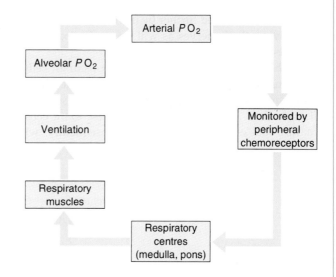

Figure 11.4
Control of arterial PO_2.

to lose appreciable amounts of O_2 (see Fig. 7.22). Above this, haemoglobin is more than 90% saturated with O_2, but below it, the supplies of O_2 are increasingly threatened.

It is important to note that the chemoreceptors monitor the concentration of O_2 dissolved in the interstitial fluid, which is related to the PO_2 of blood and not to the total O_2 content. The total O_2 content depends on the number of red cells and their content of haemoglobin. Consequently, the chemoreceptors are not stimulated in anaemia or in carbon monoxide poisoning (see Carbon monoxide poisoning; p. 154). In both cases, arterial blood PO_2 is normal although the total amount of O_2 carried in blood is reduced (see p. 221).

Stimulation of breathing

When the chemoreceptors are stimulated, impulses pass along autonomic sensory nerve fibres to the respiratory centres in the medulla to stimulate breathing (Fig. 11.4). The increased ventilation of the alveoli raises the alveolar PO_2 and increases the diffusion of O_2 into the blood. At the same time, the concentration of CO_2 in the alveolar air decreases and the elimination of CO_2 is increased. This reduces the concentration of CO_2 and hydrogen ions in blood, which then inhibits the chemoreceptors (see Ch. 12) and makes the increase in ventilation caused by the arterial hypoxia smaller than it would otherwise be.

At high altitude, blood PO_2 is reduced because of the fall in barometric pressure. Some of the changes that occur in the respiratory and cardiovascular systems are depicted in Figure 11.5. As the chemoreceptors are stimulated by the lack of O_2 experienced at high altitude, ventilation is stimulated immediately and then increases further and more gradually over 3 to 4 days. The gradual increase occurs because the inhibitory effect of the lowered CO_2 concentration is slowly overcome (see Ch. 12). This is part of the process of *acclimatisation*.

CARBON DIOXIDE NARCOSIS

In healthy people when CO_2 levels rise the respiratory rate increases. This increase allows excess CO_2 to be blown off by the lungs. However, in chronic obstructive airways disease (COAD; see Ch. 7), where chronic ventilatory problems result in constant high levels of arterial CO_2, this mechanism becomes blunted and eventually PCO_2 has no effect on the respiratory centre in the brain (see Ch. 12). With severe CO_2 retention the respiratory drive is created by the low PO_2 stimulating the carotid and aortic bodies. This is known as the *hypoxic drive*. High concentration of O_2 will suppress this hypoxic drive and if PO_2 is raised even to normal, breathing becomes shallow, more and more CO_2 is retained, further depressing the respiratory centre, and a condition known as carbon dioxide narcosis develops. This is characterised by increasing drowsiness and eventual death.

The hypoxic drive must always be considered when O_2 is prescribed for patients with COAD. Usually this is not more than 24% of O_2 – slightly more than the 21% in room air – which is enough to improve oxygenation without eliminating the hypoxic drive. Prior to, and during, O_2 therapy it is essential to determine ABG levels and to prescribe O_2 accordingly. Correct percentage is ensured by using controlled flow O_2 masks and other appliances.

Q: How would you explain the hypoxic drive to a patient with COAD who is about to be sent home on O_2 therapy.

CONTROL OF RED CELL PRODUCTION

Erythropoietin

The production of red cells in the bone marrow is regulated by erythropoietin (Fig. 11.6), a hormone formed by the kidneys (see Ch. 10). Its secretion is stimulated by O_2 deficiency, which may be due to:

- a lack of O_2 in the blood arriving at the kidneys
- a decrease in renal blood flow.

Secretion is increased further by increased activity in the renal sympathetic nerves as will occur, for example, in response to haemorrhage.

Erythropoietin acts on the primitive precursor cells in the bone marrow that are destined to become red cells and stimulates them to develop and divide (see Ch. 4). It takes 2 to 3 days for the first of these extra cells to mature and enter the circulation. Consequently, when

O_2 deficiency is experienced on ascending from sea level to a high altitude in the mountains, several days elapse before the total number of red cells in the blood increases noticeably (Fig. 11.5). On return to see level, the secretion of erythropoietin decreases and red cell numbers gradually readjust to the new conditions. ③

Some erythropoietin is normally present in blood all the time to maintain the normal rate of production of

③
Athletes who live and train at high altitudes have been shown to have an increased red blood cell count. How might this affect their performance?

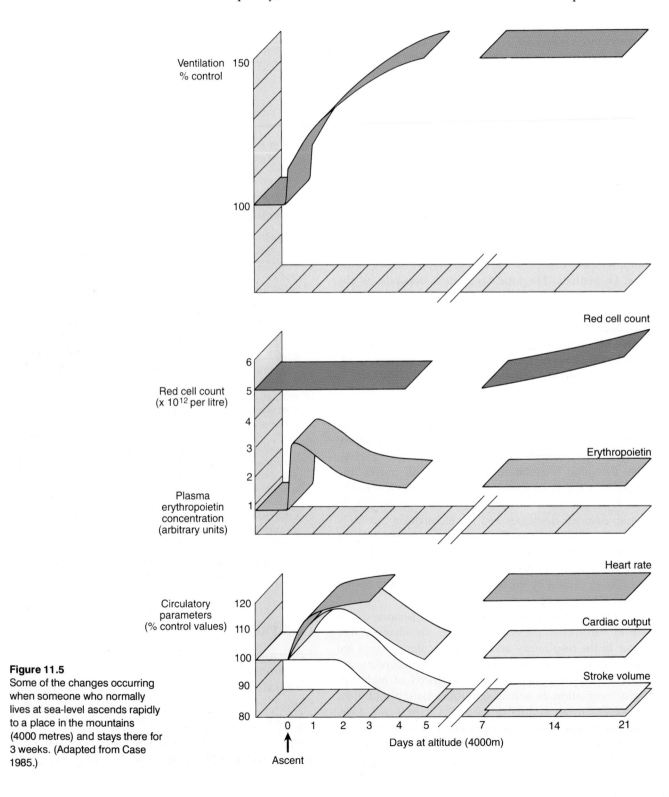

Figure 11.5
Some of the changes occurring when someone who normally lives at sea-level ascends rapidly to a place in the mountains (4000 metres) and stays there for 3 weeks. (Adapted from Case 1985.)

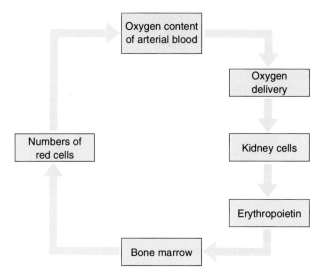

Figure 11.6
Control of arterial oxygen content by regulation of red cell numbers.

SECONDARY POLYCYTHAEMIA

Chronic tissue hypoxia due to COAD (see Ch. 7) or heart disease stimulates the production of erythropoietin by the kidneys, which in turn increases the production of red blood cells (RBCs) by the bone marrow. Erythropoietin may also be produced by tumours of the kidney, liver, uterus and cerebellum with the same end result.

Because of the increase in RBC mass the patient looks *plethoric* (skin has a purplish tinge) and may complain of symptoms due to increased blood viscosity. In addition to the chronic tissue hypoxia, circulation is slowed down and blood vessels are more easily blocked by atherosclerotic plaques, which can lead to the formation of clots and emboli. If cerebral perfusion is compromised this can manifest in headaches, dizziness, confusion and transient ischaemic attacks (TIAs).

A normal person can cope with an increase in packed cell volume but in patients with COAD the hard work of pumping blood through chronically congested lung tissue is made even more difficult by increased viscosity (see Ch. 5). This puts an additional strain on the heart and some people with COAD go on to develop right-sided heart failure (*cor pulmonale*).

If the cause of the condition is a tumour then it may be possible to remove it; otherwise venesection may be performed with removal of 200 to 300 ml of blood, which may be replaced by low molecular weight dextran or the patient's own plasma after the cells have been spun off. This treatment can be repeated weekly until the packed cell voume (PCV) is nearer normal and cerebral perfusion is improved.

The patient should be monitored regularly by his physician and advised on ways of improving oxygenation within the lungs, thus preventing further stimulation of erythropoietin. Such advice would include:

- avoiding cigarette smoke and other pollutants
- avoiding chest infections or seeking early treatment
- taking regular appropriate physiotherapy
- adopting body positions that maximise chest expansion.

---

red cells. If the number of red cells in blood is increased by the transfusion of packed cells (essentially red cells only; see Ch. 4), the secretion of erythropoietin decreases and fewer cells are manufactured by the bone marrow. ④

Other hormones

Other hormones that influence the production of red cells include:

- glucocorticoids (see Ch. 10)
- thyroxine (see Ch. 10)
- androgens (see Ch. 34)
- oestrogens (see Ch. 34).

The first three promote production, whereas oestrogens have a small inhibitory effect.

CONTROL OF THE DISTRIBUTION OF BLOOD

The maintenance of a sufficient blood supply to every tissue of the body depends on:

- the pumping action of the heart (see Ch. 5).
- distribution of the cardiac output according to need.

Distribution of cardiac output at rest

At rest, the needs that have to be met include the requirement of all cells for O_2 as well as the requirements created by the specialised functions of certain tissues, such as temperature regulation in the skin (see Ch. 16) and urine formation in the kidneys (see Ch. 8).

The blood flow that some tissues receive matches their O_2 requirements quite well (Table 11.2). For example, liver, brain and skeletal muscle consume about 60% of the O_2 used by an individual at rest and receive about 60% of the cardiac output. The skin and the kidneys, however, receive a much larger blood flow than is required by their needs for O_2 because a high flow is needed for their specialised functions.

Control of the circulation

The O_2 requirements of different tissues change according to their activity. Adjustments need to be made to the flow and distribution of blood so that the specific needs of individual tissues are met without threat to other areas. This control occurs at two levels:

- local – guarantees individual supplies
- central – sets an order of priorities.

Local control

When the metabolic activity of any cell increases, changes occur locally in its chemical environment. For example, if O_2 is being used up, the PO_2 will decrease and the PCO_2 will increase as CO_2 is generated. If

④
Which conditions benefit most from an infusion of packed red blood cells? Why?

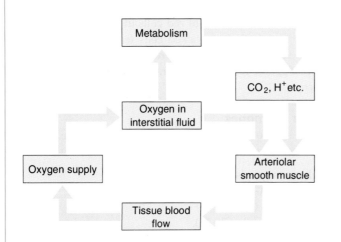

Figure 11.7
Control of oxygen concentration in interstitial fluid by regulation of tissue blood flow.

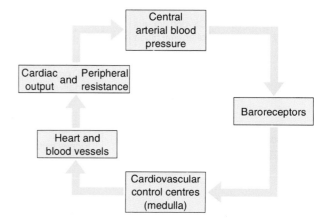

Figure 11.8
Control of arterial blood pressure.

metabolism is anaerobic, lactic acid will be formed (Fig. 11.2) and the concentration of hydrogen ions will increase. Other products of cell activity may also accumulate, including potassium, histamine (from sites of injury) and local hormones such as kinins (see Ch. 10) that are released from secretory glands.

In general, these changes in the local environment cause the smooth muscle in the walls of the arterioles to relax (see Ch. 5). The arterioles dilate and blood flow increases, which helps to wash out the waste products and improve the supply of O_2. Hence, metabolic activity acts as its own regulator of local blood flow and therefore of O_2 supply (Fig. 11.7).

If the blood supply to an area is occluded for a short while and then released the blood flow through the area is vastly increased temporarily after the circulation is restored. This response to occlusion is called *reactive hyperaemia* and is caused by the build-up of metabolites such as CO_2, H^+ and lactic acid during the period of occlusion. Reactive hyperaemia is what causes reddening of skin that has been compressed for a while and is then released (for example the red patch that appears on the legs of someone who has been sitting with them crossed).

Central control
The distribution of blood flow to different parts of the body is also governed by an order of priorities that is set and coordinated largely by the autonomic nervous system. At the top of this list of priorities comes the flow of blood to:

● brain (cerebral circulation; see Ch. 20)
● heart (coronary circulation; see Ch. 5).

Blood flow to priority organs. Blood flow to the brain and heart is protected through a control system that monitors and maintains central arterial blood pressure

(Fig. 11.8; see also Ch. 5). As long as an adequate pressure is maintained, any change in the requirements of the brain and heart can be met by local control mechanisms. In both cases, when the need for O_2 increases, local factors act as potent vasodilators.

Central arterial blood pressure is monitored continuously by the baroreceptors of the aortic arch and the carotid sinuses. Those located in the carotid sinuses are conveniently sited to detect any change in the pressure of blood going to the brain. If a decrease in blood pressure is detected, then both cardiac output and peripheral resistance are reflexly increased to maintain an adequate pressure. The increase in peripheral resistance is caused by increased activity in the sympathetic nerve fibres, which causes widespread vasoconstriction.

Central arterial pressure is threatened whenever the local needs of one part of the body provoke appreciable vasodilation. Vasodilation lowers peripheral resistance and therefore reduces arterial blood pressure. For example, when a meal is being digested and absorbed, local factors and gastrointestinal hormones cause vasodilation of the splanchnic circulation (see Ch. 6), which

An increase in PCO_2 causes arterial vasodilation. First-aid treatment for central retinal artery occlusion is to lie the patient down and get him to breathe into a paper bag. In so doing he is breathing back his own CO_2 and there is a chance that the artery will dilate because of this and that with increased positional flow the embolus will be flushed into a peripheral and less critical arterial branch. With central retinal artery occlusion there is sudden and total loss of vision but, if the embolus can be flushed to a peripheral branch, there is less retinal damage and a chance to save some of the visual field. Early detection and diagnosis is imperative for the success of the manoeuvre. Sudden and total loss of vision in one eye is the clue.

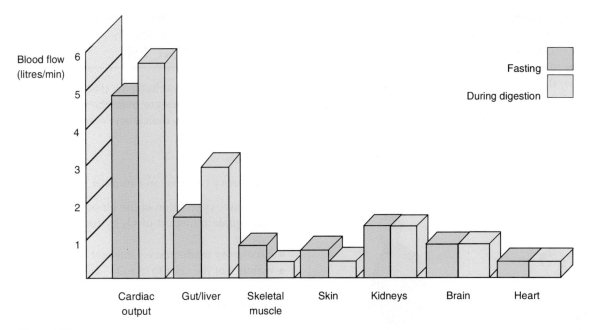

Figure 11.9
Changes in cardiac output and its distribution provoked by the digestion of a meal.

should lower blood pressure. However, blood pressure does not normally fall because the autonomic nervous system makes adjustments in the supply and distribution of blood to the rest of the circulation at the same time (Fig. 11.9). If this did not happen, fainting would be liable to occur after each meal! In fact, this can happen in *autonomic neuropathy*, a condition in which reflex control of the circulatory system is disordered.

Priorities set by sympathetic nervous system. All arterioles are innervated by sympathetic nerve fibres, but the effect of sympathetic excitation is not the same in all places. The arterioles that are least affected are those of the cerebral, coronary and pulmonary circulations. Blood flow to these areas is thus maintained at times when the flow of blood to other areas is cut down by sympathetic vasoconstriction.

Organs and tissues in which blood flow is appreciably reduced by sympathetic vasoconstriction include the skin, digestive system, skeletal muscle and kidney. The degree of vasoconstriction depends on:

● the severity of the threat to central arterial blood pressure
● the demands that are being made on each tissue at the time.

If the threat to arterial blood pressure is modest, as in standing up (see Ch. 17), blood flow is likely to be reduced to the skin, the digestive system and skeletal muscle in a non-active person. If the threat is more severe, as in an acute haemorrhage, then blood flow to the kidney is also reduced. This is likely to decrease

glomerular filtration rate (see Ch. 8) and, if prolonged, can cause renal damage.

If the metabolic requirement of a tissue is high, then the vasodilator action of the local metabolites will conflict with the vasoconstrictor effect of the sympathetic nerves. The balance between the two will determine the effect on blood flow. If a meal is being digested, for example, the flow of blood to the digestive system cannot be reduced to the same extent as in fasting.

SHOCK

Shock occurs when there is a severe threat to central arterial blood pressure due to malfunction of the heart or circulatory system, or to a drastically decreased blood volume. It may be classified as cardiogenic, distributive or hypovolaemic and is characterised by inadequate tissue perfusion leading to tissue hypoxia and altered cellular metabolism.

Although some clinical signs of shock vary depending on the underlying cause, all types of shock are characterised by a falling blood pressure, an initial increase in pulse rate and a pale, cool and clammy skin.

Early response by the sympathetic nervous system to the fall in blood pressure and to tissue hypoxia leads to an increase in heart rate and to generalised vasoconstriction in order to shunt blood to the heart and brain, which take priority over other less vital organs. This is manifest in pale, cool and clammy skin. Blood pressure will continue to fall if compensatory mechanisms or medical intervention fail.

Q: Why is application of peripheral warming devices contraindicated in patients suffering from severe shock?

Limits of control

If demand (need for blood flow) exceeds the supplies available (cardiac output), arterial blood pressure cannot be maintained and the flow of blood to the vital organs is threatened, with the brain being the first affected. When arterial pressure falls, consciousness is lost and fainting occurs (*syncope*).

A set of everyday events that could provoke this is depicted in Figure 11.10.

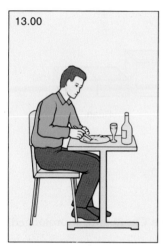
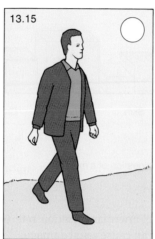
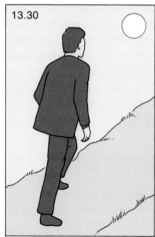
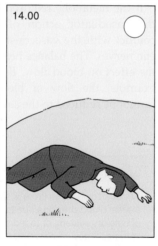

Figure 11.10
A circulatory challenge. Blood vessels in the digestive system and in skeletal muscle will be dilated by metabolic products generated by digestive activity and physical activity. Cutaneous blood vessels in the skin will be dilated because of the need to eliminate heat (see Ch. 16). The volume of fluid in the circulation is likely to be reduced because of losses of water and electrolytes in sweating (see Ch. 13). All these factors are a threat to the maintenance of arterial blood pressure. The 'central controller' stimulates the activity of the sympathetic nervous system, increasing the pumping action of the heart and reducing blood flow to lesser priority tissues wherever possible by vasoconstriction. Significant vasoconstriction can occur in the renal circulation, but elsewhere the smooth muscles of the arterioles cannot contract very much because of the opposing factors, such as vasodilator metabolites, making them relax. Cardiac output increases but if it is insufficient to maintain adequate blood pressure fainting is inevitable.

HYPOXIA: CAUSES AND CONSEQUENCES

When the control mechanisms that ensure adequate O_2 delivery to all tissues are overwhelmed, for example by disease, hypoxia (O_2 deficiency) results.

CAUSES

O_2 deficiency can arise in a number of ways:

- deficient oxygenation of the blood – *hypoxic hypoxia*
- inadequate transport of O_2 by haemoglobin – *anaemic hypoxia*
- circulatory inadequacy – *stagnant* or *ischaemic hypoxia*
- inability of the cells to use O_2 – *histotoxic hypoxia*.

CONSEQUENCES

In all forms of hypoxia, the capacity of the body to form ATP is reduced. Consequently, the cellular processes that rely on this source of energy cannot be maintained at the same level.

Specific effects of O_2 deficiency depend on the tissues affected by it:

- in brain, disorientation and drowsiness may be experienced
- in muscle, weakness will occur
- in kidneys, erythropoietin secretion will increase and eventually there may be tubular necrosis.

The consequences of hypoxia also vary depending on its cause:

- the skin may have a bluish tinge (*cyanosis*)
- there may be circulatory changes
- there may be an increase in ventilation.

Because of these differences, it is helpful to consider the four categories of hypoxia individually (Table 11.3).

TYPES OF HYPOXIA

Hypoxic hypoxia

Causes
The feature that distinguishes hypoxic hypoxia from all the others is that the arterial PO_2 is below normal (*hypoxaemia*). It can be caused by:

- low PO_2 of the air breathed
- inadequate ventilation of the lungs
- deficient gas transfer between alveolar air and blood
- inequalities of ventilation and perfusion
- shunts between the right and left heart.

At high altitude, the PO_2 of the air breathed is low because of the low barometric pressure. Although the

Table 11.3   Types of hypoxia: summary of distinctive features

Type	Arterial PO_2	Cyanosis	Arterial O_2 content	Tissue blood flow
Hypoxic	Low	Yes (central)	Low	Increased
Anaemic	Normal	No	Low	Increased
Stagnant (ischaemic)	Normal	Yes (peripheral)	Normal	Decreased*
Histotoxic	Normal	No	Normal	Normal

* May be general decrease if cardiac output is low; or limited to specific circulations where blood flow is hindered.

per cent composition of the air is the same as at sea level, the partial pressures of the constituent gases are all reduced in proportion to the decrease in barometric pressure. As the air breathed has a low PO_2 to start with, both alveolar and arterial PO_2 will be low.

Inadequate ventilation of the lungs may be due to depression of the respiratory centres by drugs (such as barbiturates and derivatives of morphine) or by damage to the medulla or the respiratory motoneurones. It may also be caused by defects in the respiratory muscles (as in progressive muscular dystrophy) or thoracic cage, or by bronchial obstruction. ⑤

The transfer of gases is impaired by anything that causes thickening of the alveolar–capillary barrier. This can occur in fibrosis, asbestosis, interstitial pneumonia and pulmonary oedema. The impairment of gas transfer may not be obvious when someone is resting but becomes evident on exertion.

The cause of the hypoxaemia created by imbalances in ventilation and perfusion of the lungs and by shunts is explained in Chapter 7.

Consequences

If hypoxaemia is severe enough, it will lead to cyanosis, a bluish colouration of the skin and mucous membranes. In hypoxaemia, the bluish colouration is caused by the presence of large amounts of deoxygenated haemoglobin in the blood.

> As a rule of thumb, cyanosis is usually noticeable when the concentration of deoxygenated haemoglobin in blood exceeds 50 g/litre.

The consequences of hypoxaemia depend upon its severity and its cause. Unless the cause is inadequate ventilation (Fig. 11.4), the low arterial PO_2 will stimulate the peripheral chemoreceptors and increase ventilation, as at high altitude.

The peripheral chemoreceptors also excite the vasomotor centre and reflexly provoke vasoconstriction in circulations in which the sympathetic nervous system

controls blood flow – skin, for example. Elsewhere, the hypoxaemia acts locally to cause vasodilation. The only exception is the pulmonary circulation, where hypoxaemia provokes vasoconstriction (see Ch. 7). A low PO_2 also stimulates the secretion of adrenaline by the adrenal medulla, which stimulates the heart and increases heart rate (Fig. 11.5).

If tissue PO_2 becomes too low to sustain aerobic metabolism, cells that can will increasingly use anaerobic glycolysis to produce ATP. The lactic acid produced in turn disturbs acid–base balance (see Ch. 12). Eventually, chronic hypoxaemia will stimulate the production of red cells (Fig. 11.5).

Anaemic hypoxia

Causes

In anaemic hypoxia, arterial blood PO_2 is normal, but the total amount of O_2 in the blood is low. This can be due to:

- lack of haemoglobin (too few red cells or too little haemoglobin in each cell; see Ch. 4)
- inability of haemoglobin to carry O_2 in the usual way (because of binding of carbon monoxide, for example; see Ch. 7).

Consequences

Because arterial PO_2 is normal, the peripheral chemoreceptors may not register any O_2 deficiency, so ventilation may not necessarily increase. However, other tissues do experience O_2 deficiency, which can cause vasodilation, a decrease in peripheral resistance and a compensatory increase in cardiac output.

If the decrease in O_2-carrying capacity is due to a lack of red cells, blood viscosity will be decreased, which will also increase blood flow.

The total amount of O_2 that can be delivered to the tissues is reduced in proportion to the degree of anaemia and may be sufficient for undemanding activities but inadequate on exertion. Hence, those who are anaemic may tire easily and generally feel weak and lacking in energy.

⑤ *What significance does depression of the respiratory centre by drugs have for pre- and postoperative observations and nursing care?*

Stagnant hypoxia

Causes

In stagnant hypoxia, the arterial PO_2 and the O_2 content of blood are normal, but the delivery of O_2 to the tissues is reduced because of a sluggish circulation. This may be restricted to one part of the body (because of a thrombus (see Ch. 4) or cutaneous vasoconstriction in cold exposure (see Ch. 16), for example) or it may be generalised as in circulatory shock.

In shock, the cause of inadequate perfusion of the tissues with blood may be:

- a decrease in blood volume (such as occurs in haemorrhage or with burns)
- cardiac failure
- massive vasodilation (as caused by endotoxins or histamine, for example).

Consequences

Because blood is flowing more slowly through the tissues, a greater proportion of the O_2 bound to haemoglobin is released to maintain O_2 supplies to the cells. Consequently, more deoxygenated haemoglobin is formed. If circulation through the skin is sluggish, cyanosis may appear. The cyanosis of stagnant hypoxia is referred to as *peripheral cyanosis* to distinguish it from that of hypoxic hypoxia, known as *central cyanosis*.

The two forms of cyanosis can be distinguished by inspection of the tongue and mucous membranes of the eye in addition to the skin. The amount of O_2 extracted by the former two tissues is relatively small in relation to their blood flow and, therefore, even when blood flow is sluggish, cyanosis does not usually develop at these sites. If they look pink when the skin is blue, the cyanosis is peripheral. If they also appear blue, the cyanosis is central.

In stagnant hypoxia, the consequences of an inadequate blood flow include the effects of O_2 deficiency as well as those caused by the local build-up of cellular waste products and secretions.

Histotoxic hypoxia

This is a rare form of hypoxia in which the tissues, though plentifully supplied with O_2, are unable to make use of it. One cause is poisoning by cyanide. This chemical inhibits the flavoprotein cytochrome system and prevents ATP formation. Cells such as neurones that rely on aerobic metabolism will be seriously affected and eventually irreversibly damaged.

> The difference between peripheral and central cyanosis is an important distinction and should always be determined. In addition, be aware that cyanosis may be a late sign of hypoxia and should not be relied upon as an early indicator.

OXYGEN THERAPY

O_2 therapy can be used to improve the oxygenation of blood and therefore is of value in the treatment of almost all forms of hypoxic hypoxia except that caused by cardiac shunts. It is, however, of little or no benefit in other forms of hypoxia.

O_2, though vital to life, can be damaging to the body if administered in too high a concentration for too long. The reasons for this are not clear, but it is known that O_2 inhibits alveolar macrophages (see Chs 4 and 15) and reduces the secretion of surfactant (see Ch. 7). Irritant effects have been detected after ventilation with 100% O_2 for as little as 8 hours, and overt lung damage after 1 to 2 days' exposure.

KEY POINTS

What you should now understand about the maintenance of oxygen supplies:

- why oxygen is needed
- what control systems are involved in maintaining oxygen supplies
- how the control systems work
- how oxygen deficiency (hypoxia) can occur
- what the consequences, and therefore signs, of oxygen deficiency are
- why oxygen therapy is of use in some, but not all, forms of hypoxia.

REFERENCES AND FURTHER READING

Bard P (ed) 1961 Medical physiology, 11th edn. Mosby, St Louis
Case R M (ed) 1985 Variations in human physiology. Manchester University Press, Manchester
Dirix A, Knuttgen H G, Tittel K (eds) 1988 The Olympic book of sports medicine. Blackwell Scientific Publications, Oxford, vol 1
Ganong W F 1991 Review of medical physiology, 15th edn. Appleton & Lange, East Norwalk, Connecticut, p 625
Heath D, Williams D R 1981 Man at high altitude, 2nd edn. Churchill Livingstone, Edinburgh (Specialist book for reference)
Minors D S 1985 Abnormal pressure. In Case R M (ed) Variations in human physiology. Manchester University Press, Manchester (Useful source of further information on high altitude)
Royle J A, Walsh M (eds) 1992 Watson's Medical–surgical nursing and related physiology, 4th edn. Baillière Tindall, London
Stryer L 1988 Biochemistry, 3rd edn. W H Freeman, New York
West J B 1992 Pulmonary pathophysiology – the essentials, 4th edn. Williams & Wilkins, Baltimore (Clinical companion to *Respiratory physiology* by West – see Ch. 7 – includes useful chapters on respiratory failure, oxygen therapy and artificial ventilation)

Chapter 12
ACID–BASE BALANCE

Acids are substances which in solution produce hydrogen ions (*hydrions*). Hydrions interact very readily with many chemical substances. The structure and properties of proteins, for example, are affected by the hydrion concentration of the body fluids. For these reasons it is important that the concentration of hydrions in body fluids is kept within acceptable limits. Many systems contribute to this but especially important roles are played by the respiratory system and the kidneys. If regulation is defective then acidosis or alkalosis results, and these conditions alter body function.

DEFINITIONS

ACIDS

Any substance which in solution yields free hydrogen ions (H⁺ or hydrions) is defined as an *acid*. Some physiological examples include:

- hydrochloric acid (HCI) produced by the stomach (see Ch. 6)
- carbonic acid (H_2CO_3) formed by all cells
- lactic acid ($CH_3.CHOH.COOH$) from anaerobic glycolysis (see Ch. 11).

In solution each of these molecules splits up (*dissociates*) to give two ions, one of which is a hydrion (Fig. 12.1).

Hydrions are also sometimes referred to as *protons*. This is because a hydrogen atom consists only of a proton and an electron. There are no neutrons. The loss of the electron to form the ion leaves just the proton (see Ch. 2).

Strong and weak

HCI is referred to as a *strong acid* because in solution almost all the HCI splits up into the free ions (Fig. 12.1). Carbonic acid is classified as a *weak acid* because in solution most of it remains in the undissociated form as H_2CO_3 and only a few ions are present. ①

ALKALIS

An *alkali* is any substance which in solution yields free *hydroxyl ions* (OH⁻). Magnesium hydroxide (present in milk of magnesia, sometimes prescribed for stomach upsets) is one example (Fig. 12.2). Some substances, such as ammonia, make solutions *alkaline* because they react with water molecules to form hydroxyl ions (Fig. 12.2).

Water itself can be defined as an acid and an alkali, although exceedingly weak, because it can dissociate to yield hydrions and hydroxyl ions (actually 1 molecule in every 550 000 000 molecules).

① *How is the stomach wall protected from this strong hydrochloric acid? What are the factors which might reduce this protection, and what might be the results?*

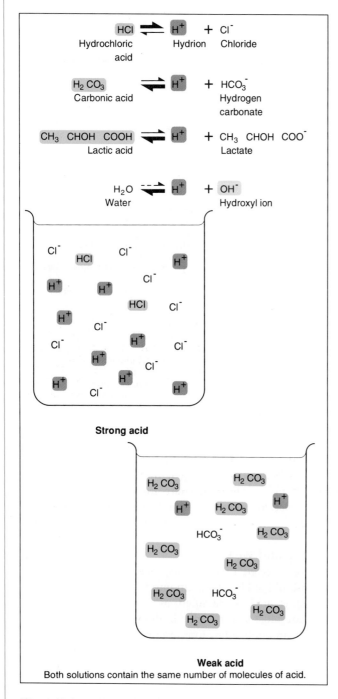

Figure 12.1
Examples of strong and weak acids.

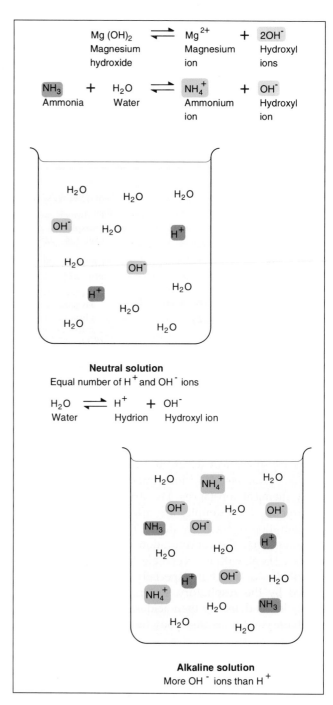

Figure 12.2
Neutral and alkaline solutions.

Patients with gastric or duodenal ulcers are sometimes prescribed 'antacids' such as magnesium hydroxide or aluminium hydroxide. As the term antacid suggests, these alkaline substances counteract the strongly acid environment in the stomach because the hydroxyl ions 'mop up' the hydrogen ions present in the gastric hydrochloric acid. One problem, if these antacids are taken to excess (they are available without a prescription), is that they can bring about an alkalotic state (see p. 234).

BASES

Any substance which in solution can *accept* hydrions is defined as a *base*. Thus Cl^-, HCO_3^-, lactate, OH^- and ammonia are all bases. Like acids, bases can be either strong or weak. Chloride is a weak base as it is a reluctant acceptor of hydrions, whereas hydrogen carbonate (HCO_3 or bicarbonate) is a stronger base as it holds on to hydrions more tightly, and OH^- is even stronger.

The terms alkali and base are sometimes used interchangeably. This is correct for any substance that reacts with water to produce hydroxyl ions, such as ammonia (Fig. 12.2B), as it is *both* a hydrogen acceptor and a hydroxyl producer. Magnesium hydroxide, however, is *only* a hydroxyl producer and is therefore an alkali, whereas the hydroxyl ion, as a hydrogen acceptor, is a base.

BUFFERS

Weak acids and bases have an important role to play in stabilising H^+ concentration in body fluids because the amount of H^+ that they release or accept depends on the concentration of H^+ in the fluid at that time. For example the dissociation of carbonic acid into hydrions and hydrogen carbonate can be represented thus:

$$H_2CO_3 \rightleftarrows H^+ + HCO_3^-$$

The symbol linking these substances indicates that the chemical reaction could go in either direction. A solution of carbonic acid will contain all three substances. If a few more hydrions were added to the solution, some of them would combine with some of the HCO_3^-, and a little more carbonic acid would be formed. Conversely, if a few molecules of another base were added to the solution they would combine with some of the hydrions. Because of this the chemical equilibrium would be displaced and a few more molecules of carbonic acid would dissociate and replace some of the hydrions that had been mopped up by the base.

Either way, the concentration of free hydrions in solution does not change as much as would be expected from the amounts of acid or base added to the mixture. The concentration of free H^+ ions is said to be *buffered*; in other words, the impact of the added acid or base on the total free H^+ concentration of the solution is lessened. Chemicals which act in this way are referred to as *buffers*. There are many examples in the body. Some will be described below.

Table 12.1 Different units used to describe the concentration of hydrions

mol/l	pH	nmol/l
1	0	
0.1	1	
0.01	2	
0.001	3	
0.0001	4	
0.00001	5	
0.000001	6	1000
0.0000001	7	100
0.00000001	8	10
0.000000001	9	1
0.0000000001	10	0.1

pH

The concentration of most substances in the body is usually quoted as grams per litre, millimoles per litre or as quantities greater or smaller than this on the decimal system (i.e. kg, mg, μg, ng etc.). However, the concentration of H^+ ions has traditionally been quoted differently (in *pH units*) partly because of the techniques used to measure it and partly because of the very wide range of H^+ concentrations encountered in biological systems. For example, the hydrogen ion concentrations of three body fluids are listed below:

Pancreatic juice	0.00001 mmol/l
Plasma	0.00004 mmol/l
Gastric juice	100 mmol/l

It can be seen that there is a 10 000 000-fold difference in hydrion concentration between pancreatic juice and gastric juice. The numbering system is simplified if a logarithmic scale is used. For example gastric acid has a H^+ concentration of 0.1 mole per litre. The logarithm of 0.1 is –1. Similarly, pancreatic juice has an H^+ concentration of 0.00000001 mole per litre, and the logarithm of this is –8. By convention the minus sign is dropped. Thus on a logarithmic scale the above concentrations are noted as follows:

	pH
Pancreatic juice	8.0
Plasma	7.4
Gastric juice	1.0

On this scale, an increase of one unit from 1 to 2 or from 5 to 6 denotes a 10-fold change in H^+ concentration, whereas an increase of two units denotes a 100-fold change, three a 1000-fold change, and so on (Table 12.1).

Pancreatic juice is alkaline because it contains sodium hydrogen carbonate. Food in the stomach is mixed with hydrochloric acid as part of the digestive process (see Ch. 6). In the duodenum, the next part of the gastrointestinal tract to receive the food, the mixture is neutralised by pancreatic juice in order to bring the pH to a level which is suitable for the pancreatic enzymes to work (pH 6.5).

ACIDS AND BASES IN THE BODY

NORMAL CONCENTRATIONS

Hydrions

The normal concentration of hydrions in arterial plasma usually ranges between 36 and 44 nmol/l (pH 7.44 to

7.36). A broader range of concentration can be tolerated under extreme circumstances: the limits are 22 to 140 nmol/l (pH 7.65 to 6.85) at the very most. Intracellular fluid is usually slightly more acid (pH 7.2) than extracellular fluid.

Bases

There are many different bases in body fluids. Two important ones for acid–base balance are hydrogen carbonate (HCO_3^-) and hydrogen phosphate (HPO_4^{2-}). Their normal concentrations in extracellular fluid are 26 and 1 mmol/l respectively. ②

SOURCES

Acids and bases are gained in the diet and produced in body metabolism.

Diet

The dietary component varies. Diets rich in fruit and vegetables tend to raise the base content of the body, whereas meat diets lead to a net gain of acid.

Fruits actually contain weak organic acids like citric and malic acid but their metabolism within the body generates bases like hydrogen carbonate. A standard meat diet yields roughly 80 millimoles of acid products (sulphuric and phosphoric acids) per day from the metabolism of proteins.

Metabolism

Even if no food is ingested, acids and bases are generated by body metabolism (Table 12.2). Acid production is the greater of the two by far and therefore there is a continual need for acid to be eliminated. The chief product giving rise to acid is carbon dioxide formed largely in the citric acid cycle (see Ch. 11). CO_2 combines with water to form carbonic acid:

$$CO_2 + H_2O = H_2CO_3$$

② Can you state the normal range of commonly occurring electrolytes (such as sodium, potassium and chloride) in the body? (By remembering these normal values, you will be able to asssess the significance of blood test results more easily.)

KETO-ACIDOSIS

During periods of prolonged starvation, the body's energy requirements are met by the breakdown of stored fats and proteins, rather than by a continuing intake of carbohydrates. Similarly, in the new diabetic (or one who is poorly controlled) a deficiency of effective insulin prevents the use of glucose by body cells for energy production. Consequently, fats and proteins are used instead. (It will be recalled that, even when a person is 'resting', the body is still using energy – for example, for new cell production, tissue repair, enzyme and hormone production, maintenance of muscle tone and respiration.)

Metabolism of fats under such conditions – starvation (see Ch. 14) or uncontrolled diabetes mellitus – leads to the accumulation of ketone bodies in the bloodstream and, consequently, in the urine, where they may be detected by the use of dipsticks. Ketone bodies consist of beta-hydroxybutyric acid, aceto-acetic acid and acetone, the first two being acids. Keto-acidosis, or ketosis – the accumulation of large quantities of these ketone bodies in the blood – is a form of metabolic acidosis (see p. 234).

The equivalent of about 13 moles of acid is formed in this way each day. It is a major function of the respiratory system (see Ch. 7) to transport and eliminate this acid-producing substance.

By comparison, the amounts of other acids, such as lactic acid and butyric acid, formed within the body are usually relatively small. Some may be transformed into other products – for example lactic acid is converted into glucose by the liver. Others, such as butyric acid, are excreted in the urine. When no food is ingested, and body metabolism is being maintained by the usage of stores, proteins may be broken down (*catabolised*) as well as glycogen and fats (see Ch. 14). Protein catabolism yields acid products, such as sulphuric acid, as in the metabolism of a meat diet.

Table 12.2 Acids and bases formed in body metabolism

Acid	Source	Chapter reference	Base
Carbonic acid	Carbon dioxide	11	Hydrogen carbonate
Lactic acid	Anaerobic glycolysis	11	Lactate
Aceto-acetic acid / Beta-hydroxybutyric acid	Ketone bodies from fat metabolism	14	Aceto-acetate / Beta-hydroxybutyrate
Sulphuric acid	Sulphur-containing amino acids	2	Sulphate
Phosphoric acid	Nucleic acids	2	Phosphate
Uric acid	Purines in nucleic acids	2	Urate
Acetic acid / Propionic acid / Butyric acid	Metabolism of dietary fibre by colonic bacteria	6	Acetate / Propionate / Butyrate
Ammonium	Protein metabolism	14	Ammonia

BUFFERS IN THE BODY

Buffers help to prevent big changes in the H^+ concentration of the body fluids from occurring whenever acids and bases are gained in the diet or produced in metabolism. Of the many buffer systems in the body, three are especially important (Fig. 12.3);

- hydrogen carbonate/carbonic acid system (HCO_3^-/H_2CO_3)
- phosphate buffers
- proteins.

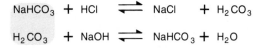

$$NaHCO_3 + HCl \rightleftharpoons NaCl + H_2CO_3$$
$$H_2CO_3 + NaOH \rightleftharpoons NaHCO_3 + H_2O$$

A **Sodium hydrogen carbonate/carbonic acid**

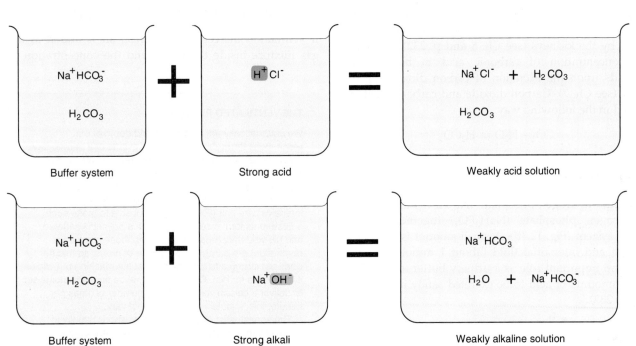

B **Disodium hydrogen phosphate/sodium dihydrogen phosphate**

$$\underset{\text{Strong acid}}{Na_2HPO_4 + HCl} = \underset{\text{Weakly acid}}{NaH_2PO_4} + NaCl$$

$$\underset{\text{Strong alkali}}{NaH_2PO_4 + NaOH} = \underset{\text{Weakly alkaline}}{Na_2HPO_4} + H_2O$$

Buffer system

C **Acidic and basic amino acids in proteins**

Figure 12.3
Three important buffer systems of the body.

HYDROGEN CARBONATE/CARBONIC ACID

Hydrogen carbonate/carbonic acid (Fig. 12.3A) is an important buffer system both in the plasma and interstitial fluid. It is important quantitatively as normally there is a lot of HCO_3^- (26 mmol/l) in these fluids to mop up hydrions. It is also important functionally because the concentrations of hydrogen carbonate and carbonic acid are regulated by the kidneys and the respiratory system respectively.

The amount of hydrogen carbonate in blood depends on how much is lost in the urine or returned to the blood by the kidneys (see Ch. 8 and p. 232). Likewise, the concentration of carbonic acid in body fluids depends upon the excretion of carbon dioxide by the lungs (see Ch. 7). Carbon dioxide and carbonic acid are related in the following way:

$$CO_2 + H_2O \rightleftarrows H_2CO_3$$

PHOSPHATE

Disodium hydrogen phosphate (Na_2HPO_4) and sodium dihydrogen phosphate (NaH_2PO_4) together form a buffer system (Fig. 12.3B). A small amount is present in plasma and interstitial fluid (about 1 mmol/l). It also plays an important role as a urinary buffer and enables large amounts of acid to be excreted safely in the urine (see p. 233). ③

③
Contrast the pH of acid urine with the pH of hydrochloric acid produced by the stomach.

PROTEINS

Proteins can bind and release hydrogen ions, and therefore act as buffers because they contain some amino acids like aspartic acid that are acidic and some like lysine that are basic (Fig. 12.3C; see also Ch. 2, Fig. 2.5 and Table 2.1).

Proteins act as buffers both outside and inside cells. The plasma proteins (see Ch. 4) act as buffers in blood plasma. Of the huge variety of intracellular proteins, haemoglobin in the erythrocytes (see Chs 4 and 7) is of note. It buffers the hydrions derived from carbonic acid and thus facilitates the transport of carbon dioxide in blood (see Ch. 7).

When hydrogen ions are bound or released by proteins the structure of the protein molecule alters, and this changes the properties of the protein be it an enzyme, transporter or structural element. Sometimes this is detrimental to cell function as, for example, when the binding of hydrions by proteins inside muscle cells (see Ch. 22) inhibits contraction. Sometimes, however, it is used to drive other processes. For example the binding of hydrions to haemoglobin (see Ch. 7) is one of the factors that releases oxygen from haemoglobin in the capillaries of active tissues. ④

④
What acid is produced by muscles as they become exhausted?

RESPIRATORY REGULATION OF pH

The large amount of carbon dioxide produced in metabolism is a continual threat to the maintenance of pH. However, carbon dioxide is efficiently excreted by the lungs and the amount excreted can be altered by changing the ventilation of the lungs.

EFFECTS OF VENTILATION ON pH

If ventilation increases, more fresh air is added to the gas mixture inside the lungs, and the concentration of

---

THE VENTILATED PATIENT

We automatically adjust the rate and depth of our respirations throughout the varying events of a normal day – walking to work, running up stairs, relaxing after a meal, and sleeping. Unless our breathing becomes very fast or laboured, we are probably quite unaware of the changes which occur. By contrast, a patient on a ventilator in an intensive care unit (ICU) is usually unable to make such adjustments for himself. Often, such a patient is sedated, and his voluntary muscles (including those involved in respiration) are paralysed by means of drugs, so that he does not struggle to breathe against the machine but allows it to breathe for him. Consequently, once the ventilator is set to deliver a certain volume of air a number of times per minute, this 'minute volume' does not vary.

The anaesthetist (the senior doctor who is usually in overall charge of ICU patients) will undertake regular analysis of arterial blood gases, in order to ascertain that PO_2, PCO_2 and pH are within normal limits. If, for example, blood levels of CO_2 rise, and the pH falls, the anaesthetist may adjust the ventilator to deliver a slightly greater volume of air at each stroke, or a higher number of strokes per minute, or both. (Note that increasing the oxygen intake would not bring down a raised PCO_2 level.) The danger is that prolonged ventilation of a patient, together with infrequent blood gas analysis, may lead to a rise in PCO_2 and a fall in pH (that is, an acidotic state).

Patient restlessness may sometimes (but not always) be attributable to changes in CO_2 levels. For example, if the PCO_2 rises because of, say, inadequate ventilation, this will stimulate the patient's respiratory centre, causing him, if under-sedated, to breathe against the ventilator. (That is, he attempts to breathe for himself, his own respiration rate going against the rhythm of the ventilator.) Raising the ventilator's minute volume may help calm the patient by reducing his CO_2 level and, therefore, his respiratory drive. Patient restlessness is likeliest to occur when his sedation and paralysing drugs are wearing off.

Similarly, when a patient is being 'weaned off' a ventilator, the anaesthetist sometimes allows the patient's PCO_2 to rise by, for example, reducing the ventilator's stroke volume or decreasing its rate per minute. Consequently, when the effects of sedative and paralysing agents have worn off, the patient's respiratory drive is enhanced by the increased carbon dioxide level.

carbon dioxide in alveolar air decreases. As a result, the gradient for the diffusion of carbon dioxide from the blood to the alveolar air gets steeper and more carbon dioxide is eliminated from the blood per minute. Thus, the concentration of carbon dioxide in body fluids decreases and the amount of carbonic acid (and thus H⁺) in the body fluids decreases also. In other words, the pH increases.

Hyperventilation

Voluntary over-ventilation of the lungs, or over-breathing, can decrease the hydrion concentration of blood from 40 to 32 nmol/l (pH 7.4 to 7.5) within a matter of seconds. You can become quite dizzy by doing this, a fact which many children have discovered. The dizziness is caused by the increase in pH and decrease in carbon dioxide concentration. These changes provoke a variety of effects including cerebral vasoconstriction and a decrease in the concentration of free calcium in body fluids. Both of these effects influence nerve cell function indirectly and directly.

Hypoventilation

Conversely under-ventilation, or breath-holding, leads to the retention of carbon dioxide, and therefore of acid, within the body. Consequently the hydrion concentration increases (pH decreases). Most people can hold their breath for at least half a minute. In this time, blood pH decreases from 7.4 to 7.35.

CONTROL OF VENTILATION BY pH AND PCO_2

Normally, ventilation of the lungs is reflexly adjusted by the nervous system in such a way that arterial blood pH and arterial PCO_2 are stabilised at 7.4 and 40 mmHg (5.3 kPa) respectively. The effects of arterial pH and CO_2 on

---

CORRECTING SEVERE ACIDOSIS

In the event of cardiac arrest, the victim's respirations will cease within a short time of the heart stopping. (Indeed, cessation of breathing may have been the cause of cardiac arrest.) As a consequence, the concentration of CO_2 in the patient's body fluids will rise, and the pH will fall. This is because carbon dioxide is no longer being blown off from the lungs at each expiration. Instead, it is accumulating in the body. At the same time, the lack of delivery of oxygen to the tissues results in the formation of lactic acid by anaerobic glycolysis. This makes the pH fall even further and depletes hydrogen carbonate in the body fluids.

First-aid measures consist of mouth-to-mouth resuscitation and cardiac massage until more effective artificial ventilation can be attempted using an endotracheal tube, through which high levels of oxygen can be delivered. Further resuscitation measures will include the administration of drugs and/or direct current electric shocks but, unless the patient's acidotic state is reversed, these will be to no avail. The longer the patient remains without adequate ventilation and circulation, the deeper will be his acidotic state.

High levels of oxygen delivered via an endotracheal tube, together with effective cardiac massage, should be successful in achieving circulation of well-oxygenated blood, an increase in the PO_2 of the body fluids and, because CO_2 is now being blown off, a fall in PCO_2. The pH should rise and the patient's acidotic state will be reversed. In the event of extended resuscitation measures, intravenous sodium bicarbonate (sodium hydrogen carbonate) 8.4% will be given to counteract the patient's low pH. However, this infusion should not be required if successful resuscitation is achieved quickly.

---

ventilation are illustrated in Figure 12.4. Even small changes in PCO_2, above and below the normal arterial value of 40 mmHg (5.3 kPa), cause significant changes in the rate and depth of breathing. This is strikingly different from the effects of oxygen (see Ch. 11), and makes

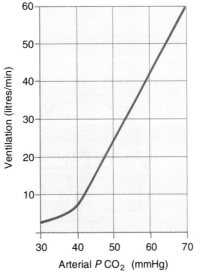
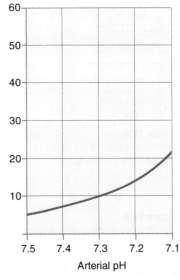

Figure 12.4
Relationships between blood PCO_2 and pH, and ventilation of the lungs. CO_2 is a more effective stimulant of breathing than is blood pH. (Adapted from Guyton 1986.)

clear how important CO_2 is as a regulator of breathing in health.

The respiratory centres (see Ch. 7) are influenced by impulses from chemoreceptors, some of which monitor the composition of the arterial blood (*peripheral chemoreceptors*), and some the extracellular fluid in the brain (*central chemoreceptors*).

Peripheral chemoreceptors

The peripheral chemoreceptors are the same as those that respond to the PO_2 of blood (see Ch. 11). They are sensitive to arterial PCO_2 and hydrion concentration (pH) as well. If CO_2 and/or hydrion concentration increases (i.e. pH decreases), the chemoreceptors are stimulated, and ventilation of the lungs reflexly increases. As a result, the elimination of carbon dioxide is enhanced, the concentration of carbonic acid in body fluids decreases and hydrion concentration is stabilised (Fig. 12.5).

Central chemoreceptors

The central chemoreceptors are situated close to the front (ventral) surface of the medulla oblongata, near to the respiratory control centres (Fig. 12.6 and Ch. 7). The receptors are sensitive to the hydrion concentration of the extracellular fluid surrounding them, which is linked with the cerebrospinal fluid (CSF) (Fig. 12.7).

If the extracellular fluid becomes more acid (i.e. pH decreases) the receptors are excited and ventilation is stimulated. This increases the excretion of carbon dioxide, and reduces the concentration of carbonic acid (and therefore hydrions) in the body fluids as a whole, including the brain extracellular fluid and the CSF. In this way the pH of the fluid bathing the neurones of the brain is stabilised.

Effects of arterial PCO_2

The pH of brain extracellular fluid decreases when the concentration of carbon dioxide in blood increases. This is because carbon dioxide diffuses easily into the fluid from the blood (Fig. 12.7). The carbonic acid formed from it is not as well buffered as it is in the blood because the concentration of proteins in the brain extracellular fluid is much lower than in the plasma. Consequently, only a small increase in arterial PCO_2 is needed to change the pH sufficiently to excite the central chemoreceptors.

Effects of arterial pH

The pH of the brain extracellular fluid is, however, not directly affected by the hydrion concentration of the blood. This is because the blood–brain barrier restricts the movement of many substances, including H^+ ions, between the blood and the brain (see Chs 5 and 20). The

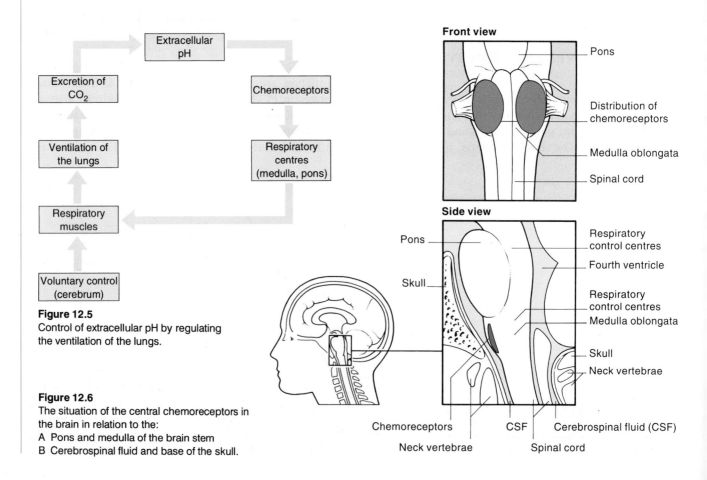

Figure 12.5
Control of extracellular pH by regulating the ventilation of the lungs.

Figure 12.6
The situation of the central chemoreceptors in the brain in relation to the:
A Pons and medulla of the brain stem
B Cerebrospinal fluid and base of the skull.

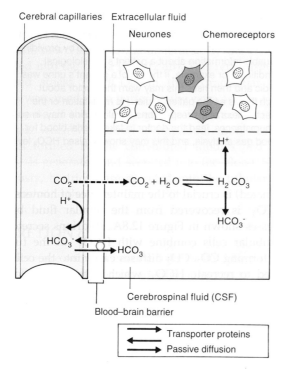

Figure 12.7
Relationships between cerebral capillaries, cerebrospinal fluid, and neuronal extracellular fluid. The central chemoreceptors are excited by an increase in hydrion concentration in the extracellular fluid, but not by an increase of H^+ in the blood. H^+ ions cannot easily cross the blood–brain barrier but CO_2 can. CSF H^+ concentration is regulated in the long term by the transport of hydrogen carbonate across the blood–brain barrier.

central chemoreceptors therefore respond much more vigorously to changes in blood pH caused by carbon dioxide than to the same changes in blood pH caused by acids and bases like lactic acid and hydrogen carbonate for example.

Long-term regulation of CSF pH
If the concentration of carbon dioxide in blood is chronically lowered, as it is at high altitude, or raised, as in some respiratory diseases such as chronic bronchitis, the pH of the CSF is maintained at a normal level by adjusting the CSF concentration of the base, hydrogen carbonate. The hydrion concentration of the CSF is increased by evicting base from the CSF and decreased by accumulating it (Fig. 12.7).

These changes take place slowly, as evidenced by the changes in ventilation that occur at high altitude. When someone ascends rapidly to a high altitude ventilation is stimulated by hypoxia (see Ch. 11). The increased ventilation increases the loss of carbon dioxide from the body, reduces the concentration of carbonic acid in body fluids and increases their pH. The raised CSF pH inhibits the central chemoreceptors, and this partly counteracts the stimulatory effects of hypoxia on ventilation mediated by the peripheral chemoreceptors.

ACCLIMATISATION TO HIGH ALTITUDES

Himalayan mountaineers attempt to overcome the problems of 'altitude sickness', brought on by rapid change of altitude, by undertaking long approach marches for the purpose of acclimatisation. Gaining altitude too quickly (such as being air-lifted to a high basecamp) would cause hyperventilation, tachycardia and dizziness. Acclimatisation enables climbers partly to overcome these problems because they gain altitude over a period of days.

Hyperventilation, triggered by high altitude hypoxia, brings its own problems. One is that, in order to drag in as much oxygen as possible during the hard physical effort of climbing, the climber uses his accessory muscles of respiration – diaphragm, abdomen and shoulders. These use up part of the oxygen inhaled, so that less is available for the skeletal muscles. Another problem is that hyperventilation leads to loss of additional fluid from the lungs – the more breaths are taken, the more water vapour is lost into the cold, dry air. This, combined with the increased excretion of urine at high altitudes, leads to a reduction in the plasma content of blood by as much as 20 to 30% (Steele 1988). One reason that more urine is excreted is that the urine contains more hydrogen carbonate – the body's way of excreting alkali in order to compensate for the low PCO_2.

If the process of acclimatisation fails (and it varies greatly between individuals) the only answer is to assist the sufferer to a lower altitude as quickly as possible.

However, over a few days, as hydrogen carbonate is pumped out of the CSF, the CSF pH is returned towards normal, and the central chemoreceptors increase their firing rate. Consequently, ventilation of the lungs increases (see Ch. 11, Fig. 11.5).

RENAL REGULATION OF pH

The excretion of acid and base by the kidneys inevitably occurs over a longer period of time than the minute to minute adjustments made by the respiratory system. The kidneys contribute in three main ways to acid–base balance. They:

- allow the excretion of bases such as HCO_3^-, SO_4^{2-}, HPO_4^{2-}
- recover and manufacture HCO_3
- excrete H^+.

EXCRETION OF BASES

The filtration of between 150 and 200 litres of fluid per day allows many compounds to be cleared from the blood, including bases gained in the diet or produced in metabolism. Provided that there are no specific uptake mechanisms which retrieve them from the tubular fluid, and provided they do not escape from the tubular fluid

conditions require the conservation of acid and the excretion of an alkaline urine, ammonium disappears from the urine.

URINE pH

The pH of the urine can range between 4.5 and 8.4. Most often the pH is acid, simply because the consumption of diets containing meat inevitably generates acid for excretion. During fasting, the pH of urine will be acid also because of the catabolism of endogenous proteins. On a vegetarian diet, however, urinary pH may be alkaline because the metabolism of such diets may yield an excess of base.

⑥
Vomiting leads to the loss of hydrochloric acid (i.e. gastric acid) and, if prolonged, may bring about an alkalotic state. What effect will prolonged diarrhoea have on the body's acid–base balance, and why?

ACIDOSIS AND ALKALOSIS

DEFINITIONS

A fluid is referred to as *alkaline* or *acid* depending on whether its pH is greater or less than 7. An alkaline urine is one that has a pH > 7, and an acid urine is one of pH < 7 (Fig. 12.10).

However, when referring to the pH state of the blood, a slightly different terminology is used. This takes account of the fact that the normal arterial blood pH lies between 7.36 and 7.44. Physiologically and clinically this is taken as the reference point. Thus if blood pH is less than 7.36 a state of *acidosis* is said to exist; and if the pH is greater than 7.44 this is referred to as *alkalosis*.

Acidosis and alkalosis can arise temporarily as a result of a short-term imbalance in the net gains and losses of acid and base by the body. They also occur as a consequence of disorder.

TYPES

Acidosis and alkalosis are classified as either *respiratory* or *metabolic*.

Respiratory

In respiratory disturbances of acid–base balance, changes in the PCO_2 of blood occur, caused by over- or under-ventilation of the lungs. For example *respiratory alkalosis* (low PCO_2) occurs at high altitude because of the hyperventilation provoked by hypoxia. A *respiratory acidosis* (high PCO_2) can be induced temporarily by breath-holding. Any respiratory disorder that alters the ventilation of the lungs (e.g. emphysema, chronic bronchitis) will disturb acid–base balance in a similar way.

Metabolic

All other forms of acidosis and alkalosis are termed *metabolic*, or *non-respiratory*. The HCO_3^- concentration is

lowered in acidosis and raised in alkalosis. These disturbances may arise through:

- excessive ingestion of acids or bases (e.g. indigestion powders containing sodium hydrogen carbonate can cause alkalosis)
- increased production of acids and bases metabolically (e.g. lactic acid in strenuous exercise)
- losses of acid and base in body fluids (e.g. losses of gastric acid in prolonged vomiting)⑥
- renal disease (e.g. inability to excrete acid).

COMPENSATORY ADJUSTMENTS

When the disturbance of acid–base balance is prolonged then compensatory adjustments occur in the remaining systems.

Renal compensation

For example, if ventilation is chronically depressed through a respiratory disorder, the raised blood PCO_2 stimulates the formation of HCO_3^- by the kidney, and

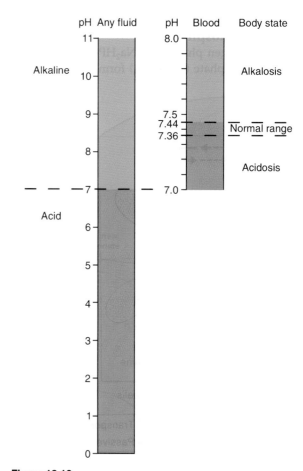

Figure 12.10
Definition of the terms 'alkaline' and 'acid', and 'alkalosis' and 'acidosis'.

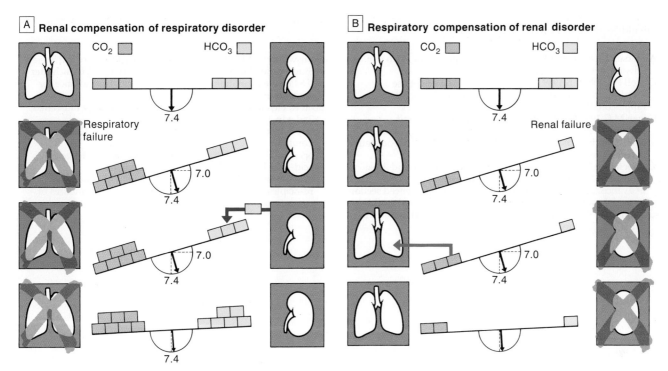

A Renal compensation of respiratory disorder

B Respiratory compensation of renal disorder

Figure 12.11
How respiratory and renal failure disturb acid–base balance, and how compensatory changes in the remaining healthy system minimise the disturbance.

the plasma concentration of HCO_3^- increases above normal. The increase in base cancels out some of the increase in acid caused by the retention of CO_2, and the pH of blood is kept close to normal levels (Fig. 12.11A).

Respiratory compensation

Similarly, if the primary disturbance is metabolic, the secondary effects include changes in respiration. Thus, in renal failure the HCO_3^- concentration of plasma decreases as acid accumulates. The decrease in blood pH stimulates the peripheral chemoreceptors and the rate and depth of breathing increase. This enhances the elimination of carbon dioxide and lowers the amount of carbonic acid in the blood. Again the loss of acid balances in part the loss of base and the result is that the pH of the blood does not change very much (Fig. 12.11B).

'AIR HUNGER' IN DIABETIC KETO-ACIDOSIS

Air hunger is a form of dyspnoea, where the patient entering a keto-acidotic or hyperglycaemic coma takes rapid, deep sighing breaths. It can be distressing both for the patient (if conscious) and the relatives. An alternative name for air hunger is *Kussmaul respirations*. In keto-acidosis, respirations increase in both rate and depth in order to blow off carbon dioxide, thus compensating for the metabolic acidosis. Kussmaul respirations are the body's way of increasing the pH of the blood. The nurse observing a diabetic patient entering such a condition may notice another characteristic of his respirations: the patient's breath may have a peculiar sweet smell. This is caused by ketones being excreted from the lungs.

KEY POINTS

What you should now understand about acid–base balance:

- what acids, alkalis and bases are
- the meaning of the terms buffer, pH, acidosis and alkalosis
- the chief acids and bases that may be gained by and lost from the body
- how the pH of body fluids is normally stabilised
- why acid–base balance is disturbed by disordered respiratory function and by inappropriate artificial ventilation
- why acid–base balance is disturbed by renal failure
- why breathing pattern and renal function change when acid–base balance is disturbed.

REFERENCES AND FURTHER READING

Anderson J R (ed) 1980 Muir's Textbook of pathology, 11th edn. Edward Arnold, London, p 869

Carroll H J, Oh M S 1989 Water, electrolyte and acid–base metabolism – diagnosis and management, 2nd edn. J B Lippincott, Philadelphia

Cogan M G 1991 Fluid and electrolytes – physiology and pathophysiology. Appleton & Lange, East Norwalk, Connecticut (Clear and informative, clinically oriented textbook. Good source of further information)

Goldberger E 1986 A primer of water, electrolyte and acid–base syndromes, 7th edn. Lea & Febiger, Philadelphia (Advanced, clinically oriented text. Large well referenced section on acid–base balance. Useful for following up original work)

Guyton A C 1986 Textbook of medical physiology, 7th edn. W B Saunders, Philadelphia, p 508

Hainsworth R (ed) 1986 Acid–base balance. Physiological Society Study Guide No. 1, Manchester University Press, Manchester (Detailed explanation of all aspects of acid–base balance for students and teachers)

Scott R, Fletcher Deane R, Callander R 1982 Urology illustrated, 2nd edn. Churchill Livingstone, Edinburgh

Steele P 1988 Medical handbook for mountaineers. Constable, London

Workman L M 1991 Introduction to fluids, electrolytes and acid–base balance. W B Saunders, Philadelphia (Clear basic text describing and explaining fundamental principles as well as examining causes and consequences of common disturbances)

Chapter 13
WATER AND ELECTROLYTE BALANCE

60% of the average person consists of water. The volume of water in the body and its distribution between cells and tissues affects many physiological processes including:

- the circulation of the blood
- the diffusion distances between blood and cells
- cell activity.

Dissolved in the water are many substances including glucose, amino acids, and electrolytes such as sodium chloride, potassium hydrogen carbonate, and calcium sulphate. In water, electrolytes dissociate into ions. Ions fulfil many roles in the body, and some such as sodium, potassium and calcium are especially concerned with the maintenance and regulation of cell activity.

Water and electrolytes are gained in food and drink, and lost in body fluids such as urine and sweat. Fluid and electrolyte balance is maintained by control systems that monitor the composition of the interstitial fluid and the volume of blood, and which adjust the gains and losses of water and ions accordingly.

> Although 'electrolyte' actually means any substance that forms ions when it dissolves in water, in biology it has become usual to use it to describe the major inorganic ions in body fluids (Table 13.1). Ions that are present in body fluids in much smaller amounts, such as iron, copper and iodide, are classed as trace elements (see Ch. 14).

WATER

DISTRIBUTION

Compartments
Water is present both inside and outside cells. Water in the body can be thought of as being contained within several different compartments, each of which differs from the others in its composition (Fig. 13.1 and Table 13.1).

Sometimes the water in the compartment is liquid, as it is in blood plasma. Mostly it is held within a gel in

Table 13.1   Approximate composition of several body fluids (mmol/l)

Electrolytes	Other constituents	Blood plasma	Interstitial fluid	Intracellular fluid
Sodium (Na⁺)		145	140	10
Chloride (Cl⁻)		110	115	3
Hydrogen carbonate (HCO₃⁻)		24	25	10
	Glucose	5	5	*
	Organic anions	5	5	*
Potassium (K⁺)		4	4	150
Calcium (Ca²⁺)		2.5	1	0.001†
	Proteins	2	0.3	8
	Amino acids	2	2	*
Magnesium (Mg²⁺)		1	1	15
Phosphate PO₄²⁻)		1	1	50
Sulphate (SO₄²⁻)		0.5	0.5	1

* Wide range in different cells according to metabolic activity.
† Free (ionised) calcium. In addition to this, some calcium inside cells is bound to proteins.

association with other molecules, such as proteins (see Ch. 2). This is the form in which it is present inside cells and in the interstitial space.

The distribution of water between the compartments is determined by two forces:

- osmotic pressure
- hydrostatic pressure.

Like any other molecule which is free to move, water diffuses from a region of high water concentration (dilute solution) to one of low water concentration (concentrated solution). If this diffusion occurs across a barrier which is permeable to water but not to dissolved solutes water will move from one compartment to the other. This is called *osmosis* (see Ch. 5). It is osmosis that makes dried fruit swell when placed in water. Similarly, fluid compartments swell and shrink by osmosis.

Water is also forced from one compartment to another by a difference in *hydrostatic pressure* between the two compartments (see Ch. 5). The process is filtration. It is hydrostatic pressure, due to gravity, that drives water through a coffee filter.

For osmotic and hydrostatic forces to be effective in driving water from one place to another the intervening barrier must be permeable to water molecules. Capillary endothelia (see Ch. 5), cell membranes and many, but not all, epithelia are very permeable.

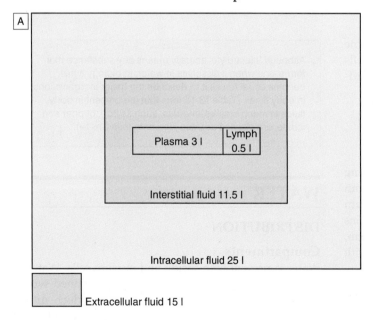

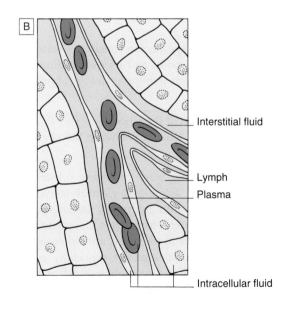

Figure 13.1

Major fluid compartments. Total body water (40 litres) is divided into two compartments: intracellular fluid (25 litres) and extracellular fluid (15 litres).

Osmotic pressure

Significant shifts of water occur between the interstitial fluid and the blood plasma depending on the balance of hydrostatic pressure on either side of the endothelium and the differences in osmotic pressure (see Ch. 5, Figs 5.27 and 5.28).

Effective osmotic pressure

Although there are many substances dissolved in the blood plasma and in the interstitial fluid, some, such as sodium chloride, do not contribute to the osmotic forces that shift water between the interstitial space and the plasma. This is because the endothelium is highly permeable to them too. They therefore do not exert an *effective* osmotic pressure across this barrier. If the concentration of sodium chloride in plasma increases, as it does if you eat very salty food, there would initially be a net shift of water out of the interstitial fluid into the blood. But then, as the sodium chloride diffuses down its concentration gradient out of the plasma, it would redistribute itself within the extracellular fluid as a whole, taking water with it. However, water would be drawn out of the cells by osmosis because cell membranes are not very permeable to sodium ions. The volume of the extracellular fluid (plasma *and* interstitial fluid) therefore expands at the expense of the intracellular fluid (Fig. 13.2). ①

Plasma expanders

Substances in the plasma that do exert an effective osmotic pressure are macromolecules that normally cannot escape easily from the vascular compartment,

---

INTRAVENOUS FLUIDS

Intravenous fluids may be given to replace fluids lost from the body – in haemorrhage, vomiting or diarrhoea, and in burns. The type of intravenous fluid chosen by the doctor will depend on the patient's condition. Where there is haemorrhage from a large wound, whole blood will be given. Where a patient has severe anaemia, an infusion of packed cells is preferable, because each infusion contains less fluid than whole blood, though its value in red cell content is the same.

Intravenous fluids can also be given where a patient is unable to take food and drink orally. In this case, the drip must include glucose, fats, amino acids, vitamins and minerals.

Sometimes drugs are given diluted in intravenous fluids, for example certain antibiotics and some cardiac drugs. Potassium chloride, when given directly into the vein, is well diluted by normal saline (0.9%) or 5% dextrose. Drugs are never added to a blood transfusion because of the high risk of contamination, blood being an ideal medium for bacteria to survive and divide in.

During and following surgery there can be severe loss of fluid from the body – not just blood. The patient will have been denied drink for several hours before the operation; his illness may have caused him to become dehydrated, as in prolonged vomiting, or in a perforated peptic ulcer where there is withdrawal of fluid from the blood into the inflamed tissues of the viscera; there may be an ileostomy or a fistula, or nasogastric drainage of the gut, leading to loss of intestinal secretions from the body.

---

such as plasma proteins and *dextran* (a polysaccharide not found in the body which is used clinically as a plasma expander). If their concentration in blood

① *As a nurse in an accident service, you are warned by Ambulance Control to expect a patient with severe internal bleeding. One item of equipment you would get ready would be an infusion line. What intravenous fluid might be ordered by the Casualty Officer?*

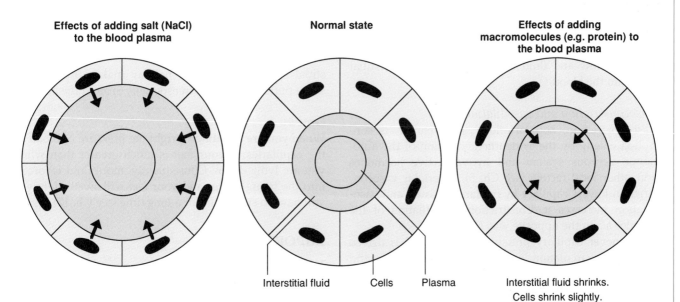

Effects of adding salt (NaCl) to the blood plasma   Normal state   Effects of adding macromolecules (e.g. protein) to the blood plasma

Interstitial fluid   Cells   Plasma

Interstitial fluid shrinks.
Cells shrink slightly.
Plasma volume expands.

Figure 13.2
Effects of adding different solutes to the blood plasma on the distribution of water between the plasma, the interstitial fluid and the cells.

② *Cell volume decreases to some extent too. Can you work out why?*

③ *Why will there be fluid loss from severe burns? From which fluid compartment will there be the most loss – intracellular or extracellular? What sort of replacement fluids will be ordered by the doctor, and why?*

④ *What signs in a patient may suggest to you that blood volume is high or low?*

increases, then fluid is drawn from the interstitial fluid into the plasma (Fig. 13.2). ②

However, if the permeability of the capillary endothelium increases, as it does in *anaphylactic shock*, and macromolecules leak out more readily, their effectiveness as an osmotic force helping to retain fluid in the circulation is reduced. They become more like sodium. Consequently, there is a shift of *fluid* (water plus dissolved substances to which the endothelium is permeable) from the plasma into the interstitial space (*oedema*). ③

A little protein does normally leak out into the interstitial space, the amounts varying from one circulation to another, according to the nature of the capillaries (see Ch. 5). This is returned to the circulation via the lymphatic capillaries which act as an important means of retrieving these macromolecules.

Isotonic fluids

Fluids which do not cause cells to either swell or shrink are said to be *isotonic* with body fluids. They have the same *effective* osmotic pressure. These include:

- 0.9% saline
- 5% dextrose.

Hydrostatic pressure

The second factor which is important in shifting fluid between the blood and the tissue spaces is the hydrostatic pressure of the blood in the capillaries. This is affected significantly by:

- blood volume
- arteriolar and venular constriction and dilation
- gravity.

Blood volume

The greater the blood volume the greater is the mean capillary pressure. After a haemorrhage, capillary pressures are low and fluid is drawn from the interstitial fluid into the blood. ④

Vasoconstriction and vasodilation

Vasoconstriction, both arteriolar and venular, is controlled chiefly by the sympathetic division of the autonomic nervous system and by vasoactive hormones and other local factors (see Ch. 5). Arteriolar vasoconstriction lowers capillary hydrostatic pressure and vasodilation increases it. Constriction and dilation of the venules act in the opposite way (Fig. 13.3).

Whenever capillary pressure is high, fluid is driven from the circulation into the tissue spaces and accumulates there gradually. This shift of fluid is evident in holiday makers from a temperature climate who spend some time basking in the sunshine of Mediterranean and tropical regions. Vasodilation occurs in the vessels of the cutaneous circulation, capillary pressures increase and fluid accumulates in the inter-

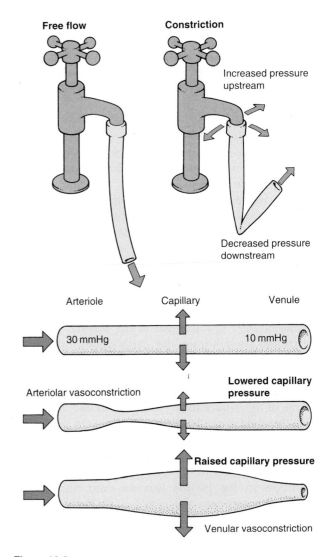

Figure 13.3
Effects of vessel constriction on fluid pressures upstream and downstream.

stitial space. As a result, holiday makers may notice some puffiness of the skin especially around the ankles.

Gravity

When you are standing upright the pressure of blood in the capillaries of your feet is much greater than when you are lying down. Consequently, more fluid is forced into the tissue spaces and your feet will swell slightly if you have to stand still for a long time (see Ch. 17).

IMPORTANCE

Volume

The volumes of water in the different compartments matter. They affect:

- circulatory pressures
- diffusion distances
- cell volume.

Circulatory pressures

Although arterial blood pressure is stabilised by control mechanisms (see Ch. 5) the more fluid that is present within the vessels of the circulation the greater will be the mean circulatory pressure. Blood volume may be increased either by an increase in the number of cells or by an increase in the volume of plasma, which consists largely of water (see Ch. 4).

Diffusion distances

The volume of water in the interstitial space affects the distance that substances have to diffuse between the blood plasma and the cells. This influences the rate at which oxygen, nutrients and waste products are exchanged (see Chs 5 and 7). If fluid accumulates in the interstitial space (oedema) the cells will not be as well nourished and their activity will deteriorate, as happens for example in varicose ulcers.

Cell volume

Cells expand if water is drawn into them and shrink if it is drawn out. These changes in volume affect the position and size of intracellular organelles (see Ch. 2) and consequently alter their activity.

Solvent for polar molecules and ions

The unique chemical characteristics of water enable it to act as a solvent for many substances including proteins, carbohydrates and ions.

Water is a *polar* molecule, which means that the electrical charges on its atoms are not evenly distributed over the molecule (see Ch. 2). One part of the molecule, the oxygen atom, has a slight negative charge, whereas the hydrogen atoms have a slight positive charge. This polarity allows water to associate very freely with other polar molecules, such as amino acids, glucose and proteins, and with ions such as Na^+, K^+, Cl^-, Ca^{2+}, and HCO_3^-. These are attracted to one end or the other of the water molecules, and are therefore easily dispersed among them.

WATER BALANCE

Gains and losses

The amounts of water lost and gained per day by an average individual living in a temperate climate are shown in Table 13.2.

Water is lost in expired air because the air taken into the lungs becomes saturated with water vapour inside the lungs. If ventilation of the lungs increases, the losses of water by this route increase too.

Although the skin is relatively waterproof (see Ch. 15), it is not impermeable and so some water continually diffuses through it and evaporates from the surface of the body. This is added to by the fluid secreted by the sweat glands (see Ch. 16) (up to 2 litres per hour in a very hot climate!).

Normally, gains and losses are kept in balance by regulatory mechanisms which monitor the amount of water in the body and which exert control over some of the ways in which water is gained and lost.

Control

The amount of water in the body is assessed physiologically in at least two ways, by monitoring:

- the concentration of water in body fluids (*osmoreceptors*)
- the volume of fluid in parts of the body (*stretch receptors*).

Osmoreceptors and stretch receptors

Osmoreceptors are neurones which are exceptionally sensitive to small changes in the osmotic pressure of

---

OBSERVATIONS OF FLUID BALANCE

The balance normally maintained by the healthy body between fluid intake and output is sometimes disturbed by certain medical conditions. These might include a patient in heart failure who is retaining fluid or someone with food poisoning who is vomiting profusely.

Sometimes a patient's condition requires that careful observation be made of his fluid balance – that is, comparison of fluid taken into the body with that excreted from it. It is an important nursing responsibility to maintain strictly accurate fluid balance records. All oral fluids taken will be recorded on a special chart. Note, the amount actually drunk by a patient is important rather than what has been poured into a glass on the locker top. Urine output is measured and recorded, as also are vomitus and diarrhoea. There are different columns on the fluid balance chart for input – oral and intravenous – and output such as urine, nasogastric drainage, surgical drains and faecal loss.

An accurately maintained chart provides the clinician with important information. He or she will make allowances for fluid loss via sweat and expired air, and will probably base the calculations of subsequent intravenous therapy on the fluid balance maintained by nursing staff, perhaps together with certain blood test results.

Table 13.2 Daily losses and gains of water*

Losses	(ml)	Gains	(ml)
Urine	1500	Drink	1250
Expired air	400	Food	1000
Diffusion through skin	400	Metabolism	250
Sweat	100		
Faeces	100		
	2500		2500

* In an adult living in a temperate climate, engaged in light activity.

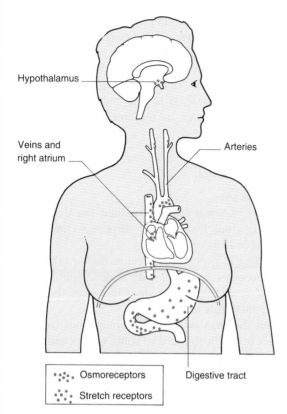

Figure 13.4
Chief locations of the osmoreceptors and stretch receptors involved in the regulation of water intake and loss.

In *diabetes insipidus*, there is decreased secretion of antidiuretic hormone (ADH) leading to the voiding of large quantities of dilute urine. Without the influence of ADH, the renal collecting ducts do not reabsorb water (see Ch. 8). Unlike *diabetes mellitus*, there is no glycosuria though, as in uncontrolled diabetes mellitus, the polyuria is accompanied by intense thirst (*polydipsia*), the body's warning signal to make good the fluid loss.

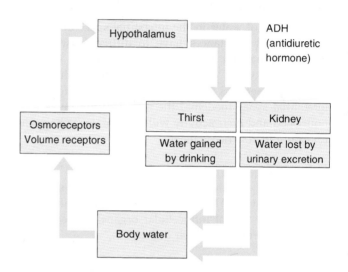

Figure 13.5
Feedback control of body water content.

their environment. Like other cells they swell or shrink depending on the osmotic pressure of the interstitial fluid in which they are bathed. In so doing they change their firing rate.

Stretch receptors respond to the expansion and contraction of the vessels and chambers in which they are found. They are located principally in the walls of some vessels in the circulation and in the digestive tract. An increase in the volume of blood in the circulation will, in the absence of any other changes, increase the pressure of blood. This in turn distends the vessels, distorts the receptors and thus excites them.

The main locations of the osmoreceptors and stretch receptors involved in the regulation of water intake and loss are shown in Figure 13.4. The receptors in the digestive tract monitor the intake of fluid and thus provide advance warning of imminent threats to the volume and osmotic pressure of body fluids. The osmoreceptors of the hypothalamus, and the stretch receptors in the circulation supply information about the actual body water state.

Effectors
All this sensory information is relayed to the hypothalamus. This controls the intake of water, through

influencing the desire to drink (see Ch. 31), and regulates loss of water mainly through the release of ADH and its action on the kidneys (see Chs 8 and 10) (Fig. 13.5). The kidneys can only conserve water that is already present in the body. They limit water losses but cannot make good any deficits. This can only be achieved by an increase in water intake in food and drink.

Disturbances

Dehydration
In *dehydration* water is lost from all fluid compartments, intracellular and extracellular. This leads to shrinkage of cells and tissues. Skin, for example, will feel 'loose'.

Rapid rehydration can be achieved safely by the infusion of a 5% dextrose solution. Water could not be given safely in the same way, as the initial decrease in the plasma osmolality would cause the red cells to swell and some would burst (*haemolyse*). As 5% dextrose is isotonic with plasma, no instant swelling occurs. Ultimately, however, the glucose is taken up into cells and used up in metabolism. When glucose enters cells, water enters too by osmosis and, so, rehydration of the intracellular fluid occurs as well.

An isotonic saline solution is on its own not as effective in rehydration because it increases the amount of non-metabolisable solute (sodium chloride) in the body and only really expands the extracellular compartment.

PATIENTS' HYDRATION REQUIREMENTS

The recommended daily intake of fluid for a normal, healthy person is 2500 ml. (How many cups or glasses of fluid make 2500 ml? It might be interesting to calculate your daily fluid intake, perhaps comparing a day on duty with a day off.) In cold weather, we may find that fluid intake rises – lots of warm drinks. The end result is more visits to the toilet. Again, if we have a holiday in the Mediterranean, the fluid intake rises – lots of refreshing cold drinks. Here, however, perspiration gets rid of much of this fluid, so that urine output remains near normal.

In certain conditions, a patient's fluid intake might be varied from what is usual. The patient with a urinary tract infection should be advised to drink at least 3 litres per day in order to keep up a good urinary output. This flushes out the urinary tract and helps prevent bacteria from ascending to the kidneys. An elderly man following prostatectomy, once he has fully recovered from the anaesthetic, should also drink at least 3 litres a day. The high urine output this produces helps wash out blood, caused by the operation, from the bladder. A patient in chronic renal failure, who is not excreting water and electrolytes, has a greatly reduced fluid intake. Further, serum potassium levels are high because potassium is not being excreted, and fruit juices, which are rich in potassium, are avoided.

Water intoxication

If more water is ingested, or administered, than can be excreted (*water intoxication*) plasma osmolality decreases, and cells swell. This disorganises cell function. Swelling of cells in the brain can cause convulsions and coma.

Where there is oedema of brain tissue, or where a forced diuresis is required (for example following poisoning), intravenous mannitol 10 or 20% is given. Mannitol is a carbohydrate which is not metabolised and so remains unchanged in the blood until excreted by the kidneys. It does not cross the blood–brain barrier easily and therefore draws fluid from tissues by osmosis into the blood and so promotes diuresis. By reducing intracerebral pressure, the risk of brain tissue damage is reduced.

SODIUM

QUANTITIES

Distribution

About half of the total amount of sodium in the body is found in the extracellular fluid. It is present chiefly

---

IS SALT GOOD FOR YOU?

Although salt is included in the cooking of many foods in this country, it is also traditionally placed on the table. Adding salt to food is such a habit with many people that they will often liberally sprinkle their food with salt before even tasting it. They might claim that unsalted food is bland and tasteless. However, people used to low-salt food would point out that they actually taste the food rather than the added salt. It is all a matter of personal taste.

Evidence is accumulating that raised blood sodium levels are linked to hypertension and coronary artery disease. Some researchers suggest that some people are salt-sensitive and produce certain pathophysiological changes more readily in the presence of raised sodium levels (Skrabal et al 1981). They suggest that a moderate salt restriction would help to reduce levels of hypertension, especially in salt-sensitive subjects.

We might be surprised at how little sodium is actually required in our diet each day. It is suggested that only 1 gram of salt (i.e. 20 mmol Na) is physiologically required daily and that little is lost from the skin except when sweating occurs (Truswell 1986). Not only does a raised sodium level cause fluid retention (water 'following' the sodium) and therefore an increased blood volume, but some sodium enters the smooth muscle cells of arterioles, increasing their tone. This has the effect of raising arterial blood pressure.

How may sodium levels be reduced? To expect someone to move immediately to a salt-free diet is over optimistic, if not impossible, since many foods contain sodium (for example bacon, breakfast cereal, biscuits and cheese). Further, there is the problem of patient compliance if the taste of food changes too dramatically. Salt may therefore be omitted initially from the cooking process and later be reduced at the table, and a move made to foods which are naturally low in sodium, such as rice, pasta, fresh vegetables and fruit.

It may be more effective to increase potassium intake at the same time as decreasing sodium intake. One reason for this is that salt substitutes in the form of potassium chloride assist compliance with salt-free diets. Another reason is that increased potassium intake prevents the rise in plasma noradrenaline which seems to occur, for no adequately explained reason, after lowering sodium intake (Skrabal et al 1981).

---

as sodium chloride (about 110 mmol/l), together with some sodium hydrogen carbonate (25 mmol/l). A little sodium (9%) is found inside cells (Table 13.1). The remainder (40–50%) is in bone.

Gains and losses

Dietary intake

Unprocessed foods usually do not contain much salt (sodium chloride). Most of the salt we consume is added to food in processing, cooking or by custom. We consume (5–25 g/day; 80–400 mmol) much more salt than we need (about 1 g/day; 20 mmol) simply out of habit. The excess has to be excreted by the kidneys. The recommended dietary intake is no more than 6 g/day.

Table 13.3 Losses of sodium			
Daily	*mmol*	*Additional*	*mmol*
Urine	150*	Diabetes mellitus	Variable
Faeces	1	Diarrhoea Ileostomy fluid	Variable + 100[†]
Sweat	0.5	Profuse sweating (heavy work in hot climates)	+ 500[†]
Milk (♀)	2		

* Amount lost depends on dietary intake.
[†] Representative values to show extent of possible loss.

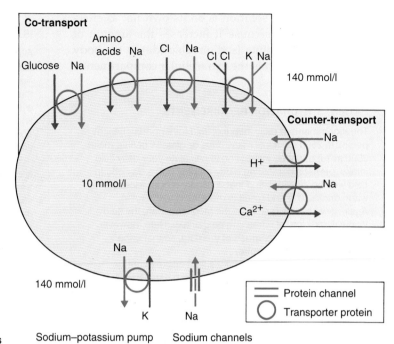

Figure 13.6
Ways in which sodium moves into and out of cells.

Losses in body fluids

As sodium is a normal constituent of all body fluids, loss of sodium occurs whenever fluids are excreted (Table 13.3). Normally, losses are relatively small but they can increase in certain circumstances:

- physically demanding work in a hot climate (sweating)
- gastrointestinal upset (vomiting and diarrhoea)
- ileostomy
- diabetes mellitus.

Whatever the circumstance, losses must be replaced by dietary intake for homeostasis to be maintained.

IMPORTANCE

The high concentration of sodium in the extracellular fluid (ECF) is important for:

- cell function
- extracellular fluid volume.

Cell function

The high sodium concentration in the ECF ($\approx$ 140 mmol/l), and low concentration in the ICF ($\approx$ 10 mmol/l) creates a natural gradient for the diffusion of sodium into cells.

Sodium enters cells through specific protein channels (*sodium channels*) and carriers (Fig. 13.6). Sodium channels play a key role in the generation and transmission of impulses in nerve and muscle cells (see Chs 21 and 22). Some sodium carriers also simultaneously transport other substances, such as glucose and amino

acids, into cells (Ch. 6). Others enable ions such as hydrions and calcium to be evicted from cells (Ch. 8).

The sodium that enters is evicted again by the sodium–potassium pump. The pump uses energy derived from ATP to drive sodium out against its concentration gradient. This maintains the low intracellular sodium concentration which is vital for cell function.

Extracellular fluid volume

Changes in extracellular sodium concentration affect the osmotic pressure of the ECF and thereby influence the movement of water into and out of this compartment. This affects ECF volume.

Effects of sodium losses and gains

If there is a net loss of sodium from the body, the osmotic pressure of the ECF decreases. In the absence of any homeostatic controls this would make water move out of the ECF into the cells, causing them to swell. However, the decrease in osmotic pressure is quickly sensed by the osmoreceptors (p. 241), the secretion of ADH is suppressed and, instead, most of the water is excreted rapidly by the kidneys (Fig. 13.5). In this way the osmotic pressure of the ECF is preserved but at the expense of its volume, and dangerous cellular swelling is avoided.

Conversely, if salt intake exceeds losses, the raised osmotic pressure of the ECF provokes retention of water and stimulates the desire to drink (see Fig. 13.5). Consequently, osmotic pressure is preserved but the volume of ECF expands.

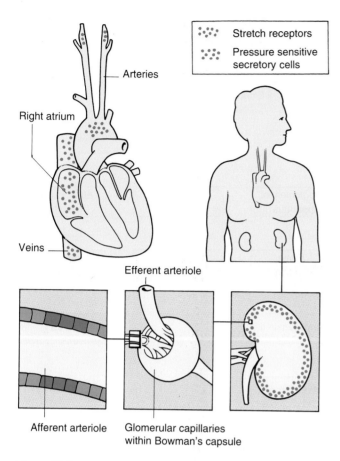

Figure 13.7
Chief locations of the sensory receptors and endocrine cells which detect changes in volume and pressure within the circulation.

These changes in ECF volume are useful in the short term in rapidly protecting the cells but if the changes are maintained they can have other potentially harmful effects.

Effects of changes in ECF volume
The volume of fluid in the ECF affects:

- cell nutrition
- blood pressure.

Cell nutrition is adversely affected when the volume of ECF, and therefore interstitial fluid, expands. There will be a greater distance between the cells and the blood and, therefore, the rate of diffusion of nutrients and waste products between them will be less (see Ch. 3).

Blood pressure is affected by increases and decreases in ECF volume, through corresponding changes in plasma volume. If volume decreases, pressure decreases; if volume increases, pressure increases.

The effects of ECF volume on blood pressure are mitigated to some extent by reflexly induced changes in the circulatory system (see p. 98 and Figs 5.25 and 5.30). These include redistribution of the blood volume between the arteries and the veins. If blood volume decreases, the veins constrict shifting more of the blood held within them into the arteries. Conversely, if blood volume expands, the veins dilate to accommodate it.

SODIUM BALANCE

Because of the link between sodium and ECF volume, the regulation of sodium balance is essentially concerned with the regulation of ECF volume.

Control of ECF volume

Volume receptors
The volumes and pressures of fluid in different parts of the circulation act as indicators of the degree of filling of the ECF with fluid. Sensory receptors and endocrine cells which detect changes in pressure and in volume are found in several places within the circulation (Fig. 13.7). Some of the detectors, namely the stretch receptors in the arteries and veins, are the same as those shown in Figure 13.4. The extra ones shown in Figure 13.7 are those specifically involved with sodium balance. These are pressure sensitive secretory cells in the atria and the kidneys which respond by secreting atrial natriuretic peptide (ANP) and renin respectively (see Ch. 10). These receptors and endocrine cells form part of control systems which:

- control arterial blood pressure (see Ch. 5)
- regulate the urinary excretion of salt and water.

Urinary excretion of salt and water
Very rapid changes in sodium excretion are brought about by changes in glomerular filtration rate (GFR). If renal arterial vasoconstriction occurs, as for example in haemorrhage as part of the baroreceptor reflex (see Ch. 5 and Fig. 13.8), then both renal blood flow and glomerular capillary pressure decrease, and GFR decreases also (see Ch. 8). As a result, less sodium and water is

---

Polyuria – the excretion of increased amounts of urine – should always be investigated when there is no obvious cause, such as excessive fluid intake. When urine volume increases (i.e. there is increased water loss from the kidneys) it is very often the case that the water is accompanied by sodium or glucose. The exceptions to this include increased water consumption and diabetes insipidus where the copious amounts of urine excreted are very dilute and contain no abnormal substances. If the kidneys need to excrete additional amounts of sodium, this draws additional water with it, just as in diabetes mellitus where the glucose in the urine is accompanied by additional water. The alternative – a prospect not pleasant to contemplate – would be to pass salt granules or sugar lumps! As a general rule, where the salt goes, water follows.

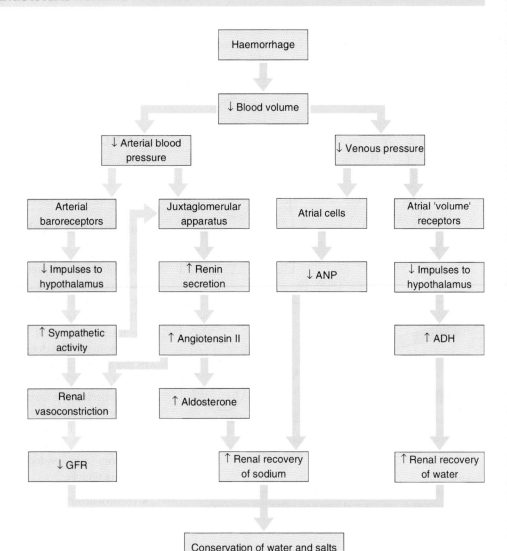

Figure 13.8
Processes and factors involved in the conservation of water and salt after a major haemorrhage.

filtered (along with other plasma constituents) and, in the absence of any other changes, less is excreted.

Conversely, once renal arterial vasodilation occurs, as blood pressure increases, in response for example to the infusion of fluids intravenously, the amount of sodium and water filtered increases and more is lost in the urine. Factors which control the renal blood vessels include the sympathetic nerves and the hormone angiotensin II.

The amount of sodium recovered from the filtrate by the renal tubules is regulated by several hormones, including atrial natriuretic peptide (ANP) and aldosterone (see Chs 8 and 10). ANP increases sodium loss. Aldosterone decreases it. ANP acts more quickly than aldosterone and enables sodium balance to be adjusted in response to relatively short-term changes in salt gains and losses. Aldosterone, however, has a longer-term effect in changing the *capacity* of the renal tubular cells to reabsorb sodium. It enables long-term adjustments to be made to changes in dietary habits or to a more persistent change in an individual's environment or activities. ⑤

Disturbances

Hypertension and hypotension

An increase in blood pressure above the normal range is referred to as *hypertension*. The retention of salt in the body is believed to be a contributory factor in some forms of hypertension. If ECF volume is low, blood pressure is likely to be low also. An abnormally low blood pressure is termed *hypotension*.

POTASSIUM

DISTRIBUTION

Most of the potassium in our bodies is present inside cells (90%) (Table 13.1). Relatively little is present in the extracellular fluid ($\approx$ 2%). The remainder (8%) is found largely in bone.

⑤
Which steroids are used in the treatment of asthma? What side effects may they have on fluid balance, and why?

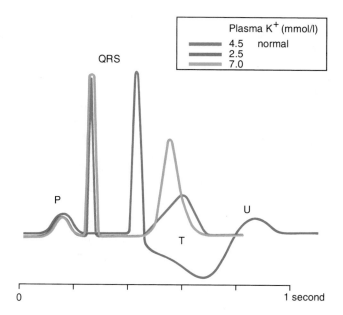

Figure 13.9
Changes in the ECG caused by changes in plasma potassium concentration (Adapted from Goldman 1986).

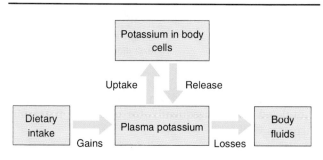

Figure 13.10
Factors affecting the plasma potassium concentration.

IMPORTANCE

The relative concentrations of potassium inside and outside cells affect the electrical state of cell membranes (see Chs 21 and 22). This is particularly important for the function of nerve and muscle cells. Some effects of a change in plasma potassium concentration on the electrical activity of the heart, as reflected in the ECG, are shown in Figure 13.9.

POTASSIUM BALANCE

The concentration of potassium in the ECF depends on the cellular release and uptake of potassium, as well as on dietary gains and losses in body fluids (Fig. 13.10).

Gains and losses

Dietary intake

As the concentration of potassium in plant and animal cells is high (Table 13.1), potassium is consumed in rela-

tively large amounts whenever plant and animal tissues are eaten. Some dietary constituents, such as fruit juice, may be especially rich in potassium. Average daily intakes of potassium are about 60 to 120 mmol.

Losses in body fluids

The two major routes of excretion of potassium are in faeces (about 15 mmol) and in urine (about 100 mmol). Faecal losses may be considerably increased in diarrhoea as potassium is normally secreted by the colon (see Ch. 6).

MAINTAINING POTASSIUM LEVELS

In health the level of potassium in the blood is maintained between 3.3 and 5.5 mmol per litre. Usually a balance is achieved between dietary intake of potassium and losses in faeces and urine. Blood potassium levels can change, however, when too much potassium is either taken into the body or retained, or when too much is lost.

Patients can lose potassium when there is severe loss of fluid from the gastrointestinal tract, as in prolonged vomiting or diarrhoea. Such a patient is not only dehydrated, and may require fluid via an infusion, but will have a low blood potassium level. Often, therefore, the drip will contain a potassium supplement.

Levels of potassium in the blood affect the function of cardiac muscle. As Figure 13.9 shows, changing levels of potassium lead to changes in the heart's electrical activity, and these show up on the cardiac monitor. A patient with a cardiac arrhythmia caused by *hypokalaemia* will require the addition of potassium in an intravenous infusion. In order to monitor the effectiveness of the infusion he may be nursed on a coronary care unit with specialised monitoring equipment, and his blood potassium levels will be estimated daily.

In all cases where an infusion contains potassium, it is important that the fluid runs into the vein strictly to time. Too fast an infusion could cause not only fluid overload but *hyperkalaemia*. Too slow an infusion would fail to correct the patient's dehydration and would not correct the hypokalaemia adequately. Sometimes a patient's condition is so critical, and achieving the correct blood potassium level is so important, that the infusion is monitored with an electronic drip counter. With this, the amount of fluid running into the vein per hour can be precisely controlled and is prescribed by the doctor. The nurse will still monitor the infusion visually from time to time, of course, in case of machinery malfunction.

Blood potassium may rise to dangerous levels in some cases of kidney failure. Cardiac changes would eventually occur, and be noticeable on an ECG, if this hyperkalaemia is not corrected. Reducing potassium levels is more difficult than raising them in hypokalaemia. Foods containing potassium are restricted – chocolate, citrus fruits, bananas and ordinary fruit juices. Calcium resonium is a cation-exchange preparation which, given either orally or rectally, reduces potassium by exchanging it for calcium.

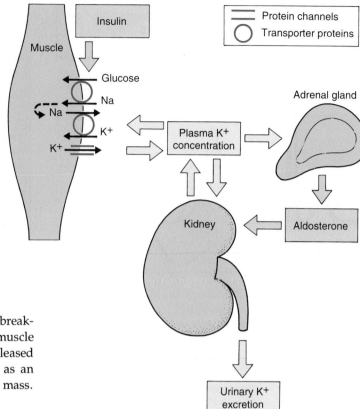

Figure 13.11
Regulation of plasma potassium concentration.

Body stores
Within the body, potassium is derived from the break-down of cells and tissues. In addition, whenever muscle and nerve cells are excited, some potassium is released into the extracellular fluid. Skeletal muscle acts as an important source of potassium because of its large mass.

Control of ECF potassium concentration
The two main ways in which the concentration of potassium in the extracellular fluid is regulated are through (Fig. 13.11):

- release and uptake from cells especially skeletal muscle
- excretion in the urine.

Cellular release and uptake
Potassium is released from muscle cells whenever the cells are activated. The local increase in potassium concentration causes vasodilation which improves the supply of nutrients and oxygen, and facilitates the removal of waste products. However, the increase in potassium concentration also affects the excitability of skeletal and cardiac muscle cells and diminishes the force developed. Re-uptake of the released potassium is thus crucial for normal activity to be maintained.

Potassium is accumulated in all cells by the sodium–potassium pump. The activity of this pump depends upon a continuing supply of ATP and is regulated by the concentrations of intracellular sodium and extracellular potassium. The pump is inhibited by decreased extracellular potassium, and stimulated by increased intracellular sodium.

Intracellular sodium concentration increases when cells take up glucose, because the carrier transports both substances (see Fig. 13.8). In many cells this uptake is facilitated by the hormone insulin (see Chs 10 and 14). When insulin concentrations are high, for example after

a meal, intracellular sodium increases, the pump is stimulated and, consequently, the uptake of potassium increases. ⑥

Renal excretion
Urinary excretion of potassium is stimulated by aldosterone which also promotes the recovery of sodium. Whenever potassium is excreted, sodium is conserved, and vice versa. The concentration of potassium in the ECF is one of the factors which regulates the secretion of aldosterone by the adrenal cortex (see Ch. 10). ⑦

Disturbances
Hypokalaemia (low blood potassium concentration) occurs if there is over-secretion of aldosterone by the adrenal cortex. It may also be provoked by overdoses of laxatives and of some diuretics, and occurs in diabetic patients treated with insulin.
Hyperkalaemia (raised concentration of blood potassium) is one of the features of renal failure. ⑧

CALCIUM

DISTRIBUTION

Altogether, just over 1 kg of calcium is present in an average person. Most of this (99%) is the calcium pres-

⑥
Why is dextrose (glucose) added to blood obtained for transfusion?

⑦
What might happen to the urinary excretion of potassium in uncontrolled diabetes mellitus, and why?

⑧
Diet plays an important part in the treatment of a patient in chronic renal failure. What sort of diet would you recommend? What foods are safe? What foods should be restricted?

ent in bone (see Ch. 28). The concentration of calcium in plasma (2.5 mmol/l) is higher than that in the interstitial fluid (1.3 mmol/l) because about half of the plasma calcium is bound to plasma proteins and, therefore, cannot easily enter the tissue space. The concentration of calcium inside cells (less than 0.001 mmol/l) is considerably less than that in the extracellular fluid.

IMPORTANCE

Calcium is another element which plays an important role in many cellular processes. Unlike sodium and potassium which are monovalent, calcium is a divalent ion which means that each ion can link with two other monovalent ions, not just one. It can therefore act as a bridge between substances and can form more complex molecules.

Thus, calcium binds to many proteins in the body and forms complexes with a variety of inorganic and organic compounds. Some of these are soluble in body fluids; some are not. Several of the functions of calcium are listed in Table 13.4.

Bone

Calcium salts make bones and teeth hard. Bone is formed by the activity of osteoblasts (see Ch. 28). The formation and breakdown of bone is influenced by several factors including:

- availability of calcium
- hormones (parathyrin, calcitonin, calcitriol and oestrogens)
- mechanical stresses.

In the process of bone formation, calcium precipitates out of solution. This can occur quite easily because of the chemical nature of calcium compounds. A delicate balance normally exists between soluble and insoluble forms. The calcium present in bone acts as a pool from which calcium may be withdrawn if plasma calcium falls.

Cell function

Although calcium is a relatively large ion it can enter cells through specific protein channels (*calcium channels*) (Fig. 13.12). Their permeability to calcium is affected by the electrical charge of the membrane and by chemical regulators. When opened, these channels allow calcium to flow into cells along its concentration gradient.

Inside cells, calcium acts as a regulator of several intracellular processes (Table 13.4 and Ch. 2). In muscle cells, calcium binds to specific proteins and activates contraction (see Ch. 22), whereas in secretory cells, such as those of the pancreas, calcium stimulates exocytosis of secretory vesicles.

The concentration of calcium in the cells is not allowed to build up because calcium is expelled again

Table 13.4 Functions of calcium		
Site	*Form*	*Function*
Extracellular	Deposits	Structure of – bone – tooth enamel – tooth dentine
	In solution	Factor involved in coagulation Influences excitability of nerve and muscle
Intracellular	In solution	Regulator of – muscle contraction – exocytosis – glycogen metabolism

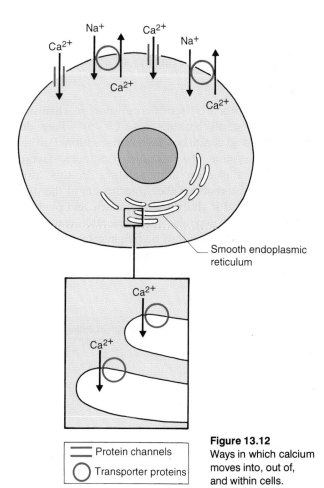

Figure 13.12
Ways in which calcium moves into, out of, and within cells.

by the action of transporter proteins in the membranes of the cell. This is vital for the cells to continue to be able to respond to future stimuli.

CALCIUM BALANCE

Plasma calcium concentration depends on the exchange of calcium between interstitial fluid and bone as well as on the balance between gains and losses (Fig. 13.13).

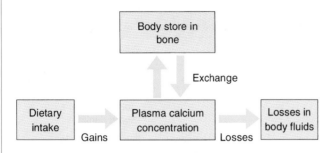

Figure 13.13
Factors affecting plasma calcium concentration.

Gains and losses

Dietary intake
The amounts of calcium ingested range between 200 and 1000 mg per day (5–25 mmol). The recommended intake is about 500 mg (12.5 mmol). Dairy products and some fish are rich sources (Table 13.5) ⑨

⑨
Are there any groups of people for whom additional calcium in the diet may be beneficial? Are there any circumstances in which dietary calcium should be restricted?

Absorption
Calcium is absorbed by specific transport mechanisms in the upper small intestine (see Ch. 6) where the slightly more acid conditions favour absorption. Further down the intestine the alkaline conditions favour precipitation of calcium from solution. In this form calcium is unabsorbable. Other constituents of the diet, such as oxalic acid in rhubarb and spinach, and phytates present in cereals, may also form insoluble complexes with calcium. A diet can thus be rich in calcium and yet not make it available for absorption. On average, about 20% of the dietary intake is absorbed.

Dietary deficiencies of calcium are made worse if there is also a deficiency of vitamin D_3 (see p. 258). This may be because of dietary deficiency or through lack of sunlight. Vitamin D_3 is manufactured in the skin by the action of ultraviolet light on 7-dehydrocholesterol (see Fig. 13.14). Growing children who are fed on cereal-based food rather than dairy products and who live in places which do not enjoy much sunlight are most likely to be at risk of calcium deficiency.

Losses
Calcium is lost in fluids such as urine and milk. Faecal loss is relatively large, but this mostly represents unabsorbed calcium (Table 13.6).

Control
Preservation of normal extracellular concentrations of calcium is achieved by the combined effects of three

Table 13.5 Amounts of various foods providing about 500 mg of calcium		
Food	*Quantity*	
Cow's milk	2 cups	400 ml
Cheddar cheese	1 piece (5 × 3 × 2 cm)	50 g
Yoghurt	2 pots	300 g
Sardines	1 small tin	120 g

Table 13.6 Approximate amounts of calcium absorbed and excreted daily by an adult person consuming a standard diet containing 750 mg calcium			
	Absorbed (mg)	Excreted (mg)		
		Faeces	Urine	Milk
	150	600	150	—
Lactating woman	400	350	150	250

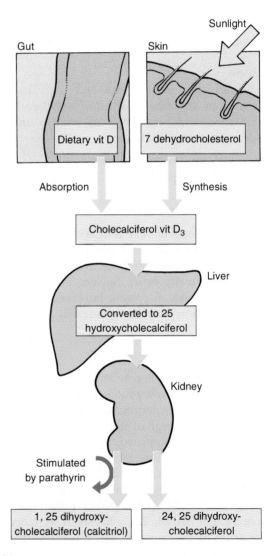

Figure 13.14
Sources of vitamin D_3 (cholecalciferol) and its conversion into the calcium-regulating factor, calcitriol.

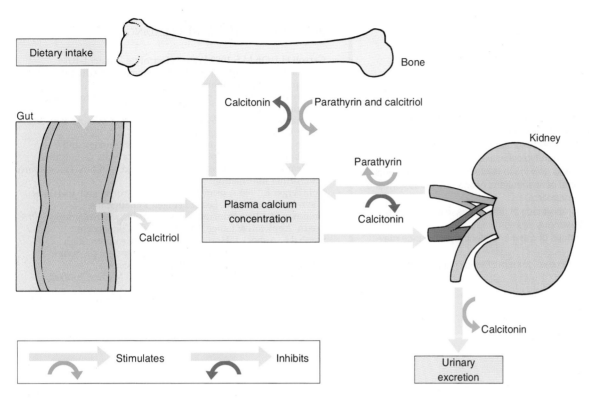

Figure 13.15
Effects of calcitriol, parathyrin and calcitonin on calcium balance.

regulatory substances: parathyrin, calcitonin (see Ch. 10) and 1,25 dihydroxycholecalciferol (also known as *DHCC* or *calcitriol*). The latter substance is formed in the kidney from a metabolite of vitamin D (Fig. 13.14). The main effects of parathyrin, calcitonin, and calcitriol on their various target organs are summarised in Figure 13.15.

Disturbances

Hypocalcaemia
The immediate effects of acute hypocalcaemia are muscle spasms (*tetany*) due to the increased excitability of nerve and muscle cells (see Chs 21 and 22). In chronic hypocalcaemia demineralisation of bone occurs.

Hypercalcaemia
Conversely, hypercalcaemia depresses nerve activity and causes muscular weakness. Also, calcium salts precipitate from solution in the urinary system forming kidney stones, especially if the urine is alkaline (see Ch. 12). Hypercalcaemia can be caused by overactivity of the parathyroid glands.

PARATHYROIDECTOMY

For the first few days following thyroidectomy it is usual for the surgeon to assess the patient's serum calcium level. It may rarely happen that, during operation on the highly vascular thyroid gland, some or all of the parathyroid glands, which are located close behind it, may be accidentally removed, or their blood supply damaged, leading to death of glandular tissue. As explained in Chapter 10, *parathyrin* (parathyroid hormone) controls the blood calcium levels within a narrow normal range (2.12–2.62 mmol/litre).

Reduction in parathyrin secretion will lead to a fall in serum calcium levels (*hypocalcaemia*) with a number of clinical features, which the nurse should watch out for. These include tetany, where increased excitability of muscle and nerve causes continuous muscle spasms. This may be noticed particularly in the wrists, where *carpal spasm* can be seen. It consists of flexion of the wrist with extension of the fingers (see illustration on p. 441 of Chilman & Thomas 1987) and the same type of muscular spasm can also affect the feet (*carpopedal spasm*). It may be accompanied by *paraesthesia* (altered feeling, such as pins and needles) and one of the first signs noticed by the nurse may be that the patient seems unsteady.

Treatment consists of supplying the missing calcium for as long as serum calcium results demand. If the parathyroid glands have inadvertently been removed – a very rare event – calcium therapy will be required for the rest of the patient's life. Initial oedema at the operation site may lead to a temporary dip in serum calcium levels, even though the parathyroid glands themselves remain intact. If this hypocalcaemia returns to normal within 2 or 3 days, without producing any clinical features, no treatment will be necessary.

KEY POINTS

What you should now understand about water and electrolyte balance:

- why water, sodium, potassium and calcium are important in body function
- the factors affecting the distribution of fluid between plasma, interstitial fluid, and cells
- how water intake and excretion is controlled
- dietary sources and typical intakes of sodium, potassium and calcium, and how these relate to daily requirements
- how the plasma concentrations of sodium, potassium and calcium are controlled
- the practical importance of differences in composition between intravenous infusion fluids
- how disturbances of water and electrolyte balance may arise
- the link between salt (sodium chloride) and circulatory pressures.

REFERENCES AND FURTHER READING

Carroll H J, Oh M S 1989 Water, electrolyte and acid–base metabolism – diagnosis and management, 2nd edn. J B Lippincott, Philadelphia
(Advanced, very well referenced text. Useful for following up original work)
Chilman A M, Thomas M 1987 Understanding nursing care, 3rd edn. Churchill Livingstone, Edinburgh
Cogan M G 1991 Fluid and electrolytes – physiology and pathophysiology. Appleton & Lange, Norwalk, Connecticut
(Clear and informative, clinically oriented textbook. Good source of further information)
Goldberger E 1986 A primer of water, electrolyte and acid–base syndromes, 7th edn. Lea & Febiger, Philadelphia
Goldman M J 1986 Principles of clinical electrocardiography, 12th edn. Appleton & Lange, East Norwalk, Connecticut
Skrabal F, Auböck J, Hörtnagl H 1981 Low sodium/high potassium diet for prevention of hypertension: probable mechanisms of action. Lancet 2(8252): 895–900
Truswell A S 1986 ABC of nutrition. British Medical Journal, London
Workman L M 1991 Introduction to fluids, electrolytes and acid–base balance. W B Saunders, Philadelphia
(Clear basic text describing and explaining fundamental principles as well as examining causes and consequences of common disturbances)

Chapter 14
NUTRITION

In order to survive cells need energy to power their activities, raw materials for renewal and growth, and a variety of supplementary substances that play small but crucial roles in cellular processes. These needs are met by the nutrients we absorb from food.

Food contains many different substances including nutrients, indigestible material and other constituents, some of which may even be harmful. Most of the food we eat is normally processed or cooked before it is eaten. This alters its nature and usually, but not always, increases its nutritional value.

Cells require nutrients all the time, not just when we happen to eat. A constant supply is maintained by control systems that regulate our intake of food, and by hormones that regulate the storage and usage of nutrients within the body in between meals.

CELLULAR REQUIREMENTS

Basically cells require:

- energy
- raw materials
- supplementary materials and factors.

Energy powers cellular activity. Raw materials are used to build cellular components and manufacture products such as enzymes and hormones. Supplementary factors including minerals and vitamins participate in cellular activities and metabolism.

ENERGY

The energy used by cells is supplied in the form of high energy phosphate compounds like ATP which are formed through the breakdown (*catabolism*) of foodstuffs (Ch. 11). The amount of energy yielded by different nutrients on breakdown can be measured by literally burning the food and measuring the amount of energy (*calories*) liberated as heat.

Calories and kilojoules

The combustion of a known quantity of a foodstuff is carried out in a sealed chamber (*calorimeter*). The heat generated raises the temperature in a water jacket which surrounds the combustion chamber. The change in the temperature of the water is recorded.

One calorie of energy is that needed to raise the temperature of 1 g of water by 1 degree Celsius.

$$1 \text{ kilocalorie (kcal)} = 1000 \text{ calories}$$

Nowadays the energy content of food is commonly expressed in SI units as *joules (J)* and *kilojoules (kJ)*.

$$1 \text{ calorie} = 4.184 \text{ joules}$$
$$1 \text{ kilocalorie} = 4.184 \text{ kilojoules}$$

Energy content of foods

Foods differ in their energy yield (Table 14.1). Protein and carbohydrate in food each yield about 400 kcal/100 g, whereas fats generate about 900 kcal/100 g. Weight for weight, fatty foods such as cheese are thus potentially richer energy sources than those such as potatoes or white fish that consist mainly of carbohydrates or proteins and water. In a calorimeter the energy yield of proteins is slightly more than 400 kcal/100 g. This

① *Additional energy is also needed if our body temperature is raised above normal. Why?*

is because proteins are completely broken down (*catabolised*) in the calorimeter but not in the body. End products of protein and amino acid metabolism in the body include urea, uric acid and creatinine all of which are eliminated in the urine (see Ch. 8). Fats and carbohydrates, however, are fully catabolised both in the body and in a calorimeter to carbon dioxide and water.

Energy needs

The amount of energy that an individual needs depends on:

- age
- activity
- environment
- physical state.

Basal metabolic rate (BMR)

The minimum energy requirement of a relaxed, awake individual who has not recently eaten a meal and who is lying down in a comfortable environment is defined as the *basal metabolic rate* or *BMR*. Under these circumstances energy is required simply to maintain cell metabolism (Table 14.2). Essentially the BMR for a particular person is determined by the:

- level of cellular activity (controlled by hormones; Ch. 10)
- mass of active cells (related to body weight)
- surface area of the body (related to heat loss; Ch. 16).

Non-basal circumstances

More energy is required over and above the basal levels to meet the demands posed by different activities and by less comfortable environments. Muscular activity of any kind increases the demand for energy. In a cold environment extra heat may be generated by shivering. The energy needed in a variety of situations is illustrated in Figure 14.1. ①

Table 14.1 Energy yielded by different foods and drinks*		
Food/drink	kcal/100 g[†]	kJ/100 g[†]
Tea (no milk or sugar)	<1	2
Coffee (no milk or sugar)	2	8
Beer	25–39	104–163
Milk (whole)	66	275
Wine (dry–sweet)	66–94	275–394
Vegetables (mushrooms–potatoes)	13–75	55–318
Fruit (melon–bananas)	19–95	81–403
Fish (cod)	76	322
Lean meat (chicken–lamb)	121–162	508–679
Eggs	147	612
Fish (mackerel)	223	926
Bread (Hovis–naan)	212–336	899–1415
Nuts (peanuts–macadamia)	564–748	2341–3082
Butter	737	3031
Vegetable oil	899	3696

* Representative values compiled from Holland et al 1991 McCance and Widdowson's The composition of foods, fifth revised and extended edition, by permission of HMSO, London.
[†] Applies to the edible part of each food. Energy depends largely on the relative proportions of fat (9 kcal/g), carbohydrate (4 kcal/g) and water (0 kcal/g) in each food and drink. Thus, tea and coffee (mostly water) yield few calories whereas butter and vegetable oil (mostly fat) yield a lot. Bread (mostly carbohydrate plus water) and potatoes (mostly water plus some carbohydrate) are intermediate.

Table 14.2 Predicted basal metabolic rates of adult men and women of different ages, each weighing 65 kg*				
Sex	Age range (years)	BMR		
		mJ/day	kcal/day	kcal/min
Male	18–30	7.07	1690	1.17
	30–60	6.82	1630	1.13
	>60	5.73	1370	0.95
Female	18–30	6.11	1460	1.01
	30–60	5.86	1400	0.97
	>60	5.32	1270	0.88

* Compiled from the report of a Joint FAO/WHO/UNU Expert Consultation 1985.

Figure 14.1
The relative energy costs of different activities undertaken by a woman as compared with her basal metabolic rate (BMR). General office work requires 1.7 times as much energy (1.7 × BMR) whereas walking with a heavy load requires four times as much (4 × BMR). Using the data in Table 14.2 you can calculate actual energy requirements in kilocalories or megajoules. (Adapted from a report of a joint FAO/WHO/UNU Expert Consultation 1985.)

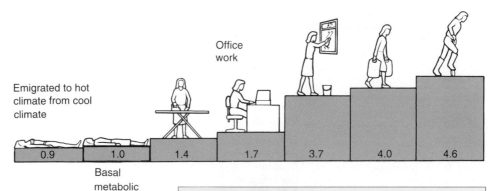

Office work

Emigrated to hot climate from cool climate

| 0.9 | 1.0 | 1.4 | 1.7 | 3.7 | 4.0 | 4.6 |

Basal metabolic rate

Dietary requirements

Ideally, the bulk of the calories needed should be supplied in the diet in the form of carbohydrates. It is wasteful in the economy of the body to use specialised molecules like proteins and amino acids as an energy souce, and it is a risk to health to consume too much fat. The caloric intakes currently recommended in several countries are listed in Table 14.3.

RAW MATERIALS

In utero and through infancy, childhood and adolescence raw materials are needed for growth (see Ch. 35). Once adulthood has been attained, the need for raw materials is normally limited to those required to replace items lost from the body. Losses include constituents of skin, hair and nails, secretions like sweat and mucus and the net losses occurring in faeces and urine. Other materials, derived from the breakdown of worn out cells and tissues, are recycled and re-used.

Cell debris is ingested and digested by phagocytic cells and the products are returned to the extracellular fluid (see Ch. 15). For example, about 20 mg of iron are derived from the breakdown of old erythrocytes each day, and this is re-used in the formation of new haemoglobin. Consequently only 1 to 2 mg of iron are required per day to replace the net losses occurring from skin cells and body fluids.

Particular circumstances in adulthood which demand greater dietary intakes, because of the net gain of body tissues, include:

- pregnancy (growth of maternal and fetal tissues; Ch. 34)
- physical activity that encourages muscle growth (Ch. 17)
- restorative stages following illness or injury (Ch. 19).

DIETARY COMPOSITION

The composition of the *average* western diet (Lask 1986) differs from that recommended by the National Advisory Committee on Nutritional Education (NACNE 1983) in several important respects. Most notable are the different contributions made by starch, sugar and fat to the total dietary intake. Whereas starch constitutes nearly half (48%) of the recommended diet, it represents less than one-third (31%) of the diet that is actually eaten. Starch is replaced by sugar, with an intake of 14% (twice that recommended), and by fat, with an intake of 38% (8% over the recommended level). Alcohol, too, is taken in excess of recommendations (5 as opposed to 4%) leaving protein as the only major component of the western diet with an intake in line with recommendations (11%).

TISSUE REPAIR AFTER SURGERY

Dangers of weight loss in surgical patients have been identified for more than 40 years but until relatively recently it was thought that nutritional problems arose in a limited number only. Many studies now indicate that nutritional assessment and appropriate nutritional intake pre- and postoperatively play a major role in patient recovery and tissue repair (Hill et al 1977, Dowding 1986).

Three factors that affect tissue repair are:

- nutrition   ● blood circulation   ● age.

Great demand is placed on the body's store of energy and protein.

Table 14.3 Daily caloric allowances recommended by different countries* for young adult (18–35 years) men and women of standard weight (by national standards†)

Country	Men		Women	
	kcal	kJ	kcal	kJ
Australia	2800	11 500	2000	8300
India	2400	10 000	1900	7900
Japan	2500	10 500	2000	8300
UK	2700	11 250	2200	9200
USA	2800	11 500	2000	8300

* Compiled from the Report of the Committee on International Dietary Allowances of the International Union of Nutritional Sciences 1975.
† The differences in caloric requirement essentially reflect differences in body build.

Table 14.4 Some of the products formed from amino acids in the human body

Product			Amino acid(s) used
Name	Function/use	Chapter reference	
Peptides	Hormones	10	All
Proteins	Enzymes Receptors Channels Cell structure	2	All
	Antibodies	4, 15	All
Purines and pyrimidines	Nucleic acids	2	Glycine Aspartic acid Glutamine
Creatine	Muscle metabolism	11	Methionine Glycine Arginine
Melanin	Pigment	15	Tyrosine
Thyroxine	Hormone	10	Tyrosine
Adrenaline	Hormone	10	Tyrosine
Noradrenaline	Neurotransmitter	3	Tyrosine
Histamine	Inflammatory response	5, 15	Histidine
Serotonin	Local vasoconstriction	4, 15	Tryptophan

Amino acids

Requirements

Amino acids are required for the synthesis of innumerable proteins and the manufacture of a variety of other products examples of which are listed in Table 14.4. For the synthesis of any given protein to occur all the constituent amino acids must be available. If one of the amino acids is deficient, synthesis is interrupted and that protein cannot be formed. 20 amino acids commonly exist in cells and tissues (see Ch. 2 and Table 14.5). Of these, in adulthood, 8 *must* be present in the diet (*essential amino acids*) because they cannot be synthesised within the human body from other sources. Recommended intakes of protein are listed in Table 14.6.

Surplus amino acids

If there are plenty of amino acids in the bloodstream, surplus ones are *deaminated*, producing ammonia and a carbohydrate molecule. The carbohydrate can be used in mebabolism to form glucose and fat. Ammonia is incorporated into urea. The losses of urea and other products of amino acid metabolism in the urine represent a daily net loss of nitrogen from the body. Thus when dietary protein intake is high, urea excretion is greater than when it is not. Urinary losses of nitrogen provide useful information about the state of protein metabolism within the body when they are compared with dietary intake.

Nitrogen balance

If an individual's intake of nitrogen in protein is balanced by urinary losses of nitrogen in waste

Table 14.5 The common amino acids found in proteins

Essential in the diet	Others
Valine*	Arginine
Leucine*	Glycine
Isoleucine*	Alanine
Threonine	Serine
Methionine	Cysteine
Phenylalanine	Tyrosine
Tryptophan	Aspartic acid
Lysine[†]	Glutamic acid[‡]
Histidine (in infancy)	Proline
	Histidine
	Hydroxyproline
	Ornithine

* Branched chain amino acids e.g. valine

$$CH_3$$
$$CH-CH_2-COOH$$
$$CH_3 \quad NH_2$$

[†] Deficient in plant proteins other than those in peas and beans.
[‡] Glutamate used in the food industry for giving meaty flavours to food.

Table 14.6 Daily intake of protein recommended for young adult men and women by different countries/organisations*

Country	Protein intake (g/day)	
	Men	Women
Australia	70	58
India	55	45
Japan	70	60
UK	68	55
USA	65	55
WHO/FAO	37	29

* Compiled from the Report of the Committee on International Dietary Allowances of the International Union of Nutritional Sciences 1975.

products he or she is said to be in *nitrogen balance*. If growth is occurring, or there is considerable repair of tissues as in recovery from illlness, then the loss of nitrogen may be less than that ingested and the individual is in *positive nitrogen balance*. Conversely, if net breakdown of tissues is occurring, then urinary losses may exceed intake and the result is a *negative nitrogen balance*. ②

Fats

Requirements

Fats are needed as an energy source and to form vital constituents of the cell. Phospholipids and cholesterol, for example, are important constituents of cell membranes. Like amino acids, fats are recycled and reused. Often during this process they are broken down and reassembled in a slightly different form, as they are during their digestion and absorption within the gastrointestinal tract (see Ch. 6). Fats are transported in the bloodstream largely in the form of *lipoproteins* (Table

HEALTH SCREENING

Screening is now carried out to identify some of the possible errors in metabolism. One such error, which is genetic, is characterised by an inability to metabolise the amino acid, phenylalanine, normally.

Phenylalanine is an essential amino acid used in the synthesis of many proteins in the body and must be supplied by the diet. Within a normal diet there is an excess to requirements.

Surplus phenylalanine is converted into tyrosine, with the aid of the enzyme, phenylalanine hydroxylase, and into phenylpyruvate (a phenylketone) with the aid of another enzyme, transaminase.

In people with phenylketonuria, phenylalanine hydroxylase is lacking and so phenylketones are formed in much larger amounts. They accumulate in body fluids and are excreted in the urine. This disorder, if undetected, is associated with nervous system abnormalities and mental retardation. Each child born has his or her urine analysed in order to detect the abnormality.

It is possible to implement a dietary control of phenylalanine until the child is 7 to 8 years old, when the brain becomes less susceptible to abnormal metabolites. Having a child on a special diet imposes many strains on a family and it is important that everyone involved in the child's care understands the diet and the reasons for the need for it.

② *Protein restriction may be advised for people with liver disorders or kidney disease. Why?*

14.7). Lipoproteins are molecular complexes consisting chiefly of:

- triglycerides
- cholesterol
- phospholipids
- specific proteins.

The complexes are dynamic structures that are being continually formed and degraded.

Small losses of fat occur daily from shed cells, in secretions and in the faeces. These losses can be made good by the dietary intake of fat and by the synthesis of fats from glucose and from amino acids.

Table 14.7 Plasma lipoproteins*

Relative size	Class	Source	% Composition				Functions
			Triglycerides	Phospholipids	Cholesterol	Protein	
◯	Chylomicrons	Intestine	90	3	5	2	Triglyceride transport
○	VLDL	Liver	55	20	15	10	
○	LDL	Plasma	8	22	45	25	Cholesterol transport
○	HDL	Various†	5	25	20	50	

* Compiled from Glickman & Sabesin 1988.
† Some HDL is secreted by intestinal and hepatic cells; some is formed in the plasma.
Key: VLDL = very low density lipoproteins; LDL = low density lipoproteins; HDL = high density lipoproteins

Table 14.8 Fat-soluble vitamins

Vitamin	Alternative or equivalent name	Major sources	Recommended* daily dietary allowance	Importance	Effects of deficiency
A	Retinol (β carotene)[†]	Butter, liver, fish liver oils, carrots	750–900 µg	Vision (see Ch. 26)	Night blindness Xerophthalmia
D	Calciferol	Action of sunlight on skin, fish liver oils, egg yolk	2.5–5.0 µg	Calcium metabolism (see Ch. 13)	Rickets Osteomalacia (see Ch. 28)
E	Alpha tocopherol	Vegetable oils, eggs	8–10 mg	Antioxidant	—[‡]
K	Menaquinone	Green leafy vegetables, bacterial metabolism (gut)	—[§]	Synthesis of some blood coagulation factors (see Ch. 4)	Bleeding disorders caused by malabsorption (see Ch. 6)

* Range of recommendations from several countries for adults. (Compiled from the Report of the Committee on International Dietary Allowances of the International Union of Nutritional Sciences 1975; and Passmore & Eastwood 1986.)
[†] Some foods such as carrots contain β carotene which is converted to vitamin A in the body. For this reason the vitamin A content of foods is quoted as 'retinol equivalents' in order to include this source of vitamin A.
[‡] Vitamin E is so widespread in foods that specific deficiency hardly arises.
[§] Production of vitamin K by intestinal bacteria makes estimation of dietary requirement difficult.

Table 14.9 Elements required in small amounts

Element	Symbol	Rich sources*	Approximate daily dietary intake (mg)	Approximate daily dietary intake (µg)	Effects of deficiency in humans
Iron	Fe	Treacle, liver, black pudding	15	—	Anaemia (see Ch. 4)
Zinc	Zn	Oysters[†], meat, whole grains, legumes	10	—	Skin disorders Poor wound healing
Manganese	Mn	Plant foods (tea)	5	—	—
Copper	Cu	Green vegetables, liver	2	—	Anaemia (rare)
Molybdenum	Mo	Plant foods	1	—	—
Fluoride	F	Drinking water, tea	1	—	Dental caries
Cobalt	Co	Leafy green vegetables	—	300	—
Iodide	I	Seafood[‡]	—	150	Hypothyroid goitre (see Ch. 10)
Selenium	Se	Fish	—	100	Uncertain
Chromium	Cr	Widespread	—	50	Insulin resistance

* Some foods that are less rich may contribute a large proportion of the dietary intake if they are eaten in large quantities. Cereals, for example, can be a significant dietary source of iron because of the amounts consumed each day.
[†] Oysters are exceptionally rich in zinc (10 to 20 times as much as in meat, legumes etc.).
[‡] In some countries (USA, Switzerland, New Zealand but not the UK) iodine is also obtained from table salt which, in these countries, is iodised.

Essential fatty acids
However, as with amino acids, certain specific fats (*essential fatty acids*) need to be included in the diet, in adequate amounts. These fatty acids are:

- linoleic acid (found in plants)
- linolenic acid (rich source in marine life).

The essential fatty acids are required for the synthesis of *prostaglandins*, which are regulators of cell function (see Ch. 10). The essential fatty acids are also constituents of some of the phospholipids in cell membranes and thereby influence membrane properties and functions.

Fat-soluble vitamins
An adequate intake of fat is required both to supply energy requirements and to provide the requisite amounts of essential fatty acids. In addition to this, an adequate intake of fats is needed to guarantee a tiny but vital intake of the compounds associated with them (*fat-soluble vitamins*) which are needed for cellular metabolism (Table 14.8).

Carbohydrates
Carbohydrates are needed to provide energy and form part of many cellular components, including DNA and RNA, and glycoproteins in cell membranes (see Ch. 2).

SUPPLEMENTARY REQUIREMENTS

Other required substances include:

- minerals
- vitamins.

Many of these are recycled in the economy of the body, but dietary intake is always needed to replace losses and to meet the additional demands posed by growth.

Minerals
Minerals are inorganic substances. They can be divided arbitrarily into two groups. Firstly there are those which are required in fairly large amounts, the *electrolytes* such as sodium, potassium, chloride, calcium, magnesium and phosphate. The need for several of these and the necessary daily requirements have been discussed elsewhere (see Ch. 13). Secondly some other elements are needed in much smaller amounts (Table 14.9). These include elements such as iron and iodine whose importance to health is well established, as well as others, often collectively termed *trace elements*, whose functions are still somewhat uncertain.

Vitamins
Vitamins are organic compounds that are required in very small amounts to maintain normal metabolism and growth (Tables 14.8 and 14.10). Vitamins come into the

Table 14.10 Water-soluble vitamins

Vitamin		Other name	Rich* sources	Recommended† daily dietary allowance (mg)	(µg)	Role	Effects of deficiency
B group	B₁	Thiamin	Yeast	1–1.5	—	Involved in various aspects of cell metabolism especially enzyme activity	Polyneuritis Beriberi
	B₂	Riboflavin	Yeast, liver	1–2	—		Inflammation of the mouth
	B₃	Niacin	Yeast	10–20	—		Pellagra
	B₆	Pyridoxine	Liver	2	—		Rare
	B₁₂	Cobalamin	Liver, kidney, eggs	—	2–3		Macrocytic anaemia (see Ch. 4)
		Folic acid	Vegetables, yeast, liver	—	200–400		Macrocytic anaemia (see Ch. 4)
		Pantothenic acid	Liver	3	—		Rare
		Biotin	Egg yolk	—	100–200		Rare
C		Ascorbic acid	Fruit, vegetables	30–60	—	Collagen formation Iron absorption Steroid synthesis	Scurvy

* Foods that are less rich may contribute a large proportion of the dietary intake because of the amounts consumed per day. Cereal based foods (such as breakfast cereals) and milk, for example, are good sources of the B vitamins.
† Range of recommended values from several countries (Australia, UK, USA) for adults.

same category as essential amino acids and fatty acids in that they are molecules that cannot be synthesised in the human body but are needed for normal health. They differ from them, however, in that the amounts of vitamins required are very much smaller.

Food contains many different substances, not all of which are available to the body. Availability is improved by processing and cooking but these have their drawbacks as well as benefits.

FOOD

The food we eat is either of animal or plant origin. It includes (Table 14.11):

- natural products
- processed foods.

COMPOSITION

Food consists of the same kinds of constituents as any living thing, namely:

- carbohydrates
- proteins
- fats
- other organic molecules (including vitamins).
- minerals
- electrolytes
- water

Table 14.11   Foods – some examples

Source	Natural products	Processed foods	
		Preserved	Manufactured products
Animal	Milk	Condensed milk	Butter, cream, cheese
	Eggs	Hard-boiled, pickled	Meringue
	Meat	Ham, bacon	Sausages, paté, lard
	Fish	Canned, smoked, salted	Fish oils
Plant	Cereals	–	Flour, bread, cakes, pasta, beer, whisky, corn oil
	Vegetables – starchy roots (potatoes, beet, cassava)		Vodka, sugar, rum, tapioca
	– legumes (peas, beans, lentils)	Tinned, dried, frozen	Soya products, soya oil
	– leafy (spinach, cabbage)		–
	Fruits	Tinned, frozen, dried	Jams, wines, brandy
	Nuts	–	Vegetable oils
	Honey	–	Mead

Table 14.12   Differences in constituents between foods of animal and plant origin

Category	Exclusively animal	Richer in animal origin foods	Present in both	Richer in plant origin foods	Plant
Carbohydrates	Glycogen (animal starch) Lactose				Amylose (starch) Cellulose Sucrose
Fats	Cholesterol	Saturated fats		Unsaturated fats	
Protein			Protein		
Vitamins	B_{12}*, D		A, B	C, E, K	
Minerals		Iron Calcium			

* Produced also by microorganisms.

However, the specific nature of the substances present and the proportions present vary between different animals and plants because of differences in metabolism. Thus some substances, such as cellulose, are chiefly found within foods of plant origin whereas others, such as cholesterol, are characteristic of animal derived foods (Table 14.12). Some constituents of food, such as dietary fibre, are indigestible; some, such as tannin and caffeine, have no nutritive value; other minor constituents are contaminants.

Vegetarian diets

All the substances necessary for normal growth and health can be derived from either a mixed diet or a balanced vegetarian diet which includes some animal products such as eggs and milk. However, some vegetarians choose not to eat any animal products at all (*vegan diet*), and this can occasionally lead to nutritional deficiencies.

A vegan diet will be deficient in vitamin B_{12} and may lack certain amino acids, iron and calcium. Care should be taken to ensure that these requirements are met, particularly in children and women of child-bearing age who have an increased need for many dietary constituents. ③

Another potential complication of a vegetarian diet is that it may consist largely of bulky, fibrous and watery foods. These easily make a person feel 'full up', but may not supply adequate amounts of energy and protein. This can be a particular nutritional risk for children. Foods of vegetable origin rich in energy and in protein, such as cereals, legumes and nuts, should be consumed in sufficient amounts to meet this need (Table 14.13).

Dietary fibre

The term *dietary fibre* is used to describe macromolecular constituents of the diet which are resistant to digestion. Fibre consists of indigestible carbohydrates (Table 14.14). Plant foods are a very rich source (Table 14.15). Although dietary fibre does not contribute to the nutrient intake of the body it is recognised as an important constituent of the diet. In Europe and the USA the daily intake is about 25 g whereas in African populations it is much larger (50–150 g). Diets low in fibre are known to be associated with an increased incidence of digestive and other disturbances. Dietary fibre:

- provides 'bulk' to a meal
- binds and adsorbs other substances
- is metabolised by colonic bacteria.

③
Which amino acids may vegetarians lack if they eat predominantly (a) beans (b) wheat?

Table 14.13   Energy- and protein-rich foods of vegetable origin*

Food		Energy kcal/100 g	Protein g/100 g
Class	Example		
Cereals	Soya flour		
	– full fat	447	36.8
	– low fat	352	45.3
	Wheat flour		
	– wholemeal	310	12.7
Cereal products	Meusli	363	9.8
	Oatcakes	441	10.0
	Bread		
	– naan	336	8.9
	– Hovis	212	9.5
	– brown	218	8.5
	– white	235	8.4
Nuts	Peanuts	564	25.6
	Almonds	612	21.1
	Walnuts	688	14.7
Nut products	Peanut butter	623	22.6
Legumes	Lentils		
	– raw, dried	297	24.3
	– boiled	105	8.8
	Peas		
	– raw	83	6.9
	– boiled	79	6.7
	Red kidney beans		
	– raw, dried	266	22.1
	– boiled	103	8.4

* Values compiled from Holland et al 1991 McCance and Widdowson's The composition of foods, fifth revised and extended edition, by permission of HMSO, London.

Table 14.14   Dietary fibre

Examples	Source	Rich dietary sources
Cellulose	Constituent of plant cell wall	All vegetables
Hemicellulose		
Lignin	'Woody' plant tissues	Cereals
Pectin	Plant sap	Fruits
Gums		

Immigrant communities retain much of their own culture, which includes eating habits. This aspect is not always addressed by institutions or hospitals. Nurses should be familiar with social and religious aspects of minority groups so that they can ensure all clients receive a diet that is both acceptable and nutritionally adequate.

Community dietitians work with health educationalists, primary health care teams and local interest groups to provide them with accurate nutritional information.

Nutrition at international level is significant in times when the world population is increasing so rapidly. Global aspects of nutrition are addressed by organisations such as UNICEF (United Nations Children's Fund), WHO (World Health Organization) and FAO (Food and Agriculture Organization (of UN)).

Table 14.15   Some fibre-rich foods

Food	Dietary fibre* g/100 g	Weight of average serving (g)
Wholemeal bread	7.4	50 (2 slices)
Muesli (Swiss style)	8.1	150
Baked beans	6.9	60
Processed peas (canned)	7.1	60
Red kidney beans (boiled)	9.0	—

* Compiled from Holland et al 1991 McCance and Widdowson's The composition of foods, fifth revised and extended edition, by permission of HMSO, London.

Bulking effect

The bulkiness of ingested food affects digestion and absorption in several ways. Firstly, in distending the stomach, a 'bulky' meal quickly evokes a sensation of 'fullness'. The desire to eat is thereby satisfied at a lower intake of available energy. Secondly, by 'diluting' the available energy in the diet, the assimilation of nutrients in the small intestine will proceed at a more measured pace (see next section on nutrient balance). Thirdly, distension of the digestive tract promotes motility and secretion, which in turn facilitate the digestive process.

Binding properties

Fibre clings to water and thus has a water-retaining effect which adds to its 'bulking' effect. This helps to make faecal residues softer and easier to evacuate. Some other substances are also preferentially adsorbed to dietary fibre. This reduces their concentration in the intestinal fluid and therefore limits their absorption. For example bile acids (see Chs 6 and 9) bind to dietary fibre. Consequently the loss of bile acids in the faeces is increased by a high fibre diet. Bile acids which are lost in the faeces are replaced by those newly synthesised from cholesterol (see Ch. 9). This contributes to the plasma cholesterol lowering effect that a high fibre diet is known to have. It has also been suggested that fibre may bind some potentially carcinogenic substances and therefore have a protective effect.

Bacterial metabolism

Although fibre is not broken down by gastrointestinal digestive enzymes, it is metabolised by the colonic bacteria, which use fibre as a source of nutrients and generate a variety of products from it including short chain fatty acids, and carbon dioxide, hydrogen and methane gases (see Ch. 6). Some of the fatty acids are absorbed. They also stimulate colonic motility and secretion.

WHY DO WE NOT EAT ENOUGH FIBRE?

Western society has become affluent; this and other sociological factors now have an effect on our dietary intake of fibre. There is:

- a variety of prepacked foods requiring minimal preparation and offering ease of presentation
- an increase in the number of working women with less time for preparation of food
- a possible lack of knowledge of the need for fibre.

Epidemiological evidence suggests that inadequate intake of fibre is a contributary factor in many disorders. The main group occurs in the large intestine and includes:

- constipation
- diverticular disease
- bowel cancer, 50% of which is found in the rectum.

Metabolic disorders include:

- obesity
- atherosclerosis
- gall-stones.

Most people need, and are able, to increase their daily fibre intake by eating more wholemeal bread, whole-grain cereals, vegetables and fruit.

Because fibre is food for colonic bacteria the numbers and the mass of bacteria increase when the dietary intake of fibre is high. This also increases the bulk of the residues in the colon. The well-known action of high fibre diets in promoting defaecation is thus likely to be due to a combination of all these factors.

Non-nutritive constituents

Any natural food may also contain tiny amounts of other substances (Table 14.16) including:

- substances peculiar to particular plant or animal species
- environmental contaminants
- bacterial contaminants.

Plants manufacture a variety of substances that are foreign to our cells. Some of these, such as caffeine, have a drug-like effect. Others such as the cyanogenetic glycosides are toxic.

Foods may also contain substances that have been taken up by the organism from the environment. Some

Cassava is the principal food of many people in the tropics. It contains a glyceride, *linamarin*, from which cyanide is released by enzymic action. Before consumption the roots are grated and dried in the sun to get rid of the cyanide. In West Africa an association has been found between the consumption of cassava and some neuropathies (disease of the nervous system; see Ch. 21). Incidentally, tapioca is produced from cassava by further processing and consists almost entirely of starch.

Table 14.16   Some non-nutritive constituents of food

Type	Examples	Sources
Natural constituents	Alkaloids	
	– solanine	Green, sprouted potatoes
	– caffeine	Tea, coffee
	– pyrrolizidine	Comfrey
	Cyanogenetic glycosides	Apricot kernels, cassava
	Flavenols	Tea
	Oxalic acid	Rhubarb
	Serotonin (5-HT)	Bananas
Bacterial contaminants	Aflatoxins	Peanuts (mouldy)
	Amines	Mould on cheese
	Ergot alkaloids	Fungus on cereals
	Mycotoxins	Moulds
Contaminants arising from human activities	Antibiotics	Animal husbandry
	Cadmium	
	Mercury	} Industrial pollution
	Lead	
	Pesticides	Agricultural practice
	Food additives (cyclamate, monosodium glutamate)	Food industry

---

FOOD AND DRUG INTERACTIONS

Tyramine is an amine formed from tyrosine by bacterial metabolism. It is, for example, formed when cheeses mature and can be found in old or fermented food products in which protein breakdown has been occurring. The older the food and the greater the bacterial contamination the greater the amount of tyramine formed. Normally, the tyramine in food is broken down by monoamine oxidase in the cells of the digestive tract and the liver so that only small amounts enter the bloodstream. When monoamine oxidase inhibitors are prescribed for the treatment of depression, this breakdown does not occur and, consequently, larger amounts of tyramine circulate in the blood.

One effect of tyramine is to promote the release of noradrenaline from sympathetic nerves, thus producing a rise in blood pressure.

Foods high in tyramine (e.g. cheeses (except cottage cheese), meat, yeast extracts, red wine) must therefore be restricted when an individual is prescribed monoamine oxidase inhibitors.

---

of these may have been used by the farmer to maximise crop yield or to restrain pests and diseases. Animal foods may contain contaminants derived from the plants which the livestock have eaten, from the drinking water or, in the case of marine fish, from the sea in areas of pollution. Some substances, such as bacteria, which are passed on in this way may be made harmless by digestion, but others, such as mercury, are retained in the food chain and passed on to the human consumer. Food may also be contaminated by bacteria that generate harmful toxins.

AVAILABILITY OF NUTRIENTS

Nutrients present in a diet are not necessarily completely available to us. Some constituents, like dietary fibre, are indigestible whereas others, like iron, may be prevented from being absorbed by conditions in the digestive tract or by other substances in the diet.

Digestibility of food

Some polysaccharides and proteins cannot be digested easily by the enzymes present in the human digestive tract. This applies to some fibrous proteins, such as keratin in skin, and to the carbohydrate cellulose in plants. In some cases, particularly proteins, cooking begins the breakdown of such macromolecules, making them more vulnerable to enzymic attack and therefore to digestion.

Lactase deficiency

After early childhood, most of the world's population (85%) have a relative deficiency of the enzyme, *lactase*, which breaks down the disaccharide, *lactose*, in milk to the monosaccharides, *glucose* and *galactose*. Consequently, lactose cannot be properly digested and, so, much of this carbohydrate in milk will be unavailable nutritionally.

Absorbability of nutrients

The absorbability of some substances, such as iron and calcium, depends on the form in which they are present in food and also on the blend of other substances in the diet, some of which may hinder their absorption.

Iron

Dietary iron, for example, is present in food in haem (from haemoglobin in meat) and exists in two inorganic forms *ferrous* (Fe^{2+}) and *ferric* (Fe^{3+}). Haem is readily absorbed whereas inorganic iron is not. However, Fe^{2+} is much better absorbed than Fe^{3+}. Conditions in the digestive tract that favour the formation of Fe^{2+}, and therefore the absorption of iron, include a low pH and the presence of reducing agents, like vitamin C, that convert Fe^{3+} to Fe^{2+}. If, however, the diet is rich in phytates (from unrefined cereals), insoluble salts of iron are formed and these cannot be absorbed. Consequently, iron deficiency can arise even though the total amount of iron in the diet appears to be adequate.

It is for these reasons that the recommended dietary intake of certain nutrients, such as iron (10–20 mg/day), far exceeds the amounts which need to be absorbed to maintain nutritional balance (iron: 1–2 mg/day).

FOOD PROCESSING AND PREPARATION

Food is usually processed before it is eaten, either during manufacture or in cooking. Only a few items, such as fruit and some vegetables, are eaten raw.

Food processing

Processing enables natural products to be:

- preserved (frozen, canned, smoked, salted, irradiated)
- made palatable (attractive to eat)
- more digestible and of greater nutrient value
- safe to eat.

Sometimes different products are manufactured by processing, for example, butter and cheese made from milk, and vegetable oils made from olives, peanuts, coconut etc.

Processing alters food. Its very real benefits, as listed above, have to be weighed against some drawbacks which may include:

- loss of fibre (in the refining of flour)
- losses of vitamins (in the heating required in canning and in thawing of frozen foods)
- undesirable effects of substances that are added (such as salt and sugar) or produced during processing (such as nitrosamines)
- changes in the chemical nature of some nutrients (such as fatty acids and amino acids) which make them less useful nutritionally.

Even 'fresh' foods may have been in transit for a time before they are purchased by the shopper and losses of vitamin C and thiamin can occur, particularly if the food is not consumed for a while. The only food that can be guaranteed as really fresh is that which is literally home-grown and eaten on the day it is picked.

The 1984 Food Labelling Regulations define an additive as 'any substance not commonly used as food which is added to, or used in, food to affect its quality, taste, appearance, alkalinity, acidity or any other technological function in relation to food.'
All prepared foods must carry an EEC additives list.

Cooking

Cooking, whether in the course of manufacture or in the restaurant and home, makes food:

- safer to eat
- appetising (usually!)
- digestible.

Safety of food

Cooking can destroy harmful bacteria, toxins and viruses. Sometimes toxic chemicals, such as cyano-genetic glycosides (Table 14.16), present in the food are rendered harmless so that the food becomes edible.

Palatability of food

Cooking makes most foods more appetising because new products are formed in the process. The blend of

---

FOOD STANDARDS

Whilst food is essential for life, it may also cause illness if it contains:

- harmful bacteria
- viruses
- parasites – tapeworms or threadworms
- poisonous chemicals – pesticides etc.

National legislation within the Health and Safety Act (1974) sets compulsory standards for production, distribution and sale of foodstuffs. Hospitals, nursing and residential homes etc. all undergo regular inspections.
Important points in relation to food handling include:

- thorough defrosting of poultry and meat before cooking
- storage of cooked food and raw food separately
- avoidance of partial cooking of meat
- rapid cooking of food that is to be subsequently stored.

Food poisoning is a statutorily notifiable disease. Organisms cause food poisoning by direct invasion of the wall of the intestine, e.g. *Salmonella* spp., or by production of an enterotoxin, e.g. *Staphylococcus aureus*, and give rise to an acute illness, which usually includes one or more gastrointestinal symptoms.

---

products depends on the form of cooking adopted, be it cooking in water or in fat, or by dry heat or radiation. Toast tastes different from bread because the charring produces dextrins from the carbohydrates. Sometimes the products generated, such as polycyclic hydro-carbons in barbecued foods, can be harmful if ingested in excess.

Digestibility of food

Cooking makes food more digestible because cells are ruptured, proteins are denatured, macromolecules are broken down and chemicals are released. Uncooked potato is not readily digestible, but cooking begins the breakdown and makes the nutrients present more available.

Minimising losses of nutrients

Losses of nutrients in cooking can be minimised by:

- avoiding the use of too much water in boiling
- avoiding too high a temperature for too long
- keeping the time between cooking and serving food to a minimum.

NUTRIENT HOMEOSTASIS

The concentration of nutrients in the blood depends upon the balance between:

- intake
- metabolism
- losses.

For many nutrients, including glucose, amino acids

and fats, dietary intake and metabolism are the key determinants of nutritional homeostasis. Both dietary intake and metabolism are regulated by neural and hormonal mechanisms in ways that maintain a supply of fuels for the production of energy and safeguard the plasma concentration of glucose.

Losses of nutrients in shed cells and tissues, faeces and body fluids are normally relatively small. Significant losses of water-soluble nutrients such as glucose and amino acids in the urine are normally prevented by their complete reabsorption from the glomerular filtrate in the renal tubules (see Ch. 8).

If more food is ingested than is needed the excess is stored chiefly as fat and weight is gained.

INTAKE

Regulation of dietary intake

The desire to eat is controlled by cells in the hypothalamus (Ch. 31). These integrate information from several sources (Fig. 14.2) about the:

- palatability of food
- 'fullness' of the digestive system
- plasma concentrations of nutrients
- individual's emotional state.

Depending on the balance of these factors at any time, a person may feel hungry and want to eat, or 'full-up' (satiated), just comfortable, or 'off their food'. In humans, social factors play a very important part in determining when food is or may be eaten. The internal controls which register when the stomach is 'full' and which note the prevailing metabolic state may be overridden by voluntary or socially conditioned factors. Thus we may eat more than we need in a way that animals generally do not.

The major internal factors involved in the control of food intake are:

- gastrointestinal
  - distension of the stomach
  - cholecystokinin
- metabolic
  - plasma glucose
  - plasma free fatty acids.

Gastrointestinal factors

A bulky meal containing a lot of fibre will give rise to a sensation of fullness more quickly than one which is more readily digestible and may in fact contain more calories.

Cholecystokinin (see Ch. 6) is released from the small intestine by the presence of amino acids and fatty acids. In addition to its functions in stimulating the pancreas

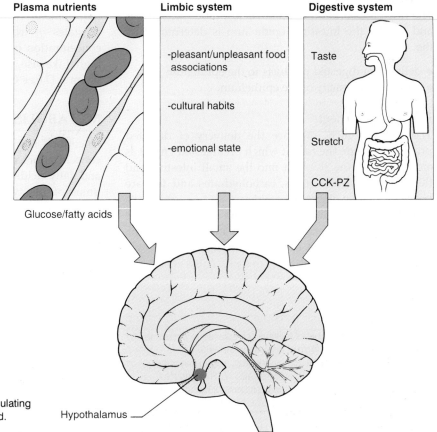

Plasma nutrients　　**Limbic system**　　**Digestive system**

Glucose/fatty acids

-pleasant/unpleasant food associations

-cultural habits

-emotional state

Taste

Stretch

CCK-PZ

Hypothalamus

Figure 14.2
Information used by the hypothalamus in regulating the desire to eat and the consumption of food.
CCK-PZ = cholecystokinin-pancreozymin.

to secrete enzymes and the gall bladder to contract, cholecystokinin also acts on the hypothalamic cells which control feeding and contributes to the feeling of satiation. In that cholecystokinin is one of the factors that slows the emptying of the stomach, it will in addition prolong the gastric distension that also contributes to the feeling of 'fullness'. Consequently, a meal rich in fats and proteins makes you feel full up for longer than a meal rich in carbohydrates.

Metabolic factors

The plasma concentrations of glucose and fatty acids are indicators of the metabolic state. High plasma glucose and low plasma fatty acid concentrations (which prevail in the fed state; see later) promote a feeling of satiation. Conversely, a low blood glucose and a high circulating concentration of free fatty acids (the state in starvation) provokes the sensation of hunger. One of the key controlling factors is the usage of glucose by the cells of the hypothalamus. This is proportional to the plasma glucose concentration provided insulin is present too. If it is not, as in diabetes mellitus, then, even though plasma glucose levels are high, the hypothalamic cells like many others in the body are in fact 'starved' of glucose. Consequently, someone with diabetes mellitus could feel hungry when they are hypoglycaemic *and* when they are hyperglycaemic.

Regulation of absorption

The rate of absorption of amino acids, monosaccharides and fats by the intestinal epithelium is determined by the:

- delivery of digested products to the epithelium
- absorptive capacity of the epithelium.

Delivery of nutrients

The factors which influence the delivery of digested products include the rate at which predigested chyme is emptied from the stomach into the small intestine and the rate at which proteins, carbohydrates and fats are broken down by digestive enzymes.

As described earlier (see Ch. 6) the rate at which the stomach empties depends on the nature of the meal. Meals containing a lot of fat are emptied more slowly than those which do not.

People who have diabetes mellitus are advised to consume carbohydrates in the form of polysaccharides (e.g. potatoes) rather than disaccharides (e.g. sugar) because polysaccharides are digested more slowly. This ensures that the flow of glucose into the bloodstream occurs at a steady rate and sudden peaks and troughs in blood glucose concentration are avoided.

INFLAMMATORY BOWEL DISEASE

Inflammatory bowel disease, predominantly Crohn's disease and ulcerative colitis, occurs as a result of a chronic non-specific inflammatory process which differs in terms of location and type of lesion. Malabsorption occurs in these disorders as the gastrointestinal tract has reduced enzyme secretion and lesions reduce the size of the absorptive area (see Ch. 6), which may lead to nutritional deficiency.

Dietary treatment of malabsorption requires an increased intake of the nutrients malabsorbed, or replacement with alternatives, concurrent with a reduction of bowel motility. A diet high in protein, calories and vitamins should be provided, with an increase in fluid intake if diarrhoea is present in order to prevent dehydration.

Absorptive capacity

The capacity of the digestive tract is such that virtually all the ingested carbohydrate and protein is digested and absorbed. Only small amounts escape into the colon to be metabolised by the colonic bacteria. Likewise, 95% of the ingested fat is also absorbed. We absorb what we are able to eat. There are no digestive controls that stop us from absorbing too much other than those that regulate gastric emptying (see Ch. 6) and that control the desire to eat (Fig. 14.2).

In the case of nutrients such as iron and calcium, which are not completely absorbed, there is scope for the amount absorbed to be regulated according to the requirements of the body. Iron absorption is increased in states of iron deficiency and decreased when the concentration of iron in the intestinal epithelial cells is high. Likewise, the absorption of calcium is regulated by vitamin D (see Ch. 13).

METABOLISM

Once food has been ingested and absorbed the plasma concentrations of nutrients such as glucose, amino acids and fatty acids are adjusted by metabolic controls. In times of plenty, surpluses are stored; in deprivation, stores are used. The nutrient whose concentration is most closely regulated is glucose. A number of different mechanisms are involved in stabilising its concentration in the face of the changing delivery of glucose to the body in feeding and fasting.

Feeding is normally an intermittent activity. In some societies food is consumed every few hours during the day so that fasting occurs only during the hours of sleep. In other societies, different cultural patterns and environmental constraints expose the body more frequently to periods of fasting, and even to starvation.

Stores

Absorbed items that are surplus to immediate requirements are stored in several ways (Table 14.17):

Table 14.17 Nutrient storage in an average well-fed resting adult

Nutrient	Form	Storage site	Amount				Daily requirement
			kg	g	mg	kcal	
Glucose	Glycogen	Liver	—	80*	—	320	1500 kcal
		Skeletal muscle	—	300*	—	1200	
Fats	Triglyceride	Adipose tissue	11†	—	—	100 000	
Iron	Ferritin	Liver mostly	—	—	500‡	—	1–2 mg
	Haemosiderin	All cells					
A, D, E, K	A, D, E, K	Liver					
B$_{12}$	B$_{12}$	Liver mostly	—	—	5	—	0.002 mg
Folic acid	Folic acid	Liver	—	—	8	—	0.3 mg

* From Astrand & Rohdahl 1986.
† From Garrow 1978.
‡ Amount varies considerably between men (1000 mg) and women (0–500 mg).

- glucose as glycogen in liver and muscle
- fats as triglyceride in adipose tissue
- amino acids are used to form proteins and surpluses are deaminated and then converted into carbohydrate or fat
- some minerals and vitamins in the liver (iron, vitamins A, D, E and K, vitamin B$_{12}$).

Some of these substances, such as the fat-soluble vitamins, simply accumulate progressively if they are ingested in excess. Vitamins, though necessary for health, can be toxic if consumed in large amounts. There are few, if any, homeostatic control mechanisms limiting the plasma concentrations of fat-soluble vitamins and some other absorbed substances, such as cholesterol, to an acceptable range. Consequently, plasma concentrations can exceed safe levels as well as fall below them. For example *hypervitaminosis* can occur if the dietary intake of any of vitamins A, D or K is too large.

Glucose

Central to the control of metabolism is the absolute requirement of some cells for glucose. These cells include red cells, neurones and cells of the testes and renal medulla. Chief among these are the cells of the nervous system. They rely almost exclusively on glucose for the formation of ATP. Hypoglycaemia is thus a grave threat to nerve cells and consequently to the body as a whole.

Normally, plasma glucose concentrations range between 4.5 mmol/l after an overnight fast to 10 mmol/l at the peak of absorption of a carbohydrate meal. Levels are normally kept within this range by metabolic adjustments which enable the surplus to be taken up after a meal and which maintain glucose supplies between meals.

After a meal – the fed state

When a meal is digested and absorbed most of the nutrients pass first to the liver before entering the general circulation (see Ch. 9). As soon as their concentration begins to increase in the arterial blood, the balance of hormones secreted by different endocrine tissues changes (see Ch. 10). The hormones enable glucose, amino acids and fatty acids to be taken up into cells and incorporated into macromolecules such as glycogen, proteins and triglycerides (Fig. 14.3).

Processing of nutrients by the liver

When food is available and digestion and absorption are proceeding the concentration of absorbed nutrients in the venous blood from the gut increases. The liver is the first organ to be exposed to the nutrients, such as monosaccharides, amino acids, some vitamins and minerals, absorbed via this route (see Ch. 6).

Glucose is taken up by the liver (Fig. 14.4A) and converted into glycogen. Galactose, from the digestion of lactose in milk, is taken up and converted into glucose. The hepatic uptake of glucose is not insulin dependent (see Ch. 10).

Amino acids are taken up too (Fig. 14.4B). Some are used to form cellular and plasma proteins. Others are interconverted so that the proportion of different amino acids leaving the liver in the hepatic vein blood is not exactly the same as that entering it in the portal blood. Unbranched amino acids are preferentially used by the liver with the result that the hepatic venous blood is relatively richer in branched amino acids (Table 14.5). Branched amino acids are used in large amounts by skeletal muscle.

Minerals such as iron, copper, and lead are also taken up by the liver cells, as are several of the vitamins including vitamin B$_{12}$ and folic acid.

Figure 14.3
The fed state: fate of absorbed nutrients and patterns of hormone secretion after the ingestion of a meal.

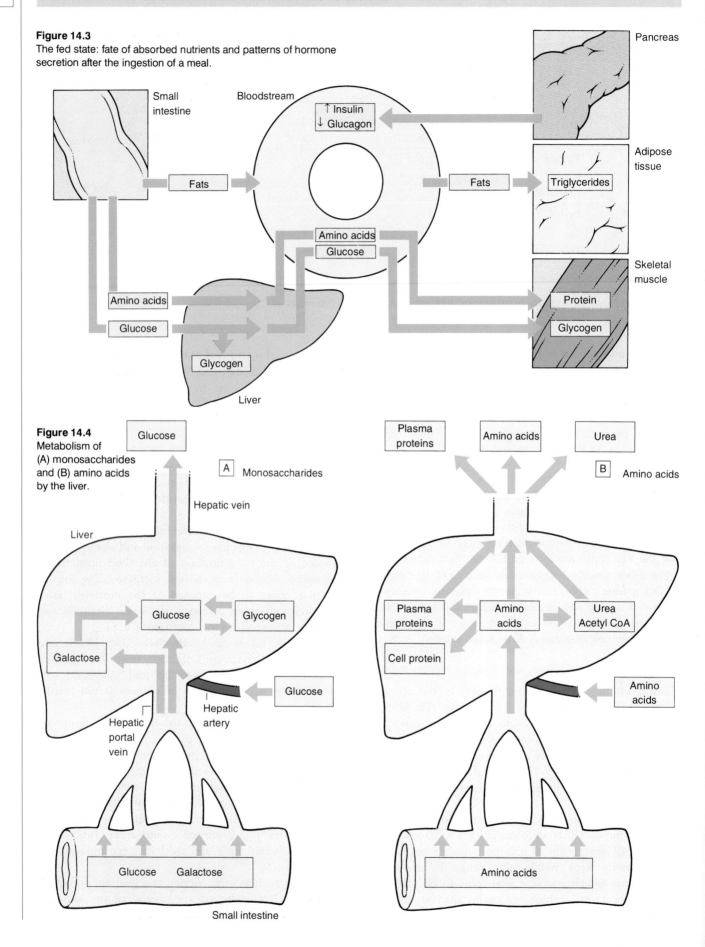

Figure 14.4
Metabolism of (A) monosaccharides and (B) amino acids by the liver.

As a result of all this uptake and metabolism, the nutrient profile in the circulation as a whole is not the same as that in the venous blood draining from the gastrointestinal tract.

Absorbed fats largely bypass the liver, by entering the lymphatic vessels of the gut in the form of chylomicrons (Table 14.7 and Fig. 14.5). The lymph flows into the bloodstream via the thoracic duct. Triglycerides in the chylomicrons are then gradually degraded by enzymes (*lipoprotein lipase*) present in the capillaries of many tissues including adipose tissue and skeletal and cardiac muscle to yield fatty acids and glycerol. Fatty acids bind to plasma proteins, chiefly albumin, and circulate in the blood in this form.

Some fatty acids and what is left of the chylomicrons (*chylomicron remnants*) are taken up and processed by the liver and used to form new triglycerides. These triglycerides are packaged with other lipids to form *very low density lipoproteins (VLDL)* that are secreted by the liver into the blood. These lipoproteins are also attacked by lipoprotein lipase in the capillaries of the circulation yielding more free fatty acids and producing *low density lipoproteins (LDL)* and *high density lipoproteins (HDL)*. LDL and HDL are good at carrying cholesterol in the blood (see Table 14.7).

Hormonal control of metabolism

The rise in the concentrations of glucose and of amino acids in the circulation enhances the release of insulin and depresses the secretion of glucagon from the pancreas. These stimuli add to the stimulatory effects of the gastrointestinal hormones and the autonomic nervous system which occur during the digestion of the meal.

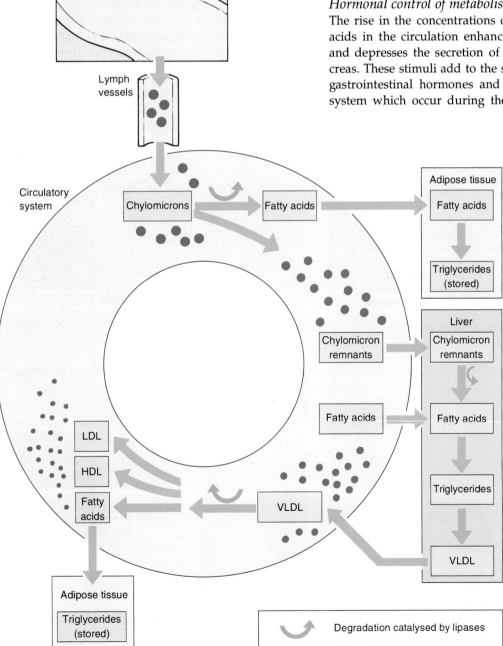

Figure 14.5
Metabolism of fats: roles of the circulatory system, adipose tissue and the liver.

The result is a substantial increase in the plasma concentration of insulin and a decrease in glucagon.

This change in the ratio of insulin and glucagon shifts the bias of metabolic activity towards the uptake of glucose, amino acids and fatty acids into cells and to their incorporation into glycogen, protein and triglycerides, respectively. This shift occurs chiefly in skeletal muscle and in adipose tissue. Some cells are not regulated by insulin in this way, including those which rely exclusively on glucose as the fuel for ATP production (neurones, red cells, kidney medulla) and the intestinal mucosa. In these cells uptake is permitted at all times.

Between meals – fasting

An average sized meal is digested and absorbed over a period of about 4 hours. Thereafter the concentration of nutrients in the blood falls gradually. As the concentration of glucose decreases, the balance of hormones secreted alters. The plasma concentration of glucagon increases and that of insulin decreases. This redirects body metabolism in such a way that the concentration of glucose in the plasma (and interstitial fluid) is protected and the supply of fuels for the production of energy is maintained (Fig. 14.6).

The concentration of glucose in the plasma is maintained in three ways:

- breakdown of liver glycogen (*glycogenolysis*)
- new synthesis of glucose (*gluconeogenesis*)
- sparing of glucose for selected tissues.

NUTRITION AND CARDIOVASCULAR DISEASE

Epidemiological studies highlight two important factors:

- cardiovascular disease (CVD) is environmentally determined (immigrant groups take on the incidence of their host country)
- there is a link between CVD and a high intake of saturated fat with a low intake of dietary fibre.

Low density lipoproteins (LDL) and high density lipoproteins (HDL) are good at carrying cholesterol in the blood, and a high intake of animal fats leads to raised serum lipids (see main text). Reducing the dietary intake of cholesterol specifically is only useful if the normal intake is high.

Polyunsaturated fats, mainly those rich in linoleic acid, tend to lower the serum LDL but their effect is only half as strong as the elevating effect of palmitic acid found in saturated fats.

Dietary fibre found in vegetables and fruit may have a positive effect of lowering blood lipids. Screening for hyperlipidaemia (high lipids in the blood) is now common. Concentrations of lipoproteins are decreased in obesity and increased by alcohol consumption.

Atherosclerosis occurs when fatty deposits rich in cholesterol develop within the inner lining of arteries, causing them to become narrow and reducing the blood flow.

When atherosclerosis occurs in the coronary arteries, ischaemic heart disease develops; when found within the cerebral arteries the individual is at risk of a cerebral vascular accident (stroke).

Much of this evidence is still under review.

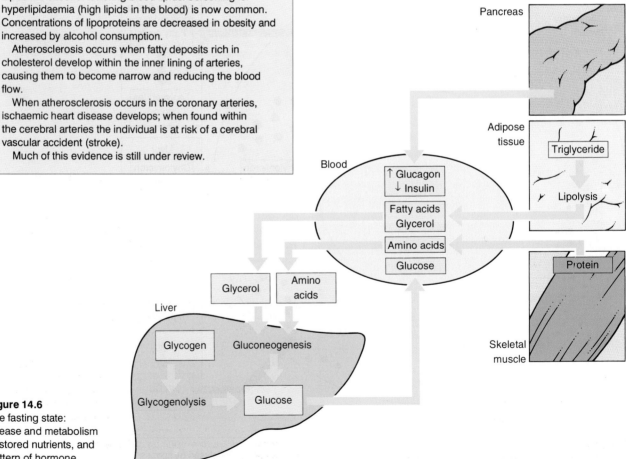

Figure 14.6
The fasting state: release and metabolism of stored nutrients, and pattern of hormone secretion.

Glycogenolysis

It has been estimated that the amount of glycogen normally present in the liver of a well-fed adult could, on its own, maintain plasma glucose concentration in a resting adult for about 8 hours, say overnight. The glycogen stored in muscle cannot be drawn upon directly in the same way. Its primary function is to supply the energy needs of muscle cells. However, lactate released from muscle cells by anaerobic metabolism (see Ch. 17) can be converted back into glucose by the liver. ④

Gluconeogenesis

While glycogen stores are being depleted, the synthesis of new glucose (hence *gluco-neo-genesis*) is stimulated by the increase in plasma glucagon and decrease in insulin. Amino acids, chiefly alanine derived from the break-down of muscle proteins, and glycerol produced by the breakdown of triglycerides (*lipolysis*) in adipose tissue are converted by the liver (and also the kidneys) into glucose.

Glucose sparing

Fatty acids released by the breakdown of triglycerides in adipose tissue are used by some tissues, including muscles, as an energy source in place of glucose. During fasting the concentration of fatty acids in the blood increases (Fig. 14.7). In this way glucose is spared for those tissues which specifically rely on it.

Starvation

If food deprivation continues, fatty acids are metabolised in increasing amounts by the mitochondria and large quantities of acetyl CoA are formed. The surplus acetyl CoA formed within the liver overloads the liver's capacity to metabolise it via the citric acid cycle and inreasing amounts spill over into the metabolic pathways leading to the formation of ketone bodies (Fig. 14.8).

Ketone bodies

Ketone bodies (or keto-acids) include aceto-acetic acid, acetone and beta-hydroxybutyric acid (also known as D-3 hydroxybutyric acid). Significant quantities of these products are detected in the blood after only a couple of days of fasting (Fig. 14.7). They can be used by various tissues, including skeletal and cardiac muscle, as an alternative fuel to glucose. In the tissues they are converted back to acetyl CoA and metabolised via the citric acid cycle (see Ch. 11). Ketone bodies have an

④

For how long before an operation are patients fasted? How long do you think is best and why?

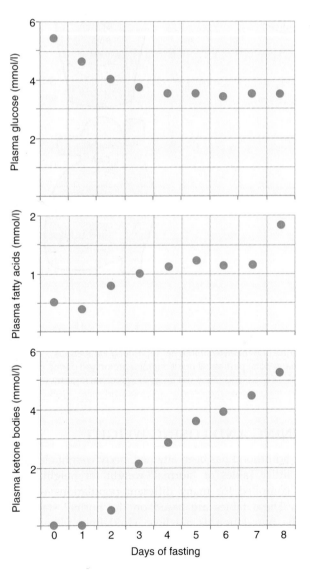

Figure 14.7
Effects of fasting on the composition of plasma: mean values from six subjects. (Adapted from Cahill et al 1966.)

PROTEIN ENERGY MALNUTRITION

Protein energy malnutrition (PEM) occurs in periods of starvation or as a result of stress associated with injury. Protein is catabolised to provide energy for the body.

Research demonstrates that no person should be without an intake of protein for longer than 5 days (Holmes 1986).

PEM is seen in the children of the Third World in two extreme forms:

- marasmus – more common where the diet is low in both protein and calories
- kwashiorkor – more common where the diet is low in protein but there is a relatively adequate energy (carbohydrate) intake.

PEM can also occur within hospitalised patients, especially following surgery and/or trauma, giving rise to a state of negative nitrogen balance. The extent of alteration in nutrient homeostasis is in direct proportion to the severity of the injury/stress and the individual's previous nutritional state. It is thus imperative that nutritional assessment is carried out prior to planned surgery and that nurses monitor, record and report on their patients' nutritional state and intake of nutrients.

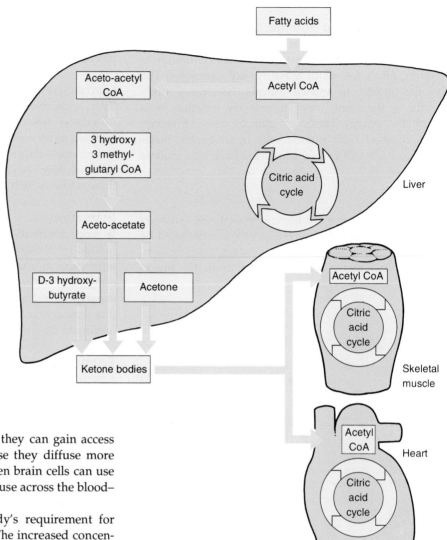

Figure 14.8
Formation and usage of ketone bodies. (Note: specific carbohydrates are needed to keep the citric acid cycle working. If these are deficient, as they are in diabetes mellitus, the concentration of ketone bodies in blood increases even more.)

advantage over fatty acids in that they can gain access to cells much more readily because they diffuse more easily through cell membranes. Even brain cells can use ketone bodies because they can diffuse across the blood–brain barrier.

As starvation proceeds the body's requirement for glucose is progressively reduced. The increased concentration of ketone bodies in the blood inhibits the release of amino acids from skeletal muscle and slows the protein breakdown occurring there.

> In *ketosis* (high levels of ketones in body fluids) an individual's breath smells of acetone. Ketones can also be detected on urine analysis.

Digestive tract

In starvation, the gastrointestinal tract atrophies. This is partly due to the general breakdown of tissues that occurs with nutritional deficiency. However, it is also caused by the lack of activity in the digestive tract and by the lack of secretion of hormones, such as gastrin and CCK-PZ, which have a growth-promoting effect (*trophic effect*) on parts of the digestive system.

Faeces continue to be formed even when no food is eaten. This is because the bulk of the faecal mass consists of bacteria. These continue to survive in the colon sustained by the nourishment they gain from shed cells and digestive secretions.

> If someone receives nutritional support by intravenous means (total parenteral nutrition) for a prolonged period of time, one consequence will be gastrointestinal atrophy.

GAINING AND LOSING WEIGHT

Once adulthood has been attained, body weight changes very little. Tables of 'normal' weight for height have been compiled for many different populations worldwide. These tables are based on the normal statistics for the population as a whole. Guidelines for acceptable weights, such as those published by the BMA (Table 14.18), represent the weights which are associated with the lowest mortality for that group (as researched for example by the Metropolitan Life Insurance Company).

Table 14.18 Guidelines for body weight in adults*				
Height without shoes (H)		*Weight (kg) without clothes (W)*		
Metres	Feet, inches	Acceptable[†]	Obese	(Grossly obese)[‡]
1.45	4, 9	42–53	64	(85)
1.48	4, 10	42–54	65	(86)
1.50	4, 11	43–55	66	(88)
1.52	5, 0	44–57	68	(90)
1.54	5, 1	44–58	70	(93)
1.56	5, 1	45–58	70	(93)
1.58	5, 2	51–64	77	(102)
1.60	5, 3	52–65	78	(104)
1.62	5, 4	53–66	79	(105)
1.64	5, 5	54–67	80	(106)
1.66	5, 5	55–69	83	(110)
1.68	5, 6	56–71	85	(113)
1.70	5, 7	58–73	88	(117)
1.72	5, 8	59–74	89	(118)
1.74	5, 9	60–75	90	(120)
1.76	5, 9	62–77	92	(122)
1.78	5, 10	64–79	95	(126)
1.80	5, 11	65–80	96	(128)
1.82	6, 0	66–82	98	(130)
1.84	6, 0	67–84	101	(134)
1.86	6, 1	69–86	103	(137)
1.88	6, 2	71–88	106	(141)
1.90	6, 3	73–90	108	(144)
1.92	6, 4	75–93	112	(150)

* Data, based partly on a report of the Royal College of Physicians 1983 and Garrow 1981, reproduced from Truswell A S 1986, ABC of nutrition, by permission of the British Medical Association.
[†] Acceptable weights are W/H^2 20–25.
[‡] Obesity is taken to start at W/H^2 30 and gross obesity at W/H^2 40.

Body weight is linked to height and size of body frame. Frame size can be ascertained by measurement of wrist circumference.

mass over and above 'normal' are not produced by overeating! As noted above, food surpluses are mainly converted into fat.

Adipose tissue

The factors that regulate the activity of adipose tissue and the storage of fat are not yet fully understood. What is clear is that, in the long term, if more calories are consumed than are required in metabolism the excess is largely converted into fat stores. It is not clear why some individuals seem more prone to obesity than others. Many factors are likely to contribute. These include:

- social and genetic factors
- emotional state
- lack of physical activity
- dietary habits
- metabolic balance
- hormonal status.

The tendency to obesity prevalent in many technologically sophisticated societies is probably associated with a lack of physical activity (born of the growth in sedentary occupations, the development of the motor car etc.) coupled with an abundance of appetising, easily assimilated, energy-rich, processed foods. Unless obesity is due to a metabolic disorder, the simplest strategy to adopt to lose weight is to limit the total number of calories ingested and to increase the amount of exercise taken.

Body weight

A change in body weight can be the result of one or more of several factors. It may represent changes in:

- total body water
- muscle mass
- adipose tissue
- a combination of these.

Total body water

The factors which affect total body water are discussed in Chapter 13. Fluid retention and fluid loss are common causes of short-term changes in body weight. The dramatic effects of some slimming regimes probably have more to do with loss of water than with loss of fat.

Muscle mass

Gain and loss of muscle mass occur as a result of a change in physical activity (see Ch. 17). Losses also occur in starvation. However, large increases in muscle

HEALTH EDUCATION

UKCC Regulations, Rule 18, states that nurses must be responsible for aspects concerned with 'the promotion of health'. It is essential, therefore, that nurses have a knowledge and understanding of the appropriate nutritional requirements of an individual during his or her life span and that they positively identify opportunites to promote healthy eating.

Education in relation to nutrition should be a priority. It can be done most successfully in maternal and child health centres but the frail 75+ age group can also benefit; simple changes to their diet may be all that are needed. Nutritional deficiencies in this age group are more usually associated with social or physical problems.

Health education authorities give advice, produce leaflets and posters, and provide teaching aids and training courses. Radio, television, and articles in newspapers and journals can all make a valuable contribution to health education and the eating patterns of society. Food should be a source of health and pleasure to us all.

KEY POINTS

What you should now understand about nutrition:

- what substances are needed in a healthy diet and why
- how foods vary in their composition and nutritional value
- how the composition of foods is affected by processing and cooking
- what biological factors influence the quantity of nutrients absorbed per day
- what happens to nutrients after they have been absorbed
- how the supply of nutrients to key tissues is preserved when no food is eaten
- key factors determining body weight.

REFERENCES AND FURTHER READING

Astrand P-O, Rohdahl K 1986 Textbook of work physiology – physiological basis of exercise, 3rd edn. McGraw-Hill, London

Atkins G L 1981 An outline of energy metabolism. William Heinemann Medical Books, London
(Useful clear summary diagrams of basic aspects of metabolism)

Barker H M 1991 Beck's Nutrition and dietetics for nurses, 8th edn. Churchill Livingstone, Edinburgh
(Clear concise, practical textbook)

Bodinski L 1989 The nurse's guide to diet therapy, 2nd edn. Delmar Publishing, Albany
(A practical book discussing therapeutic diets for specific purposes, and explaining the rationale)

Cahill G F, Herrera M G, Morgan A P et al 1966 Hormone-fuel interrelationships during fasting. Journal of Clinical Investigation 45: 1751–1769

Cliver D O 1990 Foodborne diseases. Academic Press, London
(Textbook surveying diseases transmitted by food. Examines evidence linking lifestyle diseases to diet)

Committee on International Dietary Allowances of the International Union of Nutritional Sciences 1975 Report. Nutritional Abstracts and Reviews 45: 89–111

Eastwood M, Edwards C, Parry D 1991 Human nutrition: a continuing debate. Chapman & Hall, London
(Collection of authoritative papers reviewing the scientific evidence from which dietary recommendations are made. Very useful source of reference)

Dowding C 1986 Nutrition in wound healing. Nursing 5/86: 174–176

Fieldhouse P 1990 Food and nutrition, customs and culture. Chapman & Hall, London
(An in-depth look at cultural factors determining choice of food)

Garrow J S 1978 Energy balance and obesity in man. Elsevier, North Holland

Garrow J S 1981 Treat obesity seriously. A clinical manual. Churchill Livingstone, Edinburgh

Glickman R M, Sabesin S M 1988 Lipoprotein metabolism. In: Arias I M, Jakoby W B, Popper H, Schacter D, Shafritz D A (eds) The liver: biology and pathobiology. Raven Press, New York

Hill et al 1977 Malnutrition in surgical patients: an unrecognised problem. Lancet i: 689–692

Holland B, Welch A A, Unwin I D, Buss D H, Paul A A, Southgate D A T 1991 McCance and Widdowson's The composition of foods, 5th revised and extended edn. The Royal Society of Chemistry & Ministry of Agriculture, Fisheries and Food, London

Holmes S 1986 Nutritional needs of surgical patients. Nursing Times 82(19): 30–32

James J E 1991 Caffeine and health. Academic Press, London
(Comprehensive detailed overview of findings to date)

Joint FAO/WHO/UNU Expert Consultation 1985 Energy and protein requirements. WHO Technical Report Series 724, WHO, Geneva

Lask S 1986 Nurses role in nutrition education. Nursing 8/86: 296–300

NACNE 1983 Report of the Nutritional Advisory Committee on Nutritional Education. Health Education Council, London

Newsholme E A, Start C 1973 Regulation in metabolism. John Wiley & Sons, London

Passmore R, Eastwood M A 1986 Davidson's Human nutrition and dietetics, 8th edn. Churchill Livingstone, Edinburgh
(Extremely informative, readable book on all aspects of nutrition. Very useful resource)

Paul A A, Southgate D A T, 1978 McCance and Widdowson's The composition of foods, HMSO, London. Elsevier, North Holland

Royal College of Physicians 1983 Obesity. A report of the Royal College of Physicians. Journal of the Royal College of Physicians 17: 3–58

Seely S, Freed D L J, Silverstone G A, Rippere V 1985 Diet related diseases: the modern epidemic. Chapman & Hall, London
(Interesting, readable paperback exploring the links between diet and disease)

Truswell A S 1986 ABC of nutrition. British Medical Association, London, p 37

Truswell A S 1992 ABC of nutrition, 2nd edn. British Medical Association, London
(Interesting collection of short attractive articles on many different aspects of nutrition)

Wahlqvist M L (ed) 1981 Food and nutrition in Australia. Cassell Australia, Melbourne

Chapter 15
PROTECTION, DEFENCE AND WASTE DISPOSAL

Cells need to be provided with vital materials but they also need to be shielded from anything that may distort their activity. The cellular environment must therefore be kept free of undesirable substances or, more realistically, the concentrations of such materials must be kept at tolerably low levels.

Barriers, for example the skin, and the epithelia of the respiratory tract and the digestive system, restrict the entry of substances into the body. Despite this, some penetration inevitably occurs. In addition to the entry of substances from outside, waste products generated in cell metabolism need to be eliminated. The disposal of unwanted materials originating both from outside the body (*exogenous*) and from within (*endogenous*) is dealt with by a comprehensive range of mechanisms which caters for practically all the different types of substance (gaseous, water-soluble, liposoluble and particulate) to which the body may be exposed.

Barriers to entry

The organs and tissues of the body are enclosed by a layer of tissue (*epithelium*) which acts as the first line of defence against the entry of unwanted substances. This defensive barrier includes (Fig. 15.1):

- the outer surface (the skin)
- several inner surfaces (those of the respiratory, digestive, urinary and genital tracts).

Each epithelium is specialised in ways that are appropriate to its particular functions. Each is continually renewed by the growth and development of new cells.

OUTER SURFACE: THE SKIN

STRUCTURE

The skin (Fig. 15.2) consists of two layers:

- epidermis
- dermis.

It contains glands, blood vessels, and a variety of sensory receptors and defence cells. Skin differs between different parts of the body. Skin that has hair follicles (*hairy* skin) has a thin epidermis and many sebaceous glands. Non-hairy (*glabrous*) skin, such as that on the surface of the palms, has a thicker epidermis and many more sensory receptors. There are variations between individuals, related to age, environment and ethnic origin. ①

① In people with black skin, what other differences are there between hairy and glabrous skin?

② What is the name given to cancer involving the melanocytes?

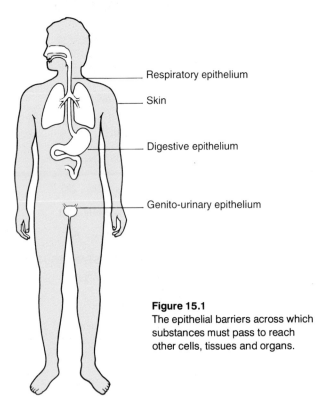

Figure 15.1
The epithelial barriers across which substances must pass to reach other cells, tissues and organs.

Epidermis

The cells of the basal cell layer (also known as the *germinal layer*) (Fig. 15.2A) act as stem cells (see Ch. 2) from which the rest of the epidermis (Fig. 15.3) is formed. From the basal layer, cells are pushed towards the surface by the formation of new cells by the stem cells. It takes about 2 weeks for the cells to reach the surface.

As the cells migrate they change in structure and activity. While still in the basal layer the cells begin the formation of fibrils of the protein, *keratin*, which continues as the cells (*keratinocytes*) move towards the surface. Eventually keratin in association with another protein, *fillagrin*, almost completely fills the cells of the outer layer (*stratum corneum*). At the same time the intracellular organelles disappear, so that the 'cells' of the stratum corneum are in effect like flattened 'bags' of protein. These 'bags' are embedded in a lipid-rich substance secreted by the keratinocytes as they near the surface, rather like bricks embedded in mortar.

Melanocytes, at the bottom of the epidermis, manufacture and secrete the pigment *melanin*. This is taken up into the adjacent keratinocytes. ②

Dermis

The dermis (Fig. 15.2A & B) consists largely of a fibrous network of two kinds of protein, *collagen* and *elastin* (see Ch. 2). These proteins are formed and secreted by cells, *fibroblasts*, scattered amongst the fibres.

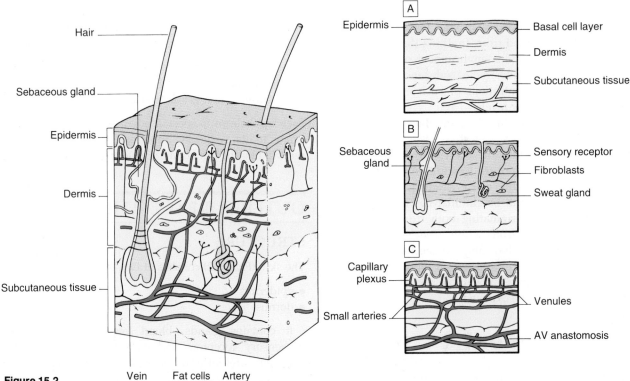

Figure 15.2
The structure of the skin: A Layers   B Component cells and structures   C Blood supply.

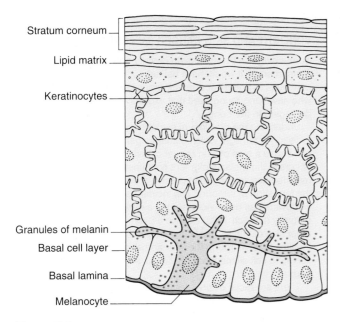

Stratum corneum

Lipid matrix

Keratinocytes

Granules of melanin

Basal cell layer

Basal lamina

Melanocyte

Figure 15.3
Structure of the epidermis.

Table 15.1 Defence cells of the skin		
Cell type	Location	Function(s)
Langerhans' cells	Epidermis	Present foreign antigens to T lymphocytes
Histiocytes	Dermis	Phagocytosis
Mast cells	Dermis	Secrete substances involved in producing the inflammatory response

There are variations in the precise arrangement and control of the cutaneous blood vessels in different parts of the body. Parts of the skin which play a large role in temperature regulation contain a large number of *arteriovenous anastomoses*, which link arteries and veins directly. These anastomoses are controlled by the nervous system, and enable blood to flow either in large quantities through superficial tissues, or to be diverted to deeper subcutaneous tissues (see Ch. 16). ⑤

Collagen fibres give strength to the skin, whereas elastin provides flexibility. ③

Situated in the dermis are secretory glands, a variety of sensory receptors, and many defence cells.

Glands
The secretory glands originate embryologically from cells of the epidermis and all secrete their products on to the skin surface. *Sweat glands*, which are widely distributed over the body, secrete a very dilute solution of salts (see Ch. 16). *Sebaceous glands* are found everywhere except in areas lacking hairs (palms, soles). These glands secrete *sebum* which contains a mixture of lipids.

Other cells
The skin contains sensory receptors of various kinds (see Ch. 24). Most of these are situated in the dermis, but some such as free nerve endings are present in the epidermis. Some receptors are involved in activating protective reflexes, for example the withdrawal reflex (pulling your hand away from a painful stimulus) (see Ch. 27).

Other cells present in the skin include *Langerhans' cells*, wandering *histiocytes*, and *mast cells*, all of which are cells of the defence system (Table 15.1). ④

Blood vessels
There are three interconnected networks of blood vessels associated with the skin (Fig. 15.2C):

- a capillary network (*plexus*) beneath the epidermis
- small arteries and venules in the dermis
- larger arteries and veins in the subcutaneous tissue.

BARRIER FUNCTION

Water-soluble substances
The stratum corneum (Fig. 15.3) is the primary barrier to the loss of water and other hydrophilic substances from the body. The lipid matrix in which the cells are embedded is not easily penetrated by these substances. Also, the protein inside the cells attracts and holds on to water molecules. This restrains the movement of water through the epithelium and restricts its loss from the body. As a result, the surface of the skin is normally fairly dry and only a small amount of water (0.5 litre) is lost from the surface per day.

If layers of the stratum corneum are stripped, as they are when adhesive tape is removed from the skin, the skin becomes much more permeable at that site. Permeability is also increased by detergents, and organic solvents such as white spirit or 'turps'. These dissolve components of the lipid matrix between the cells and allow fluid to enter the spaces, which then act as channels for the diffusion of water-soluble substances. ⑥

After a prolonged soak in water the character of the surface of the skin alters. The epidermal cells swell as they take up more water and the properties of the barrier change.

It is known that skin infections are more common in people whose skin is regularly soaked in water. The reasons for this are not entirely clear but may be related to the washing away of protective secretions.

③
How does skin wrinkle? What happens to the tissues as people get older?

④
Which irritating substance do the mast cells contain?

⑤
In assessing whether an elderly person is hypothermic, it is suggested that you feel the skin between the shoulder blades. Why is feeling a hand or an arm not as good?

⑥
Why might excessive hand washing with soap lead to skin damage?

Liposoluble substances

The lipid matrix that restricts the movement of hydrophilic substances is, however, a route for the passive absorption of liposoluble substances. The ease with which they are absorbed depends on several factors including:

- their specific chemical nature
- the thickness of the stratum corneum
- the vehicle (cream or oil) in which they are applied.

If the affinity of a substance for the vehicle is greater than it is for the lipids of the skin then absorption will be small. Creams and oils which are prepared for the topical application of medicines need to be sufficiently lipophilic to dissolve the active ingredients but not so lipophilic that they hinder absorption into the skin.

The total amount of a substance which is absorbed into the body depends also on:

- the area of exposed skin
- the skin blood flow.

The greater the area of skin and the greater the blood flow the greater is the amount absorbed. The underlying principles are the same as those governing oxygen uptake in the lungs (see Ch. 7) and the passive absorption of substances in the digestive tract (see Ch. 6). ⑦

UV radiation

The skin is an important barrier to the penetration of ultraviolet radiation. UV radiation (200–380 nm) is divided into three bands:

- UVA (320–380 nm)
- UVB (290–320 nm)
- UVC (200–290 nm).

Of these, the shortest wavelengths (UVC) are most damaging. Fortunately, they are absorbed by the ozone layer of the atmosphere so that normally the skin is exposed only to UVA and UVB. Short wavelength radiation does not penetrate very far into the tissues but it is absorbed by DNA. The radiation absorbed can cause two adjacent bases on DNA to combine (see Ch. 2) and it is this which ultimately leads to mutation and cancer.

The skin protects the body from the damaging effects of radiation in two ways, through:

- proteins in the epidermis
- the pigment melanin.

The proteins in the keratinocytes absorb some of the radiation, and also scatter some, so that not all of it penetrates to deeper layers. The pigment melanin, produced and secreted by the melanocytes, also absorbs UV light. The more pigment in the skin, the more radiation is absorbed. As a result less reaches the deeper layers of cells and tissues.

Continued exposure to sunlight provokes increased

⑦
Why might shock reduce the amount of a substance absorbed following an intramuscular injection?

⑧
How well does a balding scalp adapt to exposure?

⑨
When lying in the sun it is possible to get bad sunburn of the soles of the feet. Why may this be?

⑩
Which factors, other than pressure, could lead to reduced blood flow to the skin?

⑪
What is a corn? What causes it?

SUNLIGHT AND SKIN CANCER (MELANOMA)

Sunbathing is a truly twentieth century and western phenomenon; it would have baffled our forefathers and continues to baffle our contemporaries in hotter countries who have long recognised that excessive sunlight is damaging to the body.

Underlying the problem of sunbathing is the ultraviolet radiation in sunlight which damages genetic material and can cause a type of skin cancer called melanoma. Mutation occurs in the melanin pigment containing cells, the melanocytes, leading to excessive growth and division and the formation of tumours. The incidence of melanoma worldwide has been increasing at a rate of from 3 to 7% annually (Urbach 1983) despite a decrease in the number of other skin cancers. This is probably due to the promotion of 'healthy tans' all round the year and all over the body, which serves to sell all manner of holidays, sun creams and sun beds.

There are racial differences in susceptibility to melanoma with the darker skinned races being less susceptible. People who have black skins are much better protected against ultraviolet radiation than people with pale skins, because the skin is thicker and contains much more melanin. The development of a sun-tan by pale-skinned people is the body's defence against UV radiation but it is also a warning that the skin is being exposed to potentially damaging radiation.

Any sudden change in pigmented areas of the body such as growth and darkening of moles can be indicative of melanoma and should be investigated. The best way to avoid melanoma is to avoid the sun. Sun hats, 'modest' clothing and creams which absorb ultraviolet light can all be effective if used appropriately.

production of keratinocytes and melanocytes, so that in time the skin thickens, and darkens. ⑧⑨

RENEWAL

The skin is constantly subject to abrasion and injury. Maintenance of a normal barrier relies on the ongoing repair and renewal of the tissues. New epidermal cells are continually formed by the stem cells, so that the whole epidermis is normally renewed every 15 to 30 days. This renewal relies on an adequate delivery of nutrients in the microcirculation.

Effects of pressure

When pressure on any part of the skin displaces blood and reduces the supply, the balance between cell breakdown and cell renewal is displaced in favour of cell death (necrosis) and erosion of skin tissue occurs. If the circulation in general is sluggish or if local conditions promote vasoconstriction then blood flow is reduced further, problems are exacerbated and tissue breakdown occurs more quickly. ⑩⑪

The body's natural defence against the effects of pressure on the skin and adjacent tissues is movement. Prolonged pressure causes discomfort and this in turn

PRESSURE SORES

In the capillaries, where blood comes most intimately into contact with the cells and tissues of the body, the blood pressure is about 15 mmHg (see Ch. 5). It is not very difficult, therefore, to occlude the blood supply to a peripheral tissue such as the skin and we do so regularly in certain areas of the body by sitting down, leaning on our elbows, sleeping or wearing tight shoes. In a healthy person occlusion is eventually accompanied by discomfort which prompts a change in position and prevents damage to the tissues.

The situation is different for someone whose health is compromised, for example by hypovolaemic shock or by neurological disease such as stroke. Firstly, their tissues may not be able to withstand prolonged lack of perfusion and, secondly, they may be unable to sense when damage is imminent and take measures to prevent it. For these reasons, nurses identify patients who are 'at risk' of suffering pressure damage and take compensatory preventive measures.

Two factors dictate whether damage will occur; these are the extent of the pressure causing the occlusion and the time for which occlusion is endured. It is a combination of the two that determines the extent (both depth and area) of tissue damage.

Nursing measures to prevent pressure damage to the skin include administering positional change and putting the patients on support surfaces. The principle behind support surfaces is the physical relationship, pressure = force/area; in other words, increasing the area over which weight is distributed will reduce pressure. Positional change is used to reduce the time factor in pressure damage although the precise relationship between time and pressure is not fully understood. It is widely believed, and practice is based on the belief, that two-hourly positional change in 'at risk' patients is sufficient to prevent the formation of pressure sores.

provokes a reflex change of position (see Ch. 28), so that the pressure on one part of the body is relieved and transferred to another. Those at risk of developing pressure sores are either people whose awareness of discomfort is dulled, for example by sedation, or people whose mobility is restricted by injury, illness or weakness.

INNER SURFACES

The inner surfaces that act as the first line of defence against the entry of unwanted substances into the body include the epithelia of:

- the respiratory tract
- the digestive tract
- the urinary tract
- the genital tract (see Ch. 34).

As these epithelia are not keratinised and do not have a stratum corneum they are more permeable than the skin. However, like the skin they are continually renewed. This is vital for their barrier function.

Mechanisms which defend the body against the entry of unwanted substances at these sites include:

- protective reflexes (such as coughing and vomiting) that forcibly expel noxious materials
- secretions (such as nasal secretions and saliva) that trap and inactivate harmful substances and sweep them away
- antibacterial forces (such as leucocytes and bactericidal agents).

RESPIRATORY TRACT

The huge surface area of the alveolar epithelium (see Ch. 7) potentially offers unrestricted entry to any substance which is inhaled and can diffuse across it. Protective reflexes, secretions and macrophages all play their part in shielding this vulnerable epithelium. A key role is played by the nose. ⑫

Nose

The nose is the first part of the respiratory tract. It consists of two nasal passages, separated by the nasal septum, each of which opens independently into the upper part of the throat (*nasopharynx*) (Fig. 15.4A & B). The external part of the nose is formed mainly of soft tissue and cartilage whereas the structure of the internal passages is created mainly by the bones of the skull (Fig. 15.4B & C). The internal walls opposite the nasal septum (Fig. 15.4C) have ridges formed of bone (*conchae* or *turbinate bones*). The space between adjacent ridges is known as a *meatus*. The nasal sinuses (see Ch. 29) open into these spaces (*meati*) as do the tear ducts, which is why you have to blow your nose when you cry.

All the nasal passages are lined by an epithelium consisting of tall ciliated cells interspersed with goblet cells. The tissue beneath the epithelium has a rich blood supply, many secretory glands and much lymphoid tissue (see Ch. 4). The blood supply keeps the nasal passages warm and the secretions keep them moist. In this way, the air we breath is warmed and humidified before it reaches the rest of the respiratory tract. ⑬

When the epithelium becomes inflamed in response to an infection, the swollen tissue and extra secretions easily obstruct the flow of air through the narrow passages in the nose.

Protective reflexes

Inhalation of noxious materials is resisted by several protective reflexes, such as sneezing and coughing, which inhibit breathing and force the inhaled materials out of the respiratory tract. These reflexes are evoked by

⑫ *Relatively small amounts of glue sniffed quickly by a young person new to glue sniffing can kill. Why may the novice be especially at risk?*

⑬ *Why is mouth breathing more likely than nasal breathing to lead to respiratory infections?*

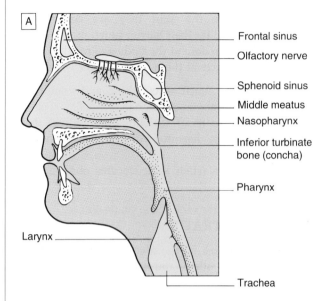

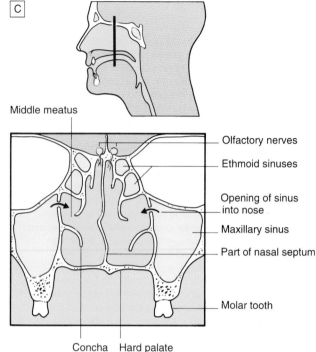

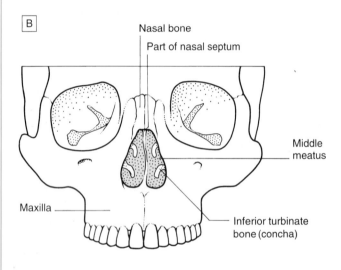

Figure 15.4
The structure of the nose:
A Related to other structures in the head
B Related to the bones of the skull
C Showing internal structures and adjacent sinuses. (The bar in the top panel shows the cross-section for the view in the lower panel.)

Concert goers are often urged to control their coughs. How controllable is a cough?

What effect does smoking have on the ciliated epithelium?

sensory receptors in the respiratory epithelium (see Ch. 7). Sneezing is evoked by stimulation of receptors in the nose whereas coughing is a vagal reflex triggered by receptors in the larynx and tracheobronchial tree. Effective stimuli include cigarette smoke and inhaled fluids. Coughing is depressed in sleep and under anaesthesia.

There are three phases to a cough:

- inspiration
- compression (forced expiration against a closed glottis)
- expulsion (sudden explosive opening of the glottis).

The forced expiration increases pressures within the thorax considerably (up to 100 mmHg) and, when the glottis is forced open, causes the rate of airflow to approach 1000 km/h. This sudden rush of air dislodges the offending substance and associated epithelial secretions and drives them out into the pharynx. Air-

flow is highest in the upper reaches of the tracheobronchial tree and, therefore, material in the upper parts of the tract is most easily dislodged. ⑭

Secretions

The whole of the upper part of the respiratory tract (nose, nasopharynx, larynx, trachea and bronchi) is lined by a ciliated epithelium, embedded in which are goblet cells and seromucous glands (see Ch. 7). ⑮

Secretions are swept continually towards the pharynx by the action of the cilia: upwards from the trachea and bronchi and downwards from the nose. Thus, particles trapped in the mucus and substances dissolving in the secretions are carried away from the highly permeable and extensive alveolar epithelium.

Secretion by the seromucous glands is reflexly stimulated through cholinergic nerves resulting in a copious flow of a watery secretion.

COMMON COLD

The biggest myth surrounding the common cold (*coryza*) is that it has something to do with either cold weather or getting caught in the rain. The common cold is viral in nature and there are several viruses known to cause it.

The viruses infect the moist passages of the nose (mucous membranes) and here they multiply and trigger localised immune responses leading to symptoms such as running nose, sneezing and coughing. Similarly to allergens in allergic reactions (see p. 289), the viral particles become attached to IgE which results in the bursting of mast cells and the release of substances such as histamine and prostaglandins which cause inflammation of the nasal passages and excessive production of nasal secretions. These protective symptoms of the common cold are the means whereby the viruses are passed on from one person to the next.

Associated symptoms, such as raised temperature (see Ch. 16), chest infection or shortness of breath, are secondary complications caused, not directly by the virus, but by bacterial infection or by an excessive immune response such as occurs in asthma (see Ch. 7).

DIGESTIVE TRACT

As the chief purpose of the digestive tract is the absorption of nutrients from the diet, this epithelium has to contend with all substances which we deliberately swallow in food and drink, some of which are potentially harmful. As in the respiratory tract the most vulnerable epithelium (intestinal) is protected by reflexes, which control access to that epithelium and evict unwanted intruders.

In the digestive tract the reflex activity which expels unwanted material, as in vomiting and diarrhoea, is almost invariably accompanied by increased secretory activity too.

Protective reflexes

Upper digestive tract
Usually we choose what we want to swallow. Information from taste buds and olfactory organs about the palatability of food either enhances our desire to eat or leads us to reject it (see Chs 14, 29 and 31).

Once material has been swallowed it may still be rejected by activation of the *vomiting reflex*. Vomiting is controlled by a group of cells in the medulla of the brain (associated with the *nucleus tractus solitarius*) that are excited by signals arising from receptors in:

- the upper gastrointestinal tract
- the chemoreceptor trigger zone (*area postrema*) in the medulla oblongata of the brain stem (see Ch. 20).

Receptors in the upper digestive tract monitor the volume and composition of ingested materials and transmit impulses via afferent neurones in the vagus,

Vomiting induced by radiation (*radiation sickness*) may be caused by the release of neurotransmitters in the gut (serotonin and substance P) which activate sensory neurones in the vagus.

whereas the cells in the brain are sensitive to blood-borne chemicals including drugs such as ipecacuanha and apomorphine.

The vomiting reflex triggers:

- relaxation of the body of the stomach
- retroperistalsis in the upper small intestine.

These events hold substances in the stomach and prevent them from passing on into the small intestine. As the same time the glottis closes, sealing off the respiratory tract. Powerful contractions of the abdominal muscles and diaphragm squeeze the stomach and forcibly expel its contents through the oesophagus and the mouth. The pressure on the stomach drives the segment of the oesophagus usually lying within the abdomen up into the thorax with the result that its sphincter function is lost (see Ch. 6, Fig. 6.6).

These events are accompanied by increased salivation and generalised activation of the sympathetic nervous system including sweating, cutaneous vasoconstriction and tachycardia. ⑯

Lower digestive tract
Irritation of the lower digestive tract also provokes secretion and contractile activity that promotes the expulsion of irritants via the rectum, as in *diarrhoea*. The responses are mediated by the enteric nervous system (see Ch. 6) and are influenced by the autonomic nervous system. Effective stimuli include bacterial toxins (including cholera toxin) and plant products used as laxatives, such as cascara and senna. ⑰

Antibacterial forces
Both saliva and gastric juice contain bactericidal agents that limit the numbers of bacteria entering the small intestine. The acid in gastric juice (see Ch. 6) is especially effective in killing bacteria.

A lack of acid gastric juice (*achlorhydria*), a condition that is more common in the elderly, makes someone more susceptible to pathogens in the diet.

The large intestine normally contains a large population of bacteria which contribute to normal functioning of the colon. Their colonisation of the small intestine is usually limited by the fact that during digestion and in fasting the normal direction of movement of food residues is from small to large intestine (see Ch. 6).

⑯
How does persistent vomiting damage the teeth?

⑰
How does diarrhoea upset the electrolyte balance in the body?

Renewal

The entire gastrointestinal epithelium undergoes continual renewal. Cells are shed constantly. They are digested along with food, and the products are absorbed. As cells are shed, more are produced from germinal tissue to replace them. The rapid replacement of cells in the stomach may be important in the protection of the stomach against erosion (*ulcers*).

Disposal and elimination of unwanted materials

Waste products generated in metabolism and unwanted items which get into the body through the protecting epithelia can be divided into several types (Table 15.2):

- gaseous
- water-soluble
- liposoluble
- macromolecules, particles and cells.

Gaseous and small water-soluble substances, such as CO_2 and urea respectively, are already in a form which allows them to be excreted easily. Gaseous molecules are breathed out in the air from the lungs (see Ch. 7), whereas water-soluble molecules are filtered from the plasma in the kidneys and eliminated in the urine (see Ch. 8).

However, other materials need to be processed before they can be eliminated. For example, redundant cells are engulfed and digested by phagocytic cells, and substances that are liposoluble, such as bilirubin from haemoglobin, are converted into water-soluble substances mainly by the liver.

Thus, unwanted materials are converted by a variety of different processes into molecules that are either re-used and recycled, or are excreted via the expired air, urine or faeces (Fig. 15.5). Some substances, such as dust particles, cannot be fully processed. These will be retained in the body and accumulate progressively over the years.

CELLS, PARTICLES AND MACROMOLECULES

The first stage in the processing of cells, particles and macromolecules is their engulfment and degradation by phagocytic cells, such as macrophages and granulocytes (see Ch. 4) and their attack by natural killer cells (NK cells). These processes are assisted by lymphocytes, cells which have the specific function of distinguishing normal items belonging to the body (*self*) from those which are foreign or abnormal (*non-self* and *altered self*).

The local release of chemicals from damaged and defending cells triggers many supporting systems that improve the blood supply locally, facilitate defensive reactions, and alert the body to potential danger. These effects are all part of the *inflammatory response*.

PHAGOCYTOSIS AND ATTACK

Cells

At least three groups of cells are involved:

- granulocytes
- macrophages
- natural killer cells (NK cells).

Granulocytes are the first cells to accumulate in large numbers at the site of injury or bacterial invasion.

Table 15.2	Categories of material for disposal and elimination		
Type	*Examples*	*Source*	*Chapter reference*
Gaseous	Carbon dioxide	Respiration	11, 7
	Acetone	Fat metabolism	14
Water-soluble	Acids, bases	Diet and metabolism	12
	Urea	Protein metabolism	14, 8
	Creatinine	Muscle metabolism	17, 8
	Ions (Na, K, Ca, Cl)	Diet and cells	13
Liposoluble	Bilirubin	Haemoglobin	4, 9
	Ammonia	Bacterial metabolism	6
	Steroid hormones	Adrenal glands/gonads	10, 34
Macromolecules	Peptide hormones	Several endocrine glands	10
Particles	Dust	Atmosphere	
Cells	Bacteria	Infection	
	Dead or abnormal cells		

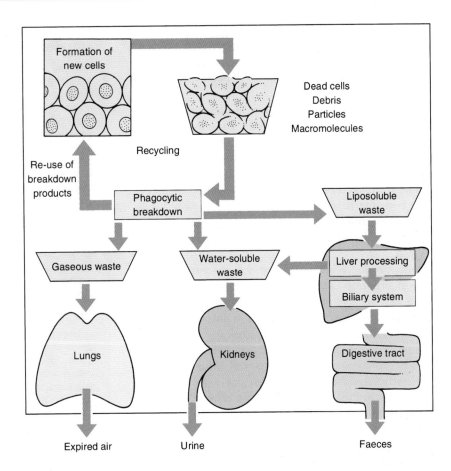

Figure 15.5
The body's recycling and waste-disposal systems.

Macrophages, which are much bigger cells (see Ch. 4), follow a little later. Both groups of cells are attracted to the site of action by chemicals produced locally. This process is termed *chemotaxis*. *NK* cells are a much smaller group. They are not phagocytic but kill target cells by the chemicals they secrete.

The numbers of phagocytic and attacking cells found at different sites within the body reflect the degree of cellular breakdown occurring there and the degree of exposure of those sites to invading cells and toxins. Thus, large numbers of phagocytic cells are normally found within the respiratory tract (*alveolar macrophages*) and lodged in the liver (*Kuppfer cells*).

Activation

The phagocytic activity of the macrophages depends upon several factors including:

- some that influence them directly
- some (*opsonins*) that make the target of their attack more attractive.

The factors that influence the macrophages directly come from several sources (Table 15.3). Many of these substances attract mobile macrophages to cell debris and foreign cells, such as bacteria, by chemotaxis. They also transform and activate cells. Monocytes, for example, are transformed into macrophages as they migrate from

Table 15.3 Factors influencing the activity of macrophages

General name	Source(s)	Chapter reference
Cytokines	Lymphocytes	15
Leukotrienes	Produced by all cells	10
Kinins	Formed in plasma from kininogens produced by the liver	10

the blood into the tissues. Within the tissues, macrophages are aroused to intense phagocytic activity by the action of cytokines, for example.

Opsonins are any factors that make substances more susceptible to phagocytosis. Antibodies secreted by lymphocytes act in this way, as does one of the products of the complement cascade (see p. 285), known as C_{3b}. Opsonins bind to the foreign cell or protein and act as 'markers' singling out that cell or protein as a target for disposal and facilitating phagocytosis (see p. 286).

Digestion

Phagocytic cells contain vesicles (*lysosomes*) (see Ch. 2) containing a variety of enzymes (*acid hydrolases*). When bacteria or macromolecules have been engulfed, the vacuole formed fuses with a lysosome, and the acid hydrolases and other bactericidal agents like hydrogen peroxide produced by the phagocyte begin the process of degradation. ⑱

Some of the products generated in digestion, such as glucose and amino acids, are used by the macrophages in their metabolism. Others are excreted by the macrophages into the body fluids and may then be taken up and used by other tissues. Iron, for example, derived from aged cells is re-used by haemopoietic cells of the bone marrow in the manufacture of new red cells. In this way, macrophages participate in the economy of the body by enabling useful waste products to be recycled.

Some products generated by the macrophages become incorporated into the cell membrane of the macrophage and act as antigens which activate lymphocytes (antigen-presenting function). This is important in the development of immunity (see p. 286).

Sometimes the material which has been engulfed by the macrophages cannot be digested. This applies to dust particles, asbestos and silica, for example. These remain within the cell for its lifespan. When the cell dies and is itself degraded and disposed of by the same system, these particles will become lodged in another macrophage. These materials are thus not readily eliminated from the body. Over a lifetime, therefore, there can be a substantial build-up of matter. ⑲

⑱ *Why are the acid hydrolases contained inside lysosomes?*

⑲ *Which occupations expose people to risk of dust accumulation in the lungs?*

RECOGNITION OF FOREIGN MATERIAL

Lymphocytes have a crucial role in identifying foreign or abnormal cells and proteins and distinguishing these from normal cells and tissues. If they fail to do this the consequences may be uncontrolled proliferation of bacteria, viruses and even aberrant cells of the body itself (*cancer*), or destruction of apparently normal cells (*autoimmune disorders*).

Lymphocytes

There are two main classes of lymphocytes:

● *T lymphocytes* (T cells)
● *B lymphocytes* (B cells).

T and B lymphocytes differ in their life histories and specialise in different activities. T cells but not B cells spend time maturing in the thymus gland after emerging from the bone marrow (see Ch. 4). Both B cells and T cells respond to a wide variety of materials, including proteins, bacteria, viruses and aberrant cells. However, T cells tend to be most effective against abnormal cells and those infected by pathogens (viruses, bacteria, fungi), whereas B cells tend to recognise pathogens encountered outside cells.

Individual lymphocytes differ from one another in the

AUTOIMMUNE DISEASE

Normally, we are aware of our immune system only when it is being used to fight infection or when it responds inappropriately, for example in allergic conditions. With the advent of acquired immune deficiency syndrome (AIDS) the consequences of an incompetent immune system have become only too apparent. For some unfortunate individuals, however, the immune system can almost be described as over competent, for example in autoimmune diseases which arise as a result of the immune system failing to discriminate between 'self' and 'non-self'. In these conditions the immune system effectively attacks and destroys body tissues.

The causes of autoimmune diseases are not known but autoimmunity has been implicated in diseases as diverse as type I diabetes mellitus and rheumatoid arthritis. A good example of the condition is autoimmune haemolytic anaemia where healthy red blood cells are removed from the circulation in the spleen and liver because immunity has been developed to an antigen on the surface of the red blood cell.

Treatment of autoimmune diseases involves administering drugs which deal with symptoms, for example the painful inflammation of rheumatoid arthritis is treated with anti-inflammatory drugs such as aspirin. Treating the underlying autoimmunity is also possible using steroids which suppress the immune response, but this raises difficulties since the action of steroids is not specific. Any general suppression of the immune system has the accompanying risk of leaving the patient more susceptible to infection.

---

specific proteins they manufacture to use in defence. These proteins, some of which are inserted into the cell membrane (*receptors*) and some of which are secreted (*antibodies*), are the molecules which latch on to foreign or abnormal cells and macromolecules. When a T or B lymphocyte encounters a cell or a macromolecule which is able to interact with the specific receptor proteins in its cell membrane the interaction stimulates the lymphocyte to:

● proliferate
● differentiate.

The specific molecule on the foreign cell or in the body fluids that triggers this response is termed the *antigen*. The events that follow differ for B and T cells (Fig. 15.6). Activated B cells secrete antibodies that disable the antigen (*humoral immunity*) whereas T cells respond in a variety of ways collectively referred to as *cellular immunity*.

Humoral immunity
Activated B cells differentiate into *plasma cells* (Fig. 15.6). Plasma cells manufacture and secrete large amounts of the specific protein which 'recognised' the cell or molecule encountered by the B cell. These secreted proteins (*antibodies*) bind to the antigen and this has

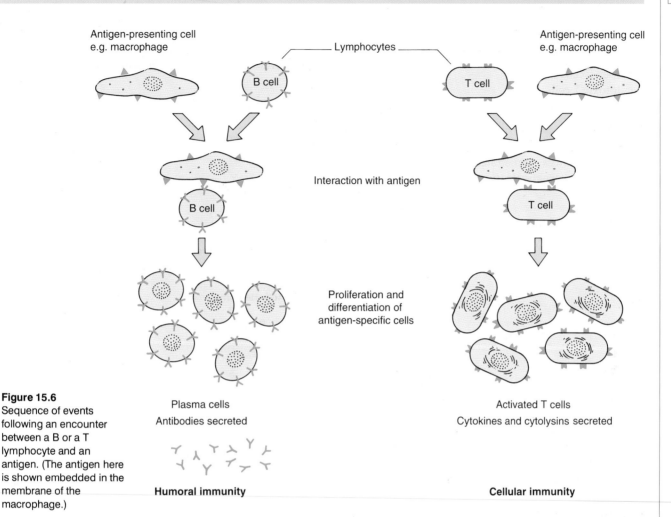

Figure 15.6
Sequence of events following an encounter between a B or a T lymphocyte and an antigen. (The antigen here is shown embedded in the membrane of the macrophage.)

several consequences each of which facilitates phagocytic attack (Fig. 15.7):

- the coating of antibody *opsonises* the antigen
- the *complement system* is activated
- antigen–antibody complexes clump together (*agglutinate*).

Opsonise means 'prepare for eating'. Antibodies prepare antigens for phagocytosis by actually linking them to the phagocyte. This triggers phagocytosis.

The *complement system* is a sequence of enzymatic reactions which generates a number of different products with wide-ranging effects including:

- inflammation (see p. 288)
- chemotaxis of phagocytic cells
- opsonisation of antigen
- cell lysis (rupture of cell membranes).

The enzymes are present in inactive form in the tissue fluids and are activated in one of two ways:

- by antibodies
- by a non-antibody system.

Agglutination creates large particles from small ones.

This limits the movement of the antigen and provides more binding sites for linkage to the phagocyte.

All antibodies have the same basic molecular structure (Fig. 15.8). Each molecule is a protein (*immunoglobulin*) consisting of four polypeptide chains linked together to form a 'stem' and two 'arms'. There are five different stems giving rise to five different families of immunoglobulins, IgA, IgD, IgE, IgG and IgM, but there are an infinite number of different 'arms' creating an infinite variety of antigen-binding sites.

Each class of antibody has a slightly different role to play in the immune response (Table 15.4). Activated lymphocytes produce IgM first before switching to the production of one of the other classes, such as IgG, the main class of antibody in plasma. Both IgM and IgG are involved in opsonising antigens. The IgA class has a different function. It tackles recognised antigens *before* they get into the body through the epithelial barriers of, for example, the respiratory and digestive tracts, or the ducts of exocrine glands. By binding to antigens, IgA class antibodies prevent their uptake into the body. IgE attaches itself to mast cells (see Ch. 4) and triggers their secretion of histamine and other chemicals of the inflammatory response.

Cell mediated immunity

There are at least three types of T cell:

- helper T cells
- cytotoxic T cells
- suppressor T cells.

Helper T cells are the first of the T cells to be activated when an antigen is encountered. In response they secrete substances, sometimes generally referred to as *cytokines* or alternatively *lymphokines* (Table 15.5), that stimulate the activity of other defence cells, including B cells, cytotoxic T cells and macrophages (Fig 15.9).

Activated cytotoxic T cells directly attack abnormal

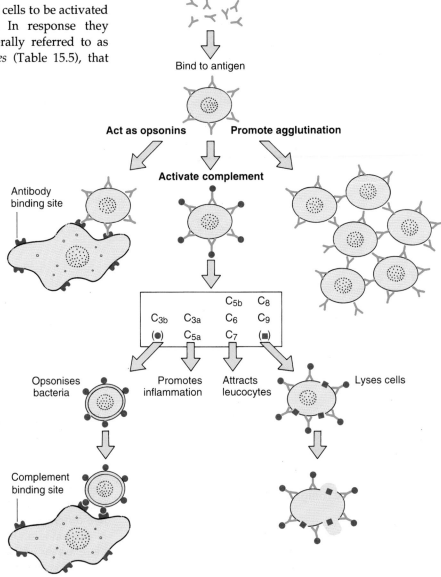

Figure 15.7
Consequences of antibodies binding to antigen.

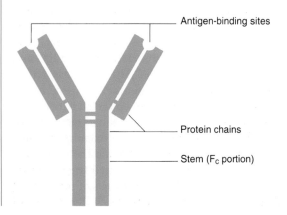

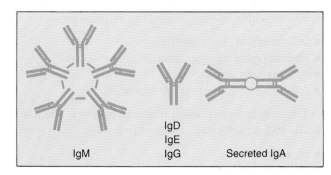

Figure 15.8
Structure of antibodies.

Table 15.4 Characteristic features of the five classes of immunoglobulins

Class	Features
IgM	Early antibodies formed by all plasma cells Effective as opsonins and in promoting agglutination; activate complement
IgG	Major class of immunoglobulin present in plasma Effective as opsonins; activate complement; disable bacterial toxins Able to cross the placenta (see Chs 34 and 35)
IgA	Secretory form secreted by epithelia (tracts and exocrine glands) Disables antigens before they penetrate the epithelial barriers
IgE	Attaches to mast cells and triggers the release of histamine Role in allergic response and parasitic infections
IgD	Distinctive characteristics uncertain

Table 15.5 Some examples of cytokines involved in the immune response

Group	Examples(s)	Source	Action(s)
Interleukins (IL)	IL 1	Macrophages	Stimulates helper T cells
	IL 2	Helper T cells	Stimulates T and B lymphocytes
Interferons	Gamma interferon	Helper T cells	Activates macrophages, cytotoxic T cells and NK cells
Tumour necrosis factors (TNF)	Cachectin	Macrophages	Kills target cells

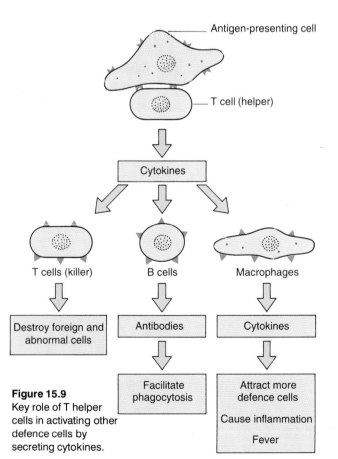

Figure 15.9
Key role of T helper cells in activating other defence cells by secreting cytokines.

cells of the body. These abnormal cells may be ones that have become disordered, as in cancer, or cells that have been invaded by viruses. The T cells latch on to the target cell and release a protein, *pore forming protein*. The protein inserts itself into the membrane of the target cell making it leaky so that the cell swells and dies.

Suppressor T cells are the last group of T cells to be activated. They appear to inhibit the immune response and may be important in preventing the response from getting out of control.

Development of immunity

The initial encounter between lymphoctyes and an antigen usually only provokes a small response (*primary immune response*) which takes several days to develop (Fig. 15.10). The sluggishness of the response is due to the time it takes for the challenged lymphocytes to multiply and differentiate into active cells producing antibodies and cytokines.

Some of the cells formed at this initial encounter continue to circulate within the blood and tissues for years after the original challenge has subsided. If the same antigen is encountered a second time, some time later, this circulating pool of cells (*memory cells*) is ready and waiting. Consequently, the response (*secondary immune response*) is quicker and more powerful than before (Fig. 15.10). On repeated exposure the number of

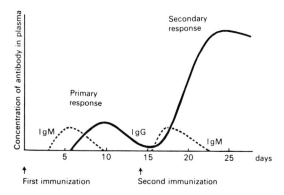

Figure 15.10
The differences in immune response between the first and the second exposure to an antigen. (Reproduced from Emslie-Smith et al (Fig. 5.9) by permission of the publishers.)

⑳

What is the difference between active and passive immunity?

cells which can specifically react against a particular antigen increases. Consequently, the immune response becomes correspondingly greater. *Immunity* has developed against that particular antigen and may swing into action speedily on any future exposure.

Immunity develops in a specific way in each individual depending on his or her exposure to antigens throughout life, and on the development of tolerance to the cells and proteins that are 'natural' to that person. Development of immunity begins in utero (see Ch. 35) and continues throughout life. ⑳

If people are exposed to bacteria or viruses which are uncommon in their natural environment, their initial defence may be inadequate to prevent illness. Thus, travellers may succumb to bacteria which are tolerated by the indigenous populations. Similarly, travellers may

import diseases which pose little or no threat at home but which are lethal in the country visited. Some protection can be conferred by *vaccination* in which a small quantity of the appropriate antigen is injected. Vaccination triggers the development of lymphocytes that can mount an attack against that antigen in the future.

SUPPORTING EVENTS

When a tissue is injured or infected many different chemicals are produced locally (Table 15.6). They originate from:

- damaged cells
- defending cells (such as macrophages and lymphocytes)
- invading cells (such as bacteria)
- plasma and interstitial fluid.

As well as influencing the activity of the defending cells they may locally:

- affect the circulation
- irritate sensory receptors
- promote tissue repair.

Circulation

Many of the chemicals released cause local vasodilation and increase capillary permeability. This improves access to the site of injury for defending cells and circulating antibodies and increases the delivery of vital nutrients necessary for the growth of new tissues.

The increased blood supply raises the temperature of the tissue, so that the inflamed area feels warm. The

Table 15.6	Chemicals produced in response to injury or infection	
Category	*Examples*	*Source*
Acute phase proteins	Fibrinogen C-reactive protein	Liver
Amines	Histamine Serotonin	Mast cells Platelets } (see Ch. 4)
Complement	$C_1–C_9$	Produced from plasma proteins secreted by the liver and macrophages
Cytokines	Interleukins Tumour necrosis factor	Activated lymphocytes and macrophages
Eicosanoids	Prostaglandins Thromboxane Leukotrienes	Many cells (see Ch. 10)
Kinins	Bradykinin	Produced from plasma proteins secreted by the liver (see Chs 4 and 10)
Lysosomal enzymes	Hydrolases	Macrophages

ALLERGIC RESPONSES

Allergy is an excessive response of the immune system to everyday substances such as house dust or pollen. Some people are unaffected by these substances but others react by having sore eyes, running nose, itching skin, sneezing and, in extreme cases, shortness of breath. Substances such as pollen have large molecules on their surfaces which are, indeed, foreign to the body (i.e. antigens). The difference in response between the allergic and non-allergic person is in the class of antibody which responds to these antigens. The 'normal' response is for the G class of antibodies (IgG) to bind and inactivate the antigen and for the other classes to play only a minor role. In the allergic person, the E class of antibodies (IgE) plays a larger role and this is at the root of the allergic response.

IgE is attached to mast cells which reside in the skin and mucous membranes of the body. When antigen binds to these cells they burst releasing histamine which is largely responsible for the symptoms of allergy. Histamine acts in several ways. It causes the muscles of the respiratory system to contract leading to shortness of breath. It causes the muscles of blood vessels to relax leading to reddening of the skin in areas where it has been released and leakage of fluid from the blood vessels producing a kind of blister called a weal. It elicits an inflammatory type of response in the tissues of the nasal passages causing soreness and excessive production of mucus. It can, in fact, be difficult to distinguish an allergic response such as hay fever from the common cold (Davies & Ollier 1989).

It is possible for people who are severely debilitated by allergy to be 'desensitised' to particular antigens by gradually exposing them to increasing doses of substances to which they are allergic. In this way, through a kind of 'immunisation' process, it is hoped to increase the amount of IgG which will respond to and bind the offending antigens, thus preventing their binding by IgE. Alternatively, the allergic person can take drugs such as antihistamines, which block the action of histamine, to lessen the symptoms of the condition.

increase in capillary permeability and the raised capillary pressure increase the formation of tissue fluid and result in swelling (see Chs 5 and 13).

Sensation

Sensory receptors that respond to noxious stimuli (*nociceptors*) (see Chs 24 and 32) are stimulated by chemicals such as histamine, prostaglandins and bradykinin (see Ch. 10). This results in discomfort ranging from an irritating itch, such as that produced by an insect bite, to pain (see Ch. 32).

The pain associated with inflammation can be reduced by inhibiting the action of the local mediators or by inhibiting their production. For example, antihistamines soothe the irritation associated with an insect bite by inhibiting the action of histamine, and aspirin reduces the pain of arthritis probably by inhibiting the synthesis of prostaglandins.

Tissue repair

Tissue repair involves:

- formation of a connective tissue scaffold
- growth of new blood vessels
- replacement of specific tissue cells.

Soon after an injury a temporary scaffold of interlacing strands of fibrin is formed which seals off blood vessels and forms a crust over the wound (see Ch. 4). This is gradually replaced by a connective tissue scaffold formed by fibroblasts (see Ch. 2). The connective tissue knits the wound together forming strong *scar tissue*, walling off the injury from uninjured areas and providing a framework to guide the growth of the specialised tissue cells. Later on, macrophages clear away some of this scaffolding. This is why scar tissue formed after surgery becomes less prominent after months or even years.

If the connective tissue completely envelops a region of inflammation, so that bacteria and defending cells are completely walled off, the result is an *abscess*.

Delivery of vital supplies to the tissue under repair is guaranteed by the growth of new capillaries (*angiogenesis*). These sprout from existing vessels. Capillary endothelial cells, stimulated by factors released

WOUND HEALING

The objective in caring for any type of wound is, at the very least, to 'do no harm'. While there is speculation that it may someday be normal practice to accelerate wound healing by the addition of growth factors it has not yet been convincingly demonstrated and it may not even be possible.

Wound healing is a precise series of physiological events which follow tissue damage (Johnson 1988). The events, some of which may overlap, begin with *inflammation*, which is an immediate and localised response to injury. Its purpose is to deal with local infection and mobilise the cells which will be required for wound healing. Following inflammation there is a phase of *proliferation* in which there is rapid growth of dermal tissue. *Remodelling* then takes place whereby the wound obtains its optimal strength by rearrangement of the collagen. Finally, and concurrently with the other phases, *epithelialisation* takes place in order to cover the wound with a new layer of epidermis.

The right environment for wound healing is one where moisture and warmth are maintained, using dressings that are occlusive or semi-occlusive. These prevent moisture loss from the surface of the wound and allow the activity of the different cell types involved in healing, for example macrophages and fibroblasts. Macrophages, in addition to scavenging debris, have a role in controlling the function of fibroblasts and, therefore, have a key position in the wound healing process (Auger 1989). The exclusion of air from a wound encourages the growth of new blood vessels by lowering the oxygen concentration at the wound surface. Otherwise, 'doing no harm' involves, basically, doing nothing to wounds.

locally, grow out from the capillary wall and penetrate the connective tissue.

New cells replace the lost specialised cells if the tissue is capable of regeneration (see Ch. 2). This is not always possible, in which case connective tissue acts as infill (*fibrosis*). As the repair is completed and scaffolding is removed many of the new capillaries regress and the redness of the scar fades.

LIPOSOLUBLE SUBSTANCES

The liposoluble substances that need to be cleared from the body come from many different sources (Table 15.7). Some, such as bilirubin, are generated by the breakdown of cells and their components whereas others are passively absorbed through epithelia such as those of the skin and digestive tract. Liposoluble substances tend to be retained in body tissues because they associate with lipids in cell membranes, and with lipophilic proteins inside cells and in the plasma (see Ch. 2). In order to be eliminated they must be degraded or made water soluble.

All cells have the potential to metabolise liposoluble substances but those having the major role are in the liver, kidneys and intestine. Of these organs, the liver is by far the most important because of its large blood flow (see Ch. 9) and high concentration of specific enzymes.

METABOLISM

Liposoluble substances are metabolised by a variety of enzyme systems located in the smooth endoplasmic reticulum (see Ch. 2). Two major systems are:

- mixed function oxidases
- conjugases.

Table 15.7   Examples of liposoluble substances for disposal

Source	Examples
Produced endogenously	Cholesterol, steroids, bilirubin, ammonia
Ingested in the diet	
– animal origin	Cholesterol, steroids
– plant origin	Tannins, alkaloids, alcohol
– smoked foods	Polycyclic hydrocarbons
Generated by bacteria	Indoles, phenol
Taken as drugs	Phenobarbitone, morphine
Absorbed through the skin	Benzene, white spirit

Mixed function oxidases

The mixed function oxidases are a group of enzymes, including one known as *cytochrome P450*, that modify molecules in a modest way by adding new parts or by altering the existing components (Fig. 15.11). The product formed is more versatile chemically than its precursor and is usually more water soluble. These minor changes may be sufficient to allow the molecule to be eliminated.

The products generated are usually less of a threat to the cells and tissues of the body than the original substance. They are said to be less *toxic*. This is because their increased water solubility makes it more difficult for them to penetrate cells and this limits their scope of activity. However, sometimes products are formed that are more potent than the original substance. The drug phenacitin for example is converted to the more potent analgesic, paracetamol. For this reason it can be misleading to refer to the general process as *detoxification*. It is mostly but not always true.

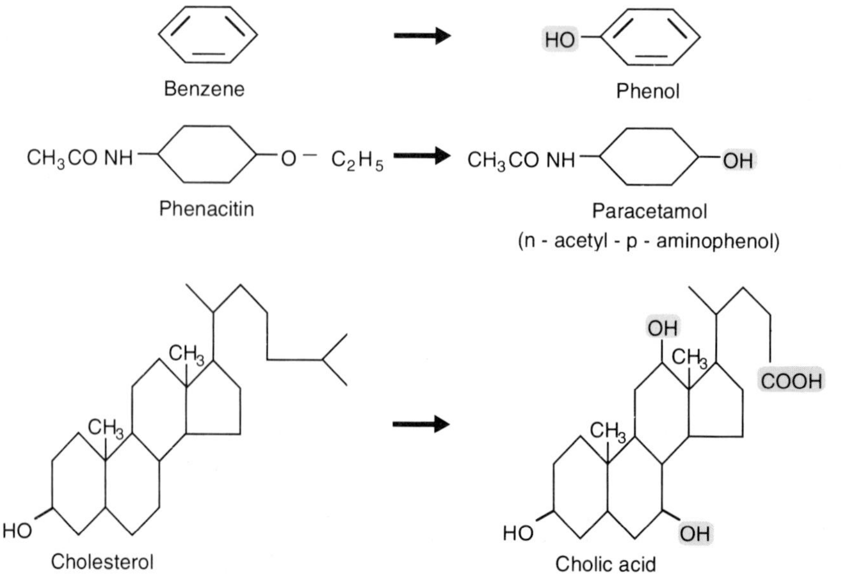

Figure 15.11
Metabolism of several substances by the mixed function oxidases. Differences between the original substance and its metabolite are highlighted. The OH (hydroxyl) and COOH (carboxyl) are polar groups. They make the molecule more water soluble (see Ch. 2).

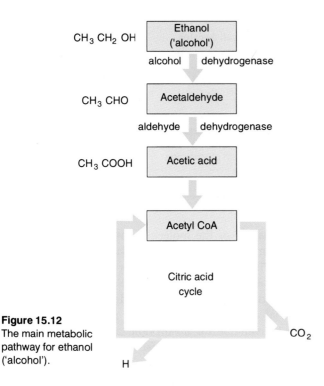

CH₃ CH₂ OH — Ethanol ('alcohol')

alcohol dehydrogenase

CH₃ CHO — Acetaldehyde

aldehyde dehydrogenase

CH₃ COOH — Acetic acid

Acetyl CoA

Citric acid cycle

CO₂

H

Figure 15.12
The main metabolic pathway for ethanol ('alcohol').

PARACETAMOL POISONING

Paracetamol is a very available analgesic. It can be bought 'across the counter' in pharmacies, supermarkets and at the corner shop. It is also incorporated into a great many other preparations. For this reason it is regularly abused by the public, sometimes in an unsuspecting way but, increasingly, deliberately. Paracetamol poisoning is one of the commonest forms of overdose (Henry & Volans 1987) and is often encountered by nurses, particularly among young girls, on medical wards and intensive care units.

Paracetamol is conjugated in the liver with glucuronic acid and most of it is metabolised in this way. A small proportion is oxidised to a reactive intermediate and this, in turn, is conjugated with glutathione before disposal via the kidneys. If too much paracetamol is present, glutathione soon becomes depleted and the reactive intermediate accumulates causing damage and death to liver cells. In fact, paracetamol poisoning is the most common cause of liver cell damage in the United Kingdom (Henry & Volans 1987). If the correct dosage for an adult of 1000 mg every 4 hours is adhered to then the liver can cope with metabolising paracetamol. If, on the other hand, an overdose is taken then the consequences are dangerous and can be fatal.

In addition to the mixed function oxidases there are a variety of other enzymes in the liver, such as *alcohol dehydrogenase* (Fig. 15.12) which also process liposoluble substances such as ethanol.

Conjugases

Conjugases link up (literally 'marry') the liposoluble compound to another molecule which is highly water soluble (Table 15.8). The product formed is much more water soluble than the original compound and is easily excreted either in the urine or in bile.

In some cases the mixed function oxidases pave the way for the conjugases to work by inserting an OH (hydroxyl) group to which the highly water-soluble substance can be linked (Fig. 15.11). Because the processing of liposoluble molecules may thus have two stages, the preliminary processing by the mixed function oxidases and other enzymes is sometimes referred to as *phase I* reactions and the conjugation reaction as *phase II*. However, not all compounds need to be processed before being conjugated. They may already posses the right chemical nature for conjugation to occur as, for example, is the case for paracetamol and for phenol (Fig. 15.11 and Table 15.8).

EXCRETION IN URINE AND BILE

The water-soluble products formed by these reactions are secreted by the cells into the interstitial fluid. They equilibrate with the plasma and are then filtered by the glomeruli of the kidney and excreted in the urine. However, products generated by the liver cells have another possible exit route, namely the digestive tract, by being secreted in bile.

Biliary excretion

The molecules excreted mainly in bile, such as the antibiotic rifampicin used in the treatment of tuberculosis, tend to be larger than those excreted in urine (Table 15.9), and chemically they are partly liposoluble and partly water soluble, (amphipathic; see Ch. 2). They are concentrated in the gall bladder along with other

Table 15.8 The marriage (conjugation) of liposoluble and water-soluble substances

Liposoluble substance	Water-soluble substance	Conjugate
Phenol	Sulphate	Phenylsulphate
Paracetamol*	Glucuronic acid	Paracetamol glucuronide
Bilirubin	Glucuronic acid	Bilirubin glucuronide
Cholic acid	Glycine	Glycocholic acid

* Strictly a trade name for n-acetyl-p-aminophenol.

Table 15.9   Chief route of excretion of some substances processed by the liver hepatocytes

Urine		*Bile*	
Substance	Molecular weight	Substance	Molecular weight
Urea	60	Glycocholic acid	466
Phenyl sulphate	174	Rifampicin	823
Paracetamol* glucuronide	328	Bilirubin glucuronide	937

* Trade name for n-acetyl-p-aminophenol.

organic constituents of bile before being expelled into the duodenum. The molecular size and water solubility of the excreted substances prevent their being reabsorbed to any significant extent either within the gall bladder or in the small intestine (see Ch. 6). Consequently, they pass on through the digestive tract and are excreted with digestive waste in the faeces.

Enterohepatic recycling

However, in the large intestine, bacteria can metabolise the excreted substances and generate products which are again more liposoluble (see Ch. 6). These products of bacterial metabolism are absorbed to a small extent by passive diffusion (see Ch. 6).

The small amounts reabsorbed pass into the venous blood from the large intestine and are returned to the liver in the hepatic portal blood. Here they are re-extracted, possibly reprocessed, and then resecreted into either the plasma (urinary excretion) or into the bile. The recycling of products between the liver and the digestive system is referred to as *enterohepatic circulation* (Fig. 15.13A). The consequences of this process for the metabolism of bilirubin are shown (Fig. 15.13B).

The greater the degree of enterohepatic recycling of a particular substance the slower is the elimination from the body. Key factors influencing the extent to which recycling occurs include:

- bacterial activity
- colonic absorption.

Bacterial activity varies with diet (see Chs 6 and 14) and is reduced by antibiotics. Colonic absorption depends on the nature of the molecules involved as well as on colonic motility and the time that residues may stay there. With a sizeable bacterial population and a slow transit of residues through the colon, recycling is promoted and excretion is reduced. Conversely if bacterial activity is decreased by antibiotics or if little time is available for absorption (as in diarrhoea) then recycling is reduced and faecal excretion is increased.

WATER-SOLUBLE SUBSTANCES

Many of the water-soluble substances to be excreted are products of metabolism (Table 15.10). Their fate depends upon their size. Very large water-soluble molecules, such as proteins, are degraded to smaller units, whereas smaller molecules are simply filtered by the kidneys and excreted in the urine.

ENDOCYTOSIS OF PROTEINS

Proteins in the plasma are removed by endocytosis by endothelial cells in some parts of the circulation, such as the liver (see Ch. 9). They are then degraded intracellularly to amino acids and the products are recycled and re-used in the synthesis of new proteins.

The enterohepatic recycling of substances can have important implications for the metabolism of drugs and other substances. For example oestrogens, as used in contraceptive pills, are partly excreted in bile and undergo some enterohepatic recycling. If a woman is given a course of antibiotics that reduce colonic bacterial activity, more oestrogen is excreted, plasma oestrogen concentrations decrease and the contraceptive power of the pill may be reduced.

Table 15.10   Water-soluble substances

Example	*Source*
Inorganic ions Na^+, K^+, Cl^-, SO_4^{2-}	Diet
Urea	Surplus amino acids
Creatinine	Muscle metabolism
Uric acid	Nucleic acid metabolism
Hippuric acid	Benzoic acid in plants (diet)
Drug metabolites	Medication/treatment
Peptides/proteins	Plasma proteins Enzymes Hormones

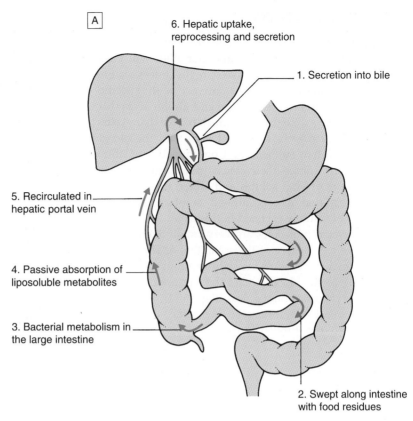

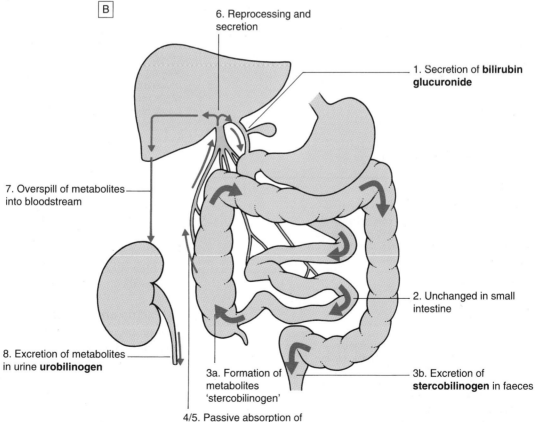

Figure 15.13
The enterohepatic circulation of
substances secreted in bile:
A Sequence of events in the circuit
B Consequences for the elimination of bilirubin glucuronide.

URINARY EXCRETION

Any water-soluble molecules that are smaller in size than the pores in the renal glomerular filter will pass through into the tubular fluid (see Ch. 8). Unless water-soluble molecules are able to interact with specific proteins in the tubules (as glucose and amino acids do) or unless, like urea, they are not much bigger than water molecules, they do not easily get back into the blood across the tubular epithelium. Consequently, as they pass along the tubule their concentration increases as large amounts of vital solutes and water are absorbed. The result is that a concentrated solution of waste products is eventually excreted in the urine.

If the excreted molecules are very small, like urea, or if they have any degree of liposolubility, as some acids and bases may have, some may diffuse from the tubular fluid back into the blood so that the amount eliminated in the urine is corresponding less (Fig. 15.14).

A few selected substances, including drugs, are excreted into the tubular fluid by specific transport mechanisms.

Urea

Urea is absorbed passively across the tubular epithelium, but the amount absorbed depends upon the urinary flow rate and especially the permeability of the collecting ducts.

If urine flow rate is low, as it is in the presence of ADH when water is being conserved (see Ch. 8), the concentration of urea in the fluid in the collecting ducts

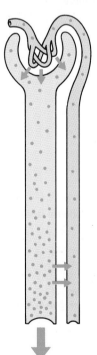

1. Urea filtered at glomerulus

2. Urea concentration in tubular fluid increases as other solutes and water are absorbed

3. Urea diffuses from tubular fluid back into the blood

4. Remaining urea excreted in the urine

Figure 15.14
Urinary excretion of small water-soluble substances such as urea.

---

will be relatively high. Consequently, the gradient for diffusion of urea back into the blood will be large and less urea is excreted. Conversely, if there is diuresis, urea is not concentrated to the same extent, the gradient for back-diffusion is low and, as a result, less urea is absorbed and more is excreted. These principles apply to any molecule filtered at the glomerulus that has similar chemical characteristics.

Weak acids and bases

The excretion of water-soluble substances that are acidic or basic in nature is influenced by the pH of the urine. This is because pH affects the amount of the substance that is present in either its dissociated or undissociated form (see Ch. 12). An acid, for example, dissociates as follows:

$$HA \rightleftharpoons H^+ + A^-$$

If the pH of the urine is low (H$^+$ concentration is high) the above equilibrium shifts in favour of the formation

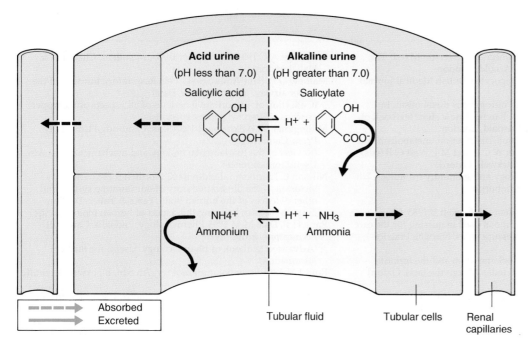

Figure 15.15
Effects of the pH of urine on the excretion of weak acids (e.g. salicylic acid) and weak bases (e.g. ammonia).

of HA and the amount of A⁻ is reduced. As the un-dissociated acid (HA) is able to diffuse across the epithelium, absorption occurs leaving just a little A⁻ in the tubular fluid to be excreted.

However, if the urine pH is high (H⁺ concentration is low) the equilibrium shifts in the opposite direction and more of the substance exists as A⁻ and less in the form of HA. As A⁻ cannot diffuse easily across the epithelium very little is absorbed and most remains in the tubular fluid and is excreted.

Thus, the urinary excretion of weak acids, such as salicylic acid in aspirin, is favoured by the formation of an alkaline urine (pH > 7) because salicylate is formed. Conversely, the excretion of weak bases, such as ammonia, is favoured by an acid urine (pH < 7) (Fig. 15.15) because ammonium is formed.

These properties can be used to good advantage should it be necessary to hasten the clearance of a drug, such as salicylate or barbiturates, from the body, as for example after an overdose. Sodium bicarbonate (hydrogen carbonate) may be used in a gastric lavage. It is absorbed in the digestive tract and excreted in the urine, making it alkaline. This promotes the elimination of any salicylate or barbiturate that remains within the body.

Thus, both urine flow rate and urine pH affect the speed with which some water-soluble substances such as drugs can be eliminated from the body. This in turn affects their plasma concentration and thus their efficacy and/or toxicity.

Tubular secretory mechanisms

Some water-soluble molecules, for example penicillin, are specifically secreted into the tubular fluid by the cells of the proximal convoluted tubules (see Ch. 8). The mechanisms appear to be similar to those involved in the biliary secretion of waste materials, except that the cells of the kidney specialise in handling low molecular weight (mol. wt. < 400) highly water-soluble molecules.

KEY POINTS

What you should now understand about the protection and defence of the body, and the disposal of redundant materials:

- how internal organs and tissues are protected against environmental hazards by the barrier functions of epithelia
- the key features contributing to the barrier functions of the skin and how these may change
- what immunity is, and how it develops and is maintained
- what is happening when tissues become inflamed
- what happens when tissues are injured
- how the body's own components are degraded, recycled and, if necessary, eliminated
- how drugs and other foreign substances (xenobiotics) are metabolised and eliminated
- what types of substances accumulate in the body in hepatic or renal failure and why
- how disturbances of the immune system can result in the proliferation of aberrant cells (cancer) or the destruction of the body's own cells (autoimmune diseases).

REFERENCES AND FURTHER READING

Alderson M 1982 The causes of cancer. In: Alderson M (ed) The prevention of cancer. Edward Arnold, London

Auger M J 1989 Mononuclear phagocytes. British Medical Journal 298: 546–548

Baron D N et al 1988 Protein and nitrogenous metabolism. In: Baron D N, Whicher J T, Lee K E (eds) A new short textbook of chemical pathology. Edward Arnold, London

Bowman W C et al 1975 Absorption, distribution, metabolism and excretion of drugs. In: Bowman W C, Rand M J, West G B (eds) Textbook of pharmacology. Blackwell, Oxford

Cooke E M 1991 Hare's Bacteriology and immunity for nurses, 7th edn. Churchill Livingstone, Edinburgh
(Clear basic text)

David J A, Chapman R G, Chapman E J, Lockett B 1983 An investigation of the current methods used in nursing for the care of patients with established pressure sores. Nursing Practice Research Unit, Harrow

Davies R, Ollier S 1989 Allergy, inflammation and the immune response. In: Davies R, Ollier S (eds) Allergy the facts. Oxford University Press, Oxford

Eley A 1992 Microbial food poisoning. Chapman & Hall, London
(What food poisoning is, what causes it and how it may be controlled)

Emslie-Smith D, Paterson C, Scratcherd T, Read N W (eds) 1988 Textbook of physiology, 11th edn. Churchill Livingstone, Edinburgh

Henry J, Volans G 1987 Analgesic poisoning: paracetamol. In: Henry J, Volans G (eds) ABC of poisoning. Part 1: drugs. British Medical Association, London

Johnson A 1988 Natural healing processes. The Professional Nurse 3(5): 149–152

Leveridge A C 1991 Therapy for the burn patient. Chapman & Hall, London

Mathew O P, Sant'Ambrogio G 1988 Respiratory function of the upper airway. Marcel Dekker, Basel
(Collection of authoritative reviews of all aspects of the upper airways written for and by specialists)

Millington P F, Wilkinson R 1983 Skin. Cambridge University Press, Cambridge
(Review of the fundamental biology and mechanics of the skin. Useful for reference)

Nilsson L, Lindberg J, Lindqvist K, Nordfelt S 1987 The body victorious – the illustrative story of our immune system and other defences of the human body. Faber & Faber, London
(Superb pictures bringing this aspect of human biology to life)

Rang H P, Dale M M 1991 Pharmacology, 2nd edn. Churchill Livingstone, Edinburgh
(Advanced textbook of pharmacology. Useful for further information)

Roitt I M 1991 Essential immunology, 7th edn. Blackwell Scientific Publications, Oxford
(Beautifully presented, advanced textbook. Useful for further information)

Thody A J, Freidman P S 1986 Scientific basis of dermatology. A physiological approach. Churchill Livingstone, Edinburgh
(Specialist text for reference)

Trounce J 1990 Clinical pharmacology for nurses, 13th edn. Churchill Livingstone, Edinburgh
(Describes the drugs commonly used in practice and how they work)

Urbach F 1983 Cancer of the skin. In: Urbach F (ed) The epidemiology of cancer. Croom Helm, London

Chapter 16
MAINTENANCE OF BODY TEMPERATURE

People live in the Arctic and in the desert. Even in less extreme climates individuals experience environmental temperatures ranging between 0°C and 28°C. We tolerate such a wide range of air temperatures simply because the inner temperature of our bodies is maintained close to 37°C by a number of temperature regulating mechanisms. These include behavioural responses, such as choice of clothes and environment which affect the gains and losses of heat by our bodies, and a variety of reflex responses, such as cutaneous vasoconstriction and sweating. If these mechanisms are inadequate for the circumstances we encounter, or are disordered, body temperature cannot be maintained and *hyperthermia* or *hypothermia* results.

BODY TEMPERATURE

Normal body temperature, measured orally in adults under comfortable environmental conditions, ranges between 36.3 and 37.1°C.

CORE AND SURFACE

Oral temperature is close to the temperature of the core of the body. The temperature of the surface of the body is almost always lower than this (Fig. 16.1). The size of the core, held at 37°C, is not constant but varies with the environmental temperature. In a cold environment the core consists just of the internal tissues and organs of the head, thorax and abdomen. The temperature of the tissues of the arms and legs is much less. Fingertips and toes are coldest of all. Under warm conditions the core expands to include most of the body.

A patient returning to the ward from theatre is sometimes found to be shivering from cold. It needs to be remembered that an operating theatre is kept relatively cool for the comfort of staff and that the patient has been lying on the operating table covered only by a thin, sterile sheet. The temperature of the surface of the patient's body will have decreased accordingly.

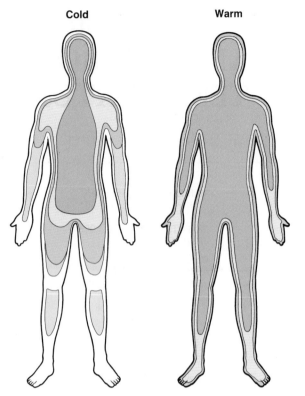

Cold   **Warm**

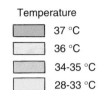

Temperature

	37 °C
	36 °C
	34-35 °C
	28-33 °C

Figure 16.1
Diagram to show how the temperature of different parts of the body varies in cold and warm environments. A central core is maintained at 37°C but the temperature of the periphery varies according to environmental temperature. (Adapted from Aschoff & Wever 1958 by permission of Springer-Verlag, Heidelberg.)

normally agree quite closely. But in a cold environment, oral temperature is probably nearest to that of the core. Oral temperature is easy to take but can be misleading if hot or cold drinks or food have been consumed shortly before body temperature is measured. Sufficient time must be allowed after a drink for the temperature of the mouth to return to that of the core. ①

HEAT BALANCE

The temperature of the core represents the balance struck between the gains and losses of heat by the body (Fig. 16.2). Many of these gains and losses are regulated by neural and hormonal control mechanisms.

① *Which patients should not have their temperatures taken orally?*

MEASUREMENT

Under warm environmental conditions body temperatures recorded in the mouth, the armpit and the rectum

---

TAKING A PATIENT'S TEMPERATURE: ROUTINE TASK OR INDIVIDUALISED CARE?

It used to be the case (and perhaps still is in some hospital wards) that towards the end of a night duty shift – at about six in the morning – all patients on a ward had their temperatures recorded. (This is a good example of task-oriented nursing, as opposed to individualised care.) Because there were only two nurses on each ward caring for about 30 patients, and because of additional tasks, the time allowed for the thermometer to remain in each patient's mouth was between 30 and 60 seconds. Consequently, every patient except the most pyrexial had a recorded early morning temperature of about 35°C. Curiously, neither the Ward Sisters nor the Consultants commented adversely on this. Trouble only arose if a recording was forgotten, and the temperature chart showed a blank. Recordings which were obviously inaccurate, even taking into account the normal early morning dip in body temperature, were apparently acceptable!

Since taking temperatures is probably one of the most frequently performed nursing tasks, it is perhaps worth asking how accurately it is done. Assuming that the nurse is able to read the mercury level correctly from a clinical thermometer, is that reading an accurate reflection of the patient's body temperature? The answer to this question will depend principally on another question: how long should the thermometer be kept in a patient's mouth (or under the axilla, or in the rectum) to attain the correct level?

In an attempt to answer the second of these questions,

a group of 12 student nurses planned and performed a small research project. They carried out a literature search and devised an experiment – using themselves as subjects – which they later wrote up for publication (Goodall 1986). The literature search revealed times (all referring to oral temperature recordings) which varied from 1 minute to as much as 20 minutes. The students found that thermometer readings in their study had ceased to rise after 7 minutes. They suggested that 4 minutes might be a suitable time to choose, from both clinical and practical viewpoints.

Whatever time is chosen, however, should be communicated to and maintained by all nurses. In this way, any variation in reading may be attributed to the patient's condition, rather than to alterations in nursing practice. Similarly, the site chosen for the thermometer should be agreed. A confused patient should not have the thermometer placed in his mouth; and even when it is placed under the axilla the nurse should be in constant attendance. Axillial readings are likely to be less accurate in the extremely thin patient, since the thermometer bulb is not in close proximity to the skin.

This brief research project, with all its limitations, not only showed the students involved the importance of the research process to nursing practice, but also demonstrated flaws in the current nursing procedures. It showed that, had this particular procedure been evaluated, such obviously inaccurate recordings could not have occurred.

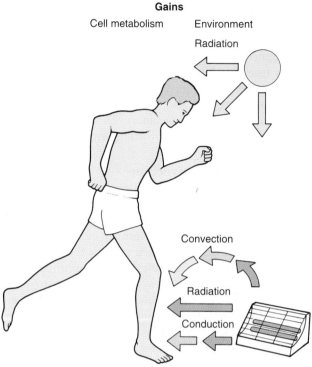

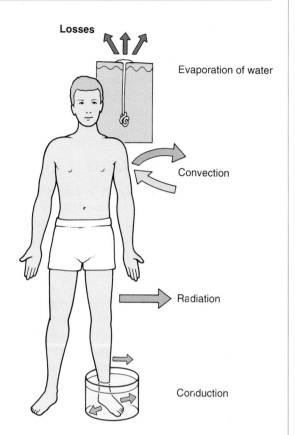

Figure 16.2
Ways in which we gain and lose heat.

HEAT GAINS

Heat is gained from:

- cellular metabolism
- the environment.

CELL METABOLISM

All cells produce heat as an incidental consequence of metabolism, but some, such as muscle cells and brown fat, play specific roles in temperature regulation.

Incidental metabolic gains

The generation of heat (*thermogenesis*) by cells is a side-product of metabolism. The metabolism of a resting individual in a comfortable environment (basal metabolic rate; see Ch. 14) creates about the same amount of heat as a light bulb (300 kJ of heat per hour ≡ 83 watts). The level of cellular activity is regulated by hormones such as thyroxine and adrenaline (see Ch. 10). ②

Any increase in the activity of a part or parts of the body, over and above the basal rate, creates more heat. Examples include:

- skeletal muscle contraction (in movement and maintenance of posture)
- secretory and absorptive activity (feeding)
- cell division and hypertrophy (growth).

Specific metabolic gains

Heat is also produced by some tissues solely for the purposes of temperature regulation. This includes heat production by:

- skeletal muscle in shivering
- other tissues including brown fat (non-shivering thermogenesis).

Shivering

In shivering, skeletal muscles are stimulated to contract involuntarily, in an uncoordinated way. The contractions are not involved in maintaining posture or controlling movement. Shivering can increase heat production by about fivefold over resting levels.

Non-shivering thermogenesis

Any other form of heat production which is not secondary to specific cell activities, and which is not associated with shivering is termed *non-shivering thermogenesis*. This is controlled by the sympathetic nervous system releasing noradrenaline. In infants and small mammals the major source of this extra heat is *brown fat*. Brown fat cells contain many small droplets of fat and mitochondria and have a very high potential for heat production. They too are innervated by noradrenergic sympathetic nerves which stimulate the cells and increase heat production. The maximum amount of heat generated is about 500 watts/kg of brown fat.

②
Which organs (not tissues) contribute most to resting heat production?

The importance of brown fat in adults is uncertain. Small amounts (about 50 g in total) are present, scattered in adipose tissue around the kidneys and heart and in between the shoulder blades. Maximal stimulation of this small amount of tissue could produce an extra 25 watts of heat (an increase of almost 30% above basal levels).

ENVIRONMENTAL GAINS

In addition to the heat which is internally generated, heat is gained from the surrounding environment by radiation, conduction and convection and, to a small extent, by conduction through the ingestion of hot drinks and foods.

Radiant energy

Radiant energy is electromagnetic energy released from an object or body and beamed to surrounding objects (Fig. 16.3). It excites the objects which absorb it and increases their energy and, therefore, their heat. In turn, these hot objects radiate electromagnetic energy at a lower level to objects in their surroundings.

We receive much radiant energy from the sun so that, even when the temperature of the air is cold, we are warmed by the sun's energy. It is this which enables skiers to sunbathe in the snow, *and* to become severely sunburnt.

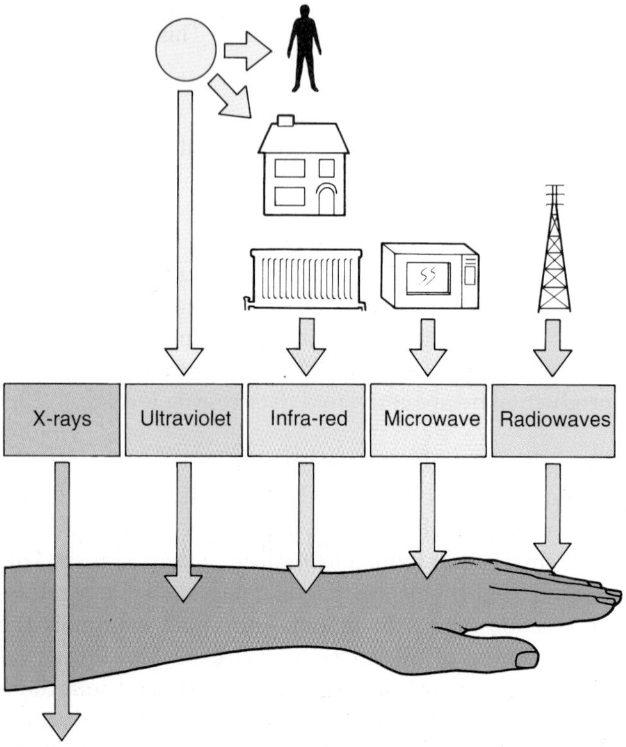

The sun's radiant energy is short wavelength (ultraviolet range). Pale skin absorbs only half as much of this as a very dark highly pigmented skin, but in dark skin the pigment *melanin* absorbs much of the ultraviolet energy (see Ch. 15) and reduces the amount of radiation which reaches and heats deeper tissues.

Radiant energy is also derived from other sources around us such as hot machinery. This can significantly influence the comfort of the working environment.

Conduction and convection

In *conduction*, energy is passed on from one molecule to the next, rather like a ripple of excitement passing through a crowd of people. In *convection*, molecules of air or water that have been warmed by contact with a hot object move away and their place is taken by cooler molecules. A flow of molecules (*convection current*) is set up. The warmed molecules take their heat to other objects and the cooler molecules which replace them are warmed up in their turn.

Whenever the temperature of the environment (air, water or hot object) is greater than the temperature of the surface of your body (outer clothing, hair and exposed skin), you will gain heat by conduction and convection.

Air is not a very good conductor of heat. Convection currents, caused for example by an electric fire within a room, and radiant heat are usually more important in delivering heat through the air to our bodies. Gains by conduction are, however, much greater from hot objects in contact with our bodies, such as a hot water bottle or a mug of tea. ③

③
Many elderly people use a hot water bottle in bed. In hospitals, however, this practice is not allowed. How would you explain to a patient that she cannot be provided with a hot water bottle at night? What reason would you give, and what alternatives might be offered?

Figure 16.3
Radiant energy: sources, types and relative extents of tissue penetration.

HEAT LOSSES

We lose heat from our bodies (Fig. 16.2) by:

- conduction, convection and radiation
- using it to evaporate water.

CONDUCTION, CONVECTION AND RADIATION

Whenever the temperature of the outer surface of our bodies (skin or clothing) is greater than that of the environment we lose heat by conduction, convection and radiation. The amount of heat lost depends on:

- the body surface – temperature and area
- the environment – air or water.

Losses of heat from key organs such as the brain and heart are minimised by the insulation provided by the tissues around them.

Body surface

Temperature

The bigger the temperature difference between the surface and the environment the greater is the heat loss. If you lower the temperature of the surface, for example by wearing clothing that does not pick up heat very easily from your body, you reduce heat loss and *insulate* the body core. Conversely, if the temperature of exposed skin is raised by cutaneous vasodilation, bringing warm blood close to the surface, then losses increase. ④

Surface area

The larger the surface area of your body in relation to your mass of metabolically active cells and tissues, the greater is your heat loss. If you are tall you will lose slightly more heat than someone else of the same weight who is shorter and stouter (Fig. 16.4). A tall person, particularly one who is thin and lacks insulation (see p. 303), needs to generate more heat in order to maintain body temperature than someone who is short and fat.

Environment

Air

Air is not a very good conductor of heat and therefore losses by conduction are normally very small. We lose much more heat by convection and this is greatly increased by draughts and wind.

Losses of heat by radiation are determined by the temperature of the body surface and the temperature of

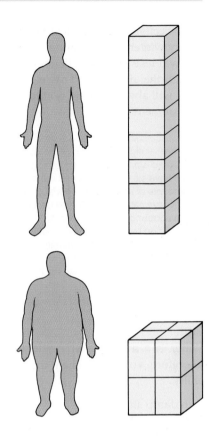

Figure 16.4
For the same total mass of tissue, surface area is greater for a tall thin object compared with a short squat one. Each of the objects on the right of the Figure is built from eight cubes of equal size. Calculate the total surface area of each object and compare your answers.

④ A sip of whisky or brandy when we are cold may well give us rosy cheeks and make us feel warmer. But why is a drink of spirits not to be recommended for someone feeling chilled, or suffering from hypothermia?

ACCIDENTAL HYPOTHERMIA IN MOUNTAIN CLIMBING

Hospitals in mountainous regions of Britain are well accustomed to treating casualties suffering from hypothermia or exposure. This is a condition which, it should be emphasised, can occur in temperatures above freezing as well as below. It more often affects the young, for example members of school parties, than the well-equipped and experienced mountaineer.

In the valleys, the sun may be shining and a gentle breeze blowing so that a light sweater seems adequate protection against the elements. But, for every 500 feet climbed, the still air temperature falls by 1°C so that, for example, there is a difference of 8°C between Fort William and the summit of Ben Nevis. More significant to the hill walker, however, is the wind chill factor. On a mountain top, in cold still air in the sunshine, a person can sit comfortably in shirt sleeves. A moderate wind, however, will greatly reduce the apparent temperature.

Heat loss from the unprotected or ill-protected body to the air is by conduction and convection. Conduction transfers heat from the skin to clothing and the surrounding air; convection disperses heat from around the body into the atmosphere. The higher the wind speed and the less effective the protection provided by clothing (and the wetter that clothing is), the greater is the loss of heat.

Mountain rescuers stress that exposure is more likely when the climber is tired and frightened. After a hard physical climb, the body's energy stores are diminished and, if high energy replacement is not available (chocolate, hot sweet drinks or glucose tablets), the risk of hypothermia is increased. Symptoms include dizziness, weakness, blurring of vision, feeling cold and, perhaps, muscle cramps. Clinical signs which may be observed by the climber's companions could be stumbling, slow responses to questions and irrational behaviour such as sudden irritation or loss of temper.

First-aid treatment consists of:

- resting the victim out of the wind (this may involve seeking shelter behind a boulder or constructing a stone windbreak)
- placing him in a sleeping bag, preferably with a healthy member of the party
- reducing his anxiety by reassurance
- providing hot fluids and food.

Unless the casualty responds well to this first-aid treatment, he should be evacuated from the mountain on a stretcher. All these measures, of course, presuppose experience and appropriate equipment. Sadly, exposure most often strikes members of parties that are ill-prepared and do not have hot drinks, high energy foods and warm sleeping bags.

the object(s) to which heat is being radiated. If, on a snowy winter's day, you are seated alongside a window you will lose heat by radiation to the snow outside even though the air temperature in the room is warm. A hot body will always radiate heat to other cold objects in the environment.

> A familiar sight at the end of the London Marathon is of massed runners, all wearing shiny space blankets. They will have exercised hard and will be radiating increased amounts of heat from the surface of their bodies. The highly reflective nature of the space blanket limits loss of heat to the surrounding air (which may be comparatively cool, the Marathon being run in April). Despite their light weight, these blankets are an extremely good protection against heat loss; they can be used in mountaineering, in ambulances and in nursing the hypothermia victim in hospital.

Water

Water is a much better conductor of heat than is air. Therefore you lose much more heat and easily feel chilly:

- in damp air
- wearing wet clothes
- immersed in water.

It has been calculated that the minimum water temperature at which it is possible to generate sufficient heat by metabolism (mainly through shivering) to match heat loss is about 24°C. Water temperatures below this cannot be tolerated for more than a few hours and core body temperature eventually decreases (Fig. 16.5). The colder the water the more rapidly hypothermia occurs. At 0°C it takes only a few minutes (15 at most). The decrease in core temperature happens even more quickly, particularly if you are lean, when you move

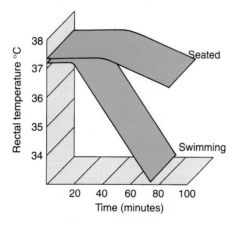

Figure 16.5
Changes in core temperature in a lean person sitting immersed in a bath of cool water (16°C), and swimming in water at 16°C. (Adapted from Pugh & Edholm 1955.)

> ### REWARMING THE CORE TEMPERATURE IN MOUNTAIN RESCUE
>
> Rewarming victims of hypothermia in mountaineering accidents, just like rewarming people rescued from the sea, is not simply a question of applying as much heat as possible as quickly as possible. *Gradual* warming is the key – along with prevention of further heat loss – so that blood from the body core is not transferred to the skin surface too quickly.
>
> A relatively new method of rewarming the body core is the use of heated, humidified oxygen (or air) supplied through a face mask. With this equipment, which is portable, the deep tissues of the lungs, and thus the major vessels of the chest and neck, are warmed. (To appreciate the effectiveness of this method, consider which vessels return blood to the heart from the lungs, and how that blood is then pumped to the thorax, neck and head.) This method is of use only in conjunction with effective methods of preventing further heat loss from the victim's body.

around in the water or swim (Fig. 16.5). By moving, you increase convective losses of heat and you also raise skin temperature by increasing the flow of warm blood to the active muscles. Shivering does not increase muscle blood flow to the same extent.

Care needs to be exercised in rewarming someone who has been rescued from very cold water. This must be done slowly. Rapid heating only really warms the surface (like defrosting a chicken too quickly) and may in fact cool the core by causing blood to be diverted from the core to the surface when the skin blood vessels dilate.

Insulation

The core of the body is shielded from the environment by two forms of insulation:

- clothing (and bedding)
- tissues forming the outer shell.

Both forms of insulation are adjusted, according to the environmental conditions, by behavioural and autonomic reflexes respectively.

Clothing and bedding

The insulation offered by different types of clothing is illustrated in Figure 16.6. It is scaled in units of *clo*. Really warm comfortable clothes (and bedding) are those that trap a lot of air between different layers and among the fibres of which they are made. The fibres conduct heat but the air, being poorly conducting and immobile, acts as an effective insulator.

If, however, the same clothes (or bedding) become wet, for example through perspiration, rain or incontinence, then their insulating effect is considerably reduced because water is such a good conductor of heat.

Tissues as insulators

Natural insulation of the body core is provided by the shell of tissues surrounding it.

The depth of this shell depends mainly on the distribution of blood flow between the superficial and the deeper layers of tissue. It is also affected by the amount of subcutaneous fat. People who are fat are somewhat better insulated than those who are lean.

The distribution of blood flow between superficial and deeper layers is controlled by the sympathetic nervous system. If warm blood is diverted away from the superficial vessels of the skin to the deeper vessels below, the depth of the layer of natural insulation increases, and vice versa. Thus, when you are cold, vasoconstriction occurs in cutaneous blood vessels. This reduces cutaneous blood flow, cools the surface of the body and helps to retain heat within the core.

Cutaneous arteries and veins are richly supplied with $alpha_2$ receptors (see Ch. 3). These receptors are unusual in that when they are cooled their vasoconstrictor effect, triggered by sympathetic stimulation, is enhanced. In other blood vessels, in which $alpha_1$ receptors predominate, cooling causes vasodilation.

In Raynaud's disease, a condition in which fingers and toes turn blue or white very easily in response to cold, it has been found that the proportion of $alpha_2$ to $alpha_1$ receptors in skin blood vessels is greater than normal. This may explain why the vasoconstrictor responses are triggered so easily (Flavahan 1991).

A great deal of heat may be lost via the limbs. This is because their surface area is very large in comparison with their mass. The particular arrangement of blood vessels in the limbs (Fig. 16.7) allows blood to be brought to the surface vessels or to be diverted to deeper veins according to need.

EVAPORATION OF WATER

Heat is also lost from the body as a result of the energy used up in evaporating water. The amount of water evaporated (and therefore heat lost) depends on:

- the humidity of the air
- the airflow over the surface.

If the atmosphere is dry evaporative losses of water increase but, if the atmosphere is humid (contains a lot

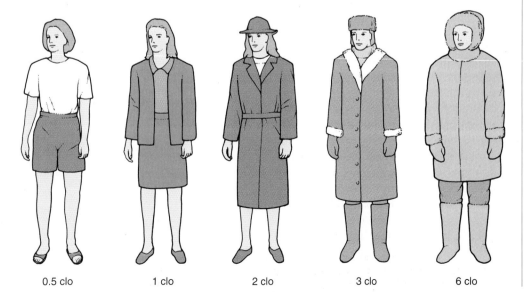

Figure 16.6
Approximate amounts of insulation provided by different types of clothing. The unit of measurement for insulation is the clo. (Adapted from Aucliems & Hare 1973.)

| 0.5 clo | 1 clo | 2 clo | 3 clo | 6 clo |

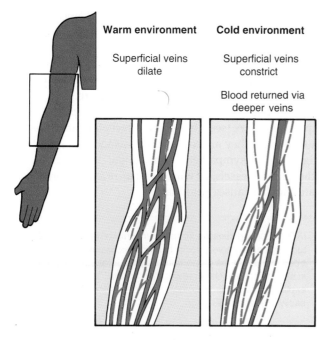

Figure 16.7
Arrangement of blood vessels in the forearm showing how blood may be brought to superficial layers or diverted to deeper veins according to environmental temperature. (Adapted from Emslie-Smith et al 1988, based on Krog 1974.)

of water vapour already), losses are less. In a dry atmosphere the evaporation of water from the surface of the body is enhanced by a breeze. This sweeps away the air that is saturated with water vapour and replaces it with dryer air.

The sources of the water for evaporation are:

● incidental
  – water content of skin
  – wet clothing/bedding
● specific
  – fluid secreted by sweat glands.

Incidental losses

Water normally evaporates continually from the surface of the skin (0.5 litres per day) and from the respiratory tract (0.4 litres per day). Losses of heat by incidental evaporation of water are increased enormously if you are wearing damp or wet clothes, or if you have just stepped, wet and dripping, out of the shower or bath.

Losses increase if there are draughts or if it is windy when you are outdoors. Similarly, more water and heat are lost from the respiratory tract when you ventilate your lungs more as, for example, when running.

Specific losses: sweating

Water is secreted on to the surface of the skin by sweat glands (see Ch. 15). These are widely distributed over the body. When maximally active they can secrete up to

Normally when we breathe, the air we take in is warmed and moistened by its passage through the nose or mouth. (Think of the blood supply to the membranes lining the nose.) When a patient is ventilated via an endotracheal tube (which delivers air to the trachea, near the bifurcation of the two main bronchi) the air supply needs to be both humidified and warmed because the upper respiratory passages have been bypassed.

When a patient is breathing through a tracheostomy, the incoming air similarly bypasses the upper respiratory tract and is prevented from picking up moisture. It is very important, therefore, that a means of humidifying air is provided, especially in the days soon after tracheostomy formation when secretions need to be aspirated by suction catheter. If humidification is not adequate, these secretions become dry and crusted and are difficult to remove.

about 2 litres of fluid per hour. The composition of the fluid secreted varies with flow rate (Table 16.1) but the total concentration of solutes is usually less than that in plasma, so sweat is normally hypotonic. The fluid formed by the cells at the base of the gland is similar to interstitial fluid but it changes in composition as it passes through the duct. Some sodium chloride is reabsorbed, unaccompanied by water, and so the fluid becomes dilute (Fig. 16.8).

Heat can be lost by sweating only if the water secreted can evaporate. When the air is fully saturated with water vapour (very humid) this cannot happen and so there is no heat loss even though sweating may be profuse.

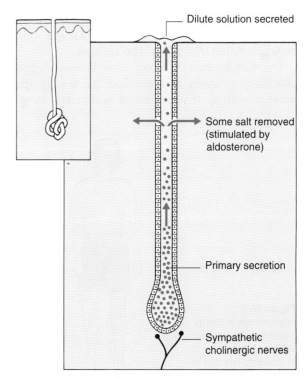

Figure 16.8
How sweat is formed and its secretion controlled.

Table 16.1   Composition of sweat (mmol/l)

	Slow flow	Fast flow
Sodium	20	100
Potassium	4	4
Chloride	20	80

Our environmental comfort depends not just on the temperature, but on the humidity of the climate. Tourists often claim that a Mediterranean summer is more comfortable than a warm British one, because in Britain humidity is usually high. Dry heat is more comfortable because we are able to lose heat by the evaporation of moisture from the skin. In a very humid atmosphere, sweat is less likely to evaporate and we feel 'sticky'.

The sweat glands are innervated by sympathetic nerves (see Ch. 3), but these are cholinergic (secrete acetylcholine) rather than adrenergic (secrete noradrenaline). Blood flow to the glands increases when they are active, due, it is thought, to the local vasodilator effect of bradykinin (see Ch. 10).

Figure 16.9
Central role of the hypothalamus in the control of core temperature.

CONTROL

MAINTAINING BODY TEMPERATURE

Core temperature is maintained close to 37°C by effector mechanisms coordinated by the hypothalamus. These effector mechanisms adjust the gains and losses of heat in response to signals from sensory receptors monitoring the temperatures of the core and the surface of the body (Fig. 16.9).

Effector mechanisms

Hot environment

In a hot environment which threatens to raise body temperature above normal (*hyperthermia*), heat balance is maintained by reducing the gain of heat as far as possible, while at the same time increasing the amounts of heat lost. Thus, in a hot environment, heat gain can be reduced by:

- minimising activity (movement, feeding etc.)
- shading the body by choice of clothes or shelter.

Simultaneously, losses of heat can be increased by:

- cutaneous vasodilation (bringing heat from the core to the surface)
- choosing circumstances which lead to surface cooling (cold shower, fan)
- sweating.

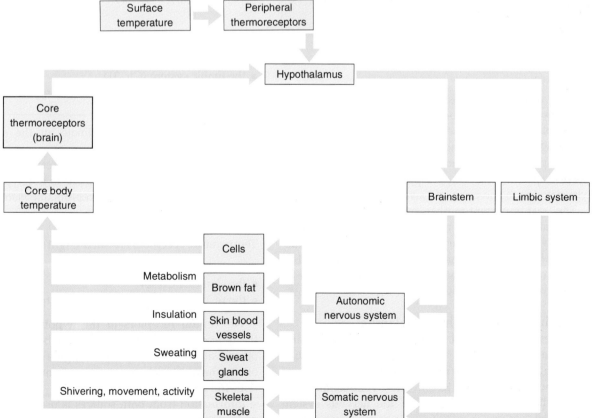

Cold environment

Conversely, in a cold environment, which threatens to reduce body temperature below normal (*hypothermia*), balance is maintained by increasing the production of heat, and by minimising losses. Thus, the production of heat can be increased by:

- shivering
- stimulating metabolism (non-shivering thermogenesis)
- increasing appetite and physical activity.

Simultaneously, losses of heat are reduced by:

- cutaneous vasoconstriction (increases insulation of the core)
- putting on clothing (increases insulation of the body)
- choosing a warmer place to be!

Altering one's environmental conditions to increase or decrease heat loss is not a measure open to the newly born infant, the young child, the unconscious and some disabled, elderly or mentally handicapped people. Such individuals have to rely on the response of other people. A paralysed person may not be able to reach for another sweater, or discard the one he is wearing. A mentally handicapped man living in the community may not think of taking a cold drink or switching on a heater unless someone reminds him. We need to remember that actions which for us are almost automatic can be impossible for others, the most vulnerable in our society.

Q: What are the particular problems – physiological and social – faced by the elderly in coping with changes in environmental temperature?

Relative importance

Of the various mechanisms listed above arguably the most important ones for us are those affecting our behaviour. We control the microclimate of our bodies by choosing our clothing and activities, and by controlling the temperature of our homes and places of work. And we are motivated to do this partly by the discomfort associated with shivering and sweating.

The least important mechanisms for us are those that specifically control cell metabolism. In response to a cold environment we barely increase our heat production in this way, unlike small mammals, such as gerbils and hamsters, which produce large amounts of heat by non-shivering thermogenesis.

Coordinating centre: hypothalamus

All these physiological responses are driven and coordinated by specific clusters of cells (*temperature regulating centres*) in the preoptic and anterior parts of the hypothalamus (Fig. 16.10). The hypothalamus has links with several other parts of the nervous system including:

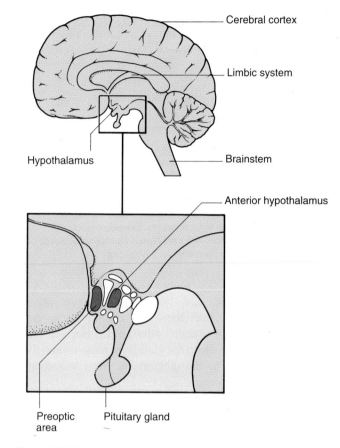

Figure 16.10
Position of the temperature regulating centres within the brain.

- the autonomic nervous system and the pituitary gland (Chs 3 and 10)
- the limbic system (Ch. 31)
- the parts of the brain stem controlling muscle contraction (Ch. 28).

It is therefore able to coordinate all the autonomic, hormonal and behavioural responses.

Information about the temperatures of the core and the surface of the body is supplied to the hypothalamus by a variety of temperature receptors (*thermoreceptors*).

Thermoreceptors

Temperature receptors are sited (Fig. 16.11) in:

- the hypothalamus
- the skin (see Ch. 24)
- the respiratory and gastrointestinal tracts.

The central receptors in the hypothalamus monitor the temperature of the 'core' of the body, whereas the others, situated in the periphery, give advance warning of any threat to body temperature from the environment (Fig. 16.11).

Information from both sources is used to regulate the various mechanisms which control heat gain and loss.

In general, a change in core temperature activates sweating or shivering whereas alterations in skin temperature provoke changes in cutaneous blood flow.

MAINTAINING COMFORT

People living in sophisticated technological societies have become increasingly reliant on technology to maintain heat balance and less reliant on intrinsic mechanisms of temperature control. Individuals who lose the opportunity to regulate their personal environment and their activities, through illness, injury or disability, have to rely on intrinsic mechanisms of temperature control (chiefly, control of cutaneous blood flow, shivering and sweating) to maintain heat balance. Body temperature can be maintained within safe limits by shivering when you are cold and sweating when you are hot but only at the cost of some discomfort.

Thermoneutral zone

A comfortable environment can be defined as one in which body temperature can be maintained without recourse to shivering or sweating and without extreme vasoconstriction or vasodilation. The range of environmental temperatures over which neither increased heat production nor increased evaporative loss is used to maintain temperature is termed the *thermoneutral zone* (Fig. 16.12). Within it, the effects of small fluctuations in environmental temperature can be compensated simply by changes in skin blood flow. The thermoneutral zone for someone wearing a lightweight suit (1 clo) in a temperate climate is around 18 to 22°C and for a naked person is 26 to 30°C. Skin temperature under these conditions is about 33°C.

In water the thermoneutral zone is exceedingly narrow and high (around 36°C). Below this, body temperature can only be maintained by shivering.

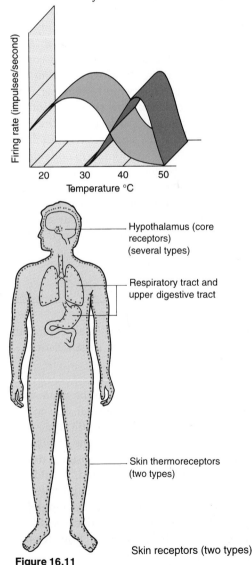

Figure 16.11
Thermoreceptors: distribution and types. The graph shows the way in which skin receptors respond to a change in temperature. (Adapted from Kenshalo 1976.)

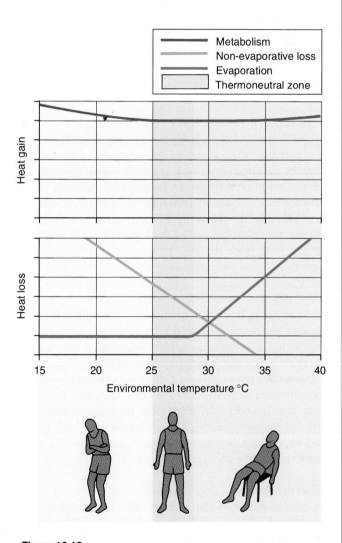

Figure 16.12
The thermoneutral zone. Gains and losses of heat at different environmental temperatures in someone wearing vest and shorts. (Adapted from Gagge et al 1938.)

EFFECTS OF ALTERED BODY TEMPERATURE

CORE TEMPERATURE

Hypothermia

The first part of the body to become significantly disordered when the core temperature falls is the nervous system. At first a person becomes unresponsive, sluggish and confused. Below a core temperature of 33 to 35°C thermoregulatory mechanisms themselves become increasingly ineffective and the rate of fall of temperature is accelerated. Below 30°C consciousness is lost. As the temperature continues to fall cardiac function becomes disordered, cardiac arrhythmias occur and eventually death is caused by ventricular fibrillation. On average 25°C is the lowest survivable core temperature for an adult.

> The normal clinical thermometer does not provide an accurate reading for the patient whose body temperature is below 35°C. Special low-reading thermometers should be used.

Hyperthermia

Hyperthermia threatens body function in at least two ways. It affects the structure and activity of proteins and thereby disturbs many aspects of cell metabolism. It also creates additional threats to homeostasis because of the effector mechanisms used to regulate body temperature. For example the lowering of peripheral resistance by cutaneous vasodilation and the losses of water and salts in sweating both threaten blood pressure (see Chs 11 and 13).

Heat stroke

In heat stroke there is a runaway, potentially lethal rise in core temperature. This occurs when the temperature regulating mechanisms fail or when they are unable to cope with the conditions encountered. Once core temperature rises above 41°C the temperature regulating system itself becomes less effective and core temperature rises rapidly. An additional problem is posed by the fact that cell metabolism is stimulated by an increase in temperature. So, the more heat is produced the more the temperature goes up (see Fig. 19.8).

Heat exhaustion

In heat exhaustion the problem created is the loss of water and salts caused by profuse sweating. The loss of water causes dehydration. The loss of salt decreases the volume of the extracellular fluid even more. Blood volume decreases and this threatens blood pressure (see Ch. 13).

> Heat exhaustion is a common problem with marathon runners. Such people need to take in plenty of fluids throughout the race, but the type of fluid is important and drinks with specific levels of electrolytes are manufactured. Sodium as well as water is lost in sweat and so both need to be replaced. (Bursztyn 1990)
>
> **Q**: What is the electrolyte composition of manufactured 'sports' drinks, and how do they compare with body fluids?

Pyrexia (fever)

Substances produced by invading organisms such as bacteria and viruses (*exogenous pyrogens*) and by various cells including active leucocytes (*endogenous pyrogens*) alter the sensitivity of parts of the temperature regulating system. They may act by increasing the production of prostaglandins in the hypothalamus (see Ch. 10).

In the presence of pyrogens, heat gain and conservation (shivering and cutaneous vasoconstriction) are activated at higher core temperatures than usual. As a result more heat is produced and retained and consequently core temperature rises. Paradoxically, you feel cold even though your core temperature is rising. This may be partly due to the decrease in skin temperature caused by vasoconstriction and partly due to the way the cerebral cortex interprets the signals it receives from the hypothalamus (see Ch. 23).

When the infection subsides, the responsiveness of the temperature regulating system returns to normal. The raised core temperature now activates heat loss mechanisms. Sweating and vasodilation occur and the individual feels 'hot', even though body temperature is now falling.

PERIPHERY

Local effects of cold

The immediate effects of cold are local cutaneous vasoconstriction and decreased cellular metabolism.

Skin colour

If vasoconstriction is intense the skin will be white (in a fair skinned person) or paler than normal due to the lack of blood in the capillaries. If there is still some flow albeit small, or if blood has stagnated in the capillaries, the skin is likely to have a bluish or greyish tinge due to the presence of deoxygenated haemoglobin. A cold red skin indicates that there is blood in the capillaries but not much oxygen is being removed from haemoglobin. Less oxygen is being used because of the decreased level of metabolism and less is being released from haemoglobin (see Ch. 7).

Freezing temperatures

If skin temperature remains close to or below freezing,

CARE OF THE PYREXIAL PATIENT

Nursing measures in the care of the pyrexial patient are designed both to reduce temperature and to increase comfort.

A pyrexia of up to 38.5°C (low grade pyrexia) may be treated by reducing the amount of bedclothes, ensuring adequate ventilation in the room and encouraging fluid intake. If the pyrexia is caused by an infection, appropriate antibiotics may be prescribed. Cool washes will refresh the patient, but should largely be carried out by the nurse since muscular activity by the patient will only help to maintain his high temperature. He will be encouraged to remain on bed rest for the same reason.

Where the patient's temperature rises above 39°C, or even above 40°C (hyperpyrexia), a procedure called tepid sponging may be carried out. In some hospitals this is medically prescribed while, in others, nurses may institute such treatment if they feel it is required. The principle of tepid sponging is that body temperature is reduced by a *specified amount* within a *specified time*, for example 1°C in 1 hour. This means that the patient's temperature must be recorded both before and after the procedure.

Sponges or cloths are soaked in water at 33 to 35°C and placed on the patient's exposed body; the body heat then evaporates the water. It is important that the patient's temperature is not reduced so swiftly as to cause shivering (which would cause a rise in body temperature).

Drugs such as aspirin may be used to reduce pyrexia, if they are not contraindicated for any other reason. Aspirin, an antipyretic which inhibits the synthesis of prostaglandins, is believed to act on the hypothalamus, resetting its temperature sensitivity to a normal level.

A patient's pyrexia is telling the nurse that there is an infection or an inflammatory response. It therefore needs investigation to identify the cause. Patients, about 2 days after myocardial infarction, usually show a mild pyrexia caused by the inflamed, damaged area of heart muscle. An infant who appears flushed and distressed requires medical attention; he may have a cold, but other possibilities include otitis media. If a patient has a temperature of 39°C shortly after urethral catheterisation, what may have happened? What nursing interventions may be needed?

FROSTBITE

Frostbite is *localised freezing* of peripheral parts of the body, usually the fingers, toes, ears and nose. This is in contrast to the generalised body cooling in hypothermia. Frostbite can occur in British winter mountaineering, but is more likely in the Alps and Himalayas where temperatures are much lower. White, waxy tips of ears, nose or fingers is the typical appearance of superficial frostbite. If pain or tingling can be felt in the affected parts, nerves are still undamaged but blister formation and skin loss can occur (Steele 1988). With deep frostbite, gangrene (tissue death) can set in and toes and fingers may be lost.

Prevention is essential, since the full effects of frostbite cannot be cured – only amputated. Hands, ears and much of the face can be protected by a balaclava helmet; toes should be encased in dry woollen socks and well-fitting boots. (Boots which are too tight can restrict blood flow to the already chilled extremities leading to gangrene.)

A discredited method of treating frostbite is to rub the affected parts with snow. (Arthur Ransome, the children's author, has one of his characters – a doctor, too – give this advice in *Winter Holiday*.) It is now known that the sharp snow crystals will damage the skin, which is already at risk from a diminished blood supply.

Unlike the gradual rewarming of the whole body suffering from exposure or hypothermia, frostbitten toes and fingers should be warmed quickly. The longer cells are frozen, the greater the likelihood of permanent tissue damage. The first aider should be aware that rewarming of affected limbs may cause the victim severe pain. (Why should this be? See Ch. 32.)

Q: High altitude mountaineers are more likely to suffer from frostbite because of the much lower temperatures they experience. What other physiological challenges might contribute to cell death at high altitudes?

skin heals more rapidly than cold skin. Vasodilation improves the delivery of nutrients, oxygen and defence cells to the tissues.

Injury

Too much heat, however, damages cells. It irreversibly alters the structure of proteins (*denatures* them). Damaged cells release intracellular constituents which in turn provoke vasodilation, increase capillary permeability and attract leucocytes (see Ch. 15).

Damage can be caused by radiant heat or by contact with a heat source. The amount of heat transferred depends on the temperature of the heat source and the contact time. Many a burn, which might have been caused by touching a hot oven or plate, has been successfully avoided by plunging the affected hand immediately under a stream of cold water. The swift cooling of tissues rapidly withdraws heat and minimises tissue injury.

periods of intense vasoconstriction may alternate with brief interludes of increased flow. It is thought that the cold reduces the effectiveness of the vasoconstrictor mechanism and the vascular smooth muscle periodically relaxes.

Whether freezing occurs or not, exposure to cold can of itself cause tissue injury. Although the cause of the injury is not fully understood the release of substances locally from disrupted cells and tissues may be involved. Blood vessels and nerve endings are most affected.

Local effects of heat

Benefits

Heat increases cellular metabolism, and speeds the replication and differentiation of cells (see Ch. 2). Warm

KEY POINTS

What you should now understand about body temperature and its regulation:

- how body temperature is measured and the precautions necessary to obtain a reliable reading
- the principal ways in which heat is gained by and lost from the body
- the various mechanisms involved in the regulation of body temperature and their relative importance
- why different forms of clothing and bedding vary in their thermal comfort
- why popular activities such as hill walking and water sports can pose grave threats to the maintenance of body temperature
- why people who have limited control over their environment are at special risk of hypothermia and hyperthermia
- why the onset of a fever is characterised by feeling cold, and recovery from it by feeling hot
- what happens to cells, tissues and body systems when body temperature is raised or lowered.

REFERENCES AND FURTHER READING

Aschoff J, Wever R 1958 Kern und Schale in warmehaushalt des Menschen. Naturwissenschaften 45: 481

Aucliems A, Hare A F 1973 Visual presentation of weather forecasting for personal comfort. Weather 28: 478

Boore J, Champion R, Ferguson M (eds) 1987 Nursing the physically ill adult. Churchill Livingstone, Edinburgh, p 889–90

Bursztyn P 1990 Physiology for sportspeople. Manchester University Press, Manchester, p 184–191

Clark R P, Edholm O G 1985 Man and his thermal environment. Edward Arnold, London
(Specialist book for reference. Includes colour plates showing variations in skin temperature from head to toe in different circumstances)

Emslie-Smith D et al 1988 Thermoregulation. In: Emslie-Smith D, Paterson C R, Scratcherd T, Read N W (eds) Textbook of physiology, 11th edn. Churchill Livingstone, Edinburgh, ch 41
(Useful source of further information)

Flavahan N A 1991 The role of the vascular α_2 adrenoreceptors as cutaneous thermosensors. News in Physiological Sciences 6: 251–255

Gagge A P, Winslow C-E A, Herrington P 1938 The influence of clothing on the physiological reactions of the human body to varying environmental temperatures. American Journal of Physiology 124: 30

Garland H O 1985 Altered temperature. In: Case R M (ed) Variations in human physiology. Manchester University Press, Manchester
(Useful source of information on the effects of high and low environmental temperatures on body function)

Goodall C J 1986 Heat trials. Nursing Times 84(32): 62–63

Kenshalo D R 1976 Correlations of temperature sensitivity in man and monkey. In: Zotterman Y (ed) Sensory functions of the skin in primates. Pergamon Press, Oxford, p 309

Khogali M, Hales J R S 1984 Heat stroke and temperature regulation. Academic Press, London

Krog J 1974 Peripheral circulatory adjustments to cold. In: Borg A, Veghte J H (eds) The physiology of cold weather survival. NATO: Agard Report No: 620, p 12

Lloyd E L 1986 Hypothermia and cold stress. Croom Helm, Beckenham
(Practical, detailed and interesting book covering the prevention, treatment and effects of cold stress under a variety of conditions)

Moffat G 1964 Two star red. Hodder & Stoughton, London

Pugh L G C, Edholm O G 1955 The physiology of channel swimmers. Lancet 2: 763

Steele P 1988 Medical handbook for mountaineers. Constable, London

Vallotton J, Dubas F (eds) 1991 A colour atlas of mountain medicine. Wolfe Publishing, London

Part C
DIFFERENT BODY STATES

As we go about our daily activities, all systems continually readjust in order to maintain appropriate conditions inside the body. Indeed, readjustment happens to some extent in advance of a change in our activities, on the basis of past routine. If systems are faulty, as a result of injury or disease, or if the circumstances we face are beyond our normal capacity, the right internal conditions are not maintained and we become ill.

The chapters in this part:

- focus on the body as a whole
- look at the meaning of homeostasis in health and illness, from a broader perspective.

Chapter 17
FROM REST TO ACTIVITY

From the time we get up to the time we go to bed, our bodies have to adapt to the many challenges posed by our changing activities. The first challenge of each day for many is getting up! Whatever else the event may be, it is a physical stress. The change in position from lying down to standing up is, because of gravity, a threat to the circulation in general and brain blood flow in particular. Several homeostatic mechanisms must be engaged to prevent us from fainting each time we stand. But this is not all, for gravity also affects fluid balance and modifies lung function.

Once up, most people move around, stretch, bend, lift, walk, run etc. Additional energy is needed to power each of these activities, however minor they may be, and physiological adjustments have to be made to meet the new demands. At the very least, there will probably be a small increase in blood flow to the active muscles. As activity increases, more extensive changes will take place in the heart and circulation and in the various systems responsible for the delivery of oxygen and nutrients to the active tissues and for the disposal of carbon dioxide, waste products and heat. It really is a case of 'all systems change'.

We will begin by looking at the effects of gravity on the body and then move on to consider the challenges posed by an increase in muscular activity and how these are met.

LYING, SITTING, STANDING

GRAVITY

Astronauts living on a space station can stand up, sit down and do head stands and somersaults with relatively little ill effect. Those of us who are earthbound cannot do these things without contending with the effects of gravity.

Gravity is the force that makes objects have weight. The weight of one object on top of another exerts pressure on the one beneath. Tissues and organs have weight and consequently exert pressure on the structures below them. Some tissues, such as lungs, are relatively light, whereas those that consist almost entirely of water, such as blood, are heavier.

When you take the weight off your feet and lie down, the total weight of your body is distributed over a much larger area than it was previously. Consequently, the pressures developed at any part of the body are not as great as when you were standing with all the pressure exerted on just your feet. When lying down, the pressure of blood in the large arteries is much the same in all parts of the body (about 100 mmHg) (Fig. 17.1A). When you stand up, however (Fig. 17.1B), the pressure of blood in the arteries in your feet increases by the weight of blood in the vessels between your heart and your

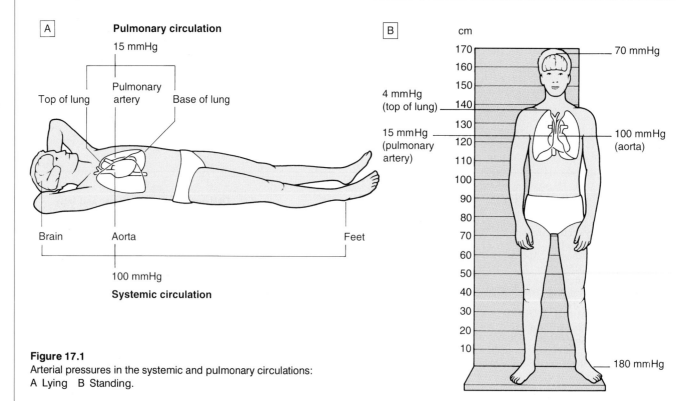

Figure 17.1
Arterial pressures in the systemic and pulmonary circulations:
A Lying   B Standing.

feet. In a person of medium height (170 cm), the increase will be about 80 to 90 mmHg. Likewise, the pressure of blood in the arteries above the level of the heart will be less by an amount depending on their distance from the heart. These differences in pressure affect the distribution of blood in the circulation and the distribution of fluid within the body. ①

The weight of other tissues also matters. For example, the weight of the lungs, even though they are relatively light, affects ventilation (see Lung function; p. 316). Also, the weight of the body as a whole pressing on some of the bones of the skeleton stimulates the growth of bone tissue.

> Demineralisation of bone occurs both in patients who are confined to bed for a long period of time and in astronauts on long space flights because their bones don't have the weight of the body pressing on them. The individual can to some extent counteract this loss of minerals by carrying out an exercise programme when possible.

Effects of gravity on the circulation

Venous pooling
The differences in pressure created by gravity in the circulatory system would not matter if blood vessels were rigid. Because they are not, the increased pressure in the vessels below the level of the heart causes them to distend and hold more blood, while those above the heart shrink. The most vulnerable vessels are the thin-walled veins (see Ch. 5). Consequently, when you stand

up there is a shift of blood volume from the top half of the body to the lower part. This shift is termed *venous pooling*. As a result, on standing, venous return is temporarily reduced, which in turn reduces cardiac output and arterial blood pressure (see Ch. 5).

If unchecked, the fall in blood pressure on standing reduces blood flow to the brain, starves the cells of O_2 and leads very quickly to loss of consciousness. As a result, fainting occurs – a helpful reaction because it instantly reverses the reduction in venous return, restores the original pressures and increases blood flow to the brain. ②

> Because of the effects of gravity on blood circulation, people who have fainted should not be encouraged to sit up very quickly but should be left lying in a comfortable position until they feel able to get up. Even then, they should get up slowly.

Circulatory adjustments
Ordinarily, the sudden drop in the pressure of blood flowing to the brain is detected by the arterial baroreceptors (see Ch. 5) and reflex adjustments are made to blood flow and cardiac output (Fig. 17.2). Arterial and venous vasoconstriction occur and heart rate increases. As a result, venous pooling is reduced and venous return and arterial blood pressure increase.

The effectiveness of this reflex in countering the threat to brain blood flow depends partly on other vasoactive substances circulating in the blood at the time. The

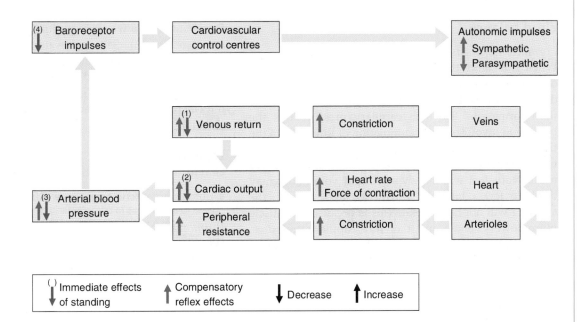

Figure 17.2
Some effects on the circulatory system of standing up.

hormone progesterone, for example, relaxes vascular smooth muscle and, if present in significant concentrations, will limit the vasoconstrictor effect of the noradrenaline released from the sympathetic nerves. Progesterone is one of the hormones secreted in large amounts during pregnancy (see Ch. 34) and is one of the factors that contribute to the episodes of faintness that a pregnant woman may experience on standing. Faintness on standing (*postural hypotension*) may also be experienced by those who have been bedridden for a while, by those who are feeling ill, or even by a healthy person who gets up too quickly after a night's sleep. In each case the baroreceptor reflex is less effective than usual, but the specific reasons for this will differ.

Muscle pump

One of the factors that help to maintain venous return and arterial blood pressure when you stand is the pressure that the contracting muscles in the limbs exert on the leg veins. This pressure compresses the vessels and massages them when you move around. Because of the valves present in the veins (see Ch. 5), when the vessels are massaged by muscle contraction, blood is pushed towards the heart and the volume of blood contained in the leg veins is reduced.

When you remain motionless, however, there is no pump action of the muscles. Although there is a steady background contraction, venous pooling is not counteracted to the same extent.

'Scrub nurses' can reduce the risk of fainting during long periods of standing immobile in theatre by wriggling their toes or shifting their weight from one foot to the other. This has the effect of contracting the calf muscles and therefore assisting venous return.

RECORDING THE LYING AND STANDING BLOOD PRESSURE

Patients suffering from hypertension may be prescribed drugs which will lower the blood pressure. Methyldopa is one such drug. By reducing sympathetic activity, it decreases vasomotor tone and hence blood pressure. Occasionally, however, a patient receiving methyldopa may find that, on rising in the morning or on standing up suddenly, he feels dizzy and may even faint. This *postural hypotension* results from the reflex increase in vasomotor tone being insufficient to prevent venous pooling of blood, and so blood pressure is no longer maintained at an adequate level.

Such patients on methyldopa may need to be admitted to a medical ward for observation. The nurse's role includes accurate recording of the patient's blood pressure while he is both lying on the bed and standing up. The two readings need to be carefully distinguished on the patient's observations chart. In this way the physician can judge the progress of drug therapy over a period of time. It may be, for example, that after the patient has been taking methyldopa for some time, the two blood pressure readings – lying and standing – which were at first disparate move closer together. This could be a sign that the patient is adapting more readily to changes in posture despite the use of the hypotensive drug.

Nurses should be aware of the safety needs of their patients (not just those on hypotensive drugs) for example when leaving a warm bath. The nurse may care to consider the effect on a person's venous return (and therefore cardiac output) of (a) lying down, and (b) being in a warm environment. These conditions are combined when a patient takes a bath. When he stands up, reflex changes in vasomotor tone are required to maintain adequate cardiac output by reducing venous pooling. The healthy glow so noticeable on the skin of someone who has just left a hot bath is a sign of peripheral arterial vasodilation. Constriction of the peripheral vessels, perhaps on meeting cooler air, will help to raise the blood pressure by increasing peripheral resistance.

Fluid balance

Formation of tissue fluid

When you stand, the pressure of blood in the capillaries of the feet increases considerably. This makes a big difference to the balance of forces that determine tissue fluid formation. The high capillary pressure tips the balance in favour of the accumulation of fluid within the tissue spaces (see Ch. 5). Consequently, over a period of time, particularly if you do not move around very much, your feet will slowly swell and your shoes may begin to feel a bit tight. If you do walk around, the swelling will not be so great. This is because the muscle pump lowers venous and, therefore, capillary pressures. Whatever posture is adopted, fluid will tend to accumulate slowly in tissues below the level of the heart (the *dependent parts*).

> In cardiac failure involving the right-hand side of the heart, oedema develops because of the increase in venous pressure (see Ch. 5). Oedema occurs around the ankles if the patient is up and about. But if he is confined to bed the site of oedema will be in the sacral region.

Fluid retention

Because of venous pooling and the gradual accumulation of tissue fluid in the lower parts of the body, the blood vessels in the upper half of the body are less full of blood. When you stand up, receptor cells within the circulation, in or not far from the heart, register this apparent drop in blood volume and reflexly influence kidney function and the desire to drink so that body fluid content as a whole is gradually increased (Fig. 17.3; see also Ch. 13). Salt and water are retained by the kidneys, fluid intake increases, and the volume of extracellular fluid expands.

On lying down, these effects are reversed, urine flow rate increases and the accumulated salt and water is gradually excreted.

Lung function

Gravity affects lung function by influencing:

- pulmonary circulation
- inflation of the lungs.

Pulmonary circulation

When you sit upright or stand, the blood pressure at the top of the lungs immediately falls almost to zero (Fig. 17.1B). This is because of the effects of gravity on the low pulmonary pressures (see Ch. 7). In consequence, in the upper part of the lung there is a decrease in:

- blood volume
- blood flow
- tissue fluid formation.

The volume of blood in the pulmonary circulation changes substantially as the pressure changes because the pulmonary vessels are very distensible (see Ch. 7). Up to 400 ml of blood may be displaced from the pulmonary to the systemic circulation when someone who has been lying down stands up. Blood flow to the upper part of the lung decreases because the lower pressures there distend the vessels less and so the resistance to blood flow through them increases. Tissue fluid formation decreases because of the lowered capillary pressure.

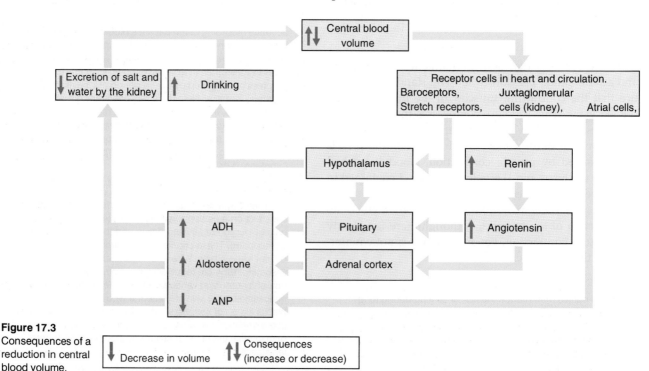

Figure 17.3
Consequences of a reduction in central blood volume.

Breathing is often easier in the sitting position for someone who has pulmonary oedema caused by left-sided heart failure. The lowering of the pressure within the pulmonary vessels reduces their engorgement, allowing more room for the lungs to expand within the thoracic cavity. Also, less tissue fluid is likely to be formed in the upper parts of the lungs.

Inflation of the lungs

In the sitting or standing position, the weight of the lung tissue presses down on the alveoli and airways at the base. The alveoli and airways at the base of the lung are thus more contracted in size than those at the top. This affects breathing in two ways. First, the resistance to airflow is greater at the base than at the top of the lungs. Thus, early in inspiration, air flows most readily into the alveoli at the top (Fig. 17.4). Later on, the airways at the bottom expand and the alveoli there fill more easily with air. Second, although the alveoli at the base fill slowly at first, they have more scope for expansion because they are smaller to begin with. Consequently, they take in more fresh air, relative to their original volume, than those at the top. In other words, once they do fill with air, they are better ventilated.

When you lie flat on your back, however, it is the ventral (anterior) parts of the lungs that are on top and which press down on the dorsal (posterior) parts below. Consequently, the ventral parts fill first, followed later and more fully by the dorsal parts of the lung.

PHYSICAL ACTIVITY

THE CHALLENGES POSED

Any form of physical activity increases the need to:

- supply ATP to power muscle contraction
- dispose of the waste products generated by muscle metabolism.

If these needs cannot be met, contraction cannot be maintained and the muscle fatigues.

Supplying ATP

For short bursts of activity (for example lifting something heavy), the ATP that is needed can be formed using the resources available on site in the muscle itself – creatine phosphate, glycogen and oxymyoglobin (O_2 bound to myoglobin). But these resources are limited. Consequently, for sustained activities such as walking, sufficient O_2 and either glucose or fatty acids have to be delivered continuously to the muscle through its blood supply to sustain the manufacture of ATP by the process of oxidative phosphorylation (Fig. 17.5 and Ch. 11).

At the start of any activity, the initial supply of ATP is always derived chiefly from the resources on site. As depletion of local O_2 occurs, metabolism shifts towards the anaerobic mode. Products generated aerobically and anaerobically (such as CO_2, lactic acid and adenosine) cause local vasodilation, which improves the oxygenation of the tissue (see Ch. 11), and muscle metabolism begins to shift back from the anaerobic to the aerobic mode. When activity ceases, the depleted resources on site are replenished. This requires O_2 and this extra requirement is known as the *oxygen debt*.

Thus, whenever physical activity occurs, additional supplies of O_2 and suitable fuels need to be delivered to the muscle cells.

Waste products generated

The products generated as a result of muscle activity include:

- lactic acid   ● CO_2 ● heat.

Lactic acid is formed when metabolism is anaerobic and CO_2 when it is aerobic. Both of these waste

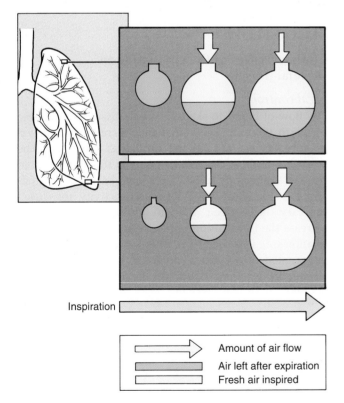

Inspiration

⇨	Amount of air flow
▭	Air left after expiration
▭	Fresh air inspired

Figure 17.4
How ventilation at the top and bottom of the lung differs in a person who is sitting upright or standing. At the beginning of inspiration the alveoli and airways at the base of the lung are less expanded than those at the top because the weight of the lung tissue above compresses them. Consequently, on inspiration, the alveoli at the base begin by filling slowly but eventually contain proportionally more fresh air than those at the top.

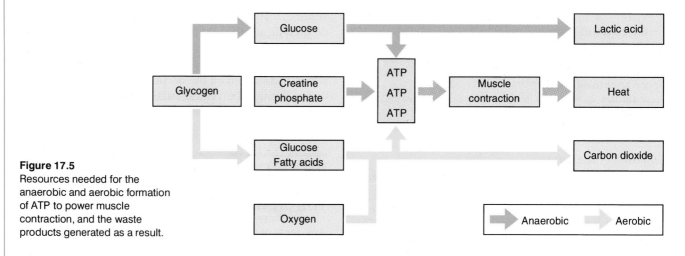

Figure 17.5
Resources needed for the anaerobic and aerobic formation of ATP to power muscle contraction, and the waste products generated as a result.

products increase the acidity of the intracellular and extracellular fluids. This disturbs cellular function and can inhibit the process of muscle contraction. A great deal of heat is produced when muscles contract (over 75% of the energy expended) and this too threatens normal function. For the process of muscle contraction to be at its best and for homeostasis to be maintained, the products generated need to be dealt with. The maintenance of an adequate blood flow through the active muscle tissue is crucial.

Fatigue

If blood flow is inadequate, insufficient ATP is formed to power contraction and the build-up of lactic acid and other metabolic products impairs neuromuscular function. The muscle *fatigues*. Contraction cannot be sustained and discomfort is experienced. ③

The point at which fatigue occurs during a specific activity varies, depending on a person's fitness, body state at the time and environmental conditions. With suitable training, muscles can develop resistance to fatigue (see Ch. 22). One of the long-term changes that contributes to this improvement is in the circulation of blood to the muscles.

③
What factors may give rise to pain during exercise?

In the text that follows, we will first look at the factors that are involved in maintaining an adequate blood flow to muscle tissue before going on to consider the processes that are specifically concerned with ensuring the delivery of O_2, glucose and fatty acids and the disposal of CO_2, lactic acid and heat. Finally, some of the long-term effects of a programme of exercise and of prolonged inactivity will be summarised.

BLOOD FLOW

Characteristics of the circulation to skeletal muscle

Local control

The flow of blood to skeletal muscle tissue can increase by 30- to 100-fold. This remarkable increase is achieved because at rest not all the capillaries are open. The smooth muscle at the terminal part of the arterioles can contract sufficiently to block off some parts of the capillary bed (see Fig. 5.26). With muscle activity, the closed capillary beds open up. In addition, local factors increase the flow through open vessels by causing vasodilation (see Chs 5 and 11). These local responses bring oxygenated blood much closer to the active cells and steepen the gradient that drives the diffusion of O_2 from the blood to the cells (see Fig. 7.17).

Sympathetic control

In addition to the usual sympathetic vasoconstrictor nerve fibres, which release noradrenaline, the blood vessels are also innervated by sympathetic vasodilator fibres, which release acetylcholine. The latter may be

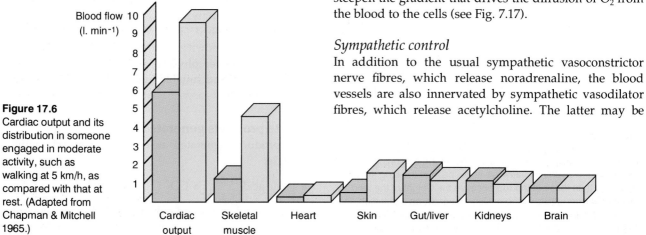

Figure 17.6
Cardiac output and its distribution in someone engaged in moderate activity, such as walking at 5 km/h, as compared with that at rest. (Adapted from Chapman & Mitchell 1965.)

activated when muscular activity is anticipated and they help to increase blood flow in the early stages of physical activity before local vasodilator factors take over. Vasodilation is also caused by adrenaline, released from the adrenal medulla, acting on beta receptors (see Ch. 3).

Intermittent flow

The blood vessels are compressed whenever muscle contraction occurs. If a powerful contraction is maintained, blood flow may be severely cut down and metabolism will shift from the aerobic to the anaerobic mode. However, if contraction alternates with relaxation, then periods of *ischaemia* (lack of blood) will alternate with surges of blood flow through the dilated capillary bed.

Muscles differ in their functions. Some, such as arm muscles, are used intermittently. Others, such as postural muscles of the neck and back, must maintain tension almost all the time during waking hours. The blood flow differs for each type. In the former, intermittency of flow will regularly occur, while, in the latter, a steady blood flow is maintained to support the

sustained contraction. Muscles that have to maintain activity for long periods have a more extensive network of vessels and a higher blood flow than those that are used only intermittently.

Role of the heart and circulation

Mild activity

If the activities pursued are mild, the needs of the active muscles can be met simply by a modest increase in cardiac output and some redistribution of blood flow between different circulations (Fig. 17.6). Some of these changes in the circulation are evoked through autonomic reflexes triggered by signals from:

- receptors in the muscles and joints (see Ch. 24)
- cardiovascular baroreceptors (see Ch. 5)
- brain areas that control posture and movement (see Ch. 27).

The increase in cardiac output is caused mainly by an increase in stroke volume (+50%) and partly by a modest increase in heart rate (+20–40 beats/minute). Venous return, and hence stroke volume, is increased by the muscle pump and the respiratory pump (see Ch. 5).

The circulations from which some blood may be withdrawn in order to meet the new demand include those of the gastrointestinal tract, the skin and non-active skeletal muscle. Vasoconstriction occurs at these sites mediated by noradrenergic sympathetic nerve fibres. Should an increased blood flow be required at any of these sites at the same time, the amount of blood that can be diverted to the muscles is reduced and cardiac output has to increase to maintain muscle blood flow and arterial blood pressure. This applies to skin blood flow, which increases during exercise if body temperature rises (see Ch. 16). ④

Strenuous activity

In more strenuous activities, the alterations in the cardiovascular system are much more drastic (Fig. 17.7). Total blood flow to active muscle can reach about 20 litres/minute at a maximum cardiac output of 25 litres/minute (a fivefold increase over resting levels). This is chiefly achieved by the excitatory effects of the sympathetic nervous system (adrenaline included) on heart rate, which increases to a maximum of 180 to 200 beats per minute. Both the muscle pump and the respiratory pump help to increase stroke volume to a maximum of 120 ml.

④
For what physiological reason does skin blood flow increase during exercise?

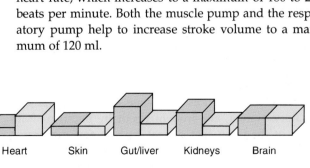

Figure 17.7
Cardiac output and its distribution in maximal exercise as compared with that at rest. (Adapted from Chapman & Mitchell 1965.)

Table 17.1 Differences in cardiac function and oxygen uptake between top athletes and other individuals

	Sedentary individuals	Top athletes (endurance events)
Resting heart rate (per min)	70	50
Maximal exercise*		
– heart rate (per min)	200	190
– stroke volume (ml)	120	200
– cardiac output (l.min^{-1})	25	40
– oxygen uptake (l.min^{-1})	3	6

* Data compiled from Ekblom 1969.

Limitations

Trained athletes can achieve higher cardiac outputs (Table 17.1) because training provokes *hypertrophy* of the heart and increases stroke volume. The resting heart rate of athletes is lower than that in untrained individuals, which means that there is more scope for heart rate to increase. Thus, trained athletes can achieve more at any given heart rate. ⑤ ⑥

The single most important factor that determines the upper limit to achievable exercise in most people is their maximum cardiac output. This determines the maximal amount of O_2 that can be picked up in the lungs and pumped to the tissues. Contrary to popular expectation, it is not the ability to breathe that limits exercise in health but cardiac function.

DELIVERY OF OXYGEN, GLUCOSE AND FATTY ACIDS

Oxygen

Oxygenation of pulmonary blood

The delivery of adequate amounts of O_2 to the active muscles depends on proper oxygenation of the blood as well as blood flow. In the healthy individual, full oxygenation of the pulmonary blood occurs in a third of the time that it takes blood to pass through the pulmonary capillaries (see Ch. 7). There is thus a safety margin that would allow blood flow through the lungs to increase threefold (equivalent to a threefold increase in cardiac output) before there is any risk of the blood not being fully oxygenated. The changes in ventilation and in the circulation occur simultaneously – full oxygenation is thus guaranteed.

Increased ventilation

Changes in ventilation, like some of those in the circulatory system, are brought about by impulses from parts of the brain that control posture and movement and from sensory receptors within the muscles and joints (Fig. 17.8; see also Chs 7 and 24). As ventilation

⑤
Hypertrophy can also occur in some heart diseases. Why might this be?

⑥
If possible, ask members of your student group to record each other's pulse rate (while relaxed). What is the range of pulse rates? Does the student with the lowest rate participate regularly in sports such as jogging and swimming?

EXERCISE AND CARDIAC REHABILITATION

Damage to the myocardium following a heart attack (*myocardial infarction*) means that the heart muscle is often weaker making the heart a less efficient pump. Cardiac output is therefore reduced. Many nurses will remember that, about 20 years ago, the nursing care of a patient following a heart attack consisted of bed rest, with the patient flat on his back and allowed to do nothing for himself for 2 or 3 weeks. Such measures might have 'rested the heart' but could have done little for the psychological state of the patient.

Modern treatment, following rest and observation on a specialised unit (Coronary Care Unit) for 2 or 3 days, consists of a carefully planned series of exercises, which take account of the patient's condition – as judged by pulse rate, blood pressure and electrocardiograms (ECG) – and are designed to prepare him for discharge. As the damaged area of myocardium begins to heal, exercise increases, but only to the extent that the patient can tolerate. Exercises might include, for example, sitting out of bed for half an hour in the morning and afternoon, then sitting for 1 hour, then walking 100 yards. Some programmes include spending 15 minutes on an exercise bicycle (with the heart monitored all the time).

Signs that a patient might be exceeding a sensible exercise limit may include tachycardia, lowered blood pressure, and angina-like chest pains. The latter are caused by the heart's demand for oxygen being greater than can be supplied via the obstructed branch of the coronary arteries to the myocardium. In such an event the patient's exercise regime will be adjusted.

A rehabilitation programme such as this increases not only the patient's strength but also his self-confidence. Nursing instructions, as the day of discharge approaches, need to be more exact than, 'Take things easy.' Clear explanation of what has gone wrong physiologically, and encouragement to persevere with the exercise regime (backed up by reassurances about its effectiveness and safety) will help the patient to take charge of his own recovery.

Stimulating ventilation for an unconscious or paralysed patient is one of the benefits of passive limb exercises performed by a nurse or physiotherapist. The stimulation of sensory receptors within the joints and muscles caused by movement of the limbs increases the rate and depth of breathing, which in turn assists in the prevention of chest infections.

increases in exercise, the partial pressure of O_2 (PO_2) in the alveolar air is maintained and even increased and the PCO_2 is stabilised. Consequently, arterial blood PO_2 and PCO_2 are maintained within normal limits. Ventilation of the lungs is made easier by a reduction in airway resistance caused by the bronchodilation stimulated by the sympathetic nerves.

Haemoglobin

The maximum amount of O_2 that can be carried in

Table 17.2 Energy stores in the human body*	
	Energy (kcal)
ATP	1
Creatine phosphate	4
Glycogen	
– liver	400
– muscle	1000
Fat	100 000

* Approximate values for an average well-fed adult. The size of glycogen and fat stores varies considerably between individuals, and according to diet and activity.

Figure 17.8
Regulation of breathing in exercise.

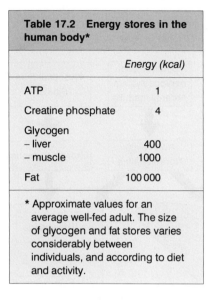

blood depends on the amount of haemoglobin available. A person who is anaemic will therefore have a lower exercise capacity than normal. Likewise, individuals who smoke and who have a proportion of their haemoglobin in the form of carboxyhaemoglobin (see Ch. 7) have a reduced O_2-carrying capacity, which will reduce their maximum exercise capacity. ⑦

Glucose and fatty acids

Glucose and fatty acids are stored in the body as glycogen and triglycerides, respectively. The fat stores are by far the larger (Table 17.2).

The glycogen on site within muscle is important in guaranteeing energy supplies at the beginning of muscular activity, particularly if the demand for ATP is high. Glycogen can be used aerobically or anaerobically depending on the availability of O_2 (see Fig. 11.2).

As cardiovascular adjustments occur and blood flow to the active muscles increases, the use of fatty acids released from adipose tissue becomes increasingly important. The improved oxygenation of the muscle tissue allows fatty acids as well as glucose to be used aerobically by the muscle cells to produce ATP.

Hormonal control

The released of fatty acids from their depot form as triglycerides in the adipose tissue is stimulated by several hormones (Fig. 17.9):

- adrenaline
- noradrenaline
- growth hormone.

Of these, adrenaline and noradrenaline are the most important in exercise. They also promote the breakdown of glycogen to glucose, both in muscle and in liver, and thus help to maintain glucose supplies for all tissues in the face of the increased demands made by the muscle cells. The secretion of growth hormone and cortisol also increases in exercise. Both help to maintain blood glucose levels by decreasing the use of glucose by tissues such as muscle that can use alternative fuels (see Ch. 10, Table 10.7 and Ch. 19, Fig. 19.6).

Choice of fuels

Fatty acids are the chief fuel used by muscle cells when activity is moderate. This allows more glucose to be available for use by other tissues, particularly those such as brain that rely almost exclusively on it.

In very strenuous exercise, when the demands of the muscles outstrip the supplies of raw materials, the stocks of glycogen on site are again used anaerobically. This is a self-limiting process because the stocks of glycogen are eventually run down. Also, the concentration of lactic acid greatly increases, which impairs neuromuscular function and inhibits the release of fatty acids from adipose tissue. The supply of ATP becomes inadequate and fatigue develops.

The diet that you consume affects the length of time for which you can exercise before feeling exhausted. A carbohydrate-rich diet increases the stores of glycogen in muscle and in liver and extends the time possible. The diet consumed regularly also affects the bias of metabolism – if the diet is rich in carbohydrate, a greater

⑦
What is the normal range of haemoglobin for men and women?

proportion of the energy produced is derived from carbohydrate regardless of the level of physical activity.

DISPOSAL OF CARBON DIOXIDE, LACTIC ACID AND HEAT

Carbon dioxide

The very large amounts of CO_2 that are generated when metabolism is aerobic are eliminated through the lungs. The increased ventilation that guarantees the oxygenation of blood also ensures the removal of CO_2. As a result, arterial blood PCO_2 in exercise hardly differs from that at rest.

Lactic acid

Lactic acid is generated during periods of anaerobic metabolism and is not eliminated but retained and reused. When activity ceases or becomes less intense, it is reconverted into pyruvic acid (see Fig. 11.2). It may then be used to form:

- ATP via the citric acid cycle
- glucose to replenish glycogen stocks in muscle and liver.

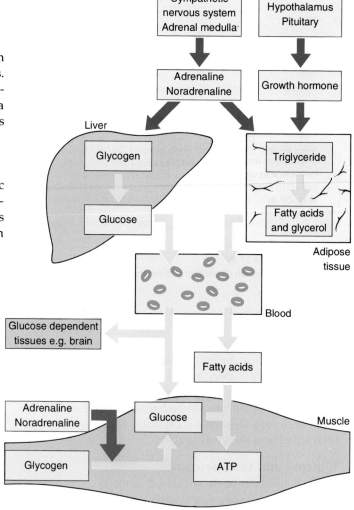

Figure 17.9
Sites of action of the hormones promoting the supply of fatty acids and glucose to muscle and other tissues in exercise.

Table 17.3   Energy costs of and heat generated by various activities as compared with some electrical appliances*

Activities			Electrical appliances	
Type	Total energy cost (kcal/min)	Heat generated (watts)	Type	Rating (watts)
Sleeping	1	70	Single electric blanket	50
Lying awake	1½	100	Light bulb	100
Office work	1½–2	100–120		
Dressing/undressing	3	150		
Walking (5 km/h)	4	200		
Making beds	3–5	150–300		
Manual labour Cycling (21 km/h) Gardening	5–10	300–500		
Playing squash Skiing	10–20	500–1000	Small fire (one bar)	1000

* Compiled from Astrand & Rohdahl 1986.

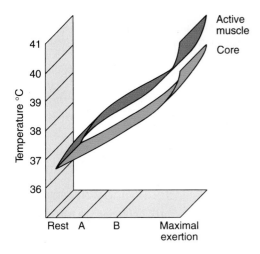

Figure 17.10
Increase of temperature of core body tissues and of active muscle at different levels of activity. Point 'A' is equivalent to walking at about 5 km/h (3 m.p.h.) and point 'B' to cycling at about 20 km/h (13 m.p.h.). Note that the temperature of active muscle is greater than that of the body core. (Adapted from Astrand & Rohdahl 1986.)

The build-up of lactic acid during periods of strenuous exercise causes the pH of muscle cells and of the blood to decrease. The hydrogen ions are buffered by hydrogen carbonate and so the hydrogen carbonate concentration decreases. The decrease in pH stimulates ventilation even more (see also Ch. 12).

Heat

Active muscles produce heat (Table 17.3 and Fig. 17.10). This can be disposed of only by conduction, convection and radiation from the surface of the body and by the evaporation of water in sweating (see Ch. 16). The increased temperature of the skin overlying the active muscles results in an increase in the amount of heat lost. This is enhanced by vasodilation of skin blood vessels. If the amount of heat produced continues to exceed the amount lost, body temperature will increase further and

sweat glands will also be activated.

Removal of the heat produced by muscular activity is vital. Even small increases in body temperature cannot be tolerated by the brain. But the temperature-regulating mechanisms that protect body temperature pose other new threats to homeostasis:

- First, the increased blood flow to the skin reduces the amount of blood that can be made available to the active muscles. This in turn may affect the supply of O_2 and nutrients and the production and disposal of metabolic products.
- Second, losses of salt and water in sweating (up to 2 litres/hour) cause a decrease in the volume of extracellular fluid and consequently of blood plasma. Because this is a threat to blood pressure, compensatory changes are provoked in the secretion of hormones such as ADH (antidiuretic hormone), atrial natriuretic peptide and angiotensin which promote the retention of salt and water (Fig. 17.3; see also Ch. 13).⑧

LONG-TERM EFFECTS OF INACTIVITY OR REGULAR EXERCISE

All in all, physical activity at its most strenuous is an enormous challenge to body systems. Maximum performance depends both on optimum function of many different parts of the body and on optimum environmental conditions. Fitness can be developed by a planned programme of activity that needs to be kept up if the improvement in condition is not to be lost. If you experience a prolonged period of inactivity, loss of strength and fitness is inevitable. Some of the changes that have been shown to occur during prolonged bed rest and during physical training are shown in Table 17.4.

The form of exercise practised determines the nature of the changes that occur both in the muscles and in the

⑧
Which electrolytes are particularly important for nerve and muscle function?

Table 17.4 Effects of bed rest (20 days) followed by training (55 days) in three normally sedentary young men*				
Conditions	Measurement	Control	After bed rest	After training
Rest	Heart rate (per min)	69	70	54
	Stroke volume (ml)	95	77	90
	Heart volume (ml)	740	690	810
'Moderate'† exercise	Heart rate (per min)	114	120	93
	Stroke volume (ml)	95	78	108
	Cardiac output (l.min⁻¹)	10.8	9.4	10.0
Exercise (maximal)	Cardiac output (l.min⁻¹)	17.2	12.3	20.2
	Oxygen uptake (l.min⁻¹)	2.5	1.7	3.4

* Compiled from Saltin et al 1968.
† Cycle ergometer set at 50 watts (equivalent to walking at 5 km.h⁻¹ or 3 m.p.h.).

SUPPORTIVE CARE OF THE LONG-TERM IMMOBILE PATIENT

Patients who are immobile for long periods of time may require the nurse to perform many of the activities of living that they cannot manage for themselves, including the provision of exercise.

Correct joint positioning and safe, regular, limb exercises (perhaps under the supervision of a physiotherapist) will help to reduce muscle wastage and joint stiffness, as well as helping to promote respiratory activity. Limb muscles maintain some of their tone, even though their movements are performed, not by the patient, but by the nurse, and venous pooling is reduced, venous return is aided and blood supply to the skin is improved. Changes in the patient's position, as often as skilled nursing deems necessary, will also reduce the risk of pressure sores forming, and will assist the ventilation of differing areas of the lungs. Lack of exercise tends to cause withdrawal of calcium from the bones leading to weakness and, possibly, pathological fractures. The calcium is then deposited within the renal tract (especially in the bladder) forming calculi. Some enormous bladder stones, which required surgical removal, have been discovered in paralysed or severely mentally disabled people.

body as a whole (Table 17.5). Very short bursts of intense activity are good at developing muscle strength, but they do relatively little for the heart and circulation. Longer periods of regular sub-maximal exercise are required to improve the function of these (Table 17.6).

Table 17.5   Components of a training programme*

Type of exercise	Effect
Bursts of intense activity (seconds)	↑ Muscle strength
Intense activity (1 min) repeated after a few minutes' rest	↑ Anaerobic power
Less than maximal activity for 3–5 min with intervening similar periods of rest	↑ Aerobic power
Sub-maximal exercise for 30 min	↑ Endurance

* Compiled from Astrand & Rohdahl 1986.

Table 17.6   Some of the long-term effects of regular sub-maximal exercise*

Feature	Effect
Mortality from ischaemic heart disease	↓ (50%)
Maximum cardiac output	↑
Stroke volume	↑
Resting heart rate	↓
Numbers of coronary capillaries	↑
Maximum oxygen uptake	↑
Muscle	
– number of capillaries	↑
– muscle blood flow (max)	↑
– aerobic metabolism	↑
Metabolism	
– use of free fatty acids	↑
– plasma triglycerides	↓
– plasma cholesterol	↓ (in some people)

* Compiled from Astrand & Rohdahl 1986.

KEY POINTS

What you should now understand about posture and physical activity:

- why someone may faint on standing
- why tissue fluid accumulates in dependent parts of the body
- why a sitting position aids respiratory function in heart failure, and how it affects ventilation of the lungs
- why cardiac function and circulatory fitness are the major factors affecting physical performance
- why someone who is anaemic tires easily
- how metabolism is adjusted in exercise to meet the increased demand for glucose and fatty acids
- how physical performance is affected by diet and environmental conditions
- what happens when muscles fatigue
- what physiological changes occur when someone is deprived of physical activity through illness, injury or disability
- why it is important to select appropriate exercises to develop fitness.

REFERENCES AND FURTHER READING

Astrand P-O, Rohdahl K 1986 Textbook of work physiology – physiological basis of exercise, 3rd edn. McGraw-Hill, London (Detailed text. Useful authoritative source of reference)
Bird S 1991 Exercise physiology for health professionals. Chapman & Hall, London (Readable book about practical uses of exercise as therapy and rehabilitation)
Chapman C B, Mitchell J H 1965 The physiology of exercise. Scientific American 212: 88–96
Ekblom B 1969 Effect of physical training on oxygen transport in man. Acta Physiologica Scandinavica (Suppl. 328)
Evans D E 1985 Exercise. In: Case R M (ed) Variations in human physiology. Manchester University Press, Manchester (Source of more information on the physiology of exercise)

Fentem P H, Turnbull N B, Bassey E J 1990 Benefits of exercise, the evidence. Manchester University Press, Manchester (Collates the evidence to date. Useful source of references)
Reilly T, Secher N H, Snell P, Williams C 1990 Physiology of sports. E & F N Spon, London (Physiology applied to individual sports, and sportsmen and women, from cyclists to sailors)
Saltin B, Blomqvist B, Mitchell J H, Johnson R L, Wildenthal K, Chapman C B 1968 Response to submaximal and maximal exercise after bed rest and training. Circulation 38 (Suppl. 7): 1–78
Whipp B J, Wasserman K 1991 Exercise. Pulmonary physiology and pathophysiology. Marcel Dekker, New York & Basel (Authoritative specialist review articles on the respiratory and circulatory systems' functioning in exercise)

Chapter 18
CIRCADIAN RHYTHMS

In previous chapters we focused on the ways in which the composition of the internal environment is maintained in the face of many different challenges. We saw how disturbances are counteracted by a host of homeostatic mechanisms.

It is important to appreciate that these reactive homeostatic mechanisms do not prevent changes in the internal environment. They simply minimise the changes that occur. Consequently there will be regular daily changes (*circadian rhythms* – from the Latin: *circa* about; *dies* day) in the level of things such as body temperature and blood glucose concentration, due to our changing patterns of activity over 24 hours.

In addition to the changes imposed by external (*exogenous*) factors, such as mealtimes and patterns of work and rest, there are other daily changes caused by a regular waxing and waning of cellular activity inside the body (*endogenous factors*) that occur even when external factors are kept constant. Endogenous factors adjust the state of the body in anticipation of daily events (*predictive homeostasis*) rather than in response to them (*reactive homeostasis*).

When we keep to a conventional routine the rhythms driven by exogenous and endogenous factors normally coincide but circumstances, such as long-distance air travel and shift work, can make them conflict, and this disturbs our well-being. Circadian rhythms may be altered in illness and influence a patient's symptoms and susceptibility to medication.

BASIS OF CIRCADIAN RHYTHMS

Circadian rhythms are created by both exogenous and endogenous factors. Some rhythms are set mainly by external events and change quickly when these alter, whereas others are driven mainly by internal factors and do not adapt as easily.

EXOGENOUS FACTORS

The regular alternation between day and night, the pattern of events during a normal working day, and the timing of meals create a number of circadian rhythms.

Examples from daily life
Whenever you change your activity, the conditions inside your body alter. For example when you lie down you alter the distribution of body fluids (see Ch. 17) and reduce your metabolic rate. As a result, adjustments are made to the cardiovascular and renal systems by neural and hormonal control mechanisms. Blood pressure changes and the rate at which urine is formed alters. If you then go to sleep there are further changes. For example the secretion of growth hormone increases whenever you go to sleep, even for a nap (Fig. 18.1).

Conversely, when you wake up and become increasingly active, patterns change. Growth hormone concentrations fall but cortisol rises (Fig. 18.1). Heart

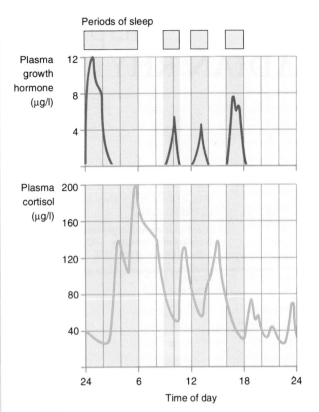

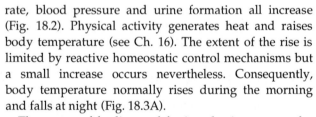

Figure 18.1
How plasma concentrations of growth hormone and cortisol fluctuate over 24 hours in relation to periods of sleep. (Adapted from Weitzman 1975 by permission of Elsevier Science Publishers BV.)

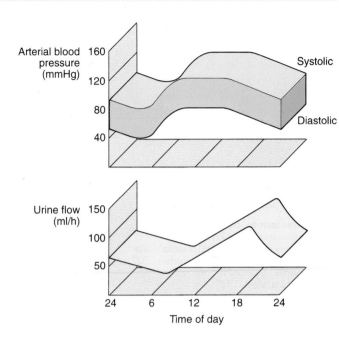

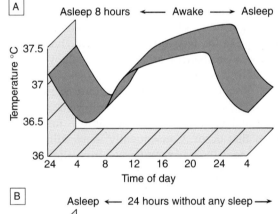

Figure 18.2
Circadian rhythms in arterial blood pressure and urine formation. (Pressure graph adapted from Millar-Craig et al 1978; urine flow rate adapted from Loutit 1965.)

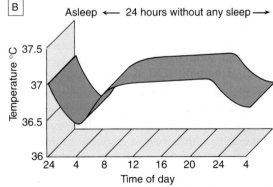

Figure 18.3
Circadian rhythm of core body temperature over 24 hours:
A With normal periods of sleep (16 h awake; 8 h asleep)
B Without any sleep.
(Adapted from Minors & Waterhouse 1981 by permission of the authors and Butterworth–Heinemann Ltd.)

rate, blood pressure and urine formation all increase (Fig. 18.2). Physical activity generates heat and raises body temperature (see Ch. 16). The extent of the rise is limited by reactive homeostatic control mechanisms but a small increase occurs nevertheless. Consequently, body temperature normally rises during the morning and falls at night (Fig. 18.3A).

The events of feeding and fasting also impose regular cycles of change in the concentration of nutrients and hormones in the blood. For example the average plasma concentrations of glucose and insulin are higher during the day than at night. The timing of meals and drinks also imposes rhythms in renal function. ①

ENDOGENOUS FACTORS: INTERNAL 'CLOCKS'

If you chose to stay awake for 24 hours and took identical small snacks every hour on the hour, you would find that various body rhythms persist despite the lack of the usual cues. Body temperature for example still drops in the early hours (Fig. 18.3B). These and other rhythms that persist are set by the activity of cells in the brain which act as an *internal clock*.

① *One of the tests for diabetes mellitus is a fasting blood glucose. What is its significance, and why should it be taken first thing in the morning? Why wouldn't a simple estimation of blood glucose at any time of the day suffice?*

Examples from experimental studies

Many studies have now been performed on volunteers who have been cut off from all external cues (daylight, clocks, radio and television etc.) by being housed for several weeks in a specially designed room. If the volunteers are allowed to follow their own natural routine, getting up, eating, and sleeping whenever they choose, they still follow a fairly regular sleep/wake cycle, and several other rhythms such as those of body temperature and blood pressure normally remain in step with this. However, this daily cycle of activity usually occcurs over a longer period than 24 hours, often about 25 hours. Thus after 24 days living in isolation people think that only 23 have actually passed!

From such studies it appears that rhythms dominated by internal rather than external cues include:

- the sleep/wake cycle
- body temperature
- cortisol secretion.

Influence of external factors

Ordinarily these endogenous rhythms are brought into step (*entrained*) with external rhythms, by the cues that are provided by environmental and social factors. External cues such as light and dark, a ringing alarm and mealtimes act as time signals and are referred to as *zeitgeber* (German for 'timegiver'). They reflexly provoke changes within us which bring the endogenous rhythms into line.

The internal clock

Site

Cells which regulate several of these endogenous rhythms are believed to be sited within the hypothalamus in the *suprachiasmatic nuclei* (Fig. 18.4). Supporting evidence in humans includes the fact that variables, such as plasma cortisol and body temperature, whose rhythm seems to be dominated by internal cues are all intimately controlled by the hypothalamus. Body temperature, for example, is controlled by cells in the preoptic and anterior regions of the hypothalamus (see Ch. 16), and cortisol secretion is regulated by CRH from the paraventricular nucleus (see Ch. 10). The activity of cells in the suprachiasmatic nuclei waxes and wanes regularly in animals and probably does the same in humans.

Number of clocks

When endogenous body rhythms are allowed free rein for a long time, by isolating a person from all the usual external time cues, different rhythms do not always remain in phase. The sleep/wake cycle, for example, sometimes adopts a different rhythm to the body temperature cycle. This suggests that other parts of the brain may also act as 'clocks'. Possibilities include

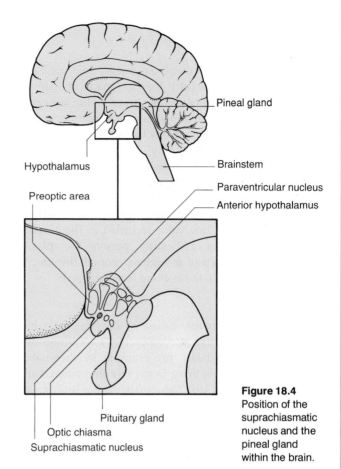

Figure 18.4
Position of the suprachiasmatic nucleus and the pineal gland within the brain.

Labels: Pineal gland; Brainstem; Paraventricular nucleus; Anterior hypothalamus; Hypothalamus; Preoptic area; Pituitary gland; Optic chiasma; Suprachiasmatic nucleus

other nuclei in the brain stem and the pineal gland (Fig. 18.4). ②

Setting the clock

It is not certain whether our internal clocks develop only as we become accustomed to regular patterns of activity, or whether they are genetically determined. Certainly babies and infants do not have very prominent circadian rhythms; neither do people who are blind or those who experience the perpetual 'day' of summer in the Arctic and the perpetual 'night' of the Arctic winter. These facts suggest that the alternation between night and day may be important in the development of some circadian rhythms. ③

A neural pathway (*retinohypothalamic tract*) links the eyes and the suprachiasmatic nuclei in the hypothalamus. It is possible that the changes in lighting between day and night experienced by the new-born infant may condition hypothalamic cells to increase and decrease their firing over 24 hours.

IMPLICATIONS FOR HEALTH CARE

Circadian rhythms are relevant to several aspects of health care for the client or patient, and for the caregiver.

② *To test this daily cycle, keep a record of your temperature every 4 hours; (a) over 3 days on duty and (b) over 3 nights on duty. How much variation in the cycle is there?*

③ *What are the sleep patterns of a new-born baby and an infant of 6 months; 12 months; 24 months?*

Client and patient

Measurements

Where regular measurements are made, such as blood pressure, it is most useful if they are made at a similar time of day. This eliminates the variation due to normal daily fluctuations and allows a better comparison of values to be made from one day to the next.

In assessing the 'normality' of a particular body measurement the circadian rhythm should be taken into account. If not, wrong judgements could be made. For example a low plasma concentration of cortisol during the morning would be a surer indication of adrenal insufficiency than a low value recorded in the evening. This is because in a healthy person the plasma concentration of cortisol is highest around the time of waking and lowest in the evening (see Fig. 18.1).

Symptoms

It is also helpful to be aware of the way in which circadian rhythms may affect a patient's condition over 24 hours. Joint stiffness, for example in rheumatoid arthritis, is worst first thing in the morning when someone has just woken up. This is due to the low plasma

concentrations of cortisol (an anti-inflammatory steroid) during the night. Similarly, someone who has asthma may experience more difficulty in breathing in the evening and night-time than during the day (Fig. 18.5) because the concentrations of cortisol and adrenaline (a bronchodilator) are lowest in the evening and highest during the morning and afternoon. Cortisol probably acts by reducing the sensitivity of tissues to histamine (a bronchoconstrictor).

> To help combat the stiffness experienced by many arthritis sufferers first thing in the morning, some non-steroidal anti-inflammatory drugs, for example indomethacin or diclofenac, can be taken in suppository form. The drug is inserted into the rectum last thing at night and is slowly absorbed throughout the night, considerably reducing early morning stiffness.

Caregiver

The condition of the caregiver also varies. Levels of alertness and skill for example vary during the day (Fig. 18.6). It is helpful if work schedules can be designed to take advantage of the times when a person works best. However, patterns differ between people: some people function best in the morning; others are best later in the day. Also some jobs, notably within industry, the emergency services, and health care, require that a person work 'unsocial' hours. It is well known that

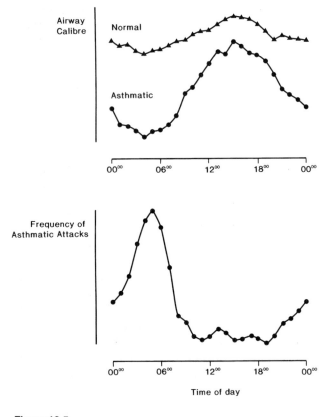

Figure 18.5
Top: Changes in airway calibre (diameter) in people with and without asthma. Bottom: Frequency of asthmatic attacks over 24 hours. (Reproduced from Waterhouse J M, Minors D S, Waterhouse M E 1990 Your body clock, Figure 14.1, by permission of the Oxford University Press.)

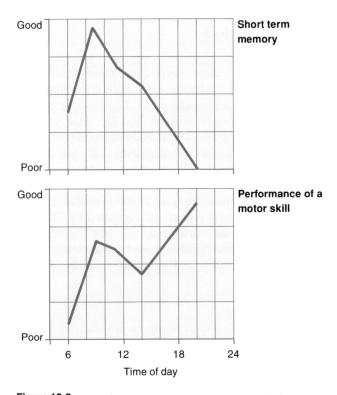

Figure 18.6
Variation in mental and motor abilities during the day. (Adapted from Folkard 1975, based on Blake 1967.)

people differ in their ability to adapt to a different daily routine. This is probably related to individual differences in the internal body clock.

EFFECTS OF ALTERED TIME SCHEDULES

In technologically sophisticated societies it is increasingly common for people to have to adjust to different time schedules. Long-distance air travel and shift work are two examples of situations where exogenous and endogenous rhythms may be brought into conflict. Whereas the jet lag experienced by air travellers passes off within a few days, the disturbances to the body caused by shift work may not be resolved and may even lead to illness.

LONG-DISTANCE AIR TRAVEL

Jet flights in an easterly or westerly direction put external cues and endogenous rhythms out of step very quickly. A flight from Britain to Australia for example in an easterly direction takes about 24 hours of real time, but, due to the time difference between the two places (Fig. 18.7), arrival time in Australia is actually about a day and a half later. Consequently, a traveller leaving Britain at 8 p.m. one evening will arrive in Australia at about 6 a.m. local time feeling ready to wind down and prepare for sleep (it being 8 p.m. by his internal clock) only to find that friends and colleagues there are just beginning their day (Fig. 18.8).

Jet lag

It takes several days for someone to adjust to the new daily pattern. Jet lag is not simply due to the effects of a long flight in an aeroplane, such as lower barometric pressure, lack of exercise and the unusual environment, because it does not occur on long flights in a north–south direction.

The symptoms experienced as jet lag include difficulties with sleep, decreased alertness and ability to concentrate, gastrointestinal upsets and general 'fatigue'. These symptoms gradually disappear as the individual's internal clock becomes geared (*entrained*) to the new schedule.

Flights east and west

The time needed to adjust to the new schedule depends for most people on whether the flight taken was in a westerly or an easterly direction. It takes about 2 days more if the flight to Australia from Britain is eastward.

The problem is that when travelling east you race through the equivalent of 1½ days in the space of 24 hours (Fig. 18.8). The schedule set by local time in the places that you stop and the meals provided by the airline force you to advance your routine. This is more

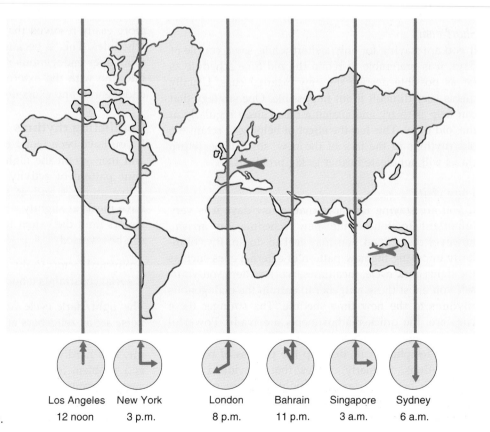

Figure 18.7
Actual time throughout the world when it is 8 p.m. (20.00) in London.

| Los Angeles | New York | London | Bahrain | Singapore | Sydney |
| 12 noon | 3 p.m. | 8 p.m. | 11 p.m. | 3 a.m. | 6 a.m. |

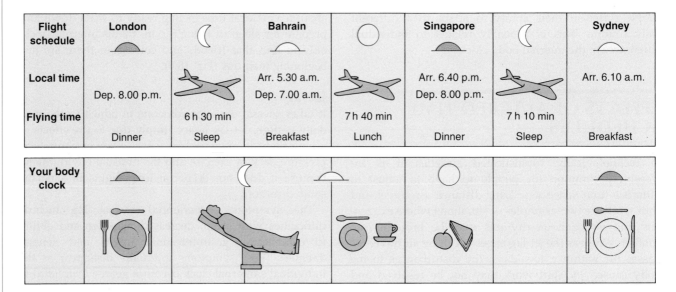

Flight schedule	London		Bahrain		Singapore		Sydney
Local time	Dep. 8.00 p.m.		Arr. 5.30 a.m. Dep. 7.00 a.m.		Arr. 6.40 p.m. Dep. 8.00 p.m.		Arr. 6.10 a.m.
Flying time		6 h 30 min		7 h 40 min		7 h 10 min	
	Dinner	Sleep	Breakfast	Lunch	Dinner	Sleep	Breakfast
Your body clock							

Figure 18.8
Two nights and two sunrises in a 24-hour eastward flight from London to Australia.

difficult to do than delaying it, which is what happens on a westward flight. Leaving in the afternoon and flying west you would experience an extended day and a very long night instead. The reason why this is easier to adjust to than a shortened day may be because most people's internal clock is set to run at more than 24 hours. Lengthening the day is therefore more natural than shortening it.

Travel tips

Short visits

If you are staying for only a short while, say a couple of days, it is preferable to retain the old time schedule as far as possible despite the new external cues. Usually this is very difficult if not impossible. One strategy that can help is to try and snatch a bit of sleep regularly at the 'old time'. This has the effect of helping to retain the old rhythms in the face of the new, so that the return travel will not create further jet lag problems.

Long visits

If you are staying for more than a few days it is very important to follow the new schedule on arrival, however disinclined you may feel to do so. By voluntarily imposing the new pattern of external cues such as the light/dark cycle, mealtimes, work pattern, on yourself you enlist these zeitgeber to entrain the endogenous rhythms to the new time shedule. The stronger these cues are, the quicker adjustments are made. Powerful auditory signals, such as a noisy alarm clock or a loud waking telephone call, do help the process of resetting the rhythms. Similarly, places that provide a sharp difference between day and night, because of bright sunlight during the day and absence of artificial light at night (for example desert places in Africa and

Australia), allow adjustments to be made more easily than places with cloudier skies and artificial lighting (for example cities in Britain). It may be that exposure to very bright artificial lights can be made to mimic the effect of sunlight as a zeitgeber and help air travellers to overcome jet lag more quickly.

DIFFERENT WORKING HOURS

The problems posed by air travel over long distances are more easily resolved than those posed by altered work schedules. This is because in travelling from one place to another endogenous rhythms are eventually brought into line with the external cues, whereas in shift work endogenous and exogenous cues continue to conflict.

Conflicting rhythms

If you have been working 'days' (8.00 a.m. to 4.00 p.m.) and then go on the night-shift (10.00 p.m. to 8.00 a.m.) your pattern of activity is, in part, reversed. You are active at night and at sleep during the day and you have meals at slightly different times. However, several factors limit the extent to which the patterns of activity can be reversed:

- physical factors (light, noise)
- social constraints (shopping hours, school times).

The light/dark cycle and the level of environmental noise act as zeitgebers and inevitably provide a conflicting set of cues to the pattern set by the new work schedule. It is hardly surprising that sleeping in the daytime is a problem for most people. Secondly, social factors, such as canteen opening hours, family commitments, and leisure pursuits, may also not key into the new schedule.

The result of all these things is that a new set of stable rhythms is not easily established. It is like being persistently 'jet lagged'. As one of the effects of this 'desynchronisation' of endogenous and exogenous rhythms is a reduction in mental alertness, it is important to know what factors can minimise the problems, or make matters worse. A key factor is sleep deprivation.

Sleep deprivation

Most people who work 'nights' experience some sleep deprivation because of the difficulties of sleeping during the daytime. This is cumulative. If lost sleep is not made up from time to time, this adds to the problems of concentration and reduced alertness. Individuals may become more irritable and touchy (see Ch. 31). It is helpful therefore to have a couple of days off after a period on 'nights' to allow the lost hours of sleep to be recouped.

Coping with shift work

Suitable schedules

The best scheme undoubtedly is for people to be permanently on the same shift whether days or nights. This allows body rhythms to develop a regular pattern. When irregular shifts are worked body rhythms cannot settle down.

However some jobs, like nursing, require people to be more adaptable and to work rotating shifts. Unfortunately there is little agreement among experts over the ideal rotating shift. Some favour a rapid rotation (change every 2 days), others a slow rotation that allows rhythms to adapt gradually to each new schedule. What is clear is that, as most of us have endogenous rhythms that have a natural period of about 25 hours, it is easier to adapt to a delay in schedules than to an advance. If a rotating set of shifts has to be worked, less difficulties are experienced by working progressively later shifts than by going from a 'normal' work day straight on to 'nights'.

Value of routine

Whatever the shift worked, it is advantageous if at all possible to adopt a regular pattern of activity, both in and out of work, and to stick to it. Meals should be taken at fixed times; an effort should be made to have some sleep at the same time each day, even if it is just a nap; and a routine should be developed for social and family commitments. All these things help to entrain and synchronise body rhythms as much as possible.

Those working nights are advised to lead a nocturnal existence as far as is possible. This means sleeping fully during the day, breakfasting in the evening, having lunch during the night shift, and arranging social activities and dinner for the morning.

PATTERNS OF SHIFT WORK

In all essential services, and in some businesses, people have to work a variety of shifts. Neither hospital wards nor fire stations can close down overnight, or at weekends or bank holidays. In most forms of nurse training there is at least one allocation of night duty so that the student can experience patient care throughout the whole 24 hours. Nursing at night offers certain challenges and requires special skills. Night duty allocation may take the form of a period of nights – 8 or 12 weeks for example – on one ward; or there may be 'internal rotation' on each ward of training, whereby the student works a short period of nights at some stage within each allocation.

Whichever system is chosen, different patterns of shift work are possible. Within a 2 week period, for example, a student may work 8, 9 or 10 nights in a row, with nights off on either side. Alternatively there may be shorter periods of nights interspersed with more frequent nights off. Each system has its advantages and disadvantages, and should ideally be suited to the preferences of the individual.

The long stretch of 8 to 10 nights apparently presents the greater challenge but, within that period, there is time for the individual's internal clock to adjust to the new shift. By the third or fourth night, the student may find that sleeping during the day is easier (depending on external factors such as noise). Where night duty is arranged in shorter spells, this period of adjustment is not possible. After 4 nights on duty, just as the 'body clock' has been reset, it is time for nights off; which means activity during the day and sleep during the night. No sooner has she got used to this, than it is time to go back on night duty again.

The problem areas are in the change-overs from night duty to day duty and vice versa. The shorter the spells of night duty, the sooner the change-overs come round, and there is less chance of adjusting to each new shift.

Nurses and other workers doing night shifts will be familiar with some problems of working against the body's internal clock. One of these is feeling cold and 'low' at about 3 in the morning, perhaps because of falls in blood pressure and body temperature (see Figs 18.2 and 18.3). There is also the risk of nodding off, even when the individual has apparently slept well during the preceding day. Conversely, the nurse may feel relatively wide awake at the end of the night shift (when blood pressure and body temperature have risen) and not particularly ready for bed.

It is noticeable, too, that bladder emptying takes time to adjust during shift work. It is usual for the bladder of the day worker to need emptying during the day, urine production falling through the night. In the shift worker, the requirements for sleep and emptying of the bladder do not coincide so well. During the first few nights on duty, he finds he must rise during the day to go to the toilet because urine flow is still raised. When he returns to nights off, and before urine flow adapts to his new pattern of activity, a full bladder tends to wake him from his virtuous rest during the night.

Individual differences

Some people seem better suited to shift work than others. Those who adjust with difficulty seem to have less stable rhythms, or ones which peak early in the day (Fig. 18.9). Those with later peaks (sometimes referred to as 'owls' in contrast to 'larks') seem to fare rather

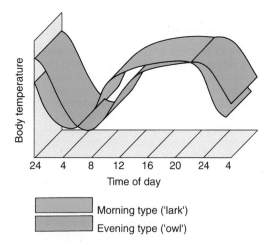

Figure 18.9
Individual differences in circadian rhythms. Some people (morning types) have rhythms that peak earlier in the day than other people (evening types).

better. Individuals who are able to alternate between the sleeping and the waking state with relative ease as the occasion demands cope better too, presumably because they do not build up the same sleep deficits. Sleep deficits may accrue more readily in older people (over 40s) as the ability to sleep continuously without waking decreases with age (see Ch. 36). Older people may therefore have more difficulty adapting to shiftwork.

CIRCADIAN RHYTHMS AND CLINICAL CARE

WARD ROUTINE AND ORGANISATION

A person admitted to hospital exchanges his own daily pattern of living for the ward routine. It is unlikely that these two will coincide. The lighting in the ward, waking and sleeping times, and mealtimes may all differ from 'normal' for that person, and this in turn may affect his well-being.

Life events, like birth and death are not geared to a nine to five work pattern. The natural onset of labour occurs most frequently just after midnight so that, if birth is determined by the body's clock and not the hospital routine, more babies will be born in the early hours of the day than later on.

Mortality, in adults and infants, is also highest between midnight and midday, with a peak around 6 a.m. This peak may be caused by both endogenous and exogenous factors: many physiological changes occur as we begin to wake up; in addition there are less likely to be people around to notice and give help in an emergency either at home or in hospital.

CHANGES IN PATIENTS' BEDTIME ROUTINE

Are hospital wards managed for the benefit of patients – or for the institution and its staff? However much we attempt to care for our patients as individuals, it is probably fair to say that there will be a certain amount of routine in the running of any ward. Meals will arrive at set times rather than when a particular patient feels ready for them. At night, lights may be switched off when most of the routine nursing work has been performed.

In the large, open, 'Nightingale' wards, patients are more likely to be affected at night by light and activity around a few patients who are seriously ill. Their individual needs – such as for television or reading late – are also less easily accommodated than are those of patients in single rooms or in bays with only a few beds. There is limited scope for the nurse to enhance the environment so that it aids patients' sleep – she cannot change the structure of the ward – but what is possible should be attempted. Simple steps like reducing noise levels by lowering voices, wearing quiet shoes and handling equipment quietly are very effective. It often takes the experience of a hospital stay as a patient for the nurse to realise how far the sound of footsteps or conversation carries.

Each person has his or her own ways of preparing for sleep. These may include a warm drink or a snack, a chapter of a book, saying prayers, yoga exercises or meditation, or listening to the last news broadcast of the day. Missing some of this routine may cause anxiety and subsequent loss of sleep.

The nurse can help the patient to sleep by encouraging, where possible, his accustomed bedtime routine. The bed may be screened so that prayers can be said in private, or the patient can read a little longer after the main lights are switched off. A telephone brought to the bedside may allow a patient to phone his wife, reassuring himself about her, and wishing her goodnight. A nurse finding time to sit and listen to a patient's worries for a few minutes, may be more beneficial than a sleeping tablet. And how many patients will remember with gratitude that welcome cup of tea – medical condition permitting – and the comforting presence of the nurse brightening an apparently endless hospital night?

Sleeplessness is not only annoying, it can affect a person's moods and concentration. Research results are not always consistent but mood changes following sleep deprivation seem to include irritability and a feeling of fatigue. Occasionally hallucinations have been reported (Canavan 1984).

If sleeplessness affects a person's feelings of well-being, it seems reasonable for nurses to try as far as possible to help their patients achieve a restful night's sleep. Sometimes a sleeping tablet may help; but good communication with the patient, effective pain relief, reassurance and, where possible, the maintenance of a patient's accustomed bedtime routines are preferable.

NURSING OBSERVATIONS

Nursing observations may differ in their significance according to the phase of body rhythms.

Body temperature

For example the waxing and waning of core body

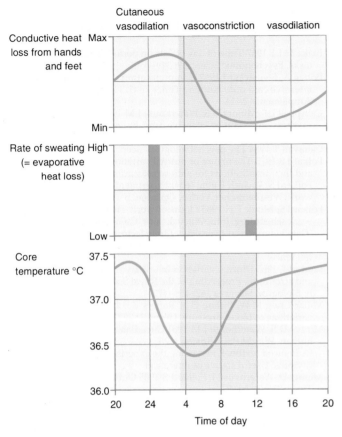

Figure 18.10
The relationship between circadian rhythms in skin blood flow and rate of sweating, and core temperature. When skin blood vessels dilate, the skin becomes warmer, more heat is lost and body temperature falls. When vessels constrict, the skin cools, heat is conserved and body temperature rises. (Adapted from Minors & Waterhouse 1981.)

temperature, brought about by the internal clock, is caused by the individual rhythms of different temperature regulating mechanisms, such as control of skin blood flow and sweating (Fig. 18.10).

In the morning, when sympathetic activity to the skin blood vessels increases under the influence of the internal clock, vasoconstriction occurs, skin temperature falls, and heat is conserved (see Ch. 16). Consequently, core temperature rises. A patient's skin is likely to feel cool to the touch even though his core body temperature is increasing. The early stages of a fever could therefore be missed unless core temperature is measured by thermometer at the same time. However, if the skin *does* feel hot a fever is very likely to be present.

Conversely, late in the evening, when the body clock causes cutaneous vasodilation to occur, skin temperature rises, more heat is lost and core temperature falls. At this time a patient's skin is likely to feel warmer, and he himself will feel hotter, even though core temperature is actually falling. It is important to note if someone

should feel chilly very late in the day because it is likely that something is then wrong.

ILLNESS

It is known that illness itself alters body rhythms. Some specific alterations may be of use in diagnosis. For example changes in the rhythms of skin temperature have been found in the female breast if there are tumours present. The growing tumour generates heat, but in addition its blood supply is not under the same control as normal tissue. Simultaneous recordings of skin temperature from both breasts can reveal differences in the pattern of rhythms between a diseased and a healthy breast.

Abnormalities of circadian rhythms also occur in some forms of psychiatric disorder, such as endogenous and manic depression. Temperature rhythms of less than 24 hours have been found in some people who suffer from regular mood swings over several days. The episodes of emotional disturbance seem to coincide with times when the temperature rhythm is most out of line with the normal body clock. Treatment of the psychiatric disturbance with drugs such as lithium sometimes causes both the mood swings and the temperature rhythm to become more normal.

DRUGS

One complex area of clinical relevance is the optimum timing and dosage of drugs. Because of the underlying circadian changes in body function, there are significant changes during the day in the uptake and elimination of drugs, in their effectiveness on their target tissues, and in the potency of their undesirable side effects. As a result, the same drug may differ in its usefulness depending on the time of day at which it is given.

For example synthetic corticosteroids are used to reduce inflammation in arthritis or to suppress an overactive adrenal gland by inhibiting the secretion of ACTH by the pituitary (see Ch. 10). When treating a person with arthritis it is probably better to give the steroids first thing in the morning. This helps to relieve the stiffness experienced at that time (Fig. 18.11) and is less likely to have the unwanted side effect of adrenal suppression because the pituitary is then least sensitive to steroids. Conversely, if steroids are being given to suppress an overactive adrenal gland the best time of administration may be the evening because the pituitary is then more sensitive. ④

PROSPECTS

It is clear that a knowledge of circadian rhythms has important implications for health, both for health workers and for those they advise or who are in their

④
Why is stiffness a particular problem for the arthritic patient first thing in the morning?

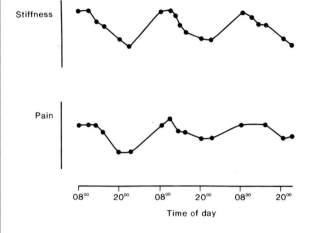

Figure 18.11
Relationship between time of day and subjective ratings of stiffness and pain over 3 successive days in a patient with rheumatoid arthritis. (Reproduced from Waterhouse J M, Minors D S, Waterhouse M E 1990 Your body clock, Figure 14.2, by permission of the Oxford University Press.)

care. As more information becomes available about the effects of altered rhythms in health and disease this aspect of homeostasis is likely to become more important in the delivery of appropriate health care.

KEY POINTS

What you should now understand about circadian rhythms:

- what circadian rhythms are and how they may develop
- why it is best to take daily measurements (such as blood pressure and temperature) at the same time each day
- why circadian rhythms are relevant to clinical care and treatment
- why shift work disturbs body function
- what workers and managers can do to minimise the adverse effects of shift work on health and well-being
- what jet lag is and what causes it
- what a traveller, making a long flight east or west, can do to minimise the effects of jet lag.

REFERENCES AND FURTHER READING

Blake M J F 1967 Time of day effects on performance in a range of tasks. Psychonomic Science 9: 349–350
Börsig A, Steinacker I 1982 Communication with the patient in the intensive care unit. Nursing Times 78 (12) (Intensive Care Supplement): 2–11
Campbell J T, Minors D S, Waterhouse J M 1986 Are circadian rhythms important in intensive care? Intensive Care Nursing 1: 144–150
Canavan T 1984 The psychobiology of sleep. Nursing 2(23): 24–25
Folkard S 1975 The nature of diurnal variations in performance and their implications for shift work studies. In: Colquhoun P, Folkard S, Knauth P et al (eds) Experimental studies of shift work. Westdeutscher Verlag, Opladen, p 119
Folkard S, Monk T H 1985 Hours of work – temporal factors in work scheduling. John Wiley & Sons, Chichester
(Detailed practical overview of time factors determining performance at work. Useful source of information and reference)
Loutit J F 1965 Diurnal variation in urinary excretion of calcium and strontium. Proceeding of the Royal Society of London Series B: Biological Sciences 162: 458–472
Millar-Craig M W, Bishop C N, Raftery E B 1978 Circadian variations of blood pressure. Lancet 1: 795–797
Minors D S, Waterhouse J M 1981 Circadian rhythms and the human. Wright PSG, Bristol, p 26
(Advanced textbook reviewing the experimental data on body rhythms. Useful source of reference)
Minors D, Waterhouse J, Folkard S 1985 Out of rhythm. Nursing Times 81(15): 26–27
Minors D, Waterhouse J, Folkard S 1985 When duty calls. Nursing Times 81(46): 27–28
Waterhouse J M, Minors D S, Waterhouse M E 1990 Your body clock. Oxford University Press, Oxford, pp 148, 151
(Very readable paperback for the traveller as well as the curious)
Weitzman E D 1975 Neuroendocrine pattern of secretion during the sleep–wake cycle of man. Progress in Brain Research 42: 93–102

Chapter 19
ILLNESS

Earlier chapters have described the mechanisms that maintain internal stability in the face of different challenges. Whilst stability is maintained we are healthy. If homeostatic mechanisms become disordered stability is lost and the range of different circumstances which we can tolerate is reduced. We become ill. We may also become ill by experiencing abnormal challenges that overload normal body systems.

Ideally, the goal of medical treatment and nursing care is to restore health, but where this is impossible the goal becomes the maximisation of well-being. This involves supporting the body's own restorative processes, managing the symptoms of illness as well as treating its cause, and developing the body's capacity to meet further challenges. Drugs are often used to support each of these strategies.

HEALTH AND ILLNESS

HEALTH

In health human beings cope with a wide variety of different circumstances such as changes in environmental temperature, activity, position and the availability of food and drink. The ordinary challenges of daily living, such as eating, fasting, sleeping, working, standing up, sitting down, and exercising, are not a problem for the person who is healthy.

People differ in their capacity to cope with such challenges but there are accepted norms of response. For example it is unusual to faint when you stand up. If you do it suggests that something is wrong. Also the ability

> The World Health Organization defines health as 'a state of complete physical and social well-being, and not merely the absence of disease or infirmity.' Health is a very individual concept; a person may be regarded as healthy within certain personal parameters. Someone with a spinal injury may be considered disabled, but would we call a wheelchair athlete in the London Marathon 'unhealthy'? Debate with colleagues the differences between chronic ill health and disability.

to cope with different circumstances changes throughout life as body systems develop, mature and eventually deteriorate (see Section 4). An average person in good health in their seventies would not be expected to be able to run for a bus like a teenager. However, a teenager who is out of breath after running up stairs at home may at best be unfit and at worst be suffering from a respiratory disorder.

Health is thus a relative term which needs to be judged against a backdrop of factors including age, sex, race, and circumstances.

ILLNESS

Illness has been defined as a 'state of insufficiency' (Neumann 1982). It may arise through:

- abnormal function of a part of the body
- abnormal circumstances.

When function is disordered a person becomes less able to cope with some aspects of normal daily living. For example if the alveolar–capillary barrier is thickened the uptake of oxygen by the lungs decreases (see Ch. 7).

① What medical conditions lead to reduced uptake of oxygen in the lungs?

Consequently that person is likely to feel out of breath (dyspnoeic) performing ordinary activities such as climbing stairs. ①

When the circumstances faced are abnormal the inherent limitations of our body systems become apparent. Tourists who have rapidly ascended the 4000 or so metres of Mt. Teidi in the Canary Islands may well feel ill, particularly if they decide to have a brisk walk. This is not due to disorder, but occurs because their body systems are not well adapted to high altitude. Consequently they experience altitude sickness.

Illness arising from either cause (abnormal function or abnormal circumstances) is due to the inability of homeostatic mechanisms to cope adequately with the circumstances faced.

② What is the source of keto-acids?

ABNORMAL FUNCTION

Each disorder has its own characteristic spectrum of effects. It is not the purpose of this chapter to consider pathophysiology in detail. However, it is appropriate in the context of the study of homeostasis to consider illness as a disturbance of that state and to analyse the consequences of such a disturbance in terms of physiological function. In any disorder there is a root problem or primary defect that disturbs body systems and has many repercussions. Several examples are given in Figure 19.1. Lack of insulin, which gives rise to diabetes mellitus (Fig. 19.1B), will be considered in more detail in order to illustrate several important principles and concepts.

THE PRIMARY DEFECT

In diabetes mellitus (type I) the primary defect may be defined as the lack of secretion of the hormone insulin from the endocrine pancreas (see Ch. 10). As insulin is an important regulator of metabolism the lack of this hormone leads to widespread disturbances in the metabolism of carbohydrates, fats and proteins. Insulin's

chief role is to facilitate the uptake of glucose into many cells of the body. Therefore the immediate consequence of an insulin deficiency is to 'starve' insulin-dependent cells of glucose.

REPERCUSSIONS

Initial effects

Cells of the body respond to the lack of intracellular glucose in much the same way as they do in health (see Ch. 14). Fat cells, for example, increase their breakdown of fat stores, releasing fatty acids into the blood just as they do in starvation. As a result keto-acids are formed in increasing amounts. However, in diabetes, unlike starvation, ketosis occurs when blood glucose concentration is high. ②

Because glucose is unable to enter many cells easily in the absence of insulin, it builds up in concentration in the blood especially after a meal. Ordinarily the increase in blood glucose concentration stimulates the secretion of insulin which in turn promotes the cellular uptake of glucose. Normally, therefore, the blood glucose con-

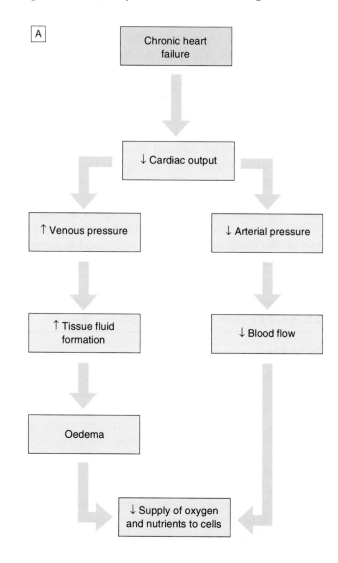

Figure 19.1 (*right and facing page*) Examples of abnormal functioning and the repercussions resulting from them:
A Chronic heart failure
B Lack of insulin
C Tumour of the adrenal medulla.

centration increases by only two- to threefold. However, in diabetes, although the absorption of sugar from the digestive tract is normal, the cellular uptake of glucose is not and, as a result, much larger increases in blood sugar concentration occur (Fig. 19.2).

Thus, when function is disordered, some of the effects produced, such as ketosis and hyperglycaemia, are an exaggeration of the normal response.

Subsequent effects

The increased plasma concentrations of keto-acids (*ketosis*) and of glucose (*hyperglycaemia*) have repercussions on other body systems.

PAINFUL JOINTS AND MUSCLE WASTING

If a joint is painful, the sufferer almost always tries to protect the affected limb by, for example, not moving it through its full range of movements or not putting his full weight on the leg. It may sometimes be noticed that muscles working the painful joint become wasted. A person's left thigh muscles may be much less bulky than those of the right thigh because of arthritis in the left hip.

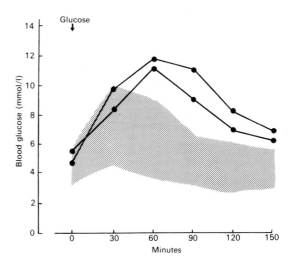

Figure 19.2
Normal range of changes in blood glucose concentration (shaded area) after the ingestion of a standard dose of glucose (glucose tolerance test). The results obtained in two people with diabetes (● — ●) are shown for comparison. (Reproduced from Emslie-Smith et al 1988, Figure 23.15, by permission of the publishers.)

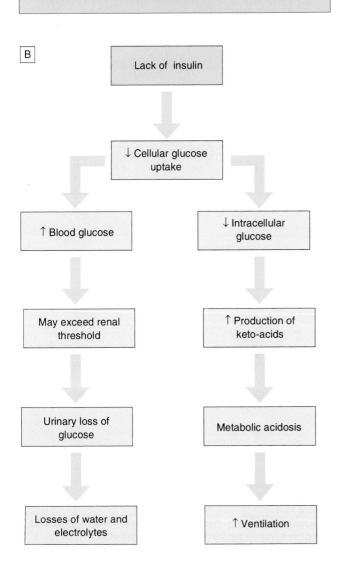

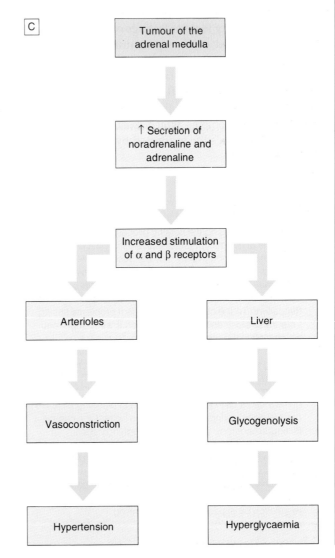

For example, more glucose is delivered to the kidney nephrons in the glomerular filtrate than can be recovered by the tubules. As a result glucose is lost in the urine accompanied by water and electrolytes (see Ch. 8). Similarly, the increased concentration of keto-acids decreases blood pH. The metabolic acidosis stimulates peripheral chemoreceptors and the rate and depth of breathing increase (see Ch. 12).

Thus, defective function of one part of the body leads inevitably to a readjustment of activity in other parts.

CLINICAL FEATURES

These and other changes in various systems of the body provide the clues from which the health worker is able to deduce the nature of the underlying problem and to make judgements as to the best course of action. The specific features which the health worker recognises as significant are *signs* of illness. In diabetes mellitus these could include a sweet smell on a person's breath and the measurable presence of glucose in the urine. Those things which the individual notices about themselves and reports to others are *symptoms* of illness. In diabetes mellitus these may include feelings of weakness or faintness, an increased need to pass urine and a persistent thirst.

Careful note should be taken of all that an individual reports. By informed questioning, further relevant information can be obtained that will help to clarify the nature of the problems which exist and the degree to which that person's life is affected by them. ③

③
What other signs and symptoms might you look for in diabetes mellitus?

PATIENT PROBLEMS

Nursing care utilising the nursing process is built on the problems of the patient rather than on the clinical features of the disease (though they may be closely related). For example, in anaemia, a reduced haemoglobin level and skin pallor may be signs distinguished by the clinician, while dizziness and lethargy may be symptoms experienced by the patient. To the nurse, it is the patient problems arising from these signs and symptoms which are important and which dictate the care provided. Thus, 'dizziness on exertion' is a patient problem calling for assistance with washing and dressing, the provision of frequent rest periods and help when taking short walks.

Patient problems need precise definition. 'Pain' is too generalised a term to assist the nurse in planning effective care. 'Pain following surgery' is a little better for it can be distinguished from, say, 'pain on coughing'. 'Pain, especially during inspiration, following cholecystectomy' is far more helpful. This tells us that we need to provide analgesia prior to breathing exercises with the physiotherapist, and that we must position the patient carefully to assist in breathing. (Incidentally, why may respiration be especially painful following cholecystectomy?)

FROM PHYSIOLOGY TO PATHOLOGY

The repercussions flowing from the primary defect are part and parcel of the controls that normally maintain homeostasis. In that sense they are physiological, but because they are much larger than normal and because they do not restore the normal state they are actually pathological.

In health, intracellular and extracellular glucose concentrations fluctuate throughout the day but stay within the normal range (see Ch. 1). It is only when concentrations fall outside this range, as they do in uncontrolled diabetes mellitus, that they are properly termed pathological.

Glucose concentrations outside the normal range will clearly produce metabolic effects not seen normally. Many of the features of advanced diabetes mellitus, such as neuropathy and vascular disease, are believed to be caused by hyperglycaemia rather than lack of insulin.

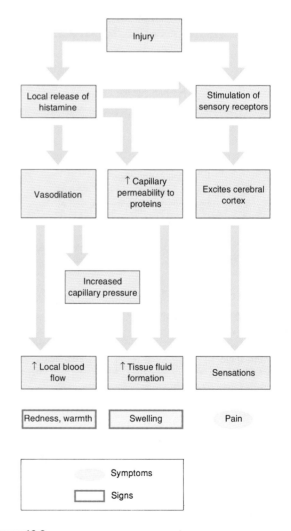

Figure 19.3
Responses to injury giving rise to the signs (outlined in blue) and symptoms (yellow background) of inflammation.

ABNORMAL CIRCUMSTANCES

The day to day challenges, or stresses, which we all face, are the ingredients that make life varied, interesting and exciting. In that sense stress is a vital part of life. However, we tend to think of stress as bad. This is because we often use the same word to describe both the challenges that we face (*stressors*) and a particular set of reactions provoked by those challenges (the *stress response*). A healthy person can tolerate a wide range of stressors but there are limits beyond which normal body systems are overwhelmed. Those limits are partly determined by the fitness we develop by being exposed to the very same stressors.

STRESSORS

Those things which disturb us, whether a change in environmental temperature, going without breakfast, or the prospect of an examination, are *stressors*. As we have seen in previous chapters, homeostatic mechanisms triggered by the disturbance produced by the stressor help to stabilise our inner environment in the face of such challenges. In response to heat, we sweat; in response to cold, we shiver. Both responses enable us to maintain an acceptable body temperature (see Ch. 16). Similarly, the responses produced by injury, such as the local release of histamine and other substances, cause inflammation which promotes the repair of the damaged tissue and defends it against further injury and infection (Fig. 19.3 and Ch. 15).

When stressors are acute or intense the normal reaction to them includes a characteristic set of responses termed the *stress response*.

THE STRESS RESPONSE

The stress response (Fig. 19.4) is normally elicited in response to life-threatening stressors such as danger, injury, and haemorrhage. Its purpose is to enable us to meet the extreme challenges posed by these situations. The stress response involves:

- activation of the sympathetic nervous system (including secretion of adrenaline)
- increased secretion of several pituitary hormones (including ACTH and growth hormone).

Activation of the sympathetic nervous system affects many different cells and tissues (Fig. 19.5) and gives rise to a familiar set of symptoms:

- increased heart rate
- sweaty hands and forehead
- feelings of queaziness
- general agitation
- dry mouth.

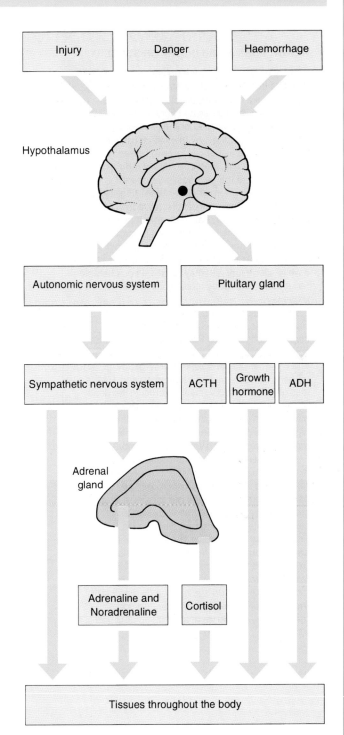

Figure 19.4
The stress response.

Simultaneous changes in metabolism caused by the hormones secreted increase glucose supplies (Fig. 19.6) and guarantee the supply of nutrients to vital tissues such as the brain.

It is the experience of these responses, together with related psychological effects that we popularly know as 'stress'. In so far as the stress response enables us to meet the actual challenge we face, as it does in injury,

WEIGHT LOSS AFTER INJURY OR SURGERY

In injury or after surgery the neural and hormonal changes that are part of the stress response (Fig. 19.4) provoke metabolic effects that flood the body fluids with glucose and fatty acids (Fig. 19.6). Glucose is conserved for the tissues such as nerves that rely upon it by the anti-insulin effect of hormones such as cortisol, growth hormone and adrenaline. Initially, metabolic rate is reduced (*ebb phase*) but then as recovery occurs it increases above normal (*flow phase*) (Fig. 19.7). After severe burns, for example, metabolic rate may double. Muscle protein is broken down and the liberated amino acids are used to form new glucose (*gluconeogenesis*) and to replenish the depleted supplies. The flow phase may persist for a while after injury and may lead to a considerable reduction in lean body mass, but it is a life preserver.

Weight loss following major surgery can be significant especially where there are complications such as infections. Elective surgery commonly leads to a loss in weight of between 4 and 8% whereas, after serious emergency surgery, the loss may be between 10 and 15%. A loss greater than 20% usually results in the death of the patient. The combination of serious injury, major surgery and septicaemia causes the highest loss of body weight, and the greatest threat to the patient's successful recovery.

If the patient is unable to eat sufficiently for an extended postoperative period, nutrients should be provided via an intravenous route (*total parenteral nutrition*). These will consist of vitamins, electrolytes and trace elements as well as carbohydrates, fats and proteins (see Ch. 14). This process is expensive, but it will enable the patient to turn around from a *catabolic* state (where there is breakdown of body proteins and fats) to an *anabolic* state, where muscle mass and fat stores are built up again. For a discussion of the effects of surgery and/or injury on body metabolism, see Boore et al 1987, pp. 393 and 742–3.

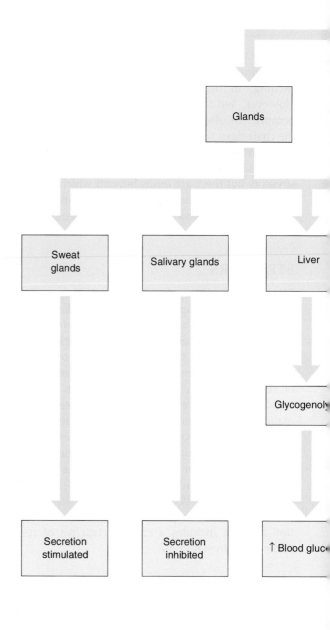

Sweating   Dry mouth

Figure 19.5 (*above and right-hand page*)
Effects of activation of the sympathetic nervous system on different tissues, and how these effects give rise to various signs (outlined in blue) and symptoms (yellow background).

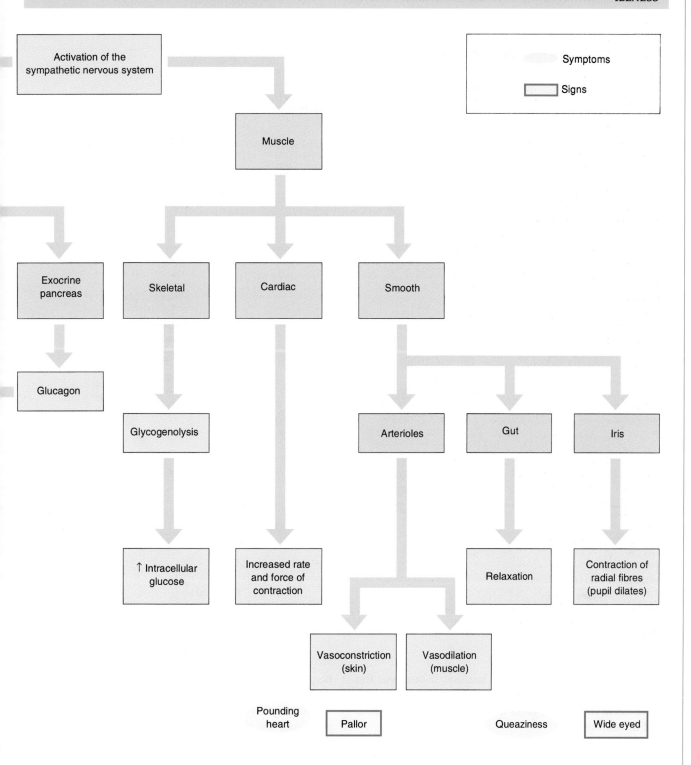

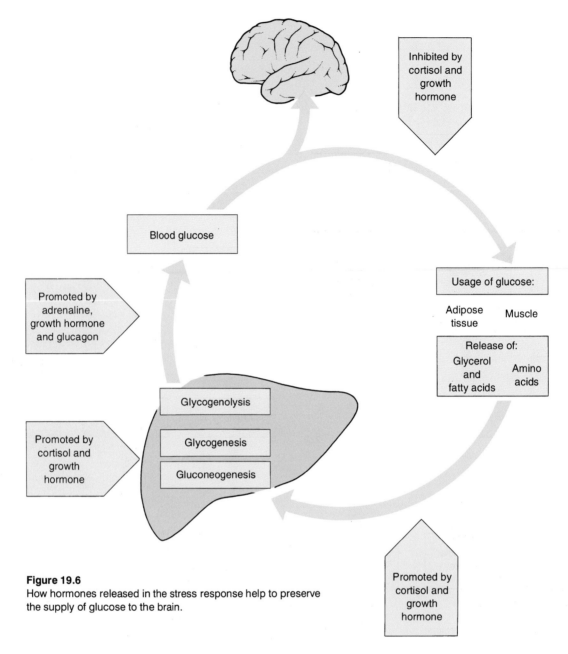

Figure 19.6
How hormones released in the stress response help to preserve the supply of glucose to the brain.

it is normal, physiological and healthy. If however the stress response is triggered by trivial events or if it does more harm to us than good it is abnormal, pathological and unhealthy. ④

OVERLOAD

There are, however, limits to the amount of disturbance that we can tolerate. If we exceed the capacity of our body systems the stability of the internal environment cannot be maintained. In heat stroke for example (see Ch. 16) the rising body temperature creates even more heat by stimulating metabolism. This is an example of positive feedback (Fig. 19.8). Once the rate at which heat is gained rapidly begins to exceed the capacity of the homeostatic control mechanisms to lose heat through

negative feedback mechanisms, body temperature rises out of control.

Similarly in major injury the homeostatic changes provoked by the stress may create further threats to stability (Fig. 19.9). There may be a reduced blood supply to many tissues (*shock*) leading to tissue hypoxia and metabolic acidosis. Problems multiply and get out

In severe cases of *septicaemia* (the presence of pathogens in the blood) there will be massive loss of fluid from the vascular compartment because of increased capillary permeability. Septicaemic shock can be severe and life-threatening, with dramatic falls in the patient's blood pressure (see Boore et al 1987, Ch. 10).

④
Can you think of healthy and unhealthy stressors in nursing? What steps might each nurse take to manage her work so as to reduce the stress response caused by some of the unhealthy stressors?

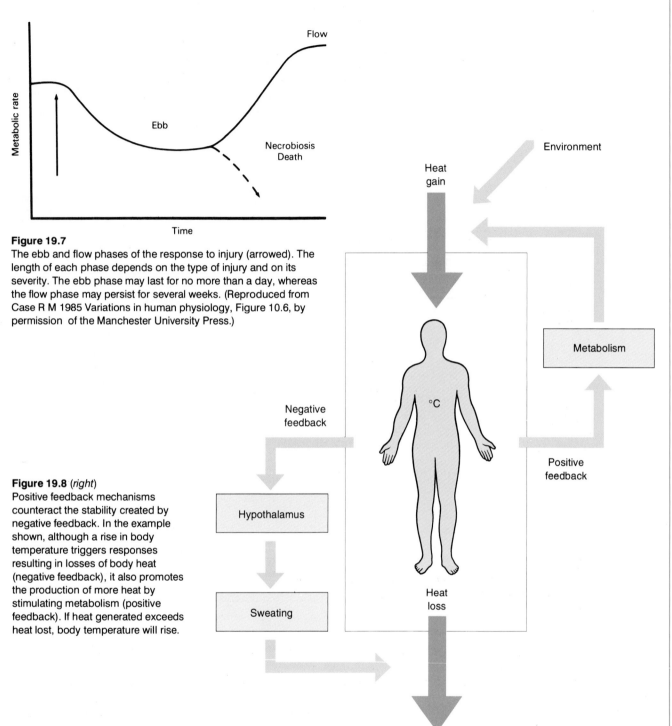

Figure 19.7
The ebb and flow phases of the response to injury (arrowed). The length of each phase depends on the type of injury and on its severity. The ebb phase may last for no more than a day, whereas the flow phase may persist for several weeks. (Reproduced from Case R M 1985 Variations in human physiology, Figure 10.6, by permission of the Manchester University Press.)

Figure 19.8 (*right*)
Positive feedback mechanisms counteract the stability created by negative feedback. In the example shown, although a rise in body temperature triggers responses resulting in losses of body heat (negative feedback), it also promotes the production of more heat by stimulating metabolism (positive feedback). If heat generated exceeds heat lost, body temperature will rise.

of control. This runaway state (*necrobiosis*) is grave and is the state usually preceding death. ⑤

FITNESS

However, stressors are not simply disturbers of homeostasis or threats to our health. They are in fact vital to our well-being because, by being exposed to stressors of various kinds, we develop a fitness of our bodies appropriate to our circumstances. For example, the formation of bone tissue is stimulated in response to pressure (see Ch. 28). If pressure is not applied, bones do not develop the same strength. Likewise, if someone is confined to bed for long periods of time, muscle wasting occurs. The tissue is only built up again if stressors are applied in the form of progressive exercise (see Ch. 17). ⑥

⑤
In which circumstances would you expect vasoconstriction to be severe?

⑥
What are the nursing implications of a patient confined to bed for long periods? How might his general fitness be maintained as far as is possible?

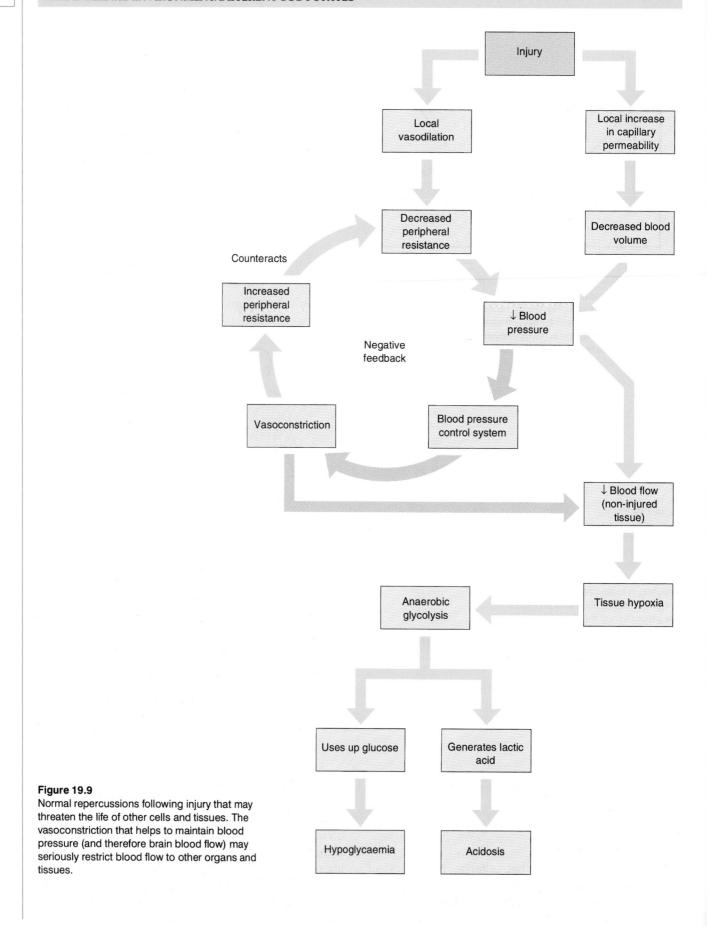

Figure 19.9
Normal repercussions following injury that may threaten the life of other cells and tissues. The vasoconstriction that helps to maintain blood pressure (and therefore brain blood flow) may seriously restrict blood flow to other organs and tissues.

ASPECTS OF CARE, TREATMENT AND THERAPY

The proper care of an ill person requires a knowledge both of the primary cause and how it may be corrected, and of the repercussions flowing from it. These may have far reaching consequences for the well-being of the individual and need to be understood in order to be managed effectively. Interventions that tackle the repercussions will make the illness more bearable and limit its extent, but only those interventions that deal with the primary cause will actually provide a cure. Whatever interventions are chosen they should assist and not hinder the body's own restorative processes.

> Nursing care needs to be based on knowledge of pathophysiology; without that background, errors can occur. A patient, 24 hours after operation, complains of pain for which you propose to give an injection of pethidine which has been prescribed. Your junior nurse points out that the patient's blood pressure is now 100/70 mmHg, a little lower than normal. She asks, 'Won't the pethidine lower his blood pressure further?' What reply would you give and what actions would you take?

ASSISTING RESTORATIVE PROCESSES

The human body itself is a primary source of healing. Thus the role of the health professional may be simply one of working *with* the body's natural defences and restorative processes to re-attain optimal functioning. Some illnesses such as those caused by infection, bacterial or viral, may just 'take their course' and the health worker chiefly acts to:

- minimise discomfort created by the patient's symptoms
- minimise further threats to recovery
- maximise conditions conducive to recovery.⑦

If the illness is more serious, a more interventionist approach may be necessary, in which the body's defences are supplemented by external means. For

CURE OR RELIEF OF SYMPTOMS

Anti-inflammatory drugs, such as indomethacin, may be prescribed for various forms of arthritis. While not providing a cure, they give relief by reducing the inflammation caused by the production of substances such as prostaglandins. Reducing the inflammation alleviates many of the symptoms such as pain and stiffness which cause discomfort. Similarly, a hip replacement for osteoarthritis of the hip, which effectively gets rid of the pain, stiffness and immobility associated with the disease process, is not a cure for the disease, though to the patient it may well feel like one.

example, in extensive sepsis of the body it has been found that the intravenous infusion of large quantities of glucose and amino acids can assist recovery. This treatment mimics the body's own 'infusion' of these substances in the flow phase of injury (see p. 340 and Fig. 19.7).

The general approach outlined above may also be appropriate for illnesses precipitated by an overload of body systems. But in these cases the immediate need to reduce the stressors precipitating the illness, in order to promote recovery, may in the longer term be replaced by a strategy in which the stressors are gradually re-introduced in order to develop fitness.

The way to overcome altitude sickness for example is to spend time acclimatising to one altitude before proceeding to the next (see Ch. 11). Similarly, people recovering from cardiac surgery need to be encouraged to increase their level of exercise gradually so that the heart may attain an optimal fitness.

MAXIMISING WELL-BEING

Not all illnesses can be cured but a person's well-being may be considerably enhanced by appropriate treatment and informed care. Treatment may itself introduce new problems which must be addressed in order to maximise wellness.

Surgery

If, for example, treatment consists of surgery to remove

A CASE OF ANAEMIA

In anaemia, the body compensates for a reduction in the oxygen-carrying capacity of the red blood cells by increasing the cardiac output. Hence, although there is a smaller amount of oxygen carried by a fixed volume of blood, the blood is circulated around the body more quickly, picking up oxygen in the lungs en route. Simultaneously, the individual's respiration rate may increase.

These adaptive mechanisms succeed for some time but, should the haemoglobin level continue to diminish (for example because of chronic haemorrhage from a peptic ulcer), the time will come when adaptation is no longer adequate. The heart will no longer be able to pump efficiently at its increased rate, and heart failure will ensue.

Medical and nursing intervention should ideally be aimed at stabilising the patient's initial physiological defect and treating the related problems. Iron supplements, together with nursing advice on diet, may improve the patient's haemoglobin level. A drug such as cimetidine may resolve the problem of the peptic ulcer and its related chronic blood loss. Nursing intervention would include advice on the avoidance of smoking, drinking spirits and eating spicy foods, and on ways of improving the response to normal stressors such as work and family life. Adequate, effective and timely intervention may prevent the problem of anaemia from developing into the more serious one of heart failure.

⑦ *Can you give examples of illnesses which fit with the three actions by the health worker?*

a part of the body which has become diseased there are bound to be some physiological repercussions. These may be minor, as in an appendectomy, or major as in a gastrectomy. Removal of the appendix results in the loss of a small part of the immune system (see Ch. 4) which may not matter in view of the enormous reserves of immune cells. However, removal of the stomach creates a variety of digestive problems and can lead to pernicious anaemia through lack of intrinsic factor (see Chs 4 and 6). Similarly, resection of a large amount of pancreatic tissue in order to treat pancreatic carcinoma may cause diabetes mellitus because of the simultaneous loss of islet cells (see Ch. 10).

Replacement therapy

Losses of function caused by surgery and by the deficient functioning of a tissue may be remedied by *replacement therapy*. This is most useful when the problem created is caused by the lack of a specific substance. For example pernicious anaemia, arising from the loss of intrinsic factor following a gastrectomy, can be treated by giving injections of vitamin B_{12}.

Replacement therapy is often used in the treatment of endocrine disorders. Diabetes mellitus became a treatable disease in the 1920s when it was shown that extracts of pancreatic tissue could be successfully injected. Before this, the life expectancy of people diagnosed as having diabetes mellitus was only a few years. One of the first people who received injections of these crude extracts was still alive and well 60 years later.

However, replacement therapy does not cure the condition. It merely compensates for defective function. It is also not as simple a treatment as it might appear. The concentration of most hormones in the body is not constant but varies during the day (see Ch. 18). Ideally, hormone replacement therapy should exactly mimic the natural state. Attempts are made to follow natural patterns of hormone secretion as closely as possible. In diabetes, for example, the timing of insulin injections is crucial and computerised injection systems are being developed.

USING DRUGS

Many drugs are chemicals that are foreign to the body (*xenobiotics*). Some are extracts of natural materials. Others have been created in the research laboratories of pharmaceutical companies. Drugs act by interfering with the chemistry of the body, and can be used to stimulate or inhibit specific cell activities, and therefore assist recovery or compensate for defective function. However, in addition to their beneficial effects on one part of the body, drugs almost inevitably disturb the

Digitalis, a drug once used in the treatment of heart failure, is extracted from the common purple foxglove (*Digitalis purpurea*). The preferred drug now in the UK is digoxin, prepared from the Australian white foxglove (*Digitalis lanata*). Digoxin is said to be more reliable in its action than digitalis, and more consistent.

Morphine and pethidine are both strong analgesics. Morphine is a natural substance derived from one of the Asian poppies. An older, and greatly abused, form of morphine was opium. Pethidine is a synthetic version of morphine; it is also highly addictive.

function of other parts (they have *side effects*) and may, if taken for a long period, cause the body to adapt to them (development of *tolerance*).

Side effects

Beta-blockers such as propranolol are sometimes prescribed to lessen the extreme anxiety of a student at examination time. Beta-blockers do this by blocking the action of adrenaline on beta receptors in the heart, thereby reducing heart rate (see Ch. 5). However, they also block the action of adrenaline on beta receptors elsewhere in the body including those in the bronchioles, thereby producing bronchoconstriction (see Ch. 7). This could be dangerous for a student suffering from asthma.

Much pharmacological research is directed at identifying side effects and developing related compounds that retain the desired therapeutic effect whilst minimising the side effects. Thus, research has led to the development of drugs such as atenolol that block beta receptors in the heart ($beta_1$) but which have less effect on beta receptors in the airways ($beta_2$).

Tolerance

Tolerance is a reduced response to repeated doses of a drug. It is caused by cells adapting to the drug. If the

WHY ANALGESIC DRUGS MAY BE TEMPORARILY WITHHELD

The administration of drugs may disguise important signs or symptoms. For example, a patient who is admitted to hospital with severe abdominal pain will have analgesia withheld until a diagnosis is made. Pain can be a vital diagnostic aid. However cruel it may seem, withholding analgesia until the patient is seen by, say, the surgical registrar may help in distinguishing between, for example, a perforated peptic ulcer and acute pancreatitis.

Analgesia is usually not given to head injury patients who are conscious. Again, it may seem kinder to rid the patient of an unpleasant headache by giving him an injection. But, should drowsiness ensue, the clinician will then have to decide whether this is caused by the injection or by the head injury itself.

drug is suddenly discontinued the cells re-adapt slowly to the new conditions and that adaptation is experienced by someone as *withdrawal symptoms*.

Adaptive mechanisms

Just as we respond to the challenge of exercise by developing fitness, so the disposal systems that deal with foreign compounds (xenobiotics; Ch. 15) may respond to the challenge posed by increased concentrations of drugs in body fluids by increasing their capacity to deal with them. An example of this is the way in which barbiturates, once commonly used as 'sleeping pills', induce the formation of more drug metabolising enzymes in the liver. As a result the drug is metabolised and eliminated more rapidly and consequently becomes less effective. Benzodiazepines, now used rather than barbiturates in the treatment of severe insomnia, do not induce the formation of more liver enzymes but still induce tolerance.

Tolerance can also develop through changes in the regulatory mechanisms controlling the number of receptor proteins (see Ch. 2) present in cell membranes. When a cell is continually exposed to a high concentration of a neurotransmitter (or hormone) it adapts by making fewer of the membrane receptors specific for it (*down-regulation*). Consequently, the cell becomes less sensitive to the same concentration of neurotransmitter. The same thing can happen in response to drugs that mimic the effect of the neurotransmitter.

The opposite process, whereby a cell adapts to a reduced level of neurotransmitter by increasing the manufacture of receptor proteins, is *up-regulation*. Up-regulation may explain the recovery of synaptic transmission occurring at synapses where the release of transmitter has been blocked by a drug.

Withdrawal symptoms

Over a period of time therefore we may adapt to a drug and come to rely upon it (*dependence*). If the drug is then abruptly discontinued our cells are again disturbed and have to re-adapt to the new environment. The experience of this re-adaptation (*withdrawal symptoms*), which takes days if not weeks to occur, can be unpleasant and severe. For this reason a staged reduction in drug dosage may be prescribed. (8)

In making use of drugs, their advantages have always to be weighed against their disadvantages. Because of the way that the body naturally adapts to new situations, the continued use of drugs in any except essential circumstances should be avoided.

KEY POINTS

What you should now understand from this chapter:

- definitions of health and illness from a physiological perspective
- how systems may become disordered leading to illness
- how the repercussions of a disturbance give rise to the signs and symptoms of disease
- the distinctions made between physiology and pathology
- what is understood by stress and what stress does
- what happens as a result of injury
- a rationale for strategies used in the prevention, management and treatment of illness
- the basis of some problems associated with the use of drugs in the treatment of disease.

REFERENCES AND FURTHER READING

Bailey R, Clarke M 1989 Stress and coping in nursing. Chapman & Hall, London
(Puts basic concepts into more complex ones used in nursing. Useful review of biological concepts of stress in Ch. 1)
Boore J R P, Champion R, Ferguson M C (eds) 1987 Nursing the physically ill adult. Churchill Livingstone, Edinburgh
Case R M 1985 Variations in human physiology. Manchester University Press, Manchester, p 221
Dornan T (ed) 1988 Diabetes care: a problem solving approach. Heinemann Professional Publishing, London
(Realistic, practical down to earth book, using case studies to illustrate problems. Good introduction to diabetes in Ch. 1)
Emslie-Smith D, Paterson C, Scratcherd T, Read N W (eds) 1988 Textbook of physiology, 11th edn. Churchill Livingstone, Edinburgh, p 295
George J (ed) 1990 Nursing theories: the base for professional nursing practice, 3rd edn. Prentice-Hall International, New Jersey
(Summarises the work of 18 nurse theorists and the background to their thinking, including Betty Neumann in Ch. 16, pp 259–278)
Little R A 1985 Injury (shock). In: Case R M (ed) Variations in human physiology. Manchester University Press, Manchester
(Useful concise review of the effects of injury on body systems)
Little R A, Frayn K N (eds) 1986 The scientific basis for the care of the critically ill. Manchester University Press, Manchester
(Collection of specialist articles. Useful for reference)
Neumann B 1982 The Neumann systems model: application to nursing education and practice. Appleton-Century-Crofts, East Norwalk, Connecticut
Pearson A, Vaughan B 1991 Nursing models for practice. Butterworth Heinemann, Oxford
(Very readable text describing six major models of nursing including 'The health care systems model' based on Neumann's work)
Trounce J 1990 Clinical pharmacology for nurses, 13th edn. Churchill Livingstone, Edinburgh
(Drugs commonly used in practice and how they work)
Watkins P J 1988 ABC of diabetes. British Medical Association, London
(Interesting, attractive collection of short articles)

(8)
What are the especial dangers of abruptly stopping steroid therapy?

Section 3
INTERACTION WITH
THE EXTERNAL ENVIRONMENT

Our lives as persons consist of all the things we are able to sense, to understand and to do. Seeing, hearing, feeling, observing, speaking, moving, making and discovering – all of these and many other activities combine to create our own unique experience of life and our personal contribution to it. Human life at its fullest involves exploring our environment, interpreting what we see, hear and feel, communicating our findings and experiences to others in word and action, and making and developing new things and ideas.

This section will focus on the structure and function of those parts of the body that affect our experiences and reactions, and what we are able to do in our work and leisure.

Part A
COMPONENT PARTS AND SYSTEMS:
structure and function

The parts of the body that are primarily concerned with our experiences and reactions and what we are able to do are:

- the nervous system
- the musculoskeletal system.

The chapters in this part of the book:

- outline the anatomy of the somatic nervous system and describe and explain how it is organised functionally
- describe the structure of nerve and muscle cells and explain how they work.

Chapter 20
THE SOMATIC NERVOUS SYSTEM: AN INTRODUCTION

The somatic nervous system controls all skeletal muscles within our bodies, and therefore determines our actions. It also creates our personal consciousness of the world about us and of our place in it. It is a complex system about which a great deal is yet to be unravelled, but it is also fascinating in that its workings determine our personality, intelligence, and skills. By knowing more about how the nervous system functions we may increase our understanding of our own experience and behaviour, as well as that of others.

During gestation, the nervous system develops from just a few primitive cells (*neuroectoderm*) to form the brain, spinal cord, and cranial and spinal nerves. Within the brain and spinal cord, neurones and their axons are grouped together to form many different structures.

Interwoven amongst the neurones are supporting cells (*glia*) that do not conduct impulses but help to maintain the function of the nervous system. Preservation of nerve cell function is also the role of the blood supply, the blood–brain barrier and the cerebrospinal fluid.

The brain and the spinal cord are both enveloped by membranes and housed within the bony chambers of the skull and vertebral canal.

> Human functions, whether physiological or psychological, are so interrelated that professional care cannot be given if disease processes are considered without taking into account their effect on the individual and his family. This is the basis of the holistic approach to nursing care.

UNDERSTANDING THE NERVOUS SYSTEM

Once the somatic nervous system is reduced to nerves, muscles and electrical events it is all too easy to lose sight of what these things mean in terms of everyday experience, particularly if psychology and physiology are viewed as completely separate subjects. Both subjects are concerned with understanding how our minds work and how we behave, but they usually approach the subject from different angles and use different methods of investigation. Often the physiologist looks narrowly at specific neural mechanisms and from this attempts to build up a model of how the brain works and how this determines behaviour. Conversely the psychologist may first observe a person's behaviour and then attempts to infer how that behaviour is brought about. For a full understanding of our minds and behaviour, both approaches are necessary and insights from each subject need to be combined. ①

PHYSIOLOGICAL FRAMEWORK

Like the autonomic nervous system (see Ch. 3), the components of the somatic nervous system may be divided into three elements:

- sensory
- motor
- integrative.

Sensory systems (Chs 23–26) are responsible for detecting changes in our external environment, for analysing

① *What is the difference between physiology and psychology?*

this information, and for selecting what is transmitted to those parts of the brain that 'make sense' of the information and power our actions.

Motor systems (Chs 27–29) control the contraction of skeletal muscle at an unconscious (i.e. reflex) and at a conscious (i.e. voluntary) level. These systems enable us to walk, run, stand, sit, make sounds, frown etc. ②

Integrative components blend information from our senses with commands issued to the muscles to produce sophisticated activities, such as thinking, writing and speaking, and other features of our personalities such as mood, emotion and motivation (Chs 30–33).

PSYCHOLOGICAL DIMENSIONS

Experience

What we experience depends in part on what our sensory receptors tell us about stimuli originating from outside and inside our bodies. Excitation of the brain provoked by activation of sensory receptors gives rise to the experience of *sensation*. For example, the absorption of light by receptors in the eye gives rise to the sensation of vision, whereas the excitation of nerve endings in the skin and elsewhere by injurious stimuli (e.g. tissue damage) gives rise to the sensation of pain. Receptors do not respond to vision or pain. Receptors stimulate the brain areas that create these sensations in our minds. These sensations in turn alert us to changes both outside and inside the body.

Intelligence

Understanding what has been sensed depends upon the links or *associations* we make between different forms of sensory experience and also between present and past experiences. There is a difference, as any student will know, between hearing the sounds of a teacher speaking and actually understanding what is being said or between looking at a drawing in a book and knowing what it means. Sensation and perception are not the same thing. In sensing something we register a change in some aspect of our internal or external environment; in perceiving it we know what it is. We think about it.

Expression

We give expression to our understanding of our experiences in various ways, by what we do and say, by our laughter, tears, smiles and frowns. We convert our thoughts into activity. We react consciously and unconsciously to the stimuli acting on us. Sometimes we react instinctively (*reflexly*). At other times we make more considered choices, weighing up different strategies and choosing what on balance seems best at the time (*voluntary behaviour*). All these things rely on nerve networks that link sensory and motor systems and on the chemical processes that allow nerve im-

pulses to be transmitted rapidly between different parts of the nervous system and ultimately to the muscles.

Emotion

Our emotions are the area of our experience that at present is least well defined. When we talk about emotion in everyday conversation we generally mean that we are talking about how we feel and the kind of mood that we are in. We talk too of what we see of other people's behaviour, whether they appear aggressive, or jolly, spirited or sad. Emotion seems to involve several systems:

- sensory systems informing us of our experience
- motor systems generating responses both somatically (somatic nervous system) and viscerally (autonomic nervous system)
- other parts of the nervous system influencing our level of alertness.

Memory and learning

Nerve impulses last for only a short time. Yet we remember skills we have learnt long after we have finished practising. We also recall names and faces, facts and figures. Sometimes just one powerful exposure to a set of events will imprint them on our minds, and overrule all others. Usually for a memory to be formed rehearsal and repetition of the stimuli will be needed to actually forge the long-term links between the brain cells concerned. Once firmly stored in the form of connections between nerve cells a new pattern of thought and action is established. ③

> Nursing practice includes many skills that are both rehearsed and repeated, for example giving injections, taking temperatures, taking blood pressures. When these skills have been used countless times they are seldom forgotten and may become mechanical. Conscious thought about the effect on the patient should always accompany the action.

STRUCTURE OF THE NERVOUS SYSTEM

TERMINOLOGY

Anatomists describe what they see, and so the various parts of the brain have usually been named according to their appearance rather than their function, rather in the way that in geography names are given to distinctive features in a landscape. Often these names are derived from Latin or Greek words so their ordinariness is not immediately obvious. *Pons*, for example, means 'bridge'

② *What is an example of a reflex action?*

③ *What is the difference between rehearsal and repetition?*

Table 20.1 Origin and meaning of some anatomical terms*

Origin	Term	Meaning
Latin	Cerebellum	Small brain
	Colliculus	A litle hill
	Commissure	A join
	Cortex	Bark, rind
	Fasciculus	A little bundle
	Foramen	A hole
	Limbic	Bordering, edging
	Nucleus	A kernel
	Ventricle	A little cavity
Greek	Arachnoid	Like a spider
	Chiasma	Greek letter 'x'
	Cranium	Skull
	Gyrus	A turn or twist
	Ganglion	Knot or swelling
	Hippocampus	Sea-horse
	Lemniscus	A strip or band
	Thalamus	Inner room
	Hypothalamus	Below the thalamus

* Source: Butterworths Medical Dictionary (1978)

and *sulcus* is a 'furrow' and so on. Some common terms and their meanings are listed in Table 20.1. Occasionally other, self-evident terms are used: the *olive*, for example, looks that shape.

Superficial structures

The component parts of the nervous system (brain, spinal cord and peripheral nerves) are shown in Figure 20.1. The central structures, namely the brain and spinal cord are termed the *central nervous system* whereas the nerves connecting these parts to the muscles form the *peripheral nervous system*. The brain consists of three parts:

● cerebrum   ● cerebellum   ● brain stem.

The surface of the cerebrum is thrown into many folds (*gyri*). There are also deep grooves (*fissures*) dividing the two halves of the cerebrum (the *cerebral hemispheres*) into sub-sections (*lobes*).

Internal structures

Nervous tissue is greyish-white in appearance because much of the nervous tissue consists of nerve axons (see Ch. 3). Axons contain relatively few organelles. They therefore do not absorb much light and consequently appear white. The whiteness is made more intense where axons are enveloped by *myelin* (see Ch. 21).

The cell bodies of the neurones contain the nuclei and other cellular organelles. These do absorb some light. Consequently, where many cell bodies are clustered together within the brain and spinal cord, the tissue appears grey.

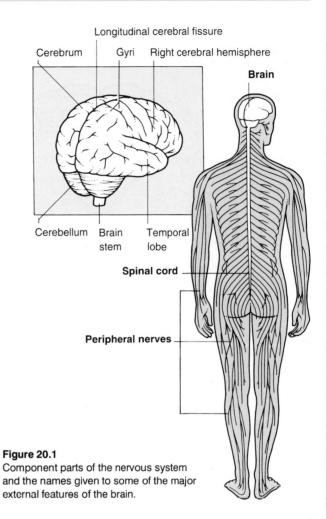

Figure 20.1
Component parts of the nervous system and the names given to some of the major external features of the brain.

Spinal cord

The appearance of the spinal cord in cross-section is shown in Figure 20.2. The grey part (*grey matter*) consists mostly of cell bodies and their dendrites whereas the whiter areas surrounding this (*white matter*) consist

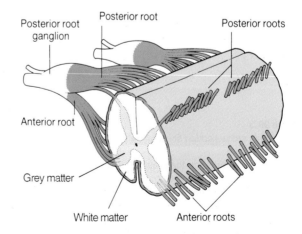

Figure 20.2
A section of the spinal cord showing the roots of the nerves carrying impulses into and out of the central nervous system, and the grey and white matter within the spinal cord. (Reproduced from Rogers 1992 (Fig. 21.14) by permission of the publishers.)

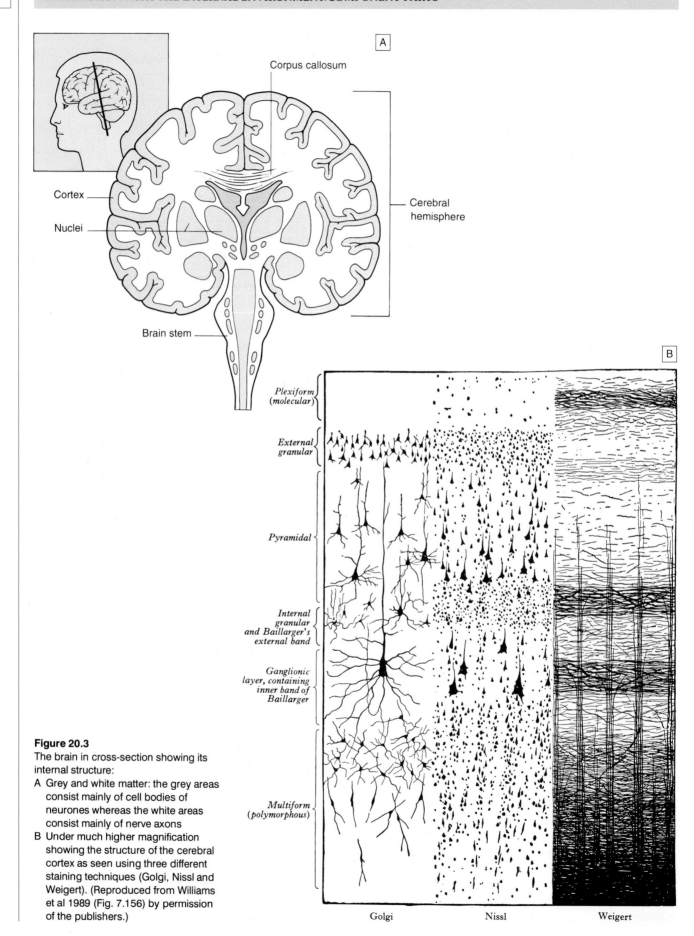

Figure 20.3
The brain in cross-section showing its
internal structure:
A Grey and white matter: the grey areas
   consist mainly of cell bodies of
   neurones whereas the white areas
   consist mainly of nerve axons
B Under much higher magnification
   showing the structure of the cerebral
   cortex as seen using three different
   staining techniques (Golgi, Nissl and
   Weigert). (Reproduced from Williams
   et al 1989 (Fig. 7.156) by permission
   of the publishers.)

of the axons of neurones carrying signals up and down the cord.

Brain

Similarly, in sections cut through the brain, some areas appear darker than others (Fig. 20.3A). Where cell bodies are grouped together to form a rounded cluster of cells the cluster is usually referred to as a *nucleus*: Some clusters are occasionally termed *ganglia* (singular = ganglion).

The outer layer (*cortex*) of the cerebral hemispheres and of the cerebellum differs in appearance from the neural tissue beneath (*sub-cortical structures*). The cortex appears greyish because there are many cell bodies, but they are arranged differently from those in the nuclei. A closer look at the cortical tissue under the high power of the microscope reveals that the cells are organised

in columns, and that cells differ in size and shape at different levels giving rise to a layered appearance (Fig. 20.3B).

The areas of the brain that appear white consist again of axons. Where axons are grouped into bundles or other structures linking one part of the brain with another they are sometimes described as *lemnisci, tracts* etc. A large band of nerve fibres (*corpus callosum*) links the two cerebral hemispheres (Fig. 20.3A).

ORGANISATION

Developmental origins

Very early in development (see Ch. 35) the primitive cells (*neuroectoderm*) giving rise to the nervous system form a hollow fluid-filled tube (*neural tube*) and the *neural crest* (Fig. 20.4A)

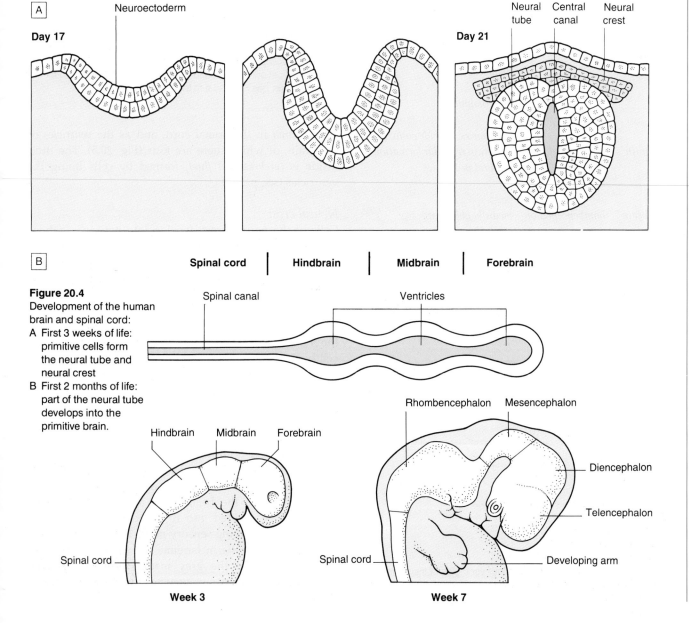

Figure 20.4
Development of the human brain and spinal cord:
A First 3 weeks of life: primitive cells form the neural tube and neural crest
B First 2 months of life: part of the neural tube develops into the primitive brain.

Neural tube

The cell bodies of the neurones in the neural tube are grouped together around the central canal. These cell bodies will form the grey matter, and axons extending from them will form the white matter on the outside of the tube. In the primitive neural tube the grey matter is divided into two layers.

- *alar lamina*
- *basal lamina.*

The alar lamina develops into sensory systems, whereas the basal lamina develops into motor systems.

Early in development, the front part of the neural tube becomes noticeably different from the rest (Fig. 20.4B). Three enlargements appear, the *forebrain*, *midbrain*, and *hindbrain*. Each develops into different parts of the mature brain:

forebrain	*telencephalon*	*cerebral hemispheres* *basal ganglia* *parts of the limbic system*
	diencephalon	*thalamus* *hypothalamus*
midbrain	*mesencephalon*	*superior & inferior colliculi* *midbrain reticular formation* *cerebral peduncles*
hindbrain	*rhombencephalon*	*pons* *medulla oblongata* *cerebellum*

The rest of the neural tube becomes the spinal cord. The hollow part of the primitive neural tube persists as the

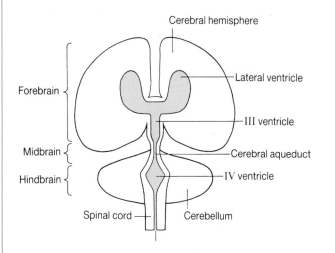

Figure 20.5
Diagrammatic representation of the four ventricles of the brain and their position in relation to other structures. (Reproduced from Rogers 1992 (Fig. 4.5) by permission of the publishers.)

In figure: Cerebral hemisphere; Lateral ventricle; III ventricle; Cerebral aqueduct; IV ventricle; Cerebellum; Spinal cord; Forebrain; Midbrain; Hindbrain.

④
What do the prefixes tel-, di-, mes- and rhomb- mean?

⑤
Which type of cell would you expect to find lining the ventricles?

central canal in the spinal cord, and as the *ventricles* of the brain, of which there are four (Fig. 20.5). The fluid inside is *cerebrospinal fluid*, formed by cells lining the ventricles (see p. 364). ④ ⑤

Neural crest

Cells of the neural crest develop into neurones, whose cell bodies lie within the peripheral nervous system (e.g. in ganglia of the spinal nerves and the autonomic nervous system) (see Ch. 3).

Spinal cord

This cord of nervous tissue (Fig. 20.1) is housed within the vertebral canal and consists of collections of nerve cell bodies (*grey matter*) and bundles of nerve cell axons (*white matter*) (Fig. 20.2). Axons, carrying nerve impulses to and from the periphery, extend from the cord as the *roots* of the spinal nerves.

Grey matter

The grey matter occupies the central part of the cord. It is here that synaptic contact is made between different cells. The cells are arranged in an ordered way in the grey matter. On the basis of its appearance the grey matter can be divided into 10 different layers (*laminae*) (Fig. 20.6A). Incoming sensory nerve fibres make synaptic contact with cells in laminae I to IV, and VI, in the posterior horn of the grey matter, whereas the cell bodies of the neurones conveying impulses to the muscles (*motoneurones*) are grouped together in the anterior

POLIOMYELITIS (ANTERIOR POLIOMYELITIS, POLIO, INFANTILE PARALYSIS)

Very few children in the UK escape being immunised against poliomyelitis. The drops, administered on a sugar lump or straight into a baby's mouth, are a recognised part of the immunisation schedule. The disease, which was prevalent world-wide 30 to 40 years ago, is now well controlled in many countries, although it still causes deaths and distressing physical handicaps in Third World populations.

The poliovirus causes a severe influenza-like illness but, if it spreads via the bloodstream to the central nervous system (CNS), it destroys motor cell bodies, particularly those in the anterior horns of grey matter in the spinal cord (anterior poliomyelitis) and in the medulla oblongata (see p. 358).

For those who survive the CNS infection, permanent disability often results. This may be anything from mild weakness of a limb to paralysis of all muscles from the neck down, the person spending the rest of his/her life in an 'iron lung' – a respirator that encases the trunk and limbs.

The severity of the disease has been forgotten by many in this country and parents are likely to ask whether immunisation is really necessary because polio is so rare. Without mass immunisation, it is possible that outbreaks would occur again. The virus circulates widely in the environment and can be ingested in drinking water contaminated with sewage and food contaminated with faeces, as well as by inhalation. Sea and river water may also become a source of virus.

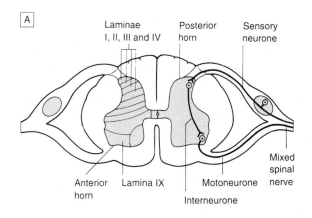

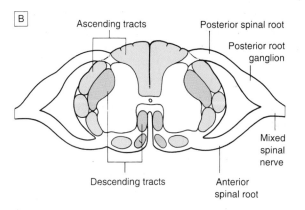

Figure 20.6
Typical structure of the spinal cord in the lumbar region:
A Grey matter: laminae and arrangement of sensory and motor neurones. (Note: the left and right halves of the spinal cord have the same basic structure. In this diagram, laminae are shown on the left and sensory and motoneurones on the right only for simplicity.)
B White matter: ascending and descending tracts.

horn in lamina IX. Many of the cells within the cord are interneurones.⑥⑦

White matter

The white matter of the cord consists of the axons of nerve fibres carrying impulses up and down the cord. The fibres are grouped into *tracts* (Fig. 20.6B). Their constituent fibres are either sensory and carry information up the spinal cord towards the brain (*afferent neurones, ascending tracts*) or they are motor and carry signals from different parts of the brain down towards the muscles (*efferent neurones, descending tracts*).

Spinal roots

Sensory information enters the cord posteriorly through the *posterior roots* of the spinal cord, and motor signals leave anteriorly through the *anterior roots*. Not far from the spinal cord the two roots merge to form a spinal nerve consisting of both afferent and efferent fibres bundled together. Included as well in this mixed nerve are autonomic fibres of the sympathetic or parasympathetic system (see Ch. 3 and Ch. 32).⑧

Spinal nerves

There are over 30 pairs of spinal nerves (Fig. 20.7). They are named according to the level of the vertebral column at which they emerge from the spine, whether cervical, thoracic, lumbar, sacral or coccygeal. Each nerve in-

nervates a group of muscles (*myotome*), and an area of skin (*dermatome*). Most also innervate some of the thoracic and abdominal organs (details in Chs 24, 28 and 32).

Anterior and posterior rami

Each of the spinal nerves divides to form two branches, the anterior and posterior rami (Fig. 20.8). The *posterior rami* innervate:

- muscles that extend the spine
- skin at the back of the body (from upper buttocks to the top of the skull)

whereas the *anterior rami* innervate:

- muscles of the
  - back that flex the spine
  - body wall
  - arms and legs
- skin of the
  - front and sides of the neck and trunk
  - limbs.

⑥
What do you understand by synaptic contact?

⑦
How would you describe an interneurone?

⑧
What might be the results of damage to a mixed nerve?

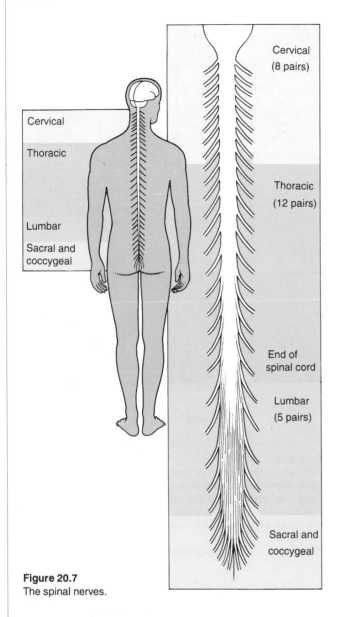

Figure 20.7
The spinal nerves.

Brain

From its external appearance the adult brain consists of three main parts (Fig. 20.1):

● brain stem
● cerebellum
● cerebral hemispheres.

Brain stem and related structures

The brain stem is the continuation of the spinal cord (Fig. 20.9A & B). It consists of:

● medulla oblongata
● pons
● midbrain.

The grey matter of the spinal cord continues up through the middle of the brain stem. The central core of this forms the *reticular formation*. Around this core are groups of cell bodies forming distinct clusters (*nuclei*).

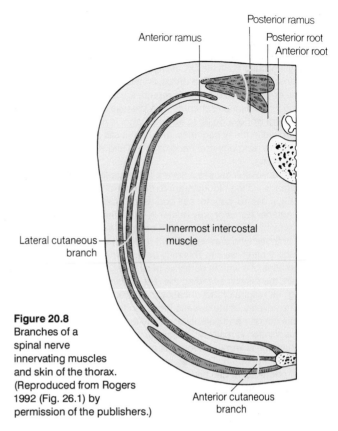

Figure 20.8
Branches of a spinal nerve innervating muscles and skin of the thorax. (Reproduced from Rogers 1992 (Fig. 26.1) by permission of the publishers.)

> Knowing what structures are innervated by each nerve enables the doctor to estimate the level at which damage to or pressure on the spinal cord has occurred. It is then possible to limit investigations to that area of the spine.

The white matter (nerve fibre tracts of the cord) also continues up into the brain stem. The nerve endings may synapse with cells of the reticular formation, or with the nuclei. Some nerve fibres cross over from one side of the brain stem to the other so that information from each side of the body is transmitted to the brain on the opposite side. A good example of this crossing over (*decussation*), but for descending rather than ascending fibres, is provided by the tracts that have an important role in controlling the movements of the fingers and toes (*corticospinal tracts*). These fibres decussate at the boundary between the medulla oblongata and the spinal cord. Because of its appearance this cross-over point has been called the *pyramids*. For this reason the corticospinal tracts are sometimes referred to as the pyramidal tracts.

Beyond the structures of the midbrain, which include the inferior and superior colliculi, is the hypothalamus.

> When the motor cortex of either of the cerebral hemispheres is damaged by injury, disease or pressure, the person is likely to have impaired movement on the opposite side of the body because of the decussation of nerve tracts.

Figure 20.9
The brain stem – component parts:
A Brain cut in half as in Figure 20.3: front view of back half
B Brain cut in half, separating the left and right cerebral
  hemispheres: side view of right half.

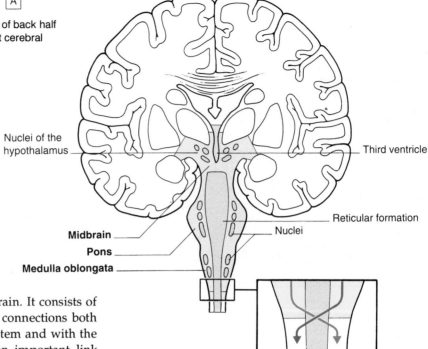

Nuclei of the hypothalamus

Third ventricle

Reticular formation

Nuclei

Midbrain

Pons

Medulla oblongata

Decussation of corticospinal tracts

The hypothalamus is part of the forebrain. It consists of several nuclei. The hypothalamus has connections both with the spinal cord below the brain stem and with the cerebral hemispheres above, and is an important link between the somatic and the autonomic nervous systems. It is involved in motivational and emotional aspects of behaviour (see Ch. 31). ⑨

Cerebellum

Straddling the pons and attached to it by the *cerebellar peduncles* (i.e. cerebral feet) is the *cerebellum* (Fig. 20.10), which has an important role in the control of movement (see Chs 27–29). The cerebellum also consists of grey matter and white matter, but the grey matter is subdivided into:

● cerebellar cortex
● nuclei.

The nuclei are embedded deep within the cerebellum, and the much folded cortex completely envelops them. The cerebellar peduncles consist of bundles of nerve axons linking the cerebellum with other parts of the brain.

Cerebral hemispheres

The two cerebral hemispheres, like the cerebellum, contain discrete clusters of cells (nuclei) enveloped by a much folded layer of cortex and traversed by numerous nerve fibre tracts (Fig. 20.11A). The nuclei include the basal ganglia, which are involved in controlling movement (see Ch. 27), and the thalamus, which has both sensory (see Ch. 23) and motor functions. Buried deep within the cerebral hemispheres are the structures forming the limbic system, which, together with the hypothalamus, is involved in motivation and emotion (see Ch. 31). The two hemispheres are linked by a massive bundle of fibres (*corpus callosum*). ⑩

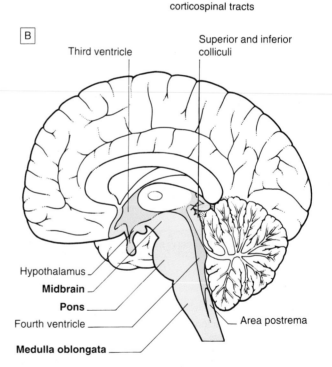

B

Third ventricle

Superior and inferior colliculi

Hypothalamus

Midbrain

Pons

Fourth ventricle

Area postrema

Medulla oblongata

The extensive folding of the cortical surface gives the brain a wrinkled appearance (Fig. 20.11B). Some of the folds dip deeply into the tissue dividing the hemispheres into several lobes:

● frontal
● temporal
● parietal
● occipital.

⑨
What differences are there between the somatic and autonomic nervous systems?

⑩
What is the common disorder associated with malfunction of the basal ganglia?

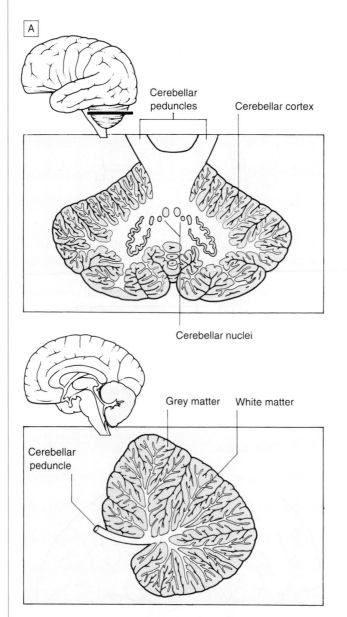

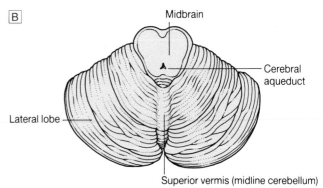

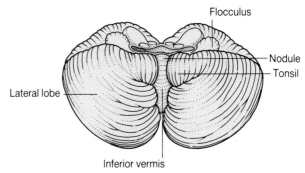

Cranial nerves

Emerging from the brain are 12 pairs of cranial nerves (Fig. 20.12). These supply various structures most of which are associated with the head and neck, although cranial nerve X chiefly innervates tissues and organs in the trunk of the body. The primary functions of each of the nerves are listed in Table 20.2.

Figure 20.10
The cerebellum:
A Internal structure
B External features seen from above (upper diagram) and from below (lower diagram). (Reproduced from Rogers 1992 (Fig. 21.9) by permission of the publishers.)

Table 20.2	The cranial nerves			
Number	Name	Functions		Chapter reference
		Sensory	Motor	
I	Olfactory	Nose	—	15
II	Optic	Eye	—	26
III	Oculomotor	—	Muscles moving eyeball	29
			Ciliary muscle, iris	26
IV	Trochlea	—	Muscles moving eyeball	29
VI	Abducens	—		
V	Trigeminal	Face, tongue, teeth	Muscles of mastication	29, 32
VII	Facial	Tongue, soft palate	Muscles of face	29
VIII	Vestibulocochlear	Balance organs, ear	—	24, 25
IX	Glossopharyngeal	Taste buds, pharynx	Salivary glands	6
X	Vagus	Tissues and organs of throat, thorax, abdomen	Tissues and organs of throat, thorax, abdomen	3
XI	Accessory	—	Muscles of head, neck, shoulders	29
XII	Hypoglossal	—	Tongue	29

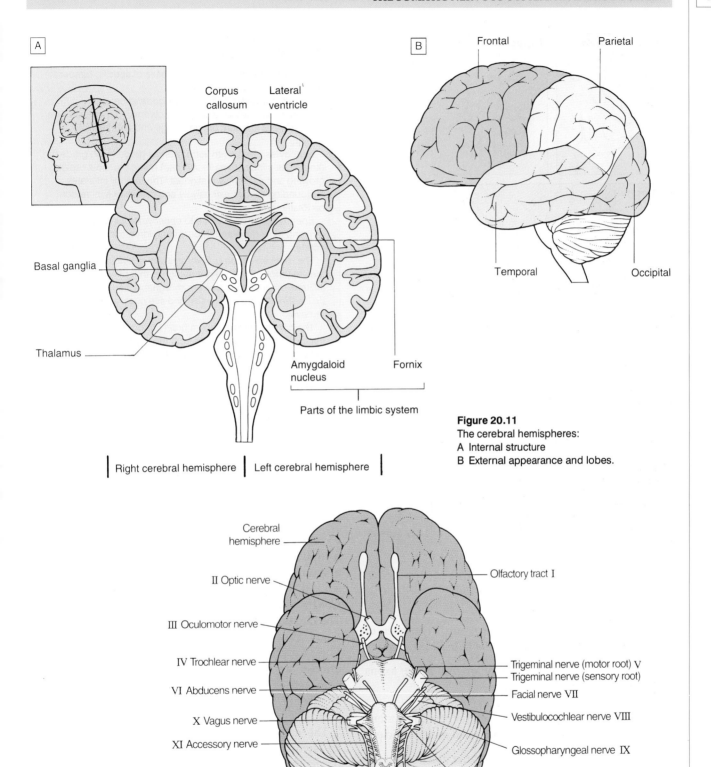

A

Corpus callosum

Lateral ventricle

Basal ganglia

Thalamus

Amygdaloid nucleus

Fornix

Parts of the limbic system

Right cerebral hemisphere | Left cerebral hemisphere

B

Frontal

Parietal

Temporal

Occipital

Figure 20.11
The cerebral hemispheres:
A Internal structure
B External appearance and lobes.

Cerebral hemisphere

II Optic nerve

III Oculomotor nerve

IV Trochlear nerve

VI Abducens nerve

X Vagus nerve

XI Accessory nerve

Cerebellum

Olfactory tract I

Trigeminal nerve (motor root) V
Trigeminal nerve (sensory root)

Facial nerve VII

Vestibulocochlear nerve VIII

Glossopharyngeal nerve IX

Hypoglossal nerve XII

Spinal cord

Figure 20.12
View of the underneath of the brain showing the 12 pairs of cranial nerves. (Reproduced from Rogers 1992 (Fig. 21.3) by permission of the publishers.)

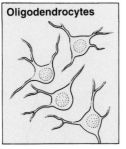

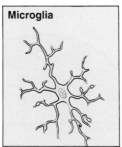

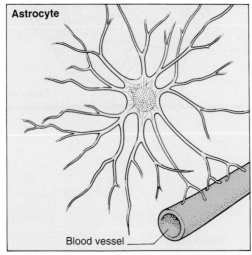

Blood vessel

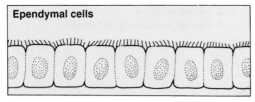

Figure 20.13 Glial cells.

⑪

What happens if the pressure of blood in the brain cannot be maintained?

SUPPORTIVE STRUCTURES

Glial cells

Present within the nervous system are a number of other cells known collectively as *glia* (Fig. 20.13):

- *oligodendrocytes* – form myelin around nerve axons (Ch. 21)
- *astrocytes* – found next to blood vessels
- *microglia* – macrophages of the central nervous system
- *ependymal cells* – lining the spinal canal and ventricles.

Much has been learnt recently about the functions of the astrocytes. These beautiful star shaped cells seem to have an important role in regulating the composition of the brain interstitial fluid. They remove some neurotransmitters (glutamate and GABA) and take up potassium from the vicinity of cells. They are also believed to act as a scaffold during the development of the nervous system. Membrane receptors have been identified on them making it clear that their function can be regulated. Defective function of these cells is likely to give rise to some neurological disorders.

Brain blood supply

The circulation of blood to the brain (*cerebral circulation*) has several distinctive features that are important in preserving a constant environment for the nerve cells:

- control mechanisms
- capillary function
- venous sinuses.

Control mechanisms

The circulation to the brain is preserved at times when blood flow to other organs is threatened (see Ch. 11). The baroreceptors located within branches of the carotid arteries are important in registering any drop in pressure and in bringing about corrective changes in the circulation that maintain the pressure of blood to the brain. ⑪

The arterioles of the brain are sparsely innervated by sympathetic nerves. Thus when vasoconstriction occurs elsewhere in the body there is little or no

Mental arithmetic

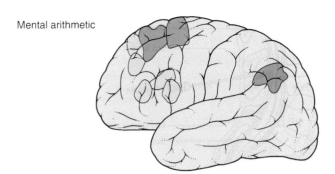

Imagining walking along a familiar route

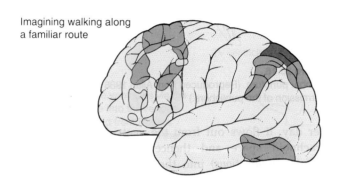

% increase in blood flow	10–19	20–29	40–49

Figure 20.14
Effects of two different mental activities on blood flow to different parts of the brain. (Adapted from Roland & Freiberg 1985.)

vasoconstriction in the brain. However, local factors, such as the concentration of CO_2, act as powerful vasodilators of the cerebral arterioles. Blood flow to different parts of the brain increases during different activities (Fig. 20.14). It appears that if blood flow increases at one site it is reduced at another so that the total blood flow to the brain hardly changes. The only notable exception is during an epileptic seizure when significant increases in total cerebral blood flow can occur.

Capillary function
Cerebral capillaries are much less permeable to many constituents of blood than are any other capillaries in the body. Molecules such as glucose, that have free access to the interstitial fluid in other tissues, have to be transported across cerebral capillaries by carrier mechanisms in order to get through to the brain interstitial fluid in adequate amounts. Many other molecules of this size and greater have difficulty diffusing passively from the blood into the brain tissue fluid. As a result the nerve cells are not exposed to as high a concentration of many potentially harmful substances as they might be. The unusual restrictiveness of the capil-

Table 20.3 Permeability of the blood–brain barrier to various substances

Very high	Intermediate	Very low
Water	Glucose	Proteins
Carbon dioxide	Amino acids	Dopamine
Oxygen	Electrolytes (e.g. Na+, K+, Cl−, HCO₃−)	Bilirubin
Ammonia	Urea	Bile salts
Gaseous anaesthetics (e.g. halothane, nitrous oxide)	L-dopa	
Alcohol		

lary barrier led scientists to coin the term *blood–brain barrier*. Substances that can cross this barrier easily are either very small molecules (e.g. water) or they are liposoluble (e.g. alcohol). Gases, such as ammonia, oxygen and carbon dioxide that are both small and liposoluble, cross very easily (Table 20.3).

In a few small areas, including the posterior pituitary and parts of the hypothalamus, the blood capillaries are much more permeable. This permits hormones secreted by these neurones to get into the blood and gives blood-borne substances, such as glucose and fatty acids, freer access to the neurones there.

The blood–brain barrier can be disrupted by infection and irradiation, and is abnormal in tumours. Because of this, if an injection of a radio-labelled marker is given, it is possible to identify areas of brain disease, as only these areas will allow the marker to get through.

DRUGS AND THE BLOOD–BLOOD BARRIER

When central nervous system infections occur, the antibiotic to which the organism is sensitive may not be able to cross the blood–brain barrier. It then becomes necessary to administer it directly into the subarachnoid space (see p. 364). This is done via a lumbar puncture needle, which is inserted between the 3rd and 4th or 4th and 5th lumbar vertebrae – the intrathecal route (Fig. 20.16).

Patients may find this treatment distressing and, apart from the normal reassurances given in such circumstances, some may require an explanation of why 'tablets won't work'. It is usually sufficient to explain that, while medicines taken in tablet form or given by injection will reach most parts of the body, some cannot reach the brain in adequate concentrations.

Some drugs do cross the blood–brain barrier. Those that are liposoluble, such as hypnotics, sedatives, analgesics and antidepressants, can diffuse across the lipid component of the membranes. L-dopa, used in the treatment of Parkinson's disease, is transported on a protein carrier. Others cross but do so less easily, for example insulin (a water-soluble polypeptide) crosses only very slowly.

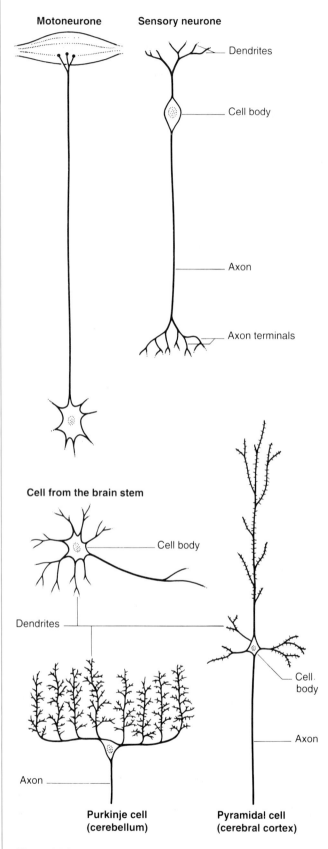

Figure 21.1
Structure of several different types of neurone.

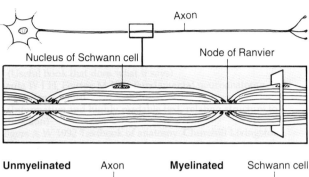

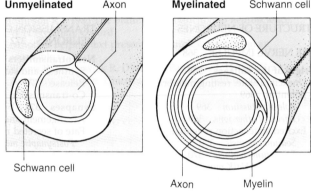

Figure 21.2
Myelinated and unmyelinated axons.

Nerves, exposed at operation or through injury, look like long white cords. They consist of bundles of nerve axons together with their supporting cells and connective tissue.

THE NERVE IMPULSE

If a very tiny probe is inserted into any cell, the small electrical charge between the inside and the outside of the cell can be measured. It ranges between 10 and 90 millivolts in different cells. This voltage can and does change depending on the stimuli acting on the cell and the effect they have on the cell membrane. However it is only in neurones, and in muscle cells, that the voltage can change abruptly from a negative value of about −70 millivolts to a positive value of +35 millivolts and back again. This distinctive change in voltage is termed the *action potential*. Cells generating action potentials are termed *electrically excitable cells*. The advantage of the action potential over other electrical changes occurring in cells is that it is a self-propagating event. Once an

Changes in electrical potential within the brain can be recorded via small electrodes placed on the scalp. This technique (*electroencephalography*) aids the diagnosis of epilepsy and the location of some lesions; it may also be used to monitor brain activity and to furnish part of the criteria for establishing brain death.

action potential has been initiated at one end of an axon this distinctive electrical event is repeated along the length of the axon so that the signal is conducted rapidly and fully from one end of the axon to the other.②

ORIGIN OF THE VOLTAGES

Unexcited state: resting membrane potential

The two main factors responsible for the presence of an electrical voltage across most cell membranes are:

- the selective permeability of the cell membrane to different ions
- differences in concentration of ions inside and outside cells.

Most cell membranes are very permeable to potassium and chloride ions and much less permeable to sodium ions. In all cells there is a carrier protein the *Na/K ATPase* which transports potassium into the cell and evicts sodium ions from it. The result of this pump activity is that virtually all cells have a high intracellular potassium concentration (about 150 mmol/l) and a low sodium concentration (about 10 mmol/l). This contrasts with the extracellular fluid which has a high sodium and a low potassium concentration (see Ch. 13).

Role of potassium

Because the cell membrane is permeable to potassium, and because there is more potassium inside the cell than outside, potassium ions have a tendency to diffuse out. Potassium ions are cations. They possess a positive charge (see Ch. 2). Therefore each potassium ion leaking out of the cell transfers one positive charge from the inside of the cell to the outside. This creates a difference in voltage between the inside and the outside of the cell (Fig. 21.3). The more potassium ions leaking out, the greater the voltage becomes. There is however a limit to this, because as the cell interior loses positive charges and therefore becomes negatively charged it increasingly exerts a restraining influence on the exit of further potassium ions. The potassium ions are being driven in opposite directions by two opposing forces:

- difference in potassium concentration (driving potassium out of the cell)
- difference in electrical charge (pulling potassium back into the cell).

Eventually a balance (*equilibrium*) is reached between these two forces. At equilibrium there is no net movement of potassium across the cell membrane, but a voltage exists, the size of which is proportional to the ratio of the concentrations of potassium inside (i) and outside (o) the cell (K_i/K_o).③

If the potassium concentration in the extracellular fluid increases, as it may do in kidney disease, the ratio K_i/K_o decreases and the size of the voltage devel-

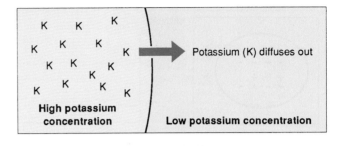

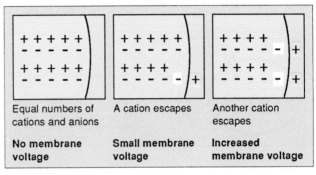

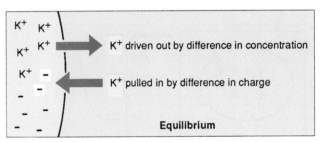

Figure 21.3
The resting membrane potential: how an electrical voltage develops across a cell membrane as a result of the diffusion of potassium ions. Potassium ions are cations (they are positively charged).

oped across cell membranes decreases (*depolarisation*). Conversely, if potassium concentration in the ECF decreases, as in hypokalaemia (see Ch. 13), the ratio K_i/K_o increases and the voltage increases (*hyperpolarisation*). This affects the function of all excitable tissues including the heart and skeletal muscle as well as nerve cells (see Chs 13 and 22).

Effects of other ions

If the cell membrane becomes very permeable to sodium ions as well, sodium diffuses in increasing amounts in the opposite direction, from the outside to the inside of the cell. As sodium ions are also cations (positively charged ions), their movement into the cell replaces the positive charges lost by the exit of potassium ions and so the voltage across the membrane decreases. If the membrane becomes fully permeable to these and other small diffusible ions the voltage virtually disappears.④

Excited state: action potential

Excitation of nerve cells is achieved by the opening of channels permeable to sodium. The action potential is

②
Is 1 millivolt less or more than 1 volt?

③
What do 'proportional' and 'ratio' mean?

④
What might make the membrane become fully permeable to sodium and other small ions?

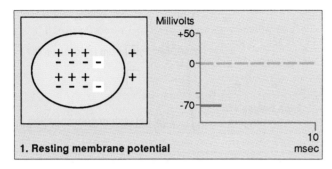

1. Resting membrane potential

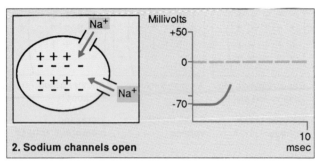

2. Sodium channels open

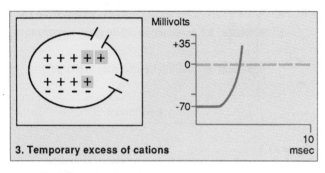

3. Temporary excess of cations

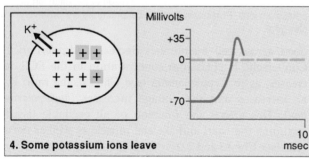

4. Some potassium ions leave

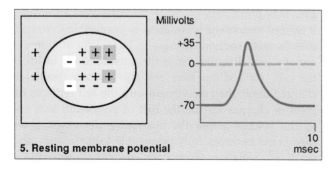

5. Resting membrane potential

Figure 21.4
The action potential: how the voltage of a nerve cell changes as a result of the opening and closing of sodium and potassium channels.

produced as a result of the fact that some cell membranes allow the membrane to momentarily become much more permeable to sodium than to potassium. Consequently, for a brief instant (about 1 millisecond), more positive ions move into the cell than leave it and the cell interior briefly becomes positively charged. The voltage recorded across the cell membrane reaches about +35 millivolts. The permeability of the membrane then swiftly returns to normal, and the voltage also returns to its unexcited ('resting') value of −70 millivolts (Fig. 21.4).

Sodium channels

The change in the permeability of the membrane is brought about through the opening and closing of specific channels in the membrane (see Ch. 2). The channels of key importance in the action potential are *voltage-gated sodium channels*. 'Voltage gating' means that the channels are sensitive to a change in membrane voltage. Voltage-gated sodium channels open when the voltage decreases. As channel opening decreases the voltage even further by letting positively charged sodium ions into the cell, even more channels open. Once a sufficient number of channels have opened there is an explosive increase in the rate of opening of the remaining channels. This point of no return is termed the *threshold*. Once it is reached the voltage across the membrane inevitably switches from being negative to being positive. This inevitability of the pattern of the response is termed the *all or nothing* property of the action potential.

The initial drop in voltage may be caused by any one of a number of things. It could be by:

- activation of a sensory receptor (see Ch. 23)
- binding of a neurotransmitter to ligand-gated channels (see p. 375)
- damage to the nerve fibre.

The size of the drop in voltage needed to open sodium channels is affected by the concentration of calcium ions in the interstitial fluid. If calcium concentration outside the neurones decreases action potentials are elicited much more easily. Conversely, if calcium concentration increases, neurones become less excitable (see Ch. 13). Hence calcium is said to stabilise membranes.

Potassium channels

The return of the membrane voltage from a positive to a negative state (Fig. 21.4) occurs because:

- sodium channels close
- more potassium channels open.

Some potassium channels are voltage gated. Like the sodium channels, they open when the membrane voltage decreases. However, they open more slowly and stay open for longer. In this way they help to bring the voltage back to its original state.

Role of the Na/K pump

The number of sodium and potassium ions entering or leaving the cell when a single action potential is generated is exceedingly small. The amounts are far too small to cause significant changes in the ionic composition of the intracellular and extracellular fluids.

However, if many action potentials are generated in quick succession the concentration of sodium inside the cell increases and that of potassium decreases. However, this change in concentration does not normally occur, even though nerves normally generate and transmit impulses continuously. This is because the Na/K pump (a transporter protein in the membrane of all cells; see Chs 2, 6 and 8) continually evicts the sodium ions entering the cells and recovers the potassium ions that leak out.

CONDUCTION OF ACTION POTENTIALS

Process

The generation of an action potential at one site in a neurone momentarily creates a difference in electrical voltage between that site and adjacent parts of the neurone (Fig. 21.5). Ions move relatively freely within the cell and within the interstitial fluid, attracted by opposite charges and repelled by those that are the same. Inside the cell therefore, potassium ions tend to move away from the depolarised site whereas chloride ions (negatively charged) tend to be drawn towards it. Similar but opposite effects occur outside the cell. The effect of all this ion movement is to reduce the voltage of neighbouring sites from the unexcited level of –70 millivolts. This drop in voltage again opens voltage-gated sodium channels. As soon as the drop in voltage is big enough to reach threshold the same explosive

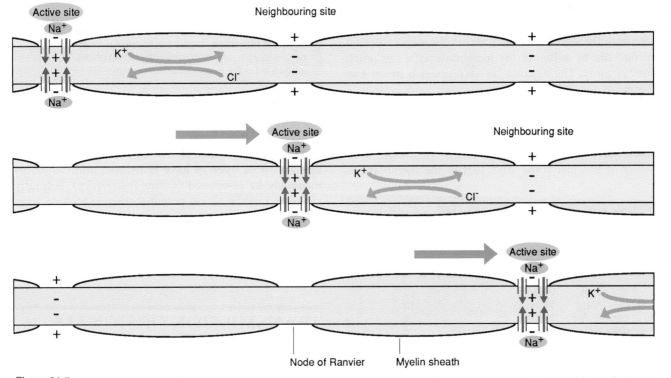

Figure 21.5
Conduction of the nerve impulse in a myelinated axon: how the movement of anions and cations between active and inactive sites depolarises the neighbouring axonal membrane, opens voltage-gated sodium channels and generates another action potential.

increase in the sodium permeability of the membrane occurs and an action potential is generated at these neighbouring sites too. These sites then activate sites further along the axon and so on. In this way the electrical impulse is conducted rapidly along the membrane of the axon until it reaches the nerve terminals at the other end.

> Impulse conduction in peripheral nerves can be blocked by pressure. Prolonged pressure on a nerve will cause a leg, for example, to 'go to sleep'. Sensation, and often movement, is impaired until nerve function and blood circulation return to normal.

Speed

Nerve axons normally conduct impulses at rates ranging between about 1 metre/second to 100 metres/second (Table 21.1), the speed of transmission depending on:

- temperature
- myelination
- diameter of the axon.

An increase in any of these, increases the speed of transmission.

Myelin makes a big difference because it restricts the sites at which an action potential has to be generated to the gaps in the myelin sheath occurring between individual Schwann cells along the axon (*nodes of Ranvier*; Figs 21.2 and 21.5). In effect the impulse 'jumps' from one node to the next (*saltatory conduction*). The myelin insulates the nerve axon and allows the depolarisation at one site to influence the membrane at a site much further away. The distance between nodes is about 1 to 2 mm.

Direction

The action potential generated at neighbouring sites does not reactivate that part of the membrane from which it has just come. This part of the membrane is

DEMYELINATION

In some diseases the myelin sheath is destroyed with the result that the nerve axon loses ability to conduct impulses quickly. Little is known about why the myelin sheath degenerates but research shows that demyelination is responsible for the symptoms of many neuropathies (*-opathy* = something is wrong but exactly what is not known).

In *multiple sclerosis*, patchy demyelination occurs within the spinal cord and brain, followed by damage to nerve fibres and the formation of plaques of scar tissue. The disease is characterised by remissions and relapses, which are unpredictable. The relapses may be very distressing for the patient. Initially, the person experiences sensations related to abnormal impulse conduction – tingling, numbness, weakness in one or both arms or legs (see Ch. 32). Visual disturbances are also common. The disease is progressive and the person eventually becomes confined to a wheelchair.

The *Guillain–Barré* syndrome develops rapidly following an often mild, pyrexial illness. Although marked demyelination of spinal nerve roots and peripheral nerves (see Ch. 20) occurs, the nerve fibre is not damaged. The myelin sheath gradually regenerates and normal function returns. The affected person suffers severe motor impairment and the muscles are very tender. It is an alarming condition due to the rapidity and severity of onset. The person requires careful nursing and much reassurance.

Symptoms of inadequate transmission of nerve impulses, such as numbness, are also experienced by some people suffering from *diabetes mellitus*. Research shows that these symptoms are caused by demyelination and axonal degeneration. When numbness affects one or both feet the risk of infection, following unfelt injury, is high. The cutting of toenails must be carried out with great care, if necessary by a chiropodist, and the feet should be inspected daily. It is advisable for the person to wear shoes that provide adequate protection. It has been known for an affected person to walk long distances with a sharp object embedded in the foot.

less sensitive to stimulation (*refractory*). There are two reasons for this. Firstly, during the action potential, there is a phase when the voltage-gated sodium channels are either open or have just closed and cannot immediately be re-opened (*sodium inactivation*). Secondly, at the end of the action potential there is a phase when the membrane hyperpolarises slightly, because extra potassium channels are still open. The membrane voltage is then further away from threshold and the membrane is more difficult to excite.

TRANSMISSION OF SIGNALS BETWEEN NEURONES

The transmission of signals between one neurone and the next occurs through the mediation of one or more chemical transmitters (*neurotransmitters*). Neurotrans-

Table 21.1	Different types of nerve fibre		
Name	*Speed of conduction* (m/sec)*	*Myelination*	*Diameter* (μm)*
A alpha (Aα)	100		15
beta (Aβ)	50	Yes	10
gamma (Aγ)	20		5
delta (Aδ)	20		4
B	10	Yes	2
C	1	No	1
* Typical values.			

mitters, released from nerve endings by the action potential, diffuse across the intervening space (*synapse*) and then excite the next cell.

NEUROTRANSMITTERS

Synthesis and storage

Transmitters are synthesised either at the nerve endings or in the cell body of a neurone. Those manufactured in the cell body are packaged in vesicles and transported along microtubules in the axon to the nerve endings (*axonal transport*) (Fig. 21.6). Much traffic occurs in both directions along the axon as has been shown by speeded up film of neurones in culture. A number of neurotransmitters are listed in Table 21.2.⑤

Two distinctive features are apparent at the nerve endings (Fig. 21.6):

- many tiny storage vesicles containing neurotransmitters
- an abundance of mitochondria.

Both features reveal the high degree of activity at this site.

Release

When an action potential reaches the nerve endings it triggers an increase in the permeability of the cell membrane to calcium ions. This causes some of the

⑤
What do you understand by 'synthesis'?

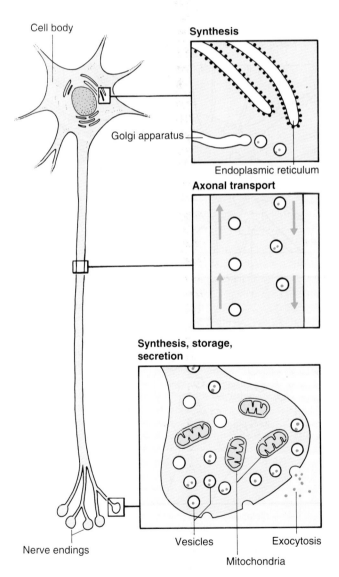

Figure 21.6
Role of different parts of the neurone in the production, delivery and storage of neurotransmitter prior to secretion.

Cell body

Synthesis

Golgi apparatus

Endoplasmic reticulum

Axonal transport

Synthesis, storage, secretion

Nerve endings

Vesicles

Exocytosis

Mitochondria

THE ROLE OF AXONAL TRANSPORT IN DISEASE

Axonal transport is used normally to move neurotransmitters between cell body and nerve endings and to carry other materials back to the cell body for recycling. However, it is also made use of by viruses and toxins. The best known of these are the herpes and rabies viruses, and the toxins produced by the organisms that cause tetanus and diphtheria.

Many people suffer from 'cold' sores on the lips and nose (*herpes labialis*). After the initial infection, usually early in life, the virus remains dormant within nerve cells. Certain circumstances, such as pyrexia, hot sunshine, cold winds and, less frequently, cosmetics, seem to reactivate the virus. Some people experience tenderness along the nerve before the lesions appear. The exudate from the blisters contains active viruses secreted by the nerve endings, and care should be taken not to transfer it to the eyes or to other people.

The rabies virus enters the body most commonly through wounds caused by dog bites. It is capable of travelling in both directions along nerve axons. The virus multiplies in ganglion cells of the brain and spinal cord (see Ch. 20) causing degenerative changes. The incubation period seems to depend on the distance of the bite from the appropriate ganglia. Thus, symptoms may appear after 2 months, or longer, if the bite is on the leg, or after less than 1 month if the bite is on the head. Great care should always be taken when approaching strange dogs and, if a stray or wild animal must be handled, protective clothing should be worn. The risk of infection is diminished if the bite is through clothing because much of the saliva is removed.

The bacillus, *Clostridium tetani*, produces a toxin that travels by axonal transport from the site of infection, giving rise to the symptoms of tetanus (lockjaw). Usually, the first symptom is pain and stiffness of the jaw muscles, progressing to rigid clamping of the jaws – hence lockjaw. Eventually severe, painful muscular spasms involve the whole body. Death may result from asphyxiation. Like rabies, the time between infection and the appearance of symptoms depends upon the time taken for the toxin to travel along the nerve axons. The bacilli, which are *anaerobic* (live without oxygen), are found in soil, particularly that which is well manured, and can survive for many years as spores, in Victorian horsehair furniture, for example, or in inadequately sterilised catgut. They enter the body via deep dirty wounds. Protection against tetanus is included in infant immunisation schedules. Adults are advised to renew immunisation every 10 years – even if one is not a gardener, road traffic accidents can happen to almost anyone.

Table 21.2   Neurotransmitters

Name	Chemical type	Example of known site of secretion	Chapter reference
Acetylcholine		Autonomic nervous system	3
Noradrenaline		Autonomic nervous system	3
Dopamine	Amine	Basal ganglia	27, 28
Serotonin		Limbic system	31
Glutamate		Cerebral cortex	30
Gamma aminobutyric acid (GABA)	Amino acid	Cerebral cortex	30
Substance P		Spinal cord	32
Enkephalins	Polypeptide	Spinal cord	32

vesicles containing transmitter to move towards the cell membrane, fuse with it and empty their contents into the interstitial fluid (*exocytosis*; see Ch. 2). The more action potentials arriving at the ending per second the more transmitter is released. The amount of transmitter released depends also on the original voltage across the membrane. This voltage can be altered by transmitters secreted by other neurones nearby (*presynaptic inhibition* and *excitation*; see p. 377).

Co-transmission

It used to be thought that each neurone manufactured only one neurotransmitter. But it is now known that two or more transmitters can be manufactured by the same cell (Table 21.3). Each substance is believed to have a different role in the overall process of synaptic transmission.

SYNAPSES

Arrangement and structure

The nerve terminals of one neurone make contact with the dendrites and cell bodies of other neurones at junctions known as *synapses*. Dendrites and cell bodies are normally smothered with nerve terminals (Fig. 21.7). A single motoneurone in the spinal cord may have about 10 000 terminals on its dendritic tree and cell body, whereas a Purkinje cell of the cerebellum (see Fig. 21.1) may be in contact with 100 000 other neurones.

Table 21.3   Examples of neurotransmitters that may coexist in the same nerve terminal

Amine		Polypeptide		Other
Noradrenaline	and	Neuropeptide Y		
		VIP*	and	Acetylcholine
Serotonin	and	Substance P	and	TRH†

* Vasoactive intestinal polypeptide (see Ch. 6).
† Thyroid releasing hormone (see Ch. 10). TRH is an example of a substance that can act both as a neurotransmitter and as a hormone (see Ch. 3).

In a typical synapse the gap (*synaptic cleft*) between the first nerve (*presynaptic neurone*) and the second nerve (*postsynaptic neurone*) is very tiny, only about 20 nanometres in width (about 1/350th of the size of a red cell).

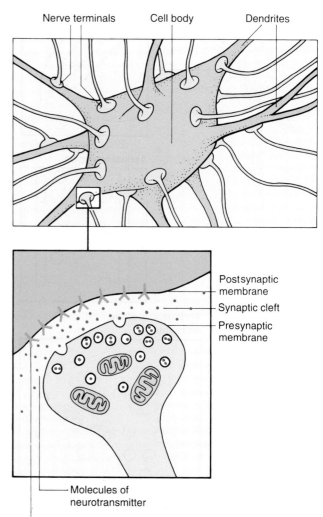

Figure 21.7
Synapses: where they are found and what they consist of. (Note: the various structures shown in the inset are not drawn to scale. If they were, the receptor proteins, for example, would be invisible.)

Fate of secreted neurotransmitters

Neurotransmitters released by the presynaptic neurone diffuse into the gap. At least one of three things may happen to them subsequently. They may:

- interact with the postsynaptic membrane
- interact with the presynaptic membrane
- diffuse away and be metabolised in body fluids.

Postsynaptic membrane

At the postsynaptic membrane neurotransmitters may bind to receptor proteins (Fig. 21.8) and activate *G proteins* in the membrane (see Ch. 2). As a result channels (*ligand-gated channels*), allowing the movement of ions across the membrane, open or close depending on the transmitters involved. The change in permeability alters the voltage across the postsynaptic membrane (see p. 376).

In some instances, enzymes in the membrane then break down the transmitter substance attached to the receptor and release the products of breakdown into the interstitial fluid. For example the enzyme *acetylcholinesterase*, located on the postsynaptic membrane of cholinergic synapses, splits acetylcholine into acetic acid and choline.

> Non-depolarising or competitive muscle relaxants used in general anaesthesia, for example tubocurarine and pancuronium, compete with acetylcholine at the receptor site, thus blocking its action. Anticholinesterases, such as neostigmine, reverse the effects of competitive muscle relaxants by combining with acetylcholinesterase to inhibit its action, thus allowing more acetylcholine to accumulate.

Presynaptic membrane

Neurotransmitter in the vicinity of the presynaptic terminal can be re-accumulated by the terminals of the presynaptic neurone, and recycled. Noradrenaline is a good example of this.⑥

Products of transmitter metabolism such as acetic acid and choline from acetylcholine may also be taken up by a specific transport mechanism into the presynaptic terminal and be re-used in the synthesis of more acetylcholine.

Some transmitter also binds to receptors on the presynaptic terminal. These receptors regulate the function of the terminal.

Tissues fluids

Some of the transmitter molecules just leak away, out of the synapse, into the surrounding interstitial fluid. They are then broken down by enzymes present in the tissue fluid and blood. For example, noradrenaline escaping into the blood is broken down by the enzyme *catechol-o-methyl transferase* (COMT).

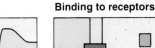
Binding to receptors

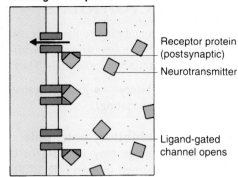

- Receptor protein (postsynaptic)
- Neurotransmitter
- Ligand-gated channel opens

Enzymic breakdown

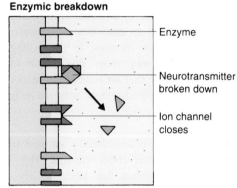

- Enzyme
- Neurotransmitter broken down
- Ion channel closes

Recovery into terminal

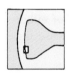
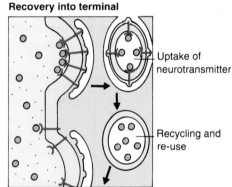

- Uptake of neurotransmitter
- Recycling and re-use

Binding to receptors

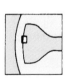
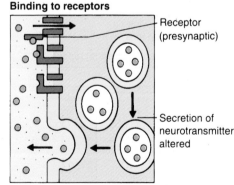

- Receptor (presynaptic)
- Secretion of neurotransmitter altered

Figure 21.8
Fate and action of neurotransmitters at postsynaptic (top two panels) and presynaptic (bottom two panels) membranes.

⑥
Where else is noradrenaline produced?

POSTSYNAPTIC POTENTIALS

The changes in membrane voltage occurring at the postsynaptic membrane (*postsynaptic potentials*) differ in several respects from action potentials. They are:

- excitatory *or* inhibitory   • graded in size
- local (not self-propagating).

Excitatory and inhibitory potentials

The membrane voltage may increase or decrease depending on the channels opened (Fig. 21.9). A decrease in voltage increases the likelihood that the postsynaptic cell will fire an action potential. This change in voltage is therefore termed an *excitatory postsynaptic potential* or *epsp*. Conversely an increase in the voltage takes the voltage further away from the threshold level and makes it less likely that an action potential will be fired. This is an *inhibitory postsynaptic potential* or *ipsp*.

Ion channels

Excitatory potentials are usually caused by the transmitter–receptor interaction causing the opening of channels that increase the permeability of the cell membrane to all small ions, including sodium. This reduces the voltage across the membrane. Inhibition, however, is caused by the selective opening of either potassium or chloride channels. This may increase the

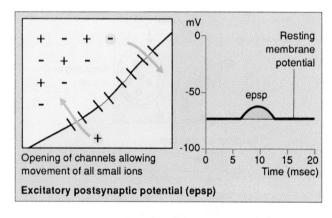

Excitatory postsynaptic potential (epsp)

Opening of channels allowing
movement of all small ions

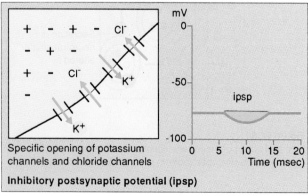

Inhibitory postsynaptic potential (ipsp)

Specific opening of potassium
channels and chloride channels

Figure 21.9
Basis of excitatory and inhibitory postsynaptic potentials.

⑦
What substances may alter the chemical environment and thus affect decisions?

voltage or simply make it more difficult for the cell to be depolarised and become excited.

Size

Postsynaptic potentials are not explosive *all or none* changes in voltage. Instead they develop and fade away relatively slowly. They may also be large or small depending on the quantity of transmitter released. If just a single action potential occurs in the presynaptic neurone then only a small quantity of transmitter is released and this results in a small postsynaptic potential. However, if a series of action potentials excites the presynaptic neurone, a series of bursts of transmitter is released from the terminal. Because postsynaptic potentials fade away relatively slowly, each succeeding pulse of transmitter may reach the membrane before it has recovered from the preceding pulse. As a result each postsynaptic potential adds on to the previous one and a much larger total change in voltage occurs. This adding together of small changes in voltage is termed *temporal summation* (Fig. 21.10A).

Location

The electrical changes produced at the postsynaptic membrane do not reproduce themselves on either side of the active site, as action potentials do. Instead, like ripples in a pond, the electrical disturbance spreads out but becomes smaller the further away it is from the initiating disturbance.

FUNCTIONS OF CHEMICAL TRANSMISSION

Impulses are transmitted from one neurone to the next by chemical means so that information from different sources can be integrated and regulated before being passed on. This is how decisions, determining our experience and actions, are made within the nervous system. ⑦

Integration of information

An action potential will be triggered in the postsynaptic neurone if the change in voltage is sufficiently large to trigger the opening of voltage-gated sodium channels. A single epsp is not big enough for this to happen. There must either be *temporal summation* or *spatial summation* of epsp's or both.

Spatial summation occurs when a number of synapses on the dendritic tree are active at the same time (Fig. 21.10B). If these are excitatory synapses, then a big enough postsynaptic potential may be generated to open voltage-gated sodium channels. Once this happens one or more action potentials are produced and, as explained above, this event is self-propagating. The signal is then passed on along the axon of the postsynaptic neurone.

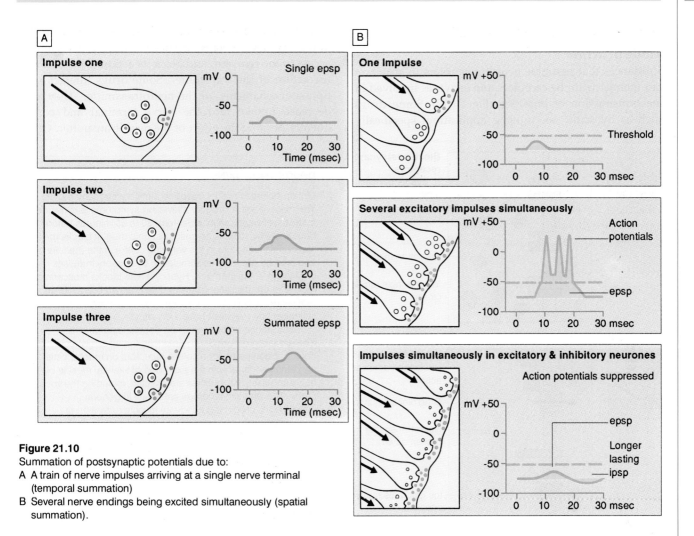

Figure 21.10
Summation of postsynaptic potentials due to:
A A train of nerve impulses arriving at a single nerve terminal (temporal summation)
B Several nerve endings being excited simultaneously (spatial summation).

However, if the synapses activated are inhibitory then the postsynaptic cell will be made less excitable. If it had been firing action potentials previously then either the frequency of firing will decrease, or the cell will be silenced.

Usually postsynaptic neurones receive a blend of excitatory and inhibitory signals. How they respond depends on the balance of excitation and inhibition occurring at any time.

Regulation of information transfer

Some nerve endings form synapses with presynaptic nerve terminals (Fig. 21.11). The transmitters released bind to receptors on the nerve terminals, and these alter the permeability of the membrane there. In so doing they change the effectiveness of the action potentials arriving at the terminal at releasing transmitter. In *presynaptic inhibition* less transmitter is released. These changes are longer lasting than postsynaptic potentials. Their usefulness lies in the fact that some inputs to the postsynaptic neurone can be selectively suppressed without affecting the sensitivity of the postsynaptic cell to other stimuli. For example when you hold on to a hot

plate that you do not want to drop, presynaptic inhibition is being used to inhibit transmission of the sensory impulses urging you to let go.

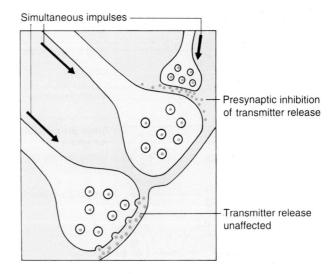

Figure 21.11
Regulation of synaptic function.

DRUGS

Mode of action

Substances that resemble neurotransmitters in structure can interact with the receptors and enzymes involved in the transmission of impulses (Fig. 21.12). Some drugs such as hyoscine (see nursing application) specifically bind to receptors on the postsynaptic membrane. By doing so they prevent the natural transmitter gaining access to the receptor, and block its action. Others mimic the action of the transmitter. Some drugs interact with uptake mechanisms for the neurotransmitter. They may decrease uptake into the nerve terminal and consequently prolong the effect of the neurotransmitter. Other

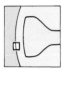
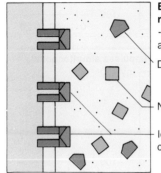

Block postsynaptic receptors
-prevents transmitter action

Drug molecule

Neurotransmitter

Ion channels remain closed

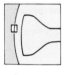
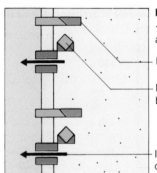

Inhibit enzymes
-prolongs transmitter action

Drug blocks enzyme

Neurotransmitter not broken down

Ion channels remain open

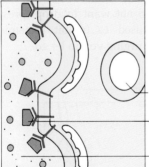

Block transmitter uptake
-prolongs transmitter action
-depletes presynaptic stores

Depleted secretory vesicle

Drug blocks receptors

Increased concentration neurotransmitters

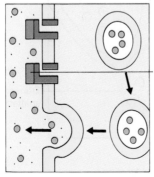

Block presynaptic receptors
-alters release of transmitter

Drug blocks receptor

Figure 21.12
Ways in which drugs can interfere with synaptic transmission postsynaptically (top two panels) and presynaptically (bottom two panels).

DRUGS AND TOXINS

Motion sickness makes travelling a misery for many people. The most effective drug for alleviating symptoms is hyoscine hydrobromide, taken in tablet form 30 to 60 minutes before travelling. Hyoscine is an antimuscarinic drug. It blocks the muscarinic receptors in the vomiting centre in the medulla and thereby prevents its stimulation by sensory impulses originating in the stomach. Hyoscine also blocks muscarinic receptors on glandular tissue and so dries up bronchial and oral secretions. Thus, if you take hyoscine for travel sickness, you may also have a dry mouth.

Tubocurarine chloride is a non-depolarising muscle relaxant derived from South American Indian arrowhead poison. It competes for nicotinic receptors on muscle cells and thus interferes with the excitation of skeletal muscle by nerve impulses. All muscles are affected, including the vocal cords. This and similar drugs are useful in general anaesthesia, producing adequate muscle relaxation to enable fairly light anaesthesia to be used and facilitating passage of an endotracheal tube between the vocal cords. Occasionally, for some reason, a patient receives insufficient anaesthetic to depress consciousness, although remaining totally relaxed, and may hear conversations between members of the operating theatre team. This also raises a note of caution for nurses caring for patients who are receiving mechanical respiration. These patients are sometimes given muscle relaxants to overcome any slight movements of the respiratory muscles that would not be synchronised with the rhythm of the respirator. The patient may become sufficiently conscious to overhear conversation without being able to communicate his awareness. It is important to talk to the patient not about him.

Toxic substances produced by bacteria may act by interfering with nerve cell transmission. *Clostridium tetani* has been described earlier (p. 373). Its toxin blocks the release of the inhibitory neurotransmitter, glycine. The consequence is overstimulation of some neurones causing muscular spasms.

The deadly toxin produced by *Clostridium botulinum* has been considered for use in germ warfare. This organism is widespread in the environment but does not normally grow inside the body. It grows and produces its toxin in food, particularly in home-processed foods, such as meat (*botulus* means 'sausage') and canned vegetables that have not been sufficiently heated to destroy bacilli and toxin. The mere tasting of contaminated food has been known to cause death. The toxin is absorbed through the intestinal wall and acts by blocking the release of acetylcholine from skeletal muscle, causing extreme weakness.

Table 21.4 Examples of drugs interfering with synaptic functions

Mode of action	Examples	Use
Block postsynaptic receptors	Hyoscine Atropine Atenolol	Travel sickness Premedication Lowers heart rate
Mimic natural transmitters	Salbutamol Morphine	Bronchodilator Pain relief
Inhibit enzymes	Distigmine	Urinary retention*
Block transmitter uptake	Cocaine	Vasoconstrictor (nasal surgery)

* In selected cases.

drugs interfere with transmitter release and some inhibit the enzymes breaking down the transmitters (Table 21.4).

Membrane receptors

Research on drugs has shown that there is usually more than one type of receptor protein for the same neurotransmitter. Acetylcholine for example interacts with at least two different receptors. These were named *muscarinic* and *nicotinic* because of the substances (*muscarine* and *nicotine*) that were first found to affect their function. At least four different receptors that can

The antimuscarinic drugs, atropine and hyoscine, are frequently used as premedication before surgery to prevent, among other things, the excessive salivation caused by intubation and inhalation anaesthetics.

interact with noradrenaline have now been identified, and at least five for opioid peptides (see Ch. 3, Table 3.7).

ESTABLISHING AND MAINTAINING SYNAPTIC CONTACTS

The synaptic contacts existing between excitable cells in the adult are established during early development. Once contacts have been formed they are preserved by use. If nerves are severed the affected nerve endings degenerate. However, provided the cell body is uninjured, axons can regrow and contacts can be re-established.

DEVELOPMENT OF SYNAPTIC CONTACTS

Once the primitive neural cells (see Ch. 20) have stopped dividing, and those that migrate have migrated to their final destination within the nervous system, extensions of the cell begin to develop. At first just one, destined to become the axon, begins to form. At its tip is a spiky enlargement (*growth cone*) (Fig 21.13). The growth cone is a highly active structure that crawls along adjacent surfaces guided by the affinity it has for

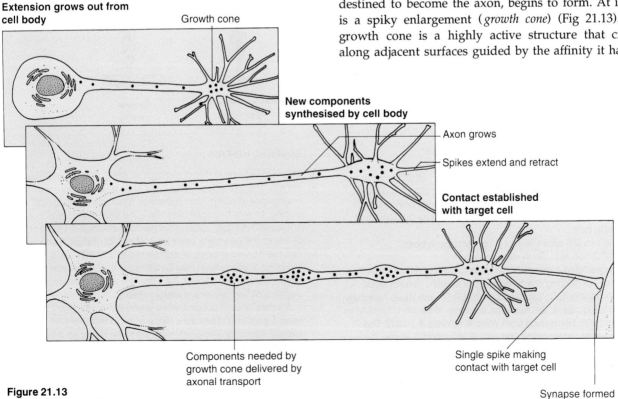

Extension grows out from cell body

Growth cone

New components synthesised by cell body

Axon grows

Spikes extend and retract

Contact established with target cell

Components needed by growth cone delivered by axonal transport

Single spike making contact with target cell

Synapse formed

Figure 21.13
Establishing synaptic contacts.

molecules nearby. The spikes extend, retract and re-form continually so that all points in the vicinity are tested for their suitability. ⑧

As the growth cone moves forward it pulls on the extension and the axon is caused to grow. The components needed for growth are synthesised in the cell body and are either built on to the existing struc-

tures or are shuttled along to the growth cone by axonal transport (Fig. 21.6).

Eventually the neurone contacts its target cell, drawn to it often by chemicals secreted by that cell. *Nerve growth factor (NGF)*, for example, is secreted by cells destined to be innervated by sympathetic neurones.

The contact point becomes transformed into a

⑧
What is the approximate size of the embryo at this stage?

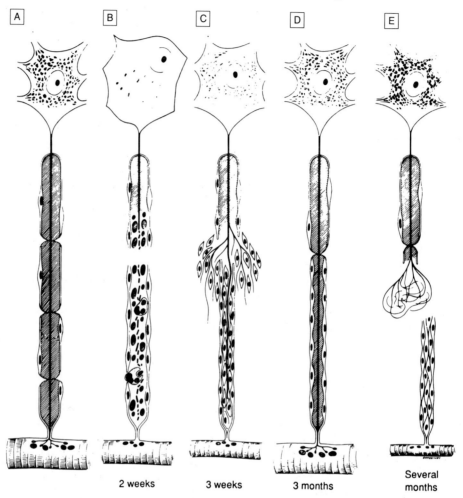

Figure 21.14
Changes taking place in a severed motoneurone:

A State prior to injury

B 2 weeks after the injury: that part of the axon cut off from the cell body is degenerating; macrophages are digesting the debris

C Cut end of the axon is sprouting; Schwann cells proliferating; axon grows back towards the muscle guided by the sheath of Schwann cells

D Several months after the injury: contacts have been re-established with the skeletal muscle

E Unsuccessful re-innervation: aimless growth of nerve fibres as a result of not 'finding' the Schwann cell sheath. (Reproduced from Junqueira L C, Carneiro J, Kelley R O 1989 Basic histology, 6th edn, Figures 9–26, Appleton & Lange, Norwalk, CT, USA, as adapted with permission from Willis R A, Willis A T 1972 The principles of bacteriology, 3rd edn, Butterworth, London, by permission of both publishers.)

SEVERED NERVES

Most people are at risk of damage to the axons of peripheral nerves. The extra-deep cut from a knife or chisel, negligence in using can openers or machinery, falling and putting an arm through a window – the possibilities are endless. The injury varies from partial division of an axon or axons to the complete severance of a limb or digit. Provided that the nerve cell body is not damaged and that there is not too large a gap (which may fill with scar tissue) between the severed ends of the axon, the axon will regrow. Varying degrees of function will gradually return.

If a limb or digit is completely severed it is important to keep it cool and make sure that it goes to hospital with the patient. Microsurgery enables limbs to be replaced and, depending on the type of injury, some degree of function to be restored. Clean cuts can be more successfully repaired than crush injuries.

synapse. If the growth cone has divided to form several extensions, a single axon may branch to form multiple synapses.

Neurones that do not contact a target cell do not survive. Substances secreted by the target cells (such as NGF) are believed to be needed to maintain neuronal function.

MAINTAINING SYNAPTIC CONTACTS

The maintenance of synaptic contacts depends partly on the transmission of impulses by the presynaptic neurone. If that neurone falls into disuse its synaptic contacts weaken and are displaced by others formed by active neurones nearby. Cells that have lost their innervation secrete factors stimulating nerve cells to sprout and make synaptic connections with them.

The properties of the synapses forged depend upon their degree of use. If for example a cell loses a lot of excitatory inputs it responds by increasing the number of receptors in the membrane that are sensitive to the excitatory transmitter (*up-regulation*). This has the effect of increasing the sensitivity of the postsynaptic neurone to the small amount of transmitter still available (*denervation supersensitivity*).

Conversely, if particular synapses are used incessantly, the postsynaptic cell adapts by reducing the number of receptors present on the postsynaptic membrane (*down-regulation*).

REGROWTH OF SEVERED AXONS

Provided the cell body of a neurone remains intact, nerve axons can regrow if they are severed through injury. The part of the axon beyond the injury deteriorates and dies, and new growth occurs from the end closest to the cell body (Fig. 21.14).

Role of supporting cells

The supporting cells (oligodendrocytes and Schwann cells) can act as a framework guiding the axon towards its normal destination. If the supporting cells that guide growth are injured the nerve may grow in different directions guided only by chemical signals in the environment.

Role of the cell body

If the cell body dies then the axon is not self-sustaining, and transmission of signals along that neurone ceases. Once nerve cells have matured they can no longer reproduce. Cells that are lost cannot be replaced. However, remaining neurones can form new synaptic contacts as more sites become available on the cells that have lost some of their innervation. Thus by making more use of the remaining neurones the effects of loss may not be as marked as expected. ⑨

Differences between parts of the nervous system

In the central nervous system, regeneration stops after about 2 weeks irrespective of whether or not contacts have been re-established. The reasons for this are not known. If the injured tract cannot be bypassed, by redistribution of function to other pathways, permanent disability may result. However, in the peripheral nervous system growth continues with the result that full re-innervation may be achieved and normal functions restored.

> **KEY POINTS**
>
> What you should now know and understand about neurones:
>
> - their basic structure
> - what is meant by a membrane potential
> - what a nerve impulse is and how it is generated
> - how nerve impulses travel along nerves
> - what a synapse is and how it works
> - how some nerve cells integrate information from different sources and how this relates to everyday experience
> - how some commonly used drugs modify neurone function
> - what happens to nerves if they are injured.

REFERENCES AND FURTHER READING

Aidley D J 1989 The physiology of excitable cells, 3rd edn. Cambridge University Press, Cambridge
(Excellent advanced textbook reviewing experimental basis of current knowledge. Extremely well referenced)
Brown M C, Hopkins W G, Keynes R J 1991 Essentials of neural development. Cambridge University Press, Cambridge
(Excellent resource for background to nerve cell growth, contact, plasticity, injury, basis of learning etc., including experimental background. Advanced, authoritative but concise. Useful for reference and further information)
Junqueira L C, Carneiro J, Kelley R O 1989 Basic histology, 6th edn. Appleton & Lange, East Norwalk, p 186
Keynes R D, Aidley D J 1991 Nerve and muscle, 2nd edn. Cambridge University Press, Cambridge
(Deceptively small, but advanced student text explaining how nerve and muscle tissues have been studied and the experimental basis of current theory)
Matthews G G 1991 Cellular physiology of nerve and muscle. Blackwell Scientific Publications, Oxford
(A friendly book providing lucid descriptions of basic principles. Includes list of further reading)
Rang H P, Dale M M 1991 Pharmacology, 2nd edn. Churchill Livingstone, Edinburgh
(Useful reference for drug action)
Turner P, Richens A, Routledge A, Routledge P 1986 Clinical pharmacology. Churchill Livingstone, Edinburgh
(Useful reference for drug action)
Willis R A, Willis A T 1972 The principles of pathology and bacteriology 3rd edn. Butterworth, London, p 32

⑨
How many causes of nerve cell death can you name?

Chapter 22
MUSCLE

Almost all cells can alter their shape by contraction of specific intracellular proteins. This enables the cell to move. White cells, for example, creep along blood vessels in an amoeba-like way, and find their way through capillary walls into the interstitial fluid (see Ch. 15). Other cells, such as those lining the respiratory tract, possess cilia which are driven to and fro (see Ch. 7). But in muscle cells this ability to contract dominates cell activity. The forces developed are harnessed in various ways: activity in gastrointestinal muscle mixes and propels food and digestive secretions; contraction of cardiac muscle drives blood around the circulation; whereas contraction and relaxation of skeletal muscle enables us to walk, write, speak and laugh.

Basically, there are three different types of muscle (Fig. 22.1):

● smooth   ● cardiac   ● skeletal.

In all three, contraction is caused by the interaction of two proteins, *actin* and *myosin*. This interaction is regulated by the intracellular concentration of calcium,

Skeletal

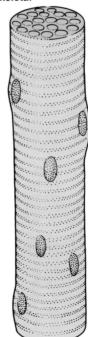

50 μm

Smooth

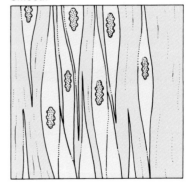

Cardiac

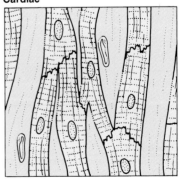

Figure 22.1 (*right*)
The three main types of muscle: skeletal, smooth and cardiac. All three are drawn approximately to scale. Skeletal muscle fibres are very long. Consequently only a short section of a single fibre is shown.

which, in turn, is controlled by stimuli acting on the muscle cells. These stimuli may be neural, hormonal or an inherent property of the muscle itself. The three types of muscle differ, however, in their structure, method of excitation and other properties, according to the roles each plays within the body.

BASIC MECHANISM OF CONTRACTION

BONDING BETWEEN PROTEINS

As explained in Chapter 2, protein molecules can change their shape through alterations in the bonds that they form internally and through interactions with other molecules and ions. In muscle cells this property of proteins is used to pull the cell into a different shape

and cause contraction. The two key proteins involved are:

● actin   ● myosin.

The protein molecules are arranged in an ordered way forming two types of protein filaments, thin and thick (Fig. 22.2). The thin filament consists of actin molecules, and the thick filament consists of myosin.

Actin and myosin have a natural affinity for one another that is controlled by other specific proteins

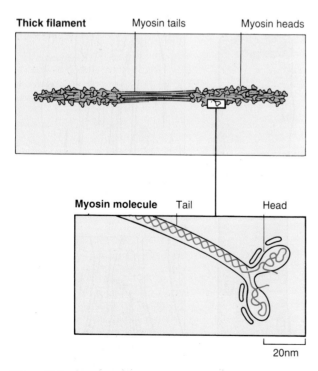

Thin filament

Actin molecule

20nm

Thick filament   Myosin tails   Myosin heads

Myosin molecule   Tail   Head

20nm

Figure 22.2
Structure of thin and thick filaments. (Adapted from Alberts et al 1983.)

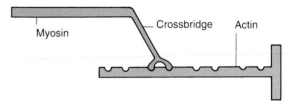

Bond forms between actin and myosin

Myosin   Crossbridge   Actin

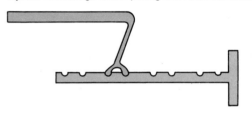

Myosin crossbridge bends pulling actin filament inwards

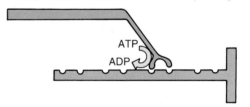

Energy released from ATP   Crossbridge straightens

ATP
ADP

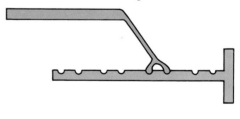

New bond forms further along actin filament

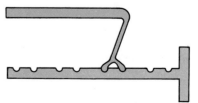

Cycle repeats

Figure 22.3
How the making and breaking of bonds between actin and myosin causes contraction.

nearby. If bonding is allowed, the myosin heads on the thick filaments are attracted to specific sites on the actin molecules of the thin filaments, forming crossbridges (Fig. 22.3). When the bond forms, the myosin cross-bridge bends. This pulls the thick filament along the thin filament. ATP then binds to the myosin head and is split with the help of the enzyme, *myosin-ATPase*. The energy released enables the myosin head to return to its original position and the bond between actin and myosin breaks. The myosin head swings to a new position further up the thin filament and bonds to the new site. The cycle is then repeated. In this way, by the forming and breaking of bonds between actin and myosin, the thick filaments are pulled along the thin filament and tension develops. But this can only happen when actin and myosin are free to associate. In the relaxed state their association is prevented by the influence of other proteins which in turn are controlled by the intracellular concentration of calcium.

CONTROL BY CALCIUM

Calcium ions carry two positive charges (see Ch. 2) and therefore can bind to negatively charged groups, such as those found on protein molecules. The proteins that regulate the interaction of actin and myosin have binding sites for calcium. When calcium is attached to these sites, changes occur allowing actin and myosin to interact and produce contraction.

The amount of calcium that binds, and therefore the degree of contraction produced, depends on the concentration of calcium in the cytoplasm (*sarcoplasm* or *myoplasm* in muscle cells). The greater the calcium concentration, the greater is the number of binding sites occupied by calcium ions. Consequently, the number of bonds formed between actin and myosin, and the

RIGOR MORTIS

For many nurses, handling the body of a patient after death produces a variety of feelings from grief to fear. Fear, in some instances, is a result of vague ideas about changes that take place in the body when death occurs. Immediately after death, the muscles are still relaxed because there is no longer any stimulation from the nervous system. It is possible to carry out 'last offices', the final care given to the patient before the body is taken to the mortuary, without any more difficulty than giving a bed bath to an unconscious patient. Because the muscles are relaxed, air will be forced out of the lungs when the patient's body is turned. The air, passing over the vocal cords, often produces a groan-like sound, which gives the impression that the patient is still alive; some nurses find this very distressing.

At the time of death, normal cell activity ceases and other chemical changes begin to take place. The majority of these are more the concern of pathologists than nurses but some knowledge of rigor mortis, the stiffness of death, is useful. Muscles remain relaxed as long as intracellular calcium concentration is low. After death, intracellular calcium concentration increases and ATP is depleted. Consequently, actin and myosin are able to associate continuously and the muscles contract. The time taken for this process to take place varies with, among other things, ambient temperature and type of illness. It is important to support the lower jaw, close the eyes and arrange the limbs in a natural position before stiffness begins. Readers of murder stories will be aware that the onset of rigor mortis gives a not very accurate indication of the time of death. Rigor mortis is not maintained indefinitely but wears off after some hours as lysosomes begin to digest cellular proteins (see Ch. 37).

degree of contraction, increases. If calcium concentration falls fewer bonds are made and contraction decreases (Fig. 22.4).

The concentration of unbound (free) calcium in the cytoplasm of relaxed muscle cells (0.1 μmol/l) is 10 000

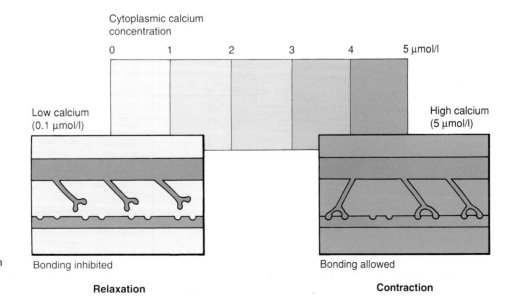

Figure 22.4
Cytoplasmic calcium concentration and muscle contraction.

times less than that outside (1 mmol/l). Intracellular concentration is affected by the amount of calcium:

- entering the cell fom the extracellular fluid
- released from intracellular stores.

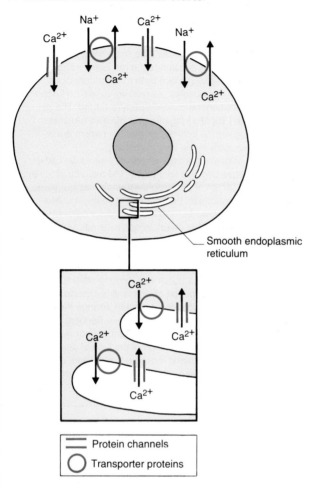

Smooth endoplasmic reticulum

Protein channels

Transporter proteins

Figure 22.5
Ways in which calcium moves into and out of the cytoplasm: ion channels allow calcium into the cytoplasm (sarcoplasm); transporter proteins eject calcium from it.

Both of these depend on pumps, carriers and channels governing the movement of calcium from one place to another (Fig. 22.5).

The entry of calcium into the cell, and its release from compartments inside the cell where it is present at high concentrations, such as the endoplasmic reticulum (*sarcoplasmic reticulum* in muscle cells), is achieved by the transitory opening of calcium channels that simply allow calcium to diffuse into the sarcoplasm. Removing the calcium from the sarcoplasm requires assistance, however, as it has to be moved from a region of low to high concentration. Carriers are present both in the cell membrane (*sodium–calcium exchangers*) and in membranes of the sarcoplasmic reticulum (*calcium pumps*).①

SMOOTH MUSCLE

Smooth muscle is present in several organs and tissues of the body including:

- blood vessels (arteries, arterioles, venules, veins)
- gastrointestinal tract, bile duct and gall bladder
- uterus and fallopian tubes
- urinary bladder and ureters
- bronchioles of the respiratory tract.

STRUCTURE

Smooth muscle is the least complex of the three types of muscle. The cells are small (50 to 700 μm in length), spindle-shaped and relatively featureless (Fig. 22.6). They are linked to one another by gap junctions (see Ch. 2), which allow electrical impulses to spead from one cell to the next. Actin and myosin filaments are scattered throughout the cell, and the sarcoplasmic reticulum is sparse.

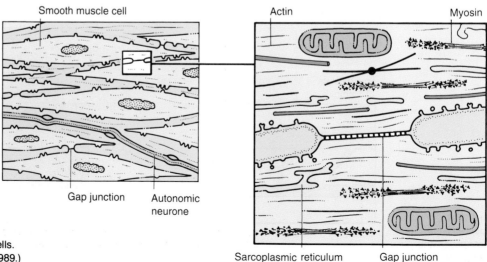

Smooth muscle cell

Actin

Myosin

Gap junction

Autonomic neurone

Sarcoplasmic reticulum

Gap junction

Figure 22.6
Structure of smooth muscle cells.
(Adapted from Williams et al 1989.)

HOW CONTRACTION IS TRIGGERED

Most smooth muscle cells are spontaneously active. They do not need an external stimulus to cause them to contract. Instead they contract and relax regularly in response to their own internal mechanism of excitation. External stimuli can make the contractions stronger or weaker but they do not initiate contraction (see below). ②

Spontaneous excitation

Contractions are triggered regularly as a result of a regular cycle of depolarisation and repolarisation of the cell membrane (*slow wave*) (Fig. 22.7). The slow wave is caused by the regular opening and closing of ion channels in the cell membrane in a set sequence. At particular phases of this cycle, action potentials are triggered. These open calcium channels in the cell membrane and calcium flows into the cell, triggering contraction.

Role of calcium

Within the cell, calcium binds to the protein *calmodulin*.

When it does so, the calcium–calmodulin complex promotes the bonding of actin and myosin, and contraction occurs. At the same time, calcium pumps in the cell membrane increase their activity and the intracellular concentration of calcium begins to decrease. As the calcium concentration falls, calcium detaches from calmodulin, the interaction between actin and myosin is inhibited and relaxation occurs. This cycle is repeated regularly, contraction occurring each time there is a burst of action potentials (Fig. 22.7).

FACTORS AFFECTING CONTRACTION

Stretch

If smooth muscle is stretched abruptly it responds by contracting. This response is said to be *myogenic* in that it originates (*genesis*) within the muscle (*myo*). Stretch is thought to depolarise the muscle and thus to excite it. Responses like this have been described in smooth muscle of the gastrointestinal tract and in the smooth muscle of blood vessels.

If, however, the stretch is maintained, it is found that

②
What external stimuli might affect smooth muscle?

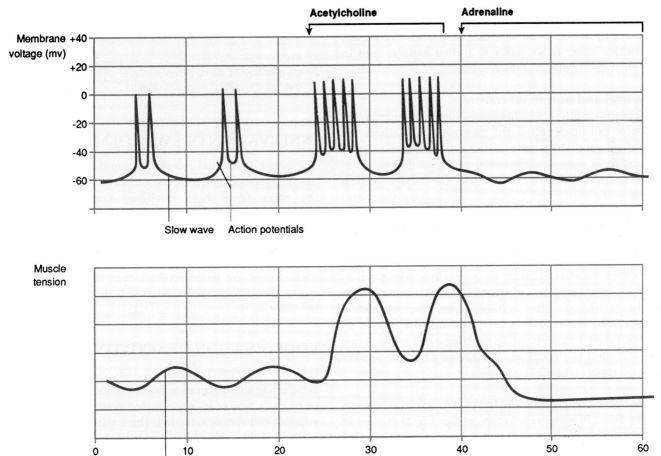

Figure 22.7
The regular cycle of depolarisation and repolarisation (slow wave) characteristic of most smooth muscle cells. The slow wave triggers action potentials (top panel) that excite muscle contraction (bottom panel). Acetylcholine stimulates the muscle whereas adrenaline inhibits it.

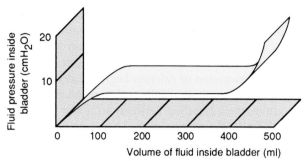

Figure 22.8
Pressure of fluid inside the human urinary bladder at different volumes (cystometrogram). Note that the pressure remains constant at about 8 to 9 cmH$_2$O as the bladder fills until the volume exceeds about 400 ml. (Adapted from Tanagho & McAninch 1984.)

after an initial contraction the muscle 'gives'. This is referred to as the *plasticity* of smooth muscle. This property of smooth muscle is seen in organs such as the bladder (see Ch. 8), and the stomach (see Ch. 6). It allows the volume of the contents of these organs to vary greatly without substantially affecting the tension in their walls, or the pressure developed within the organ (Fig. 22.8). Without this property, the stretch caused by filling would stimulate the muscle to contract, resulting either in resistance to further expansion or in premature expulsion of the contents.

Neural and hormonal control

Neurotransmitters and hormones affect the number of action potentials generated per cycle of activity by changing the excitability of the cell membrane. Some substances, such as acetycholine acting on the muscle of the gastrointestinal tract, decrease the average voltage across the membrane (*depolarisation*) making the membrane more excitable. More action potentials are fired per cycle of activity, more calcium enters the cell, and consequently the resulting contraction is bigger (Fig. 22.7).

Other substances, such as adrenaline acting on β$_2$ adrenergic receptors of gastrointestinal muscle (see Ch. 3), increase the voltage across the membrane (*hyperpolarisation*) and make the membrane less excitable. Fewer action potentials are triggered (or even none if the effect is strong) and contractions become weaker or disappear (Fig. 22.7).

Distribution of membrane receptors

The blend of membrane receptors (see Ch. 2) present in cells differs between different sorts of smooth muscle. This determines how the muscle will respond to a particular hormone as well as what hormones will affect it. For example, most arteriolar smooth muscle possesses an abundance of α adrenergic receptors that cause contraction, and therefore vasoconstriction, in response to adrenalin. However, smooth muscle in skeletal muscle blood vessels, the gastrointestinal tract and the airways has β$_2$ receptors that cause relaxation. The muscle of the uterus (*myometrium*) has some β$_2$ receptors causing relaxation but also has many receptors for the hormone oxytocin that causes uterine contraction, and has intracellular receptors for oestrogens and progesterone that influence the excitability of the myometrium (see Ch. 34).

> **SMOOTH MUSCLE RELAXANTS**
>
> Salbutamol is a widely used drug for patients with severe acute asthma and also during pregnancy to delay onset of labour. It is known as a selective β$_2$ adrenoreceptor stimulant, a sympathomimetic. During an attack of asthma, where the bronchioles are constricted, the drug acts on the β adrenoreceptors in the smooth muscle of the bronchioles. The number of action potentials is reduced so that the muscle relaxes and the patient can breathe more easily.
>
> When premature labour is threatened and it is preferable not to allow labour to progress, salbutamol may be used to relax the uterine muscle (myometrium) thus preventing further contractions. The most commonly used β$_2$ adrenoreceptor stimulant in obstetrics is ritodrine hydrochloride.

> If labour does not commence spontaneously after rupture of the membranes, an intravenous infusion of oxytocin may be given to stimulate uterine contractions.

INNERVATION OF SMOOTH MUSCLE

The nerve fibres that release transmitter onto the cells are interspersed between the muscle cells. The branching nerve fibres have swellings along their length (*varicosities*) from which transmitter is released (Figs 22.6 and 22.9). Once released, the transmitter diffuses over quite a wide area influencing any muscle cells in the vicinity. The membrane receptors to which the transmitters bind are distributed all over the muscle membrane. Blood-borne hormones reach the same receptors by diffusing through the interstitial fluid. ③

COORDINATION OF ACTIVITY

Because of the gap junctions (see Ch. 2) linking adjacent cells, if one smooth muscle cell is excited spontaneously, or by the action of locally released neurotransmitter, the adjacent cell also is activated. The activity of neighbouring cells is thus coopted and coordinated and cells work together as if they were a single unit (as a *syncytium*).

MULTIUNIT SMOOTH MUSCLE

Multiunit smooth muscle is slightly different from the smooth muscle (*single-unit* or *visceral muscle*) described

③
Can you name two blood-borne hormones that affect smooth muscle?

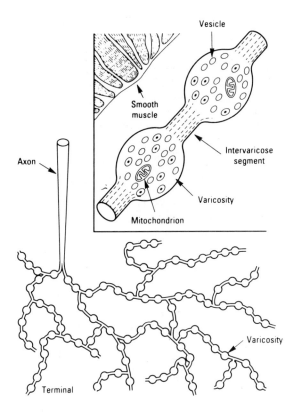

Figure 22.9
Structure of the nerve endings lying between smooth muscle cells.
(Reprinted by permission of the publisher from Kandel E R,
Schwartz J H (eds) Principles of neural science, 2nd edn, p. 140.
Copyright 1985 by Elsevier Publishing Co., Inc.)

so far. One place in which multiunit muscle is found is
the iris of the eye (see Ch. 26). Gap junctions are sparse
in this form of smooth muscle. Consequently, excitation
does not spread easily through the tissue. Also the cells
are not spontaneously active. Instead, contraction is
mainly controlled by the nerves with which it is richly
innervated. In this respect, multiunit smooth muscle is
more like skeletal muscle (see p. 395).

CARDIAC MUSCLE

The myocardium (see Ch. 5) consists of two types of
cells:

- contractile (atrial and ventricular muscle)
- conducting tissue (SA node, AV node, bundles of His,
  Purkinje cells).

Both types of cell develop embryologically from the
same precursor cells and consequently have common
features. The conducting tissue still possesses some
contractile proteins even though these cells do not play
any part in developing pressures in the heart. Conversely the atrial and ventricular muscle has similar,
though slightly different, electrical properties to the
conducting cells. The nature and properties of the
contractile cells will be described first.

CONTRACTILE CELLS

Structure
Cardiac muscle differs strikingly in its appearance from
smooth muscle (Fig. 22.10). Two of its distinctive
features are:

- intercalated discs
- striations.

Intercalated discs
Intercalated discs are specialised structures firmly linking individual cells together. Some cells branch with
the result that a closely interwoven network of cells
is formed. Gap junctions (see Ch. 2) are present in
the discs. As a result electrical events spread easily from
cell to cell as they do in smooth muscle. Both the gap
junctions and the network of firm attachments created
by the discs enable cardiac muscle cells to work together
as a unit (as a *syncytium*).

Striations
On closer inspection, the cells appear striped (*striated*).
This appearance is created by the fact that thick and thin
filaments are arranged in a very orderly way. The thick
and thin filaments are interleaved and arranged in
groups, divided by a structure called the *Z line* to form
sarcomeres. This basic arrangement is repeated many
times over to form a long *myofibril*. Each striated muscle
cell contains bundles of many such myofibrils (Fig.
22.11) extending from one end of the cell to the other.

The distinctive pattern of light and dark arises
because the places where the thick and thin filaments
overlap (*A band*) look different under the microscope
from those where they do not (*I band*). This is made
more obvious by the fact that this light and dark pattern
is in register across many myofibrils (Fig. 22.11).

Other features
Other distinctive features of cardiac muscle include the
presence of:

- many mitochondria
- sarcoplasmic reticulum
- T-tubules.

Cardiac muscle cells contain many mitochondria. These
lie between the myofibrils and generate the ATP needed
to power contraction (see Ch. 11). The *sarcoplasmic
reticulum* in cardiac muscle is more extensive than that
in smooth muscle. It is interlaced between the myofibrils
and acts as an important store of intracellular calcium.
The T-tubules consist of invaginated cell membrane

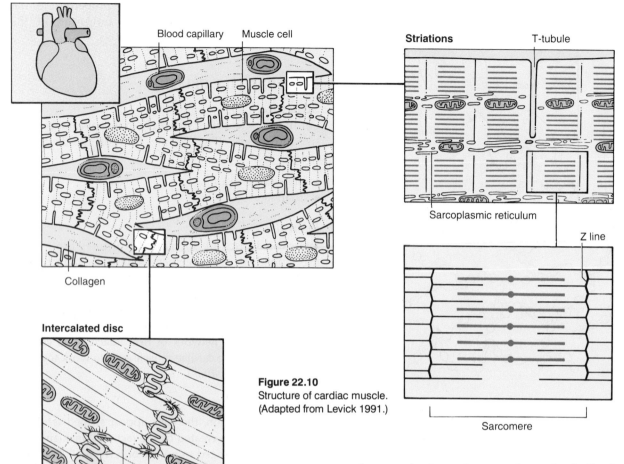

Figure 22.10
Structure of cardiac muscle.
(Adapted from Levick 1991.)

dipping deeply into the cell interior to form long narrow tubes (Fig. 22.10). These tubules transmit the impulse that excites the cell, deep into the cell interior.

How contraction is triggered

Cardiac muscle, like smooth muscle, contracts and relaxes regularly. But, unlike smooth muscle, the source of excitation is not the contractile cells but the conducting tissue (see p. 393). The conducting tissue generates action potentials, which are transmitted to the muscle cells and act as the pacemakers for the muscle cells.

Cardiac action potential

When cardiac muscle cells are excited, they generate an action potential that is conducted along the cell membrane and carried deep into the interior along the membrane forming the T-tubules. The action potential is strikingly different from that recorded in nerve axons. It lasts about 100 times longer and it has a plateau (Fig. 22.12). However, the first part, the rapid depolarisation and reversal of membrane voltage, is similar in form and basis to that in nerve axons. It is caused by the opening of voltage-gated sodium channels. The plateau that follows is caused by the opening of voltage-gated calcium channels. Because these stay open for quite a time, the membrane voltage cannot return to its unexcited state very quickly. Eventually, however, the original potential is restored as these channels close.

Role of calcium

The opening of calcium channels during the action potential allows calcium to flow into the cell from the extracellular fluid. The action potential transmitted deep into the cell via the T-tubules also stimulates the sarcoplasmic reticulum to release some calcium stored there. Cardiac cells therefore differ from smooth muscle cells in that calcium is released locally inside the cell close to actin and myosin as well as diffusing into the cell from outside (Fig. 22.5). This has the effect of shortening the time it takes for contraction to occur.

The calcium released into the sarcoplasm binds to *troponin*, a different protein from that in smooth muscle. Troponin is attached to another protein, *tropomyosin*, lying on the thin actin filaments (Fig. 22.13). The *troponin–tropomyosin* complex normally inhibits the interaction between actin and myosin. However, when calcium binds to troponin, the troponin–tropomyosin

Muscle cell

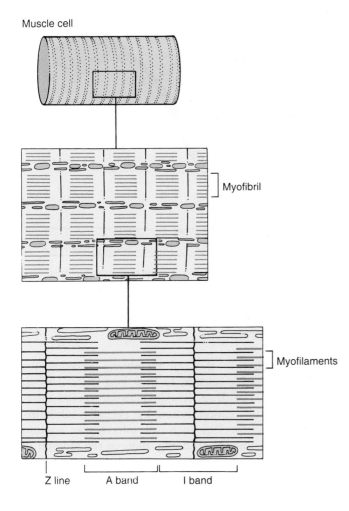

Myofibril

Myofilaments

Z line   A band   I band

Thin filament (actin)

Thick filament (myosin)

Figure 22.11
Basic structure of striated (i.e. striped) muscle: organisation of filaments and fibrils within a muscle fibre (cell) giving rise to its striped appearance.

Figure 22.13
Role of troponin and tropomyosin in the contraction and relaxation of striated muscle:
A The position of tropomysosin on the actin filament prevents bonding between actin and myosin
B Calcium binds to troponin and tropomyosin moves
C Bonding occurs between actin and myosin causing contraction.
(Reproduced from Levick J R 1991 An introduction to cardiovascular physiology, Figure 3.3, by permission of Butterworth–Heinemann.)

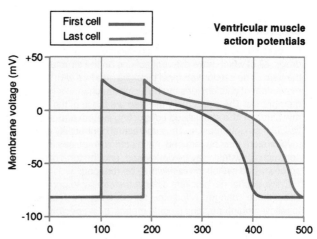

Ventricular muscle action potentials

First cell ▬▬
Last cell ▬▬

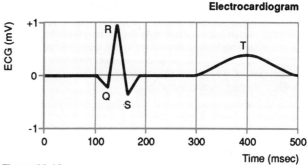

Electrocardiogram

Figure 22.12
The shape of the cardiac action potential (top panel). Two separate action potentials are shown, one from the first muscle cell in the ventricle to be excited, and the other from the last cell. The action potentials from the rest of the muscle occur between these two (shaded area). Clearly during the periods 100–180 msec and 300–500 msec there is a lot of electrical disturbance as one after the other the cells depolarise and repolarise. These two periods of electrical activity are picked up in the electrocardiogram (ECG) as the QRS and T waves respectively (bottom panel) (see Ch. 5).

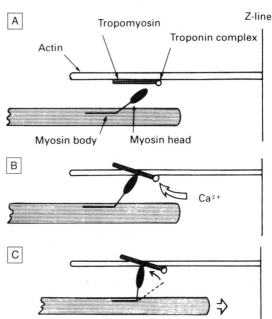

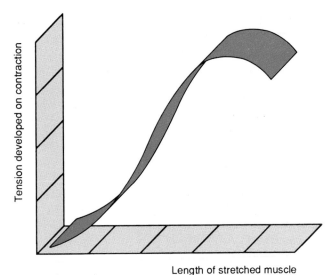

Figure 22.14
Relationship between muscle length and strength of contraction in striated muscle when muscle length is altered by stretch.

complex is displaced, enabling the myosin heads to bind to actin.

When the concentration of calcium in the sarcoplasm decreases, the inhibitory effect of troponin–tropomyosin is restored and relaxation occurs. This occurs more quickly than in smooth muscle because calcium is pumped back into the sarcoplasm as well as being transported out of the cell (Fig. 22.5).

Factors affecting contraction

Stretch

In striated muscle, the strength of contraction depends upon the extent to which the muscle is stretched. If the muscle is pulled to a greater length, the same stimulus produces a bigger force of contraction (Fig. 22.14). This property of striated muscle was alluded to in an earlier chapter (Ch. 5) as *Starling's law of the heart*. The reason for this behaviour is not fully understood. It has been suggested to be due to the degree of overlap of the actin and myosin filaments, which changes as the muscle is stretched, and the number of crossbridges which can therefore be formed. A more recent theory is that the stretching of the filaments somehow increases the affinity of troponin–tropomyosin for calcium. ④

Neural and hormonal control

The bigger the increase in calcium concentration inside the cell the bigger is the resulting contraction. The hormone adrenaline, and the neurotransmitter nor-adrenaline released from sympathetic nerves, both act

on β receptors in the cell membrane affecting the channels allowing calcium to flow into the cell when it is excited. The drug digoxin indirectly raises intra-cellular calcium concentration by partially inhibiting the Na/K pump. This increases intracellular sodium concentration and, in so doing, reduces the amount of calcium extruded from the cell by sodium–calcium exchange (see Fig. 22.5).

④
What stretches cardiac muscle? How may this vary?

Innervation

Both atrial and ventricular muscle tissue are innervated by sympathetic nerve fibres, but only atrial muscle is innervated to any extent by parasympathetic fibres. There are no specific junctions between the nerve and the muscle cells. Transmitter released from the varicosities influences several muscle cells. This is similar to the arrangement in smooth muscle (see Fig. 22.9).

Coordination of activity

Because the cells are linked to one another by gap junctions in the intercalated discs (Fig. 22.10) the electrical excitation of one cell spreads to neighbouring cells so that, once excited, cardiac muscle cells all contract almost simultaneously. This coordinated activity is helped as well by the rapid distribution of the excitatory signal to all cells by the specialised conducting tissue (see below and Ch. 5).

Metabolism of cardiac muscle

Whereas most other muscles in the body have spells of inactivity the heart beats from early in embryonic life to the day of death. This continual activity is crucially dependent on a sufficient and steady supply of ATP. The supply is guaranteed by the production of ATP by aerobic metabolism (see Ch. 11). Cardiac cells contain:

- an abundance of mitochondria to generate ATP aerobically
- myoglobin that, like haemoglobin, binds oxygen reversibly.⑤

The fuel used by the cells is chiefly fatty acids, though glucose can be used in large amounts as well, particularly after carbohydrate-rich meals. Keto-acids (see Ch. 14) are used in starvation. The supply of fuels and oxygen is guaranteed by a very rich network of blood vessels (see Ch. 5). If the flow of blood to a part of the heart muscle is reduced so that the tissue is deprived of oxygen (becomes *hypoxic*) the consequences are more serious than in skeletal muscle because the capacity of cardiac cells to generate ATP anaerobically is much more limited.

> The complete obstruction of blood flow to an area of myocardium may be caused by a clot and/or atheroma in one of the coronary vessels. Without a blood supply, the affected myocardium dies: this is known as a *myocardial infarction*.

CONDUCTING CELLS

These cardiac cells generate the impulses that excite cardiac muscle and set the pulse rate. They also carry the primary signal, generated in the sino-atrial node, rapidly to all parts of the atria and ventricles (see Ch. 5).

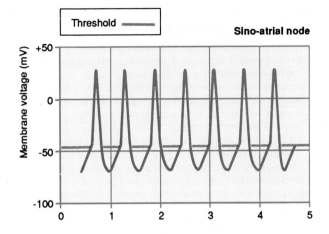

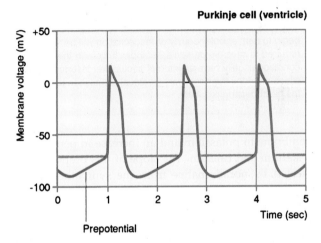

Figure 22.15
Electrical activity recorded from two different types of cell in the heart (sino-atrial node and Purkinje) when each is allowed to depolarise and repolarise at its own pace.

⑤
What does aerobic mean?

Just as in smooth muscle, impulses are generated spontaneously. The voltage across the cell membrane is never constant but continually depolarises and repolarises (Fig. 22.15).

Pacemakers

An action potential fires whenever the voltage drops below threshold. All of the conducting tissue is spontaneously active but, because the frequency of impulses fired by the SA node is higher than that of the rest of the tissue, the SA node sets the pace for the tissue as a whole. If there is a block in conduction between the atria and the ventricles, some of the Purkinje cells of the ventricles can take over as the pacemaker. Their natural rate of firing (about 40 per minute) is lower than that of the SA node (about 110 per minute) (Fig. 22.15).

Neural and hormonal control

The slow depolarisation (*prepotential*) occurring just ahead of the action potential (Fig. 22.15), is believed to be caused by a decrease in the permeability of the

⑥
Does excess plasma K⁺ (hyper-kalaemia) have any effect on the heart? If so what?

HEART BLOCK AND STOKES–ADAMS ATTACKS

There are three degrees of atrio-ventricular heart block – first and second degree, and complete (or third degree). The main text describes complete heart block (p. 393); no impulses reach the ventricles from the atria. This type of heart block may be caused by myocarditis, coronary heart disease, infarction or drugs such as digoxin. When the person's pulse rate is counted it will be 40 or lower because it is the ventricular rate that is being detected by palpation. This condition may be temporary or permanent. If it is permanent and the Purkinje cells in the ventricles establish an independent rhythm, the person may be able to live a fairly normal life. If, however, the ventricular rhythm is irregular, the person may experience episodes of *ventricular asystole* (the ventricles cease to beat). This, in turn, may progress to *cardiac syncope* (unconsciousness) otherwise known as a Stokes–Adams attack. Consciousness is lost suddenly and usually without warning although onlookers may notice a sudden pallor of the face. The heart may either begin to beat spontaneously or resuscitation will be required to save the person's life. Individuals with this condition usually have an internal pacemaker inserted, which provides the necessary electrical stimulation to keep the heart beating regularly.

membrane to potassium and an increase in permeability to sodium and calcium. The slope of this prepotential is affected by noradrenaline from the sympathetic nerve terminals, and acetylcholine from the parasympathetic fibres. Noradrenaline, acting on β receptors increases the flow of sodium and calcium into the cell and speeds up the rate of depolarisation. Threshold is reached more speedily and so it takes less time for an action potential to be fired. Repolarisation also occurs more quickly and as a result the number of impulses generated per minute increases.

Figure 22.16
Structure of a section of a skeletal muscle fibre. (Adapted from Krstic 1979.)

Intramuscular injections are commonly given into the gluteus medius muscle (the upper and outer quadrant of the buttock), the deltoid muscle and, in some instances, the lateral aspect of the quadriceps muscle. If a state of total relaxation can be achieved, by positioning and reassurance, then the injection will cause less discomfort. Even a small amount of fluid forced into a tense muscle will cause discomfort or pain.

Acetylcholine, in contrast, promotes the opening of potassium channels in the membrane. This restrains depolarisation and so it takes longer for the voltage to reach threshold. Consequently heart rate decreases. ⑥

SKELETAL MUSCLE

The amount of skeletal muscle tissue in the body is considerable (normally 40–50% of the body weight in an adult).

STRUCTURE

As compared with both smooth muscle and cardiac muscle, skeletal muscle cells are exceedingly long. Early in development they form from the fusion of many cells, end to end, to form long multinucleated fibres (Fig. 22.1). The ends of each muscle fibre are anchored in tendon which in turn is firmly attached to parts of the skeleton. There are no cross connections between adjacent muscle fibres, and no gap junctions carrying signals from fibre to fibre.

Like cardiac muscle, skeletal muscle fibres are striated in appearance. They possess a T-tubule system and an extensive sarcoplasmic reticulum that stores and releases calcium (Fig. 22.16).

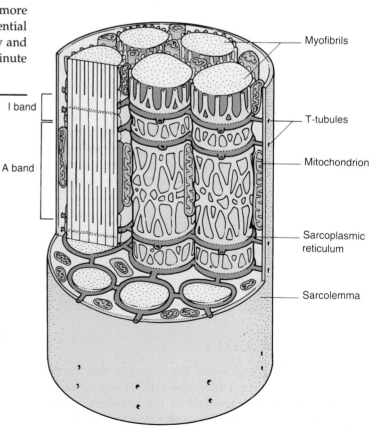

I band
A band
Myofibrils
T-tubules
Mitochondrion
Sarcoplasmic reticulum
Sarcolemma

HOW CONTRACTION IS TRIGGERED

Skeletal muscle fibres do not normally contract unless they are stimulated by impulses in the nerves innervating them. In the absence of neural excitation the fibres are completely relaxed. They lack tone.⑦

When a nerve impulse excites the fibre, an action potential is generated by the muscle membrane (*sarcolemma*) and is conducted up and down the whole length of the fibre at about the rate that a nerve impulse is transmitted in an unmyelinated nerve axon (see Ch. 21). Just as in cardiac muscle, the action potential is carried along the membrane of the T-tubules so that electrical excitation reaches deep into the cell.

> When a physician checks the function of various sections of the spinal cord by testing different reflexes (see Ch. 27) he stimulates sensory receptors that generate impulses that are transmitted to specific muscles. For example, a sharp tap on the patella tendon causes the quadriceps femoris to contract.

Muscle action potential

The muscle action potential is similar to that in nerve fibres (see Ch. 21). It is caused by the opening of voltage-gated sodium channels. Voltage-gated sodium/calcium channels are not involved. The muscle action potential therefore does not have a plateau and it lasts for only a short time (2–4 msec).

Role of calcium

The muscle action potential triggers the release of large amounts of calcium from the sarcoplasmic reticulum. Little or no calcium enters from the extracellular fluid. Just as in cardiac muscle, calcium binds to the troponin–tropomyosin complex and releases the inhibition that these proteins exert on the interaction of actin and myosin. Bonds are formed and the muscle contracts. Calcium is then pumped back into the sarcoplasmic reticulum and the intracellular concentration of calcium decreases. As a result the muscle relaxes.

FACTORS AFFECTING CONTRACTION

Stretch

Like cardiac muscle (Fig. 22.14), if the length at which skeletal muscle is held is varied, the force of contraction developed varies too. The basis of this is believed to be the same as in cardiac muscle. The relaxed length of skeletal muscle fibres in the body has been shown to be their optimum length for the development of force.

Neural control: frequency of action potentials

The duration of the muscle action potential is very much shorter than the duration of the contractile events which are triggered by it (Fig. 22.17). Consequently, it is possible for a second action potential to be generated in the muscle membrane long before the muscle fibre has completed its cycle of contraction and relaxation. As a result, more calcium is released from the sarcoplasmic

⑦
What causes the nerve impulses that stimulate skeletal muscle?

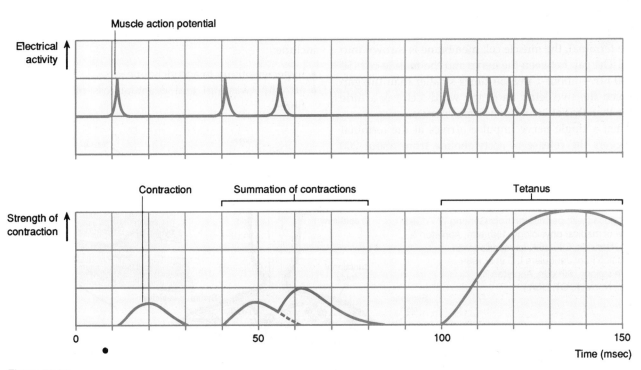

Figure 22.17
The relationship between electrical and contractile events in skeletal muscle. The contractile process outlasts the duration of the action potential. Consequently, another contraction can begin before the first one has finished, resulting in a much bigger overall contraction.

reticulum to add to that remaining from the previous impulse and a second contraction is added on top of the first (*summation*). If a whole series of impulses excite the fibre the contractions are added on top of one another so swiftly that a smooth and very strong contraction results (*tetanus*).

INNERVATION

Organisation

Skeletal muscle cells are innervated by motoneurones of the somatic nervous system. The nerve terminals form specific contacts with the fibres at a region known as the *motor end-plate* (Fig. 22.18). In the adult there is just one end-plate per muscle fibre, and this is usually situated at about the midpoint of the fibre.

However, one nerve axon branches to form several endings, so that one motoneurone in fact innervates not just one fibre but a group of fibres (Fig. 22.18). The group may be large (e.g. about 2000 fibres in calf muscles) or small (about 10 fibres in muscles of the eyeball). The motoneurone plus all the muscle fibres it innervates is termed a *motor unit*.

The force developed by a muscle, such as the biceps, depends on the size of the motor units activated. Small forces are developed by activating the small motor units. Larger forces are achieved by activating the large motor units as well (*recruitment*) (see Ch. 27). ⑧

Neuromuscular junction

The junction between the nerve terminal and the skeletal muscle fibre is intricate in structure. The nerve terminal sits in a recess in the muscle cell (Fig. 22.18). Beneath the nerve terminal, the muscle cell membrane is thrown into folds. The gap between the nerve and the muscle cell (50 to 100 nm – about 1 million times smaller than the gap between the two letter l's of the word 'cell') is a little larger than that at synapses between nerves.

When a single nerve impulse arrives at the terminal it triggers the release of acetylcholine from about 200 to 300 vesicles. The acetylcholine diffuses across the synapse and binds to *nicotinic* receptors (see Ch. 21) in the membrane. When activated these receptors increase the permeability of the membrane to sodium and potassium ions, thus depolarising the membrane. This depolarisation is termed the *end-plate potential*.

End-plate potential

In character, the end-plate potential (epp) resembles an epsp (see Ch. 21) in a nerve cell. It:

- lasts longer than an action potential
- can be summated
- fades away on either side of the end-plate.

But the epp differs from an epsp in that it is normally always big enough to generate an action potential in the muscle membrane on either side of the end-plate. One action potential in the nerve terminal therefore normally always gives rise to one action potential in the muscle fibre.

Acetylcholinesterase is present at the end-plate. Consequently acetylcholine is swiftly broken down as in other cholinergic synapses (see Ch. 21). If this enzyme is inhibited by an antichlinesterase, such as *neostigmine*, the end-plate potential increases and lasts for longer. This drug has been used to treat *myasthenia gravis*, a condition in which there is a shortage of functional nicotinic receptors at the end-plate. ⑨

Effects of denervation

If the nerves to skeletal muscle are severed, as they may be as a result of an accident, the nerve terminals degenerate, and changes occur in the muscle. These include:

- hypersensitivity to acetylcholine
- atrophy (wasting) and eventual loss of the muscle fibres.

⑧
Where is the biceps muscle situated?

⑨
What is the main symptom of myasthenia gravis?

Figure 22.18
The junction between a motoneurone and the skeletal muscle fibre it innervates (neuromuscular junction). (Reproduced with permission from Ganong W F 1991 Review of medical physiology, 15th edn, Appleton & Lange, Norwalk, CT, USA, as modified with permission from Junquiera L C et al 1989 Basic histology, 6th edn, Appleton & Lange., Norwalk, CT, USA.)

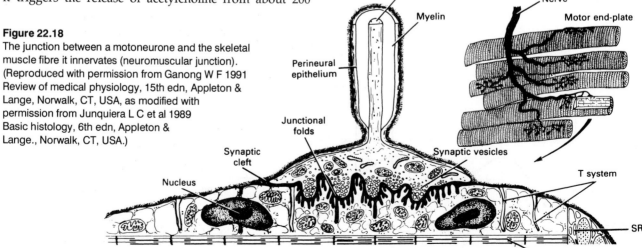

If a group of muscles are paralysed but their antagonists (opposing muscle group) are still functioning, then contraction deformities may occur. For example, 'claw hand' in untreated ulnar paralysis.

Hypersensitivity

When nerve terminals degenerate and the concentration of acetylcholine at the end-plate decreases, the muscle fibre responds by increasing the number of receptors inserted into the muscle membrane. Consequently, the muscle fibre becomes very responsive (*hypersensitive*) to small amounts of transmitter. Whereas in a normal muscle fibre the receptors are restricted to the end-plate, in a denervated muscle fibre they are inserted all over the membrane. This probably increases the chances of the cell being brought under the control of the re-growing nerve fibre.

Atrophy

At least two reasons have been suggested for the atrophy of skeletal muscle cells as a result of denervation:

- lack of use
- loss of growth factors secreted by the nerve terminals.

Muscles that are exercised can grow larger (*hypertrophy*; see Ch. 17), whereas inactivity results in wasting (*atrophy*). This may be due to the direct effects of activity of the muscle cells or may be due to factors released from the nerve. If the muscle is re-innervated within a few months through the regrowth of axons, or the sprouting of adjacent motoneurones (see Ch. 21), then the muscle also regrows (Fig. 22.19).

DIFFERENT TYPES OF SKELETAL MUSCLE

Although the basic processes are the same in all skeletal muscle cells, significant differences exist between cells in:

- metabolism
- contractile properties.

DISORDERED SKELETAL MUSCLE ACTIVITY

When muscle disorders are suspected, electromyography may be performed. In this technique, the electrical activity generated by muscle cells when they are excited is recorded. Sometimes this is done by sticking electrodes on to the skin overlying the muscle (surface electrodes) and sometimes by inserting very fine needle electrodes directly into the muscle itself. Using the latter technique, the activity from single motor units can be recorded. In either case, the voltage measured from muscle cells directly is extremely small so amplification is needed before the signal can be recorded on an oscilloscope screen. The patient needs no special preparation for electromyography other than explanation of the procedure.

Recordings are made with the muscle at rest, with slight voluntary contraction and with maximum contraction. When normal muscle with normal nerve supply is tested at rest, there is no evidence of electrical activity. However, if there has been damage to the nerve supply, some activity is present at rest due to the excitation of cells by degenerating nerve fibres. There is *fasciculation* (twitching) of the muscle due to the spontanous discharge from single motor units. Muscular fasciculation may be observed in patients with chronic degeneration of the anterior horn cells (see Ch. 20) in *progressive muscular atrophy*. Each twitch involves a group of muscle fibres, movement of which can be clearly seen under the skin. If, however, the muscle is at fault, there is no evidence of activity at rest and the main abnormality will be recorded during slight voluntary contraction and maximum contraction. The electrical activity will be less when recorded from diseased muscle because some motor units will not respond.

Two extremes are represented by *slow* and by *fast* muscle.

Slow and fast muscle

Some differences between the slow and fast types of muscle cell are listed in Table 22.1. Slow muscle is similar to cardiac muscle in that it is specialised for continual activity, its metabolism is mainly aerobic and it is resistant to fatigue. But it cannot develop very powerful forces. Fast muscle in contrast can develop very strong contractions but only for a very short period of time. It makes use of anaerobic metabolism to do this and draws on abundant stores of glycogen (see also Ch. 17).

Table 22.1 Characteristics of slow and fast muscle

	Slow	Fast
Histology	Abundant mitochondria Myoglobin content high Rich blood supply	Extensive sarcoplasmic reticulum Glycogen content high
Metabolism	Mainly aerobic (oxidative phosphorylation)	Anaerobic and aerobic (glycolysis)
Contraction	Slow response Moderate, sustained force Fatigue resistant	Fast response High, short duration force Easily fatigued

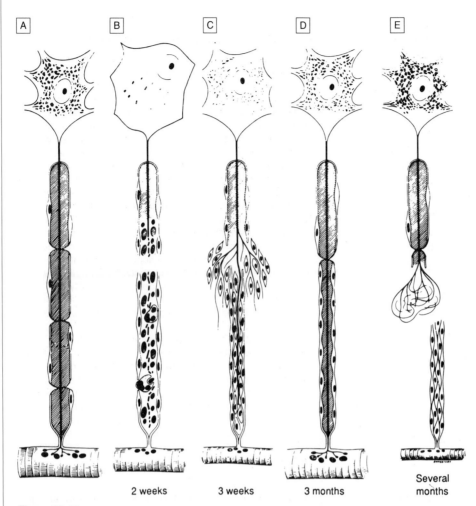

Figure 22.19
Atrophy of a skeletal muscle fibre as a result of injury to its motoneurone (A–C). If re-innervation occurs (C & D) the muscle regrows, whereas if it does not, muscle wasting continues (E). (See also the caption to Fig. 21.14.) (Reproduced from Junqueira L C, Carneiro J, Kelley R O 1989 Basic histology, 6th edn, Figure 9–26, Appleton & Lange, Norwalk, CT, USA, as adapted with permission from Willis R A, Willis A T 1972, The principles of bacteriology, 3rd edn, Butterworth, London, by permission of both publishers.)

All the muscle fibres within a single motor unit are of the same type. Muscle cells in a motor unit can be converted from one type into another by changing the pattern of impulses in the motoneurone. Intermittent bursts of impulses at high frequency over a long period convert slow muscle cells into fast fibres. Large quantities of actin and myosin are synthesised, so that the cells hypertrophy, the rate at which actin and myosin bonds are formed is increased, and the capacity of the cells to generate ATP by anaerobic means increases (see Ch. 17). Conversely, fast fibres are converted into slow ones if the cells are stimulated continually by a regular train of impulses

All muscles consist of a mixture of muscle types although the proportion of the different types does vary between muscles. Postural muscles, for example, contain a preponderance of slow muscle, whereas those that may be used intermittently to generate large forces, such as the biceps, contain more fast muscle fibres. ⑩

⑩
Which other muscles would you expect to contain more fast fibres?

GROWTH AND DEVELOPMENT OF SKELETAL MUSCLE

Early years

Once multinucleated muscle cells have developed from the fusion of myoblasts early in development, the cells then grow in length, by the addition of new sarcomeres at the ends of the fibres. Should a muscle be immobilised, for example by a plaster cast, growth is arrested. The lack of muscle growth is compensated instead by the growth of connective tissue, such as tendon. Once the cast is removed, the muscle itself will be shorter than normal and the individual fibres will be thinner.

Immobilisation affects the muscle in two ways. It:

- alters the stretching forces on the muscle
- prevents normal contractile activity.

Stretch affects the addition of sarcomeres, and activity affects how thick the fibres become. Care has to be taken therefore, when immobilising a limb in a growing child, to minimise inappropriate changes. Particularly important is the fact that if a muscle is held in a shorter than normal position not only will new sarcomeres not be added but some pre-existing ones will be lost. Once the cast is removed the shortened muscle will inevitably restrict the range of movement of that limb.

Adulthood

In the adult, activity and inactivity still influence the muscle cells. Exercise causes adaptive changes in the nature, properties and metabolism of the cells. 'Aerobic' exercises foster the development of 'slow muscle' characteristics and aerobic metabolism, whereas periods of brief, very intense exercise favour the development of 'fast muscle' characteristics, hypertrophied fibres and the build-up of glycogen reserves (see also Ch. 17, p. 323). ⑪

Bed rest predominantly causes wasting of 'fast muscle' fibres whereas, in cases of joint injury, there may be preferential wasting of 'slow' fibres. The latter is believed to be due to a reflex inhibition of the activity of 'slow' fibres triggered by stimulation of sensory receptors within the joints.

If muscle tissue is completely lost through injury in adulthood, the capacity for repair is limited. A few myoblasts persist within the muscle (*satellite cells*) but the amount of regeneration occurring is small. Lost muscle tissue is mostly replaced by fibrous tissue.

EXERCISE DURING BED REST

Immobilisation is detrimental to bones and muscles (see also Chs 17 and 28). Calcium and phosphorus are lost from bones making them brittle. Muscles soon begin to lose strength and it is said that wasting may commence as early as 48 hours after immobilisation. Many people experience a spell of bed rest as a result of back injury, and the weakness in the legs on standing for the first time usually seems out of all proportion to the time spent in bed. Patients may also develop flexion deformities if limbs are positioned incorrectly. This is because normal contractile activity is curtailed, the muscle fibres shorten through loss of sarcomeres and muscle tissue is replaced by connective tissue (*fibrosis*). The 'stiffening' of joints also commences rapidly. Research has shown that brief, less than 24 hours, immobilisation of a shoulder following dislocation causes sufficient fibrosis to require up to 18 days of physiotherapy to regain full range of movement (Perkins 1953).

Bed rest is prescribed as part of planned care and should be beneficial. During this period the patient should not develop additional problems, such as flexion deformities and pressure sores. The multidisciplinary care planning team will be aware of the purpose of the bed rest and a programme of relaxation, correct positioning, and passive and active exercise will be devised. The nurse's role may be to supervise, assist with, or carry out the programme depending on the patient's condition, as well as advising the patient and his relatives.

---

⑪
Can you think of two popular examples of these exercise types?

KEY POINTS

What you should now know and understand about muscle:

- how muscle cells differ from other cells
- the intracellular proteins involved in contraction and relaxation, how they are organised and what they do
- how calcium regulates contraction and relaxation, and how its cytoplasmic concentration is controlled
- the three main types of muscle and how they differ in structure and function
- what makes some muscles contract spontaneously whereas other do not
- the role of nerves in controlling muscle contraction and how this differs between different types of muscle
- the effects of hormones on muscle contraction and why this differs between different types of muscle
- how exercise affects the growth and development of skeletal muscle and why inactivity causes wasting
- how some drugs affecting muscle contraction work (e.g. muscle relaxants used in anaesthesia, cardiac glycosides and some antidiarrhoeal agents and antispasmodics).

REFERENCES AND FURTHER READING

Aidley D J 1989 The physiology of excitable cells, 3rd edn. Cambridge University Press, Cambridge
(Excellent advanced textbook reviewing experimental basis of current knowledge. Extremely well referenced)

Alberts B, Bray D, Lewis J, Raff M, Roberts K, Watson J D 1983 Molecular biology of the cell. Garland Publishing, New York & London, p 554, 555 & 559

Ganong W F 1991 Review of medical physiology, 15th edn. Appleton & Lange, East Norwalk, Connecticut, p 102

Jones D A, Round J M, 1990 Skeletal muscle in health and disease: a workbook of muscle physiology. Manchester University Press, Manchester
(Advanced student textbook giving useful further information)

Junqueira L C, Carneiro J, Kelley R O 1989 Basic histology, 6th edn. Appleton & Lange, East Norwalk, Connecticut, p 186, 202

Kandel E R, Schwarz J H (eds) 1985 Principles of neural science, 2nd edn. Elsevier, New York, p 140

Keynes R D, Aidley D J 1991 Nerve and muscle, 2nd edn. Cambridge University Press, Cambridge
(Deceptively small, but advanced student text explaining how nerve and muscle tissues have been studied and the experimental basis of current theory)

Krstic R V 1979 Ultrastructure of the mammalian cell: an atlas. Springer-Verlag, Berlin–Heidelberg

Levick J R 1991 An introduction to cardiovascular physiology. Butterworth, London, p 24, 26
(Useful source of further information about vascular smooth muscle as well as cardiac muscle and their control by nerves, hormones and other factors)

Matthews G G 1991 Cellular physiology of nerve and muscle. Blackwell Scientific Publications, Oxford
(A friendly book providing lucid descriptions of basic principles. Includes list of further reading)

Perkins G 1953 Rest and movement. Journal of Bone and Joint Surgery 35b: 521–539

Rang H P, Dale M M 1991 Pharmacology, 2nd edn. Churchill Livingstone, Edinburgh
(Useful reference for drug action)

Tanagho E A, McAninch J W 1984 Smith's General urology, 11th edn. Appleton & Lange, East Norwalk, Connecticut

Turner P, Richens A, Routledge A, Routledge P 1986 Clinical pharmacology. Churchill Livingstone, Edinburgh
(Useful reference for drug action)

Williams P L, Warwick R, Dyson M, Bannister L H 1989 Gray's Anatomy. Churchill Livingstone, Edinburgh, p 562

Willis R A, Willis A T 1972 The principles of pathology and bacteriology, 3rd edn. Butterworth, London, p 32

Part B
SENSING THE EXTERNAL ENVIRONMENT AND ACTING

Part Contents

We receive information about our environment, and our place within it, through sensory receptors in:

- eyes and ears
- skin, muscles and joints
- mouth and nose.

Information is processed within the nervous system, giving rise to sensations such as vision, hearing, touch, pain and proprioception, as well as reflexly evoking muscle contraction, for example turning to face an unexpected sound. Many reflex responses can be suppressed voluntarily enabling us to perform actions of our choosing.

The chapters in this part of the book:

- describe the structure of sensory organs and tissues, including the eye, ear, and skin, and explain how they function
- describe how sensory systems are organised, explaining how this determines the specific qualities of each sense
- describe the bones, muscles and joints of the musculoskeletal system
- describe voluntary and involuntary systems controlling and coordinating muscle contraction and explain how they work
- explain how various actions are performed including observing our surroundings and speaking, as well as using our hands and moving our bodies.

Chapter 23
SENSORY SYSTEMS: AN OVERVIEW

Our sensory systems enable us to detect, analyse and respond to some of the many different forms of energy to which we are exposed. The selection is made by our sensory receptors. These are attuned to respond to some energies much more readily than others.

Impulses generated by the receptors are transmitted along a variety of nerve pathways to several destinations in the central nervous system. Some sensory pathways (specific sensory systems) link up the receptors to cells of the cerebral cortex in a point to point way, so that 'maps' of sensory information are created in the brain. These pathways mediate specific sensations like those of vision, hearing, touch, taste, smell and pain. Other nerve pathways (nonspecific sensory systems) channel sensory signals to the cerebral cortex via the reticular formation of the brain stem. Part of these nonspecific systems, the reticular activating system, controls our level of alertness and consciousness.

All sensory information arrives at the cerebral cortex in the form of action potentials. From these impulses our minds create the impressions we have of ourselves and our surroundings. The impressions created depend upon the destination of the information in the brain, the number and blend of signals arriving there, and how they have been analysed en route. If sensory systems are disordered then our impression of reality alters and our responses change.

SENSORY RECEPTORS

TYPES

Sensory receptors are specialised neurones that detect and respond to changes occurring in their vicinity. These changes may be:

- mechanical (e.g. stretch, compression)
- chemical (e.g. concentration of kinins, histamine etc.)
- electromagnetic (e.g. radiation from the sun)
- thermal. ①

Although any receptor can be excited by any form of stimulus, provided it is strong enough, each receptor responds best to a particular type of stimulus. Thus receptors can be classified as:

- mechanoreceptors
- chemoreceptors
- photoreceptors
- thermoreceptors.

Within each group, receptors are specialised to respond to a particular form of that stimulus. For example in the skin (see Ch. 24) there is a variety of mechanoreceptors. Some are very sensitive and respond to the lightest of touches. Others respond only when pressure is applied. In the eye too there are four different types of photoreceptor (see Ch. 26), each of which responds best to a slightly different range of wavelengths of electromagnetic radiation.

① *What are kinins?*

SENSITIVITY

The specific sensitivity of the receptor depends in part on the specialisation of the receptor itself. For example, the four different photoreceptors in the eye each contain a different pigment (see Ch. 26). Each pigment absorbs electromagnetic radiation of a different range of wavelengths.②

But sensitivity can depend too on the *accessory structures* associated with the receptor because these determine the kind of stimuli that actually get through to it. For example, the receptors both in the ear and in the balance organs (*vestibular apparatus*) are hair cells that are excited when their cilia bend (Fig. 23.1; see also Chs 24 and 25). However, in the ear the bending is caused by vibrations (produced for example by a musi-

② What are pigments?

> When the cilia of the ear are continuously vibrated by excessive and continuous noise, permanent damage to the ear is likely to occur. This results in varying degrees of deafness. Many workers exposed to excessive noise wear ear defenders. Damage to the ear may also be caused by highly amplified disco music.

cal instrument), which are transmitted through the outer and middle ear to the fluid of the inner ear, whereas in the semicircular canals of the balance organs, bending of the cilia results from fluid movement within the canals caused by turning, lifting or lowering the head (Fig. 23.1).

STRUCTURE

Some receptors consist simply of the endings of a sensory neurone (*unspecialised nerve endings*). Other

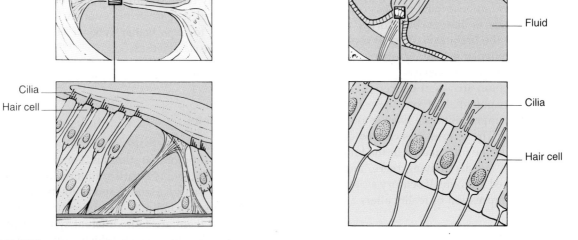

Figure 23.1
Receptor cells (hair cells) and accessory structures of the ear and of the balance organs. Note the similarities and differences between the two sense organs.

receptors have endings that are visibly adapted to form specialised structures (Fig. 23.2). If the endings are walled off from the surrounding tissues they are termed *encapsulated endings* (e.g. Pacinian corpuscles, Meissner's corpuscles in the skin; see Ch. 24).

Some receptor cells (such as photoreceptors in the eye and hair cells in the ear; Fig. 23.2) are separate from the sensory neurones transmitting signals into the central nervous system. The sensory neurones are excited by neurotransmitters (see Ch. 21) released by the receptor cells.

EXCITATION

Sensory receptors of any kind convert the energy of a stimulus into a change in the voltage (*receptor potential*) of the receptor cell membrane (Fig. 23.3A). If the change in voltage is big enough it will generate one or more action potentials which are then conducted along the sensory neurone (see Ch. 21).

In the systems in which receptor cells and sensory neurones are separate (Fig. 23.3B), excitation is passed from cell to cell by the release and action of neuro-transmitters until a cell is reached that is able to generate an action potential and carry the signal in that form into the central nervous system.

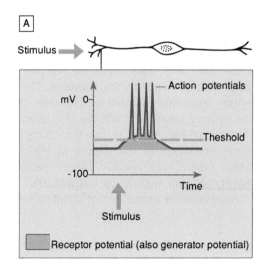

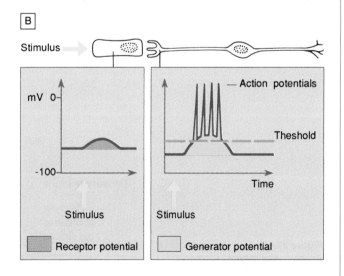

Figure 23.3
Electrical events recorded in response to a stimulus from:
A A sensory nerve ending
B A receptor cell (e.g. a hair cell) and its sensory neurone.

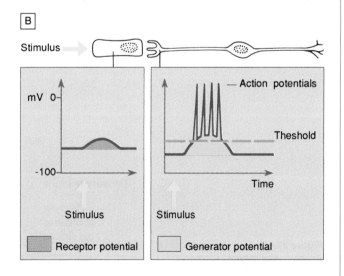

Figure 23.2
Examples of several different sensory receptors.

The change in voltage actually giving rise to the action potential is termed the *generator potential*. Unlike an action potential, it can be large or small depending on the strength of the original stimulus. Also it develops more slowly and lasts longer as can be seen in Figure 23.3A & B. Because of this, a single stimulus can produce more than one action potential. As long as the membrane voltage remains less than threshold (say at –50 mV if threshold was –60 mV) action potentials will keep on being generated. If the initial stimulus was small, the membrane at the ending will return to its unexcited state very quickly and only one or two action potentials will be generated. However, if the stimulus was large, the generator potential will be bigger and will stay below threshold for longer, and consequently more action potentials will be fired. In this way the strength of a stimulus is translated into the *frequency of action potentials* (number of action potentials per second) in a sensory neurone. ③

ADAPTATION

If the stimulus is maintained the receptor begins to get used to it. It *adapts* to the stimulus. The frequency of action potentials (number of impulses per second) in the sensory neurone gradually decreases even though the size of the stimulus has not changed (Fig. 23.4). Receptors differ in the degree to which they adapt. Some adapt very quickly (*phasic* receptors). Others adapt only very slightly (*tonic* receptors).

Adaptation is useful in that it reduces the amount of information that has to be processed by the brain at any time. If our minds have registered and stored the fact that a change has occurred in our environment, then the next thing that is important to know is when there is a further change. While all remains steady there is little point in continually receiving exactly the same, very detailed report. A note of what is going on (from tonic receptors) will do. But when circumstances change it is important to know fully the nature and extent of that change. ④

RECEPTIVE FIELDS

A sensory neurone may have several endings, or be connected to several receptor cells (Fig. 23.5). The result of this arrangement is that a stimulus that activates any of the endings or receptors will generate impulses in the same sensory neurone. The area covered by the sensory neurone in this way is termed its *receptive field*. If there are many receptors or endings spread over a wide area then the receptive field is large. If there is only one receptor per ending (as for example for cone cells in the eye; see Ch. 26) the receptive field is small.

The size of the receptive field makes a difference to the accuracy with which stimuli can be located and to the sharpness of the impression gained by our minds. If the receptive field of a sensory neurone is large our impression of the stimulus will be vague. A good example is the difference between vision at night and in broad daylight. In the daytime when the cones are used for vision the picture is much sharper than at night,

③
What do you understand by 'threshold'?

④
What common examples of adaptation can you think of?

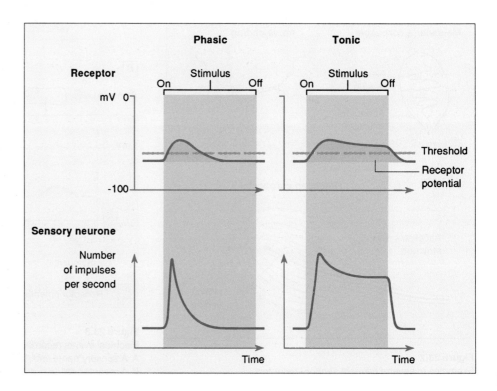

Figure 23.4
Adaptation of sensory receptors to a maintained stimulus. Some receptors (phasic receptors) adapt quickly and completely whereas others (tonic receptors) hardly adapt at all.

when the rods are used. The neurones carrying information to the brain from the rods have large receptive fields, whereas those from the cones are small (see Ch. 26).

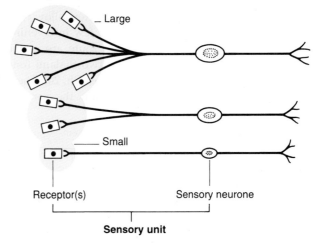

Figure 23.5
Sensory units and receptive fields. A sensory unit consists of one sensory neurone together with all the sensory receptors to which it is linked.

ADAPTING TO SOUNDS AND SMELLS

Nurses are continually adapting to sensory stimulation arising from their working environment. Two examples are sounds on night duty and unpleasant odours.

During the night in a comparatively quiet ward there are often rythmical sounds to which the night nurses will adapt fairly readily. For example there may be a piece of equipment, such as a ventilator, in use or a patient with noisy but regular breathing. When the ward has just quietened for the night, these sounds take priority over others and are often intrusive if one is trying to concentrate on something else. Eventually, the sounds are processed as being normal for that particular situation and are not consciously heard. This type of adaptation involves higher levels of sensory perception as well as receptor adaptation. It does not matter whether one notices that the pneumatic drill outside suddenly stops, but if a motor-driven piece of equipment suddenly falters or a patient's breathing changes or stops, then immediate action is required.

Night nurses also tend to adapt readily to noise created by themselves. Initially every footfall or clatter of instruments seems excessively loud in the quiet ward. Soon these sounds become part of the normal environment and are not processed – except by patients for whom they are abnormal night-time noises and cause annoyance. Some patients do not adapt to such noises, even after weeks in hospital, possibly because the noises are irregular and, in many instances, unfamiliar and liable to cause anxiety.

Olfactory receptors too adapt very rapidly although, as with other things, there are individual differences in the appreciation of smells in the first place. For example when buying perfumes or aftershave, if too many different scents are sampled, the sense of smell soon becomes saturated and confused. Most counter assistants advise leaving at least 10 minutes between trying different scents. Then, having chosen a super new perfume, you wear it continuously and find that after a few days you hardly notice it. The receptors have adapted and accepted it as part of the normal environment, leaving you free to appreciate other smells.

Adaptation to smell also has advantages. In many situations related to nursing, unpleasant smells have to be endured without allowing a patient to be aware of one's distaste. Assisting with changing colostomy bags or nursing patients whose condition produces an unpleasant odour are two examples. If you can overcome the initial powerful onslaught of the smell, then adaptation often occurs fairly rapidly. It seems unfair that one often adapts more readily to pleasant than to unpleasant smells. Many people continue to be aware (depending on the efficiency of their sense of smell) of coal gas and petrol fumes for a long time. It is not known what part the higher centres play in adaptation to smells but it is possible that where the cause of the smell is dangerous and the smell not highly concentrated then total adaptation does not always take place.

ROUTING OF SENSORY SIGNALS

Impulses generated in the sensory neurones follow several different routes to arrive at various destinations in the nervous system (Fig. 23.6). Impulses are transmitted to:

- motoneurones via interneurones to activate muscles (reflex pathways)
- chains of neurones carrying impulses to the cerebral cortex (specific sensory systems, e.g. visual, auditory etc.)
- neurones that transmit impulses to the cerebral cortex via the reticular formation (nonspecific sensory system).

REFLEX PATHWAYS

When you pick up something painfully hot, and then drop it without thinking, your instinctive response is caused by the sensory impulses generated by the *nociceptors* in your hand that reflexly excite muscles of your arm (see also Ch. 3, Fig. 3.13). Much that we do is powered by reflex responses of this kind (see Ch. 27 for more details). ⑤

In *syringomyelia* there may be a loss of temperature sense and, consequently, protective reflexes are impaired. Therefore people with this type of sensory loss need special consideration when, for example, being served with extra-hot drinks, sitting next to very hot radiators or being provided with unprotected hot water bottles.

SPECIFIC SENSORY SYSTEMS

The impulses that pass to the cerebral cortex follow relatively direct routes in which there are few intervening synapses. The main relay stations en route are in the spinal cord and brain stem, and the two thalami (one thalamus in each cerebral hemisphere; see Ch. 20). There are very ordered relationships between the sensory

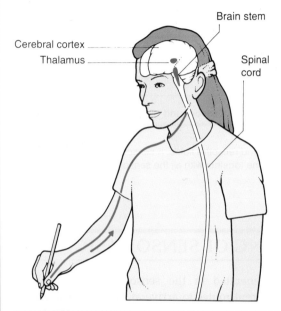

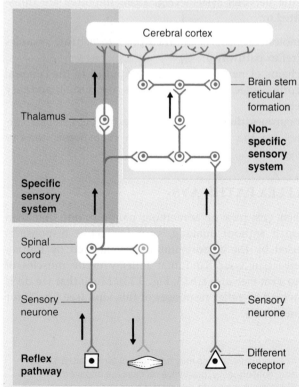

Figure 23.6
Where impulses from sensory receptors travel to within the central nervous system and how they get there.

receptors and neurones in these parts of the central nervous system resulting in three distinctive features of specific sensory systems:

- sidedness
- mapping
- proportional representation.

Sidedness

The primary sensory fibres synapse first in the central nervous system on the same side of the midline as the receptors are located. Subsequently, with only a few exceptions, the second order nerve axons cross over the midline. Thus information from one side of the body is transmitted to parts of the brain on the opposite side (i.e. *contralaterally*) (Fig. 23.7A). The second order fibres carry the impulses to the *thalami*. From here the impulses are transmitted to specific regions of the cerebral cortex (*primary sensory receiving areas*). Thus information from the right side of the body (about touch, warmth, sight etc.) is registered in the left cerebral hemisphere, and information from the left side goes to the right cerebral hemisphere. For our sense of vision it is important to be aware that the information that is registered in each hemisphere is not what is seen by the eye on the opposite side of the body, but *all* those things, seen by *both* eyes, that lie to one side or the other of the midline (Fig. 23.7B).

'Maps' of the body

Each of the neurones in the chain between the receptors and the cerebral cortex (Fig. 23.6) may be likened to a team member in a relay race. Just as the baton gets passed between consecutive members of the team, but not between members of different teams, so sensory signals get directed in an ordered way to specific places in the thalamus and then in the cerebral cortex. The relationship of adjacent neurones to one another is preserved faithfully so that adjacent areas of the cerebral cortex register information from receptors that were next to one another (in the skin or eye for example) in the same way that a geographer's map faithfully records the relative positions of different features on the land.

Scale of representation

If part of the body is richly supplied with sensory receptors, then this is matched within the central nervous system by the number of cells devoted to that part of the body. This is seen clearly in the part of the cerebral cortex receiving information from receptors in the skin and muscles (*somatosensory cortex*) (Fig. 23.7B). Large parts of the somatosensory cortex deal with information from the hands and from the face (Fig. 23.8). Both of these places are richly supplied with sensory receptors. In contrast, very much smaller areas of the somatosensory cortex are devoted to the trunk and

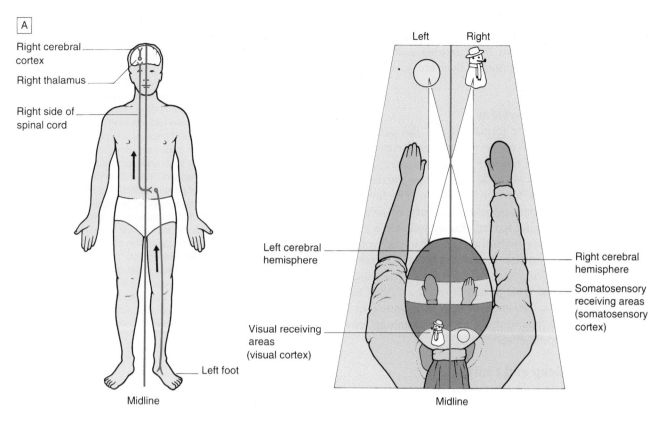

Figure 23.7
The right side of the brain receives information from the left side of the body and vice versa, for example information about:
A Pressure on the skin
B Objects to the left of the midline.

limbs, where there are fewer receptors. You can get some impression of this fact of physiology if you close your eyes, try to forget what you look like and consider how big you would think different parts of your body are just from the way that they feel. Usually one is very aware of face and hands and less so of trunk and legs.

THE NONSPECIFIC SENSORY SYSTEM

Sensory impulses are transmitted to the *reticular formation* of the brain stem via branches (*collaterals*) of the neurones in the specific sensory systems. The reticular formation is a network of neurones (hence its name – *reticulum* means 'little net') extending through the brain stem. Impulses are passed from cell to cell across many synapses. Eventually excitation is passed on to the cerebral cortex but it is not restricted to discrete areas of the cortex (such as the somatosensory cortex and the visual cortex) and it is no longer identifiable as coming from specific receptors.

What appears to happen is that information from different senses is pooled in the reticular formation (Fig. 23.6). This pooled activity generates impulses which are chiefly transmitted to the *association areas* of the cerebral cortex (see Ch. 30). This sensitises these cortical cells

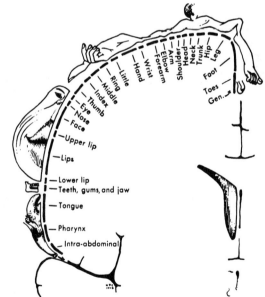

Figure 23.8
The relative sizes of the areas of the somatosensory cerebral cortex (in the right cerebral hemisphere) devoted to different areas of the body. Note how large an area is concerned with sensory information from the face and hand, and how relatively small is the area devoted to the trunk, arms and legs. (Reprinted with the permission of Macmillan Publishing Company from The cerebral cortex of man, by Wilder Penfield and Theodore Rasmussen. Copyright 1950 Macmillan Publishing Company; copyright renewed (c) 1978 Theodore Rasmussen.)

so that they respond easily to the identifiable signals reaching them via the specific sensory systems. The nonspecific sensory system thus arouses cortical cells and determines how responsive they are to incoming signals.

Reticular activating system

The cells in the reticular formation and the pathways carrying the excitation on to the cerebral cortex are collectively termed the *reticular activating system (RAS)*. When activity in this system is high we are awake and alert. When activity is low we fall asleep. The level of activity depends in part upon the amount of sensory information that is being fed into the system. On a very hot, bright, sunny day, with the noise of traffic, voices and daily activities outside it may not be easy to get to sleep even after a tiring spell of night duty. The reason for this is the raised level of activity in the RAS. Conversely, sitting in a darkened classroom listening to a monotonous voice talking dully about physiology may well have the opposite effect!

Anaesthesia, sleep and coma

Because sensory signals are passed between so many synapses in the reticular formation, this pathway is particularly susceptible to the blocking action of some drugs. If transmission at each synapse is reduced even slightly the cumulative effect, after many synapses have been traversed, will be large. So it is possible to produce *anaesthesia* by damping down the activity of the RAS, without blocking the transmission of nerve impulses everywhere else. ⑥

General anaesthesia is not the same as sleep in that

⑥
What examples can you give of drugs that block this pathway?

LYSERGIC ACID DIETHYLAMIDE

This illegal drug (acid, LSD) is known as an hallucinogen or a psychedelic. It acts specifically on receptors for serotonin. A system of serotonergic neurones is known to form part of the RAS. LSD is therefore capable of stimulating the receptors for serotonin in the RAS to produce changes in sensory perception including hallucinations. Hallucinations have been defined as mental impressions of sensory vividness occurring without external stimulus, but appearing to be located, or to possess a cause located, outside the subject. Psychiatric nurses working in drug dependency units are likely to care for people addicted to LSD, though its use is now less common. Its effect is unpredictable and highly specific to the individual using it. An adverse reaction, or 'bad trip', is usually sufficient to cause the user to seek psychiatric help. At times the alteration of consciousness may produce loss of reality orientation. The person's RAS may be so highly stimulated that a feeling of being out of control of mind and body is experienced. This alarming state may cause extremely irrational and disoriented behaviour. The effect of LSD usually lasts between 8 and 12 hours, the drug being fully excreted from the body in about 24 hours.

someone cannot be aroused easily from it. This marks the difference between a state of *unconsciousness* (not arousable) and *sleep* (arousable). Unconsciousness may be temporary, as in a faint or under anaesthesia, or it may be prolonged or even permanent, as in cases of damage to the RAS. It is then termed *coma*.

Electroencephalogram (EEG)

Different levels of consciousness are associated with different patterns of electrical activity in the brain as

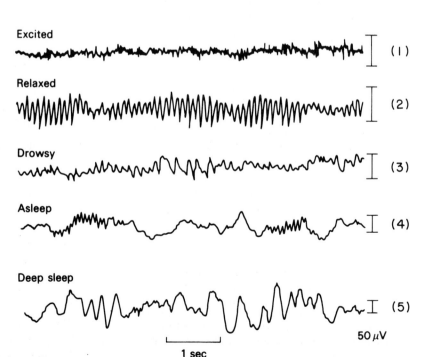

Figure 23.9
The electrical activity recorded from electrodes placed on the scalp (electroencephalogram – EEG) in a person who is: (1) awake, alert, eyes open (2) relaxed, eyes closed (3) drifting off to sleep (4) & (5) asleep. The scale of the voltage recorded is shown to the right. (Reproduced from Stein J F 1982 An introduction to neurophysiology, Figure 21.1, by permission of Blackwell Scientific Publications, Ltd.)

recorded from electrodes placed on the scalp (Fig. 23.9). The pattern of activity changes as an awake person gradually drifts off to sleep. In the awake state the *electroencephalogram (EEG)* gives a series of low voltage, fast frequency waves. As someone drifts off to sleep the waves become bigger but there are fewer of them. In the awake but relaxed state with eyes closed the pattern seen is described as the *alpha rhythm*. In deep sleep the waves are bigger and occur less frequently. In brain death no waves are seen at all. (See Ch. 31 for more about sleep and the EEG.)

MAKING SENSE OF SENSORY INFORMATION

How we create an understanding of the world about us from the action potentials that are generated and passed through our sensory systems remains an intriguing mystery. But we do know something about how sensory signals are processed and analysed, and a few of the rules that operate in sorting out this information.

KNOWING WHAT AND WHERE

A question that surfaces as soon as one has grasped the fact that all sensory information is translated into action potentials is how does the brain distinguish between action potentials originating from different sense organs, such as eyes and ears, and between different places, such as hands and feet. Answers remain puzzling but it is known that the destination of the signals in the cerebral cortex determines the sensation experienced, and that this, coupled with the way the body is mapped (*topography*), determines where the sensation is felt.

Destination

If cortical cells in the occipital cortex are excited then someone will have the sensation of vision. A blow to the back of the head can make someone 'see stars'. This is because the blow has injured that part of the head and the injury is exciting cells forming part of the visual cortex (Fig. 23.7B).

Likewise, if cells of a specific nerve pathway are excited, then someone will experience the sensations

When a limb is amputated the axons of the sensory neurones are cut across, but the cell bodies remain intact in the dorsal root ganglion. Consequently the nerves do not degenerate. The cut ends may sprout (see Ch. 21) and the nerves can still transmit impulses. If the nerves are irritated and therefore excited, impulses will be transmitted to the brain giving rise to an impression that the limb is still there.

that pathway mediates even though sensory receptors have not been excited. For example, if someone has had an arm amputated, pressure on the neurones in the stump may cause impulses to be transmitted to the somatosensory cortex creating the 'feel' of an arm (*phantom limb*).⑦

Topography

As we have seen, sensory neurones of the specific sensory pathways are very ordered and preserve that order from the receptors to the cerebral cortex. Thus when a particular cortical cell in the visual cortex is activated it is not only perceived as light but as light from a particular spot in the scene that we are viewing. Whenever, and however, that cell is excited the spot of light that is seen will always be seen as coming from the same place. In other words the sensation of the spot of light is *referred* to the same place. Neurophysiologists describe the scene that we view (*visual field*) as being *topographically* represented (i.e. mapped out) in the brain. The body is mapped out in a similar way in the *somatosensory cortex*, so that excitation of a specific cortical cell here will cause a sensation to be felt at a particular part of the body (e.g. toe, face etc.) even though sensory receptors there have not been excited.

The presence of a cerebral tumour, degeneration of the cerebral cortex, or other disease processes may stimulate cortical cells to produce abnormal sensations. The sensations might include a feeling of hot or cold water trickling down limbs, insects crawling over the skin or excessive heat. Visual disturbances occur in the form of hallucinations, including the bright, shimmering fortifications and flashing lights experienced by migraine sufferers. It is also possible to experience smells (usually unpleasant) and tastes in the absence of external stimulation.

KNOWING HOW MUCH

Sensations are perceived as strong or weak on the basis of at least three pieces of information:

- characteristics of the receptors involved
- number of sensory units excited
- frequency of action potentials in the sensory neurones.

Receptors

Receptors of the same type may differ in their sensitivity to stimuli. For example there are high threshold and low threshold mechanoreceptors in the skin (see Ch. 24). The former are excited by strong stimuli, such as a blow to the skin, whereas the latter are stimulated by weak stimuli such as the touch of a feather. In the eye, rods (receptors used in vision at night) are more sensitive than the cones (used in daytime vision).

⑦
What is the name given to these abnormal sensations?

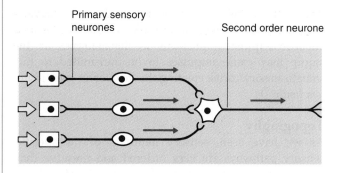

Figure 23.10
Convergence of inputs from several sensory neurones on to a single second order neurone.

Number of sensory units

The larger the stimulus the more likely it is that other units nearby will also be activated. At the synaptic relays en route there is opportunity sometimes for there to be summation of signals (see Ch. 21) because of the *convergence* of inputs from different sources (Fig. 23.10).

Frequency of impulses

The way in which the size of the stimulus is related to the frequency of impulses in the sensory neurone has been described earlier (see p. 406). The impulse frequency is then interpreted in our minds as the *intensity* of the stimulus.

DETECTING FEATURES

Although sensory neurones in the specific sensory systems were likened earlier to team members in a relay race, it is not appropriate to think of the synapses en route merely as handover points. Some processing and selection of sensory information occurs in the sensory nuclei and laminae where these synapses are.

Some cells compare the signals originating from adjacent receptors. This is made possible by the arrangement shown in Figure 23.11. The second order neurone shown in the diagram can be excited by receptors labelled 'A' and inhibited, via an inhibitory interneurone, by adjacent receptors labelled 'B' (*lateral inhibition*). If both A and B are excited at the same time the effects will cancel out. What this tells the central nervous system is that there is little to report between receptor A and receptor B.

Not all second order neurones are innervated in this way but the fact that some are permits the brain to pick out features of interest, such as boundaries between light and dark, and the edges of objects, for it is only when adjacent receptors are differently affected that the firing of the second order neurone differs from its usual rate.

In this way our nervous systems are able to pick out distinctive features in our surroundings from the mass

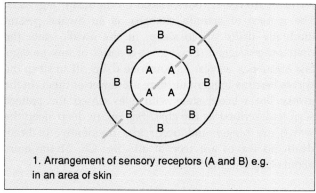

1. Arrangement of sensory receptors (A and B) e.g. in an area of skin

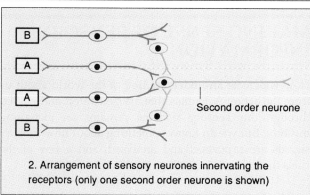

2. Arrangement of sensory neurones innervating the receptors (only one second order neurone is shown)

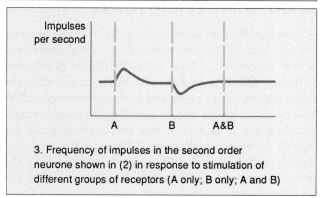

3. Frequency of impulses in the second order neurone shown in (2) in response to stimulation of different groups of receptors (A only; B only; A and B)

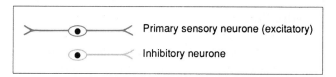

Primary sensory neurone (excitatory)

Inhibitory neurone

Figure 23.11
How sensory receptors and sensory neurones are arranged to enable second order neurones to compare information from adjacent receptors. The receptive field of the second order neurone is the whole of the coloured area in the top panel. The receptive field has an excitatory centre (red) and an inhibitory surround (purple).

of sensory information registered by sensory receptors. Through the visual system we take particular note of boundaries between different colours as well as between light and dark. These boundaries mark out the shapes of objects and symbols for us. The shape of an object is often all we need to know to be able to identify it. For example we can recognise famous people from the briefest of cartoon sketches, because what is drawn for us are some of the features that our visual systems routinely take special note of through processes like lateral inhibition. Likewise, when we handle objects we take particular note of their edges, and of any roughness that may give clues to their identity.

> The ability to recognise objects by handling them without looking provides an interesting game. A selection of small objects, some easily recognisable others more obscure, is chosen. The participant is blindfolded and allowed a specified number of seconds to identify each object. The winner identifies the most objects within the allotted time; some people are better than others at recognising objects in this way. A similar activity is used in neurological testing; impairment of discriminatory senses suggests the presence of damage in the parietal lobe of the cerebral cortex (see Ch. 30).

PAYING ATTENTION

The process described above selects for us the features of interest in what we are looking at or in what we are handling. In addition to this we can consciously or unconsciously direct our attention to particular stimuli. At a party it is possible to listen in to the music being played and not hear the conversations of people nearby, or alternatively we can join in the conversation and ignore the music. Whenever we are engrossed in something of great interest to us we can be oblivious to much else around us.⑧

This selective attention is believed to result from controls, exercised at synapses in the specific sensory pathways, which either allow or disallow signals to be transmitted. One such place of control is believed to be within the thalamus, but control also can occur at lower levels. For example it is known that the sensitivity of auditory receptors can be altered. This helps us to 'tune in' to sounds of interest to us. At both sites inhibitory

> Individual differences in ability to be selective in attention can be illustrated by the following example. The scene is a small office occupied by five health visitors; one will be writing up her notes, oblivious to everything going on around her; another will be engaged in a telephone conversation but at the same time waving to a client she has spotted passing the window; a third will be talking to a client, responding to the advances of a toddler and searching for a leaflet in her desk drawer; the fourth will also be engaged in a telephone conversation but will be 'tuned in' to the other conversations as well and will interrupt her own conversation to provide information (unasked) for her colleagues while at the same time scribbling notes for the day's activities; the fifth will be slamming things into her briefcase saying, 'I can't work in here – I'm going out.'

> **GAINING ATTENTION**
>
> When nurses are required to teach junior colleagues or patients, gaining their attention may be the most difficult part of the exercise. No matter how much knowledge the 'teacher' has acquired and wishes to impart, it will not be passed on if the 'learner's' attention is elsewhere. Some people seem to have a natural ability to gain the attention of others – we come across them in all walks of life with a group of people hanging on to their every word. It is often called 'charisma'. Some of the ingredients might be enthusiasm, interest in other people, tone of voice and so on; you can probably think of many others. These are all attributes that help others to focus their attention on the speaker. The nurse, as teacher, may wish to develop these characteristics. External distractions (sources of stimuli) may be removed as far as possible, but overcoming the internal stimuli is often more difficult. This is where showing interest in the 'learner' as a person is of importance. Learners, whether nurses, patients or clients, are often preoccupied with problems that cause short spans of attention. If the teaching is to be effective, these internal stimuli must be dealt with before teaching begins. Therefore time needs to be given to establishing rapport with the learner and to maintaining that rapport. The cocktail party situation of attention wandering between music and conversation, in this case between the teacher's pearls of wisdom and what to cook for dinner, is not conducive to learning.

interneurones can, if excited, reduce the synaptic transmission of selected sensory impulses.

The maturation of inhibitory pathways occurs fairly late in development. It may be that it is for this reason that young children are so distractable. Certainly their attention span is short. With time, practice and patience this lengthens and they become able to concentrate on one task for much longer. People differ in their ability to concentrate and this may be due to underlying differences in their ability to be selective in their attention.

REALITY AND THE 'REAL YOU'

From all the pieces of information that are collected, selected and analysed by our sensory systems, we create in our minds our own personal view of the world about us and of ourselves. If you tried, as suggested earlier, to feel the 'impression' that your somatosensory cortex has of your body, and discovered that your hands and face did feel large in comparison with your trunk and limbs, you will understand that our senses do not tell the whole truth. Inevitably, our senses give us a distorted view of the world around us because our sensory systems are highly selective in the information they detect and transmit. We do not for example have receptors sensitive to radio waves. Just imagine how your impression of your environment would change if you did!

If we rely on our senses for our view of reality then it is clear that if those systems are in any way abnormal

⑧ *What happens when you try to tune in to both conversation and music?*

Figure 23.12
Edward's drawings, aged 11:
A Self-portrait
B His mother.
Notice that (B) includes arms, trunk
and legs, whereas (A) does not,
although the self-portrait does
include hands, ears, tongue,
and feet as well as face.
(Reproduced by permission
of Edward Graves.)

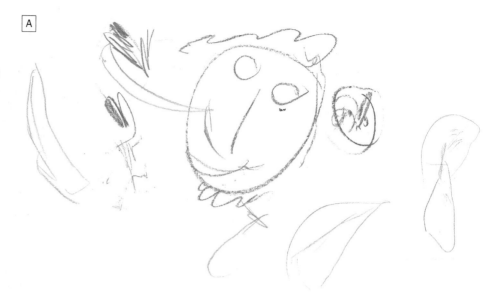

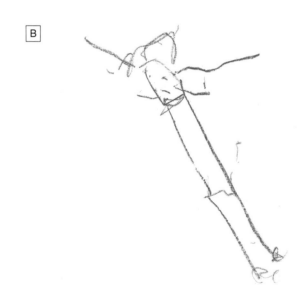

our impressions of reality will be different. A person who is totally colour blind has no way of knowing what the sensation of colour is like. Another person who has a distorted body image may believe herself to be 'fat' although her friends can see that that is not so. Another person may have hallucinations. The experiences are in each case real for the individual concerned although they bear little or no relationship to the external facts. ⑨

We cannot get inside other people's minds to see things exactly the way they do. But we can get glimpses of one another's experiences through the ways in which we express ourselves. Artwork for example can reveal a great deal. Compare the two pictures drawn by a child with Down syndrome, at the age of 11 (Fig. 23.12). The first picture is a self-portrait; the other is of his mother. The artist's impression of himself at that age is remarkably similar in its proportions to those shown in Figure 23.8, and reveals a view of himself from the inside that contrasts strikingly with his view of other people.

⑨
In what disorder does this distorted perception of body image often occur?

KEY POINTS

What you should now know and understand about sensory systems:

- what sensory receptors are and what they do
- what is meant by the terms: receptor potential, generator potential, adaptation, sensory unit, receptive field and lateral inhibition
- where impulses generated in sensory neurones travel to in the nervous system
- what is meant by the term 'specific sensory system' and how such a system is organised and works
- what is meant by the 'nonspecific sensory system', and how it is involved in determining level of consciousness
- how the impression we have of ourselves and the world about us is determined by the characteristics of our sensory systems
- why injury to the right side of the brain usually produces sensory impairment on the left side of the body, and vice versa.

REFERENCES AND FURTHER READING

Barlow H B, Mollon J D 1982 The senses. Cambridge University Press, Cambridge
(Advanced textbook for reference)
Bloch G J 1985 Body and self: elements of human biology, behaviour and health. W H Freeman, Oxford
(Useful text for linking psychology and physiology)
Clarke K A 1989 Neurophysiology: application in behavioural and biomedical sciences. Ellis Harwood, Chichester
(Easy to read text providing a bit more information, as well as further reading)
Melzack R 1992 Phantom limbs. Scientific American 266(4): 90–96
(Interesting article giving more information about this intriguing phenomenon)
Penfield W, Rasmussen T 1950 The cerebral cortex of man: a clinical study of localisation of function. Macmillan, New York, p 44
Salter M (ed) 1988 Altered body image – the nurse's role. John Wiley & Sons, Chichester
Stein J F 1982 An introduction to neurophysiology. Blackwell Scientific Publications, Oxford, p 302

Chapter 24
BODY SENSES, PROPRIOCEPTION, TASTE AND SMELL

As you sit reading this book you will be aware of a variety of sensations. You will sense the pressure of the chair under you and the touch of your clothes on your body. The room you are in may feel comfortable, chilly or warm. Your legs and feet may be out of sight under a table in front of you, but you know how they are positioned simply by how they feel. You take a drink and munch a sandwich or a biscuit and you feel the texture of the food in your mouth as well as its taste and its smell.

These sensations are created in our minds as a result of the activation of a variety of sensory receptors many of which are situated in the skin. Information from these and other receptors is carried into the central nervous system via spinal and cranial nerves, and is then routed to the cerebral cortex via specific pathways in the spinal cord and brain stem.

Awareness of the position and movement of our bodies is specifically termed proprioception. It is derived from sensory information flowing from receptors in muscles and joints, and the balance organs, as well as the skin. Proprioception is very important in posture and movement (see Ch. 27).

The sensations of taste and smell, vital to our enjoyment of food as well as our protection, are mediated by receptors in the mouth and nose.

Knowledge of the characteristics of all these systems is important in understanding someone's experience should any part of these systems be damaged through injury or disease.

BODY SENSES

RECEPTORS

Skin

Types of receptor
There are a variety of receptor endings in the skin (Fig. 24.1 and Ch. 15). Some are free nerve endings. Others, such as Meissner's corpuscles, Merkel's discs, Ruffini endings and Pacinian corpuscles (all of which are mechanoreceptors) have characteristic structures determining the stimuli that are most effective in exciting them. For example, the layers enveloping the nerve ending in the Pacinian corpuscle act as a filter so that only certain mechanical stimuli will get through.①

Most cutaneous receptors are situated in the dermis (Fig. 24.1 and Ch. 15). Meissner's corpuscles and Merkel's disks are situated at the boundary between the epidermis and the dermis. The nerve terminals of

①
*What do you
understand by
'mechano-
receptor'?*

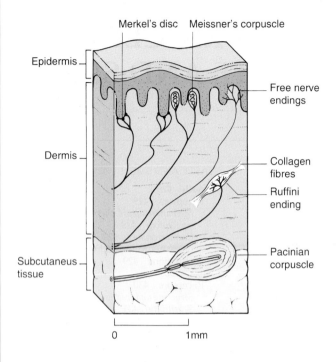

Merkel's disc   Meissner's corpuscle

Epidermis

Dermis

Subcutaneus tissue

Free nerve endings

Collagen fibres

Ruffini ending

Pacinian corpuscle

0   1mm

Figure 24.1
Sensory receptors in non-hairy skin (e.g. skin of the palms of the hands and soles of the feet).

Ruffini endings intermingle with collagen fibres in the dermis, and Pacinian corpuscles are found in deeper layers of the skin and in the subcutaneous tissue.

The position of the receptors influences the kind of stimuli that excite them. Receptors situated deeper in the skin may require a larger external stimulus to excite them whereas some receptors, such as Ruffini endings, can be excited by stimuli at a distance as a result of the forces tugging on fibres, such as collagen, in the skin. ②

Sensory units

Most cutaneous receptors do not have their own 'private line' to the brain. Usually receptors of the same type are grouped together into sensory units (see Fig. 23.5), each unit being innervated by a single nerve fibre.

For example, several Meissner's corpuscles, each tucked up in one of the papillary ridges of the dermis, are grouped together and served by the same sensory neurone (Fig. 24.1). ③

The sensory units differ in their characteristics (Table 24.1). Some have small receptive fields whereas others have large ones. Some units adapt rapidly to a maintained stimulus whereas others do not. All these features affect the quality of the sensations we experience (see Ch. 23).

Hairy and non-hairy skin

The sensory innervation of the skin is not the same all over the body. Differences exist in the numbers and types of receptor present. Some differences between

② How thick is the skin?

③ How thick are the papillary ridges?

Table 24.1	Characteristics of sensory units in the glabrous skin of the hand*			
Type†	Constituent receptors	Rate of adaptation	Breadth of receptive field (mm)	Usefulness
SA I FA I	Merkel's discs Meissner's corpuscles	Slow Fast	2–8	Outlining and locating the texture and shape of objects in contact with the skin
SA II FA II	Ruffini endings Pacinian corpuscles	Slow Fast	40–80	Broadly registering forces exerted on and in the skin (e.g. when holding an object or moving the finger and thumb)

* Compiled from Johansson & Vallbo 1983.
† Defined by characteristics of the units, such as rate of adaptation (SA – slow adapting; FA – fast adapting).

Table 24.2   Hairy and non-hairy human skin: distinguishing features

	Hairy	Non-hairy
Structure	'Thin' epidermis* Not ridged	'Thick' epidermis* Ridged
Sensory units	Less numerous	Very numerous
Sensory receptors	Many sensory endings close to hair follicles Ruffini endings Free nerve endings	Merkel's discs Meissner's corpuscles Pacinian corpuscles Ruffini endings Free nerve endings
Glands	Sebaceous (associated with hair follicles)	Sweat glands numerous

* Epidermal thickness ranges between 0.1 mm (thin) and 0.5 mm (thick). Total thickness of the skin ranges between about 1 and 5 mm in different parts of the body.

hairy and non-hairy (*glabrous*) skin are listed in Table 24.2.

The glabrous skin of the palmar surface of the hand is especially richly endowed with sensory units. The total number of mechanoreceptive sensory units has been estimated to be about 17 000. The number per unit area is very high especially on the fingertips (about 240 per cm^2).

Similarly, the skin of the soles of the feet differs from that on the top of the feet, and the skin of the trunk and limbs differs from that of the hands and feet.

> The soles of the feet tend to be very sensitive, a point worth remembering when washing or otherwise attending to normal feet. Firm rubbing for washing, drying, massaging etc. is more acceptable than trying to be gentle with light strokes. If feet are not handled reasonably firmly, the patient will tend to withdraw them from your attention.

Sensations

The different sensations that we identify, namely touch, pressure, pain, itch, heat, cold etc., do not correspond exactly to the different types of receptor seen under the microscope. Information from more than one receptor type is usually combined in our minds to create differ-

Table 24.3   Cutaneous receptors and sensations

Receptors	Sensation(s)
Nerve endings associated with hair follicles	Touch
Free nerve endings	Warmth, cold, pain
Merkel's discs	Pressure
Meissner's corpuscles	Tapping
Pacinian corpuscles	Vibration (high frequency) Tickle

> **ITCH**
>
> Itching is a sensation that is all too familiar, yet how it is mediated is still something of a mystery. What is clear is that it only occurs in the skin, the eyes and some mucous membranes. Deep tissues and internal organs do not itch. The sensation appears to be mediated by small diameter nerve fibres (C fibres) (see Ch. 21) but the nerves are probably not the same as those mediating the sensation of pain. Some of the chemicals released as a result of injury or immune mechanisms (see Ch. 15), such as histamine and the kinins, provoke itching, but how they do this is unknown.

ent feelings. Some of the receptors that are believed to contribute to the different sensations we experience are listed in Table 24.3. It is interesting that free nerve endings are believed to mediate a variety of sensations, which suggests that there are differences in the structure of the endings not revealed by histology.

Organs and tissues of the body cavities

All tissues and organs of the body are innervated by sensory receptors but not all of these contribute to the sensations we experience. For example, baroreceptors and chemoreceptors detect changes in the internal environment (see Sections 1 and 2) but we are not consciously aware of the fluctuations in blood pressure and blood composition that they detect. But there are other receptors that do give rise to a variety of different sensations, including pain, 'fullness' (of the stomach for example) and warmth.

The majority of these receptors are unspecialised nerve endings. They are found in various places including the walls of:

- blood vessels
- the gastrointestinal tract
- the bladder.

Effective stimuli for these receptors include ischaemia and distension (see also Ch. 32). ④

④ *What is ischaemia?*

In addition, free nerve endings and specialised mechanoreceptors like some of those in the skin (such as Pacinian corpuscles) are found in the epithelia and connective tissue enveloping organs in the thoracic, abdominal and cranial cavities (pleurae, peritoneum, meninges). Some of these receptors are excited by cutting, as in a surgical operation for example.

⑤
How big is a Pacinian corpuscle?

Muscles, tendons and joints

Sensory receptors in muscles, tendons and joints are very important in the control of movement (see Chs 27 and 28). They also contribute to our bodily sense especially proprioception. These receptors include:

- joint receptors
- Golgi tendon organs
- muscle spindles.

Joint receptors

The sensory receptors found in the lining surfaces of the joints include:

- Ruffini endings
- receptors similar to, but smaller than, Pacinian corpuscles
- free nerve endings.

Excitation of these cells contributes to our awareness of the angle at which joints are held and of movement. If there is inflammation, as in arthritis for example, irritation of some of the receptors contributes to the sensation of pain. ⑤

Golgi tendon organs

Golgi tendon organs are relatively simple in structure (Fig. 24.2). They consist of a set of branching nerve terminals lodged between the collagen fibres of the tendons attached to muscles. When a muscle contracts, it pulls on the collagen fibres, compresses the nerve endings and excites them. Golgi tendon organs monitor the amount of tension developed in the motor unit attached to their bundle of collagen fibres (see Ch. 22).

Muscle spindles

Muscle spindles provide information about the length at which muscles are held and how that changes as we move.

Each spindle consists of a group of tiny modified muscle fibres (*intrafusal fibres*) surrounded by a connective tissue capsule (Fig. 24.2). These tiny fibres lie in between the much larger true muscle fibres (*extrafusal fibres*). The sensory part of the spindle is in the middle portion of the intrafusal fibre. When it is stretched, impulses are triggered (Fig. 24.3A) and conducted along the sensory neurone. Thus, whenever a muscle is lengthened (for example when you extend your arm the biceps lengthens), the spindles are excited. When the muscle is made shorter, there is less stretch and fewer impulses are fired.

The sensitivity of the spindle to stretch is adjusted by

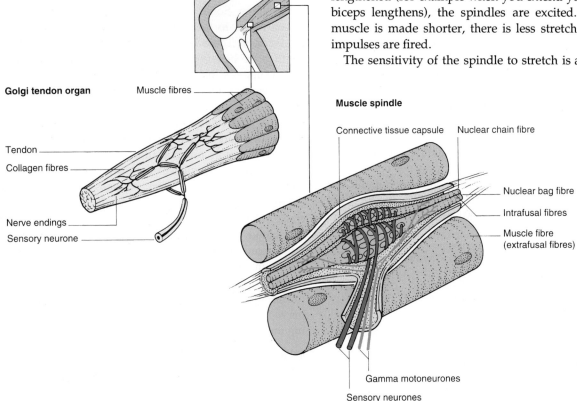

Figure 24.2
Structure of a Golgi tendon organ and a muscle spindle.

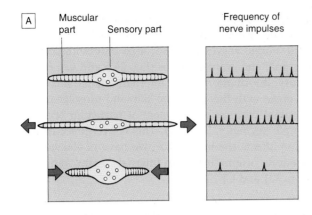

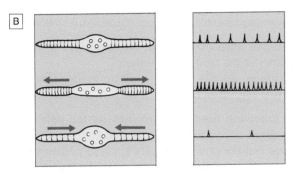

Figure 24.3
How the frequency of action potentials in the sensory neurone from a muscle spindle varies with:
A The length of the intrafusal fibre
B Contraction and relaxation of the muscular part of the intrafusal fibres.

varying the contraction of the muscular part of the intrafusal fibre (Fig. 24.3B). When the muscular part contracts it makes the sensory portion of the spindle tauter and more sensitive to further stretch. If however the muscle fibres of the spindle are completely relaxed then the sensitive part is not under tension and the spindle is not very responsive.

Contraction of the muscular part of the intrafusal fibres is controlled by the somatic motoneurones innervating them (*gamma motoneurones*) (Fig. 24.2) and these in turn are influenced by the systems in the brain and spinal cord controlling posture and movement (see Ch. 27).

There are at least two types of intrafusal fibre (Fig. 24.2):

- *nuclear bag*
- *nuclear chain*.

Each has slightly different characteristics. The bag fibres respond best to a sudden stretch (a change in length), and adapt quickly to a stretch if it is maintained, whereas the nuclear chain fibres do not adapt very quickly. Consequently, it is the chain fibres that provide information continuously to the brain about the length at which the extrafusal fibres are being held.

SENSORY NEURONES

Size and properties

The sensory neurones innervating all the receptors described so far in the skin, muscles, joints and tendons, differ in size and properties. Neurones range in size from tiny unmyelinated nerve axons of the free nerve endings mediating the sensations of pain, heat and cold, to large myelinated axons innervating the muscle spindles and the Golgi tendon organs (Table 24.4). The transmission of impulses in the large myelinated fibres is much faster than that in the small unmyelinated fibres. The fibres also differ in their susceptibility to the effects of an anaesthetic block, such as a local anaesthetic, and to ischaemia (see also Ch. 21). ⑥

Sensory neurones innervating different receptors from one part of the body are grouped together to form a *mixed nerve*. This mixed nerve also includes the axons of motoneurones supplying that region. If this mixed nerve

⑥
Why is transmission of impulses faster in large myelinated fibres?

Table 24.4	Characteristics of sensory neurones innervating somatic receptors				
Receptors	*Sensation*	*Sensory neurones*		*Susceptibility to blockage by:*	
		Diameter (μm)*	Classification	Ischaemia	Local anaesthesia
Muscle spindles Golgi tendon organs	Proprioception	13	A alpha		
Cutaneous mechanoreceptors	Touch Pressure	11	A alpha	Average	Below average
Thermoreceptors Nociceptors	Cold Pain	4	A delta		
Thermoreceptors Nociceptors	Cold Heat Pain	1	C	Below average	Above average
* Typical values.					

becomes ischaemic, and therefore hypoxic (for example as a result of pressure compressing the blood vessels), transmission of impulses in some of the fibres will be blocked more readily than in others. The consequence is that an unusual blend of sensory information will be received by the brain from that area and the part of the body served by the nerve will feel odd (*paraesthesia*). The most familiar example of paraesthesia is the curious and usually painful feelings following the numbness of a limb 'gone to sleep' (see also Ch. 32). Another relatively common clinical example is the altered sensation experienced by someone with the carpal tunnel syndrome (see Ch. 28).

⑦
Where in your back are segments?

Dermatomes and myotomes

Each spinal or cranial nerve carrying somatic sensory information transmits that information from particular areas of the body. The area of skin innervated by one spinal nerve is termed a *dermatome* (Fig. 24.4) and the muscles innervated are referred to as a *myotome*. Injury to a particular spinal nerve or to a nerve root (as for example through the compression caused by a slipped disc; see Ch. 28) therefore produces a predictable pattern of sensory loss.

Somatic and autonomic fibres

Sensory receptors in the skin, joints and muscles are innervated by somatic nerves, whereas those mediating bodily sensation from internal organs and other tissues, including blood vessels everywhere, are mostly innervated by autonomic nerves. The axons of somatic sensory neurones and autonomic neurones are bundled

together with the axons of motoneurones to form the spinal and cranial nerves.

Autonomic nerves are associated only with certain of the spinal and cranial nerves (Fig. 24.5 and Ch. 3). Thus sensory information from internal organs and tissues converges with that from the skin and muscles entering the spinal cord and brain stem at particular levels (for example segments S_2 to S_4). This convergence of information affects the impression we have of the source of sensations originating from internal organs and tissues (see p. 421 and Ch. 32). ⑦

PATHWAYS IN THE SPINAL CORD AND BRAIN STEM

Sensory axons entering the central nervous system may:

- synapse immediately with interneurones in the grey matter of the cord or brain stem
- continue up the spinal cord or brain stem before synapsing further on.

The following description focuses on the pathways in the spinal cord carrying information from the spinal nerves, but the same principles apply to pathways in the brain stem carrying information from the cranial nerves.

Pathways with an immediate synapse

Somatic

Sensory neurones that synapse immediately include those mediating the sensations of touch, pain, heat and cold. In the spinal cord these neurones synapse with interneurones in several of the laminae (see Ch. 20) that, in turn, give rise to long axons carrying the information up the spinal cord to one of three sites (Fig. 24.6):

- brain stem reticular formation (*spinoreticular tracts*)
- thalamus (*spinothalamic tracts*)
- cerebellum (*spinocerebellar tracts*).

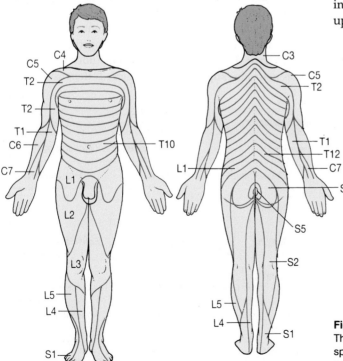

Figure 24.4
The dermatomes: areas of the skin innervated by each of the spinal nerves. (Reproduced from Rogers 1992 (Fig. 4.10) by permission of the publishers.)

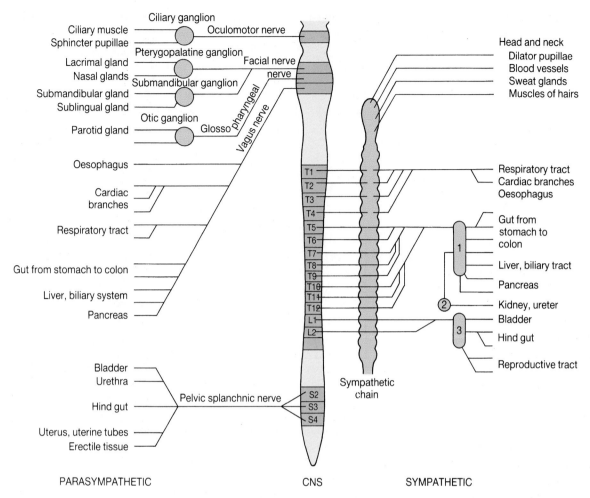

Figure 24.5
The autonomic nervous system, showing at which levels, and within which cranial and spinal nerves, autonomic fibres link with the central nervous system (1 = Coeliac ganglion; 2 = Renal ganglion; 3 = Pelvic ganglion). (Reproduced from Rogers 1992 (Fig. 4.12) by permission of the publishers.)

Sensations of touch, pain, heat and cold are mediated by the spinoreticular and spinothalamic tracts. The spinocerebellar tracts carry proprioceptive information used in the control of movement, from mechano-receptors in the joints, muscles and the skin overlying them, to the cerebellum.

The spinoreticular and spinothalamic tracts run up the spinal cord on the opposite side of the body (*contralaterally*) to that from which the sensory signals have come. Interneurones connect the primary sensory fibres with ascending tracts, which carry the signals up the opposite side of the spinal cord (Fig. 24.6). Because of this crossover of information in the spinal cord, sensory signals mediating touch, pain, heat and cold from the left side of the body are transmitted up spinal tracts on the *right* side of the cord and vice versa.

The spinocerebellar tracts differ from this. Some carry impulses up the same side of the cord as their point of entry (*ipsilaterally*) whereas others carry them up the opposite side (*contralaterally*).

Autonomic

Autonomic nerves synapse with interneurones in the laminae of the cord too. Some of the interneurones with which they synapse are the same as those used by some somatic fibres. Where this happens sensory signals from autonomic and somatic fibres *converge* on to the same neurones. The consequence is that from that point onwards the brain cannot distinguish impulses originating in an internal organ from those originating in somatic structures such as the skin. As the more usual source of sensation is the somatic one, any signals are interpreted as having originated from the skin and not from the internal organ. This is one explanation of *referred pain* (see Ch. 32), the pain caused by injury or disease of an internal organ or tissue that is felt to be coming from another part of the body such as the arm or the back.

Pathways without an immediate synapse

Some primary sensory neurones, having entered the

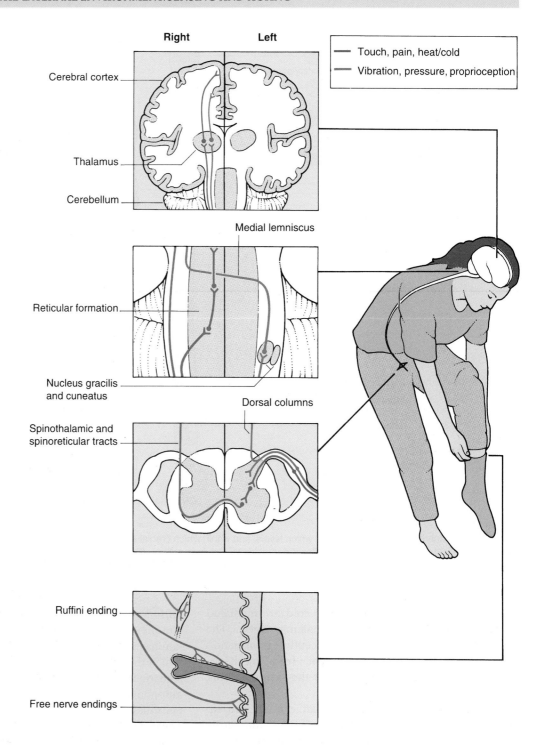

Figure 24.6
Routes through which sensory information travels from the skin to the brain.

A good example of referred pain is the pain felt in the left arm when receptors in the heart are excited by ischaemia (*angina pectoris*). Further examples are given in Chapter 32.

central nervous system, continue for a distance up the spinal cord as very long axons before synapsing. This applies to neurones mediating the sensations of pressure, vibration and proprioception. In the spinal cord, these nerve fibres form bundles of fibres (*dorsal columns*)

running up the cord on the *same* side as their point of entry (Fig. 24.6). The left dorsal column carries sensory information from the left side of the body and the right dorsal column from the right side. The primary sensory neurones giving rise to the dorsal columns do, however, also give off branches (*collaterals*) that synapse in the laminae of the grey matter. These collateral fibres are involved in influencing the transmission of signals through other pathways, for example the spinoreticular tracts, which mediate the sensation of pain (see 'gating' of pain, Ch. 32).

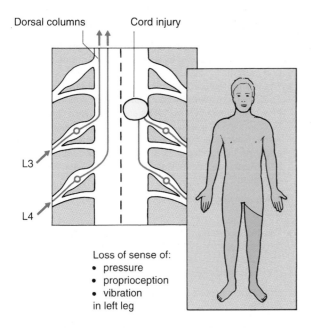

Loss of sense of:
- pressure
- proprioception
- vibration
in left leg

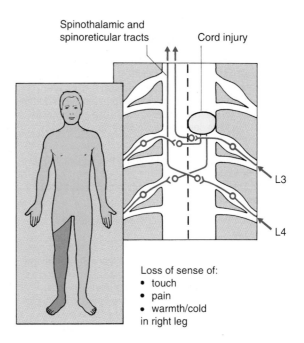

Figure 24.7
Effects of an area of injury on one side of the lumbar region of the spinal cord, on sensation in the legs. Note that both legs are affected but in different ways.

Loss of sense of:
- touch
- pain
- warmth/cold
in right leg

If there is a crush injury limited to one side of the cord, there cannot be a complete loss of sensation on one side or the other of the body. Instead, there is alteration in the range of sensations experienced on *both* sides of the body (Fig. 24.7). This is because sensory information from one part of the body gets split as it enters the cord into two separate pathways (spinothalamic and dorsal column) carrying impulses up opposite sides of the cord.

Axons of the dorsal column neurones synapse first in the medulla of the brain stem with cells of the *nucleus gracilis* and the *nucleus cuneatus*. These two nuclei in the medulla are the first place in this pathway where somatic sensory information can be analysed or modified. One of the functions of interneurones in the nuclei is to sharpen up the impression of the stimuli transmitted to the brain through this route by the process of lateral inhibition (see Ch. 23).

The neurones in the nucleus cuneatus and nucleus gracilis give rise to axons (*medial lemniscus*) that cross over the midline of the brain stem and run to the thalamus on the opposite side of the body. Eventually therefore sensory information from different receptors in the same part of the body, that has travelled up the cord on different sides in the spinothalamic tracts and the dorsal columns, is brought back together on the same side of the brain (Fig. 24.6).

DESTINATIONS IN THE BRAIN

Only sensory information reaching the thalamus and cerebral cortex gives rise to conscious sensations. That which is transmitted to the cerebellum via the spinocerebellar tracts is almost entirely involved in controlling movement (see Chs 27–29). Much of that which

travels to and through the reticular formation contributes to our general state of arousal (see Ch. 31). But that which gets to the thalamus and cortex via the spinal tracts or by the equivalent routes through the cranial nerves and brain stem creates specific 'feelings' of touch, pressure, warmth, cold, and pain.

Somatosensory cortex
The area of the cerebral cortex to which the signals are transmitted is the *somatosensory cortex* in the *post-central gyrus* of the parietal lobe (Fig. 24.8). Much of the somatosensory cortex is concerned with sensory information derived from the hands and the face. Both these areas of the body are very richly supplied with sensory receptors, and the large number of cortical neurones devoted to these areas matches this.

If there is damage to discrete areas of the somatosensory cortex, for example because of a cerebral haemorrhage (*stroke*), a patient will experience numbness of the body areas normally represented there.

CHARACTER OF SENSATIONS

The character of somatosensory sensations may be:

- discrete and well localised
- diffuse and disturbing.

The quality perceived depends upon the route through

HOW SENSATION IS TESTED

A full neurological examination cannot be carried out properly when time is at a premium. If the patient is to give reliable answers to the tests, he must feel relaxed and reassured. To gain some idea of how a patient feels during the specific assessment of sensation, ask a colleague to carry out the tests described below on you, under two conditions:

- with the tester in a hurry and urging the 'patient' to make quick decisions
- with the tester relaxed and assuring the 'patient' that there is plenty of time.

Then decide which you felt was the most accurate assessment.

Before commencing the examination, it is usual for the neurologist to enquire whether the patient suffers from any abnormal spontaneous sensation (*paraesthesia*), such as pain, numbness, tingling, 'pins and needles', 'electric shocks'. During the tests, the patient is asked to close his eyes so that sensations from the body surface are experienced without visual perception of their cause.

The integrity of the following sensory pathways is tested:

- the lateral spinothalamic pathway – chiefly mediating pain and temperature sense
- the anterior spinothalamic pathway – chiefly mediating touch and pressure sense
- the posterior (dorsal) column pathway – light touch, proprioception and vibration.

The results of these tests, though somewhat crude, indicate where a lesion might be sited and, hence, which more specific investigations are required. The development of sophisticated scanning has reduced the need for many neurological investigations, for example lumbar air encephalography and arteriography, but the crude tests are still used to indicate to the neurologist and radiologist where to look for a lesion. The tests outlined below are all performed with the patient's eyes closed.

Pain and temperature – lateral spinothalamic pathway

- Pain is tested by lightly pricking the skin with a sterile needle. The patient is asked whether he can feel anything and, if so, to describe the feeling (is the experience sharpness, pain, or both?) and its location. Areas of cutaneous numbness, for example, can be mapped by dragging a needle across the skin, the patient being

asked to indicate when the sensation changes. Deeper pain is often assessed by squeezing the Achilles tendon or a muscle.

- The test for temperature sensitivity requires two tubes. They should preferably be metal (a better conductor of heat than glass) but test tubes are often used. One is filled with ice or very cold water and the other with hot water. Care must be taken not to have the water too hot because a sensation of pain may be elicited rather than heat. Again the patient is asked to describe and locate the sensation.

Crude touch and pressure – the anterior spinothalamic pathway

- This test is carried out by touching the patient's skin with the the fingers or a blunt object, such as the end of a pen. The patient is asked whether he can feel anything and, as pressure is increased, to describe what he feels.

Light touch, proprioception and vibration – the posterior column pathway

- Light touch is tested by using a wisp of cotton wool on the patient's skin. Two point discrimination of touch should be tested with an instrument called a two-point discriminator, but ordinary dividers are often used. The two-point discriminator has blunt ends and is calibrated to measure the distance of discrimination between two points. As dividers have sharp points and no calibration, care must be taken not to elicit pain rather than touch. The patient is touched randomly with one or two points to find out whether he can appreciate the two sensations rather than interpreting them as one. Normal separation between points on the palmar surface of the thumb and fingers is 0.5 cm and much wider on, say, the back of the neck where there are fewer receptors.
- Proprioception or joint position sense. The examiner moves the patient's fingers or toes and asks him to say whether the digit is pointing up or down. Again care must be taken not to confuse sensation; if the digit is held incorrectly, the patient may guess its position from the pressure of the examiner's fingers, rather than from joint sensations.
- Vibration. A tuning fork is struck and, while vibrating, is placed on a bony prominence, such as the ankle or wrist. The patient should be able to feel the vibrations, usually described as a tingling sensation.

---

which nerve impulses have reached the somatosensory cortex.

Discrete and well localised

The sensory information reaching the cerebral cortex via pathways such as the dorsal columns and spinothalamic tracts (specific sensory pathways; see Ch. 23) is recognised by us as having come from discrete parts of our bodies. The location of the stimulus can be quite accurately defined. This is because of the highly ordered arrangement of the neurones and because the process of lateral inhibition operates at some of the synapses. At each level, in the spinal cord, the medullary nuclei, the

In areas of the body where innervation is sparse, for example on the back, it is sometimes difficult to locate the precise place of, say, an itch. Armed with a back scratcher, knitting needle or ruler, you attack the place where the itch seems to be only to find that, for relief, you have to scratch an inch or so either way. It is often more difficult to locate an itch for a patient – on occasions you may end up rubbing the whole back, having given up on the 'down a bit', 'to the left a bit' instructions.

thalamus, and the cortex, the body is 'mapped out' in the relative positions of the neurones. If the density of

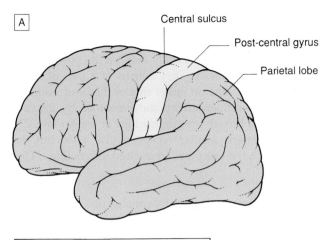

Central sulcus

Post-central gyrus

Parietal lobe

A

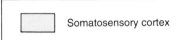

Somatosensory cortex

B

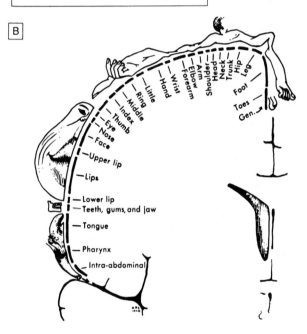

Figure 24.8
The somatosensory cortex:
A Position in the cerebrum (side view of the brain showing the left somatosensory cortex only)
B Functional divisions (brain in cross-section, viewed from the front, showing right somatosensory cortex only). Note how much of the somatosensory cortex is devoted to sensory information coming from the hand, face and tongue. The 'little man' (homunculus) constructed from this information represents the impression our minds have of the size and shape of our bodies. (Reprinted with the permission of Macmillan Publishing Company from The cerebral cortex of man, by Wilder Penfield and Theodore Rasmussen. Copyright 1950 Macmillan Publishing Company; copyright renewed (c) 1978 Theodore Rasmussen.)

innervation is high and if there is lateral inhibition, the map is very detailed and precise (as it is for the skin of the hands and face). If however innervation is sparse, then the map is less detailed and more like a sketch (as it is for the skin of the back) (see also Ch. 23). ⑧

Diffuse and disturbing

Sensory information reaching the thalamus and the cerebral cortex via the reticular formation (spinoreticular tracts) is less well ordered. This is because the transmission of the signals is not rigidly restricted to particular pathways and because lateral inhibition does not occur at all. Consequently, our sensory impressions are more diffuse though no less disturbing. Indeed because the signals tend to be more widely dispersed they may be more likely to disturb and distract us. The sensation of burning pain is mediated by this route (see Ch. 32).

PROPRIOCEPTION

When our eyes are closed, the sense we have of the position and movement of our bodies (*proprioception*) is created by sensory information derived from a variety of different receptors including the balance organs (*vestibular apparatus*) as well as receptors in the skin, the joints, the muscles and tendons already described. All these receptors are said to have a proprioceptive function. However, the term *proprioceptors* is most often

---

AWARENESS OF PROPRIOCEPTION

Can you imagine what life would be like without proprioception? Think about trying to drive a car and having to look at the pedals and gear lever every time you moved your feet and hands to change gear, brake or accelerate! We all make use of proprioception but some activities rely more heavily on it than others. For example, some people become highly skilled touch typists; they know the positions of the keys and exactly how much pressure to apply with which finger. A typist used to a manual typewriter may well take a little time to adjust to the lighter touch of an electronic keyboard, but that adjustment will be made. Nursing skills, in the main, require visual input, but with the increasing use of computerised records and computer assisted learning a new skill (typing), which depends more on proprioceptive input, may need to be developed. Prodding a keyboard with two fingers and visually searching for letters is both frustrating and time consuming.

Some people are normally less aware than others of the position of their limbs in relation to their surroundings. These are the people who are dismissed as clumsy, hamfisted, accident prone. The mug of coffee lands on the table with a resounding crash, chairs are knocked over, feet hit the stairs so heavily that the house shakes. The development of clumsiness, or an increase in awkwardness that is not normal for the person requires investigation. Messages from the proprioceptors, via the posterior (dorsal) column pathways, are interpreted at a conscious level in the parietal area of the sensory cortex of the brain. If a tumour or other lesion develops in one of the parietal lobes of the brain, one of the first symptoms noticed by the patient may be clumsiness, a tendency to knock things over and misjudge distances.

⑧
What are the advantages of high density innervation to the skin of the hands and face?

applied to the receptors present in joints, muscles and tendons (muscle spindles, Golgi tendon organs and joint receptors; see p. 418).

All proprioceptive information is important in the control of posture and movement (see Chs 27–29). Consequently, much sensory information from these receptors is directed to regions of the brain, such as the cerebellum, that are specifically concerned with motor control. Some signals do reach the sensory cortex. These are the ones that make us aware of our position and movement.

When proprioceptive information does not reach the cerebellum, varying degrees of *ataxia* become evident. Ataxia is lack of coordination of movement. A person with ataxia is, for example, unable to walk heel to toe along a straight line or to touch the tip of the nose with the index finger while the eyes are closed.

THE BALANCE ORGANS (VESTIBULAR APPARATUS)

The balance organs specifically monitor the position and movement of the head. They consist of a pair of fluid-filled labyrinths, one on either side of the head, containing receptors influenced by movement or by gravity. The system is linked with the cochlea of the ear (see Ch. 25), and contains similar receptors (*hair cells*) but the way in which the receptors are excited differs (Fig. 24.9).

Structure

Each balance organ (Fig. 24.10) consists of:

- three *semicircular ducts*
- two sacs (*utricle* and *saccule*).

The ducts and sacs form part of the *membranous labyrinth*, which lies inside the *bony (osseus) labyrinth* consisting of:

- semicircular canals
- vestibule
- cochlea.

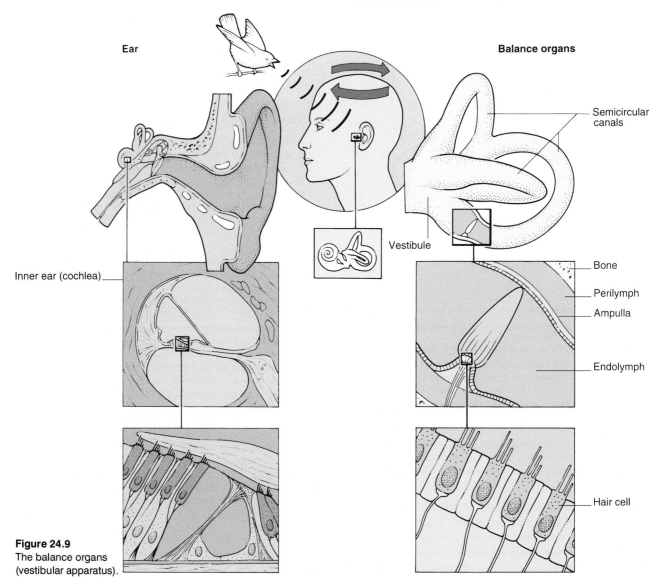

Figure 24.9
The balance organs (vestibular apparatus).

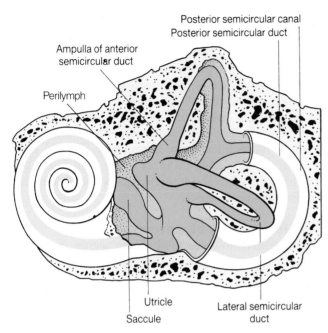

Figure 24.10
The three ducts and two sacs of the vestibular apparatus, lying within the canals and chambers formed of bone. (Reproduced from Rogers 1992 (Fig. 24.8) by permission of the publishers.)

The ducts and sacs are lined by a secretory epithelium and are filled with *endolymph* and surrounded by *perilymph*.

The sensory receptors (*hair cells*) are grouped into two different types of sensory organ (Fig. 24.11A & B):

● crista ● macula.

There is one crista in the ampulla of each of the semicircular ducts. The two maculae of each balance organ are in the utricle and saccule.

Cristae
The hair cells of the cristae possess very long cilia enveloped in a gelatinous mass known as the *cupula* (Fig. 24.11A). This plume-like structure is fixed to the top of the ampulla, but otherwise it is free to move. If the fluid in the ducts moves then the cupula bends like seaweed moving with the current and this in turn bends the cilia.

Maculae
The cilia of the maculae are shorter but they too are embedded in a gelatinous mass (Fig. 24.11B). Stuck on to the surface of this jelly-like layer are small crystals of calcium carbonate (*otoliths*). These weigh the jelly down if they are on top, or tend to exert a pull on it if they are underneath. In either case the cilia are bent and this alters the number of action potentials generated in the sensory neurones.

Excitation of the sensory receptors
When the cilia are upright (Fig. 24.12) the cells fire quite

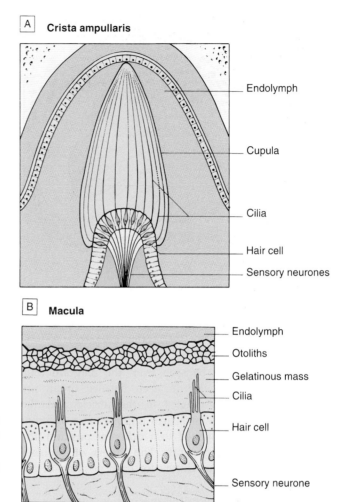

Figure 24.11
The two different types of sense organ in the vestibular apparatus.

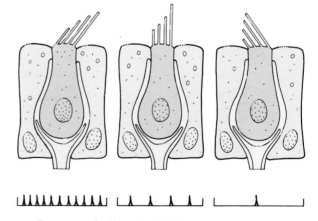

Frequency of action potentials in sensory neurone
Figure 24.12
Relationship between the bending of the cilia on the hair cell and the frequency of action potentials in the sensory neurone.

spontaneously at a steady rate. If they are then bent in one direction the cell increases its firing rate, but if they are bent in the opposite direction the firing of impulses

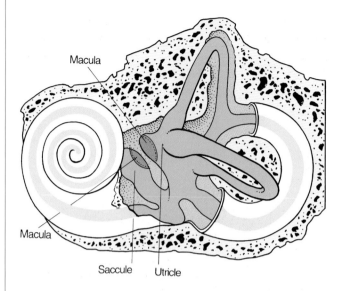

Macula

Macula

Saccule   Utricle

Figure 24.13
Position of the maculae in the utricle and the saccule. Notice that they are differently oriented. (Reproduced and adapted from Rogers 1992 (Fig. 24.8) by permission of the publishers.)

⑨ *What symptoms might occur if the labyrinth becomes inflamed?*

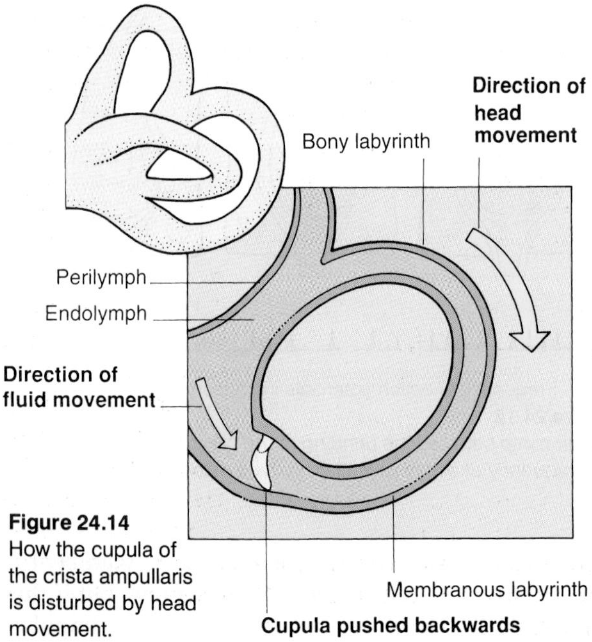

is inhibited. As can be seen from the diagram (Fig. 24.13) the two maculae in each balance organ are oriented at different angles in the utricle and the saccule. Consequently each fires impulses at a different rate. If the head is moved to a different position, the maculae alter their firing rate. The pattern of impulses from the maculae thus differs for each position of the head.

The cristae differ from the maculae in that they are best at detecting sudden movements of the head up and down, to the left and to the right, and so on. When the head is moved, the fluid in the ducts does not immedi-

ately move with it. It lags behind and so the cupula is dragged in the opposite direction to that in which the head moved (Fig. 24.14). This is just the same as the jerk backwards that you experience on a bus or train when it begins to move. When the cupula is jerked backwards the cilia bend and the cells are excited.

The different orientation of the three semicircular ducts allows us to detect swivel movements of the head in any direction. The most horizontally oriented duct canal is best at picking up turns of the head to the left and the right, while the other two are better at detecting movements up and down. ⑨

False impressions of movement

Whenever and however fluid moves within the ducts, signals are generated that are interpreted by the brain as

Direction of head movement

Bony labyrinth

Perilymph

Endolymph

Direction of fluid movement

Figure 24.14
How the cupula of the crista ampullaris is disturbed by head movement.

Membranous labyrinth

Cupula pushed backwards

THAT DIZZY FEELING

Dizzy, giddy, light headed – what exactly do we mean when we use these and similar terms? It is impossible to experience the sensations generated within another's body, so careful questioning by a doctor is essential to establish what form the 'dizziness' takes. The example in the main text of children whirling round to experience a feeling of continued movement on stopping is a realistic description of *vertigo*. Vertigo is the consciousness of disordered orientation of the body in space. Usually the person feels very insecure, frightened to move quickly, turn the head or, perhaps, look at flickering lights. When vertigo occurs without a cause that is obvious to the sufferer, for example too much alcohol, then the symptom will be treated while the underlying cause is investigated. The doctor will wish to know the nature of the dizziness and sometimes the patient may give a better description to a nurse in the course of conversation because he feels that the nurse has more time to listen. The sensations are described in the following ways:

- movement of the surroundings, rotating or oscillating
- movement of the body, rotating or a sense of falling – sometimes it is just the head that feels as if it is moving
- unsteadiness of the limbs and movement not well coordinated.

There are many known causes of vertigo and much research has been carried out, but often the underlying cause in a particular patient is not found. However, by investigation, the more worrying causes are eliminated. Not all vertigo is associated directly with the balance organs, but the causes of aural vertigo are the most numerous and probably the easiest to diagnose. It is not difficult to think of the obvious causes, such as wax in the external meatus, infection of the middle ear (otitis media), sudden changes in atmospheric pressure. Less obvious perhaps are drugs (salicylate (aspirin) and quinine in particular), impairment of blood supply, head injury, inflammation of the balance organs. These are additional to Ménière's disease, referred to in the main text. Vertigo is a very distressing and frightening symptom; the experience is actually far worse than the simulated sensation experienced by a child whirling just for fun.

movement. It is possible to create convection currents in the endolymph of the balance organs by syringeing ears with fluid that is colder or warmer than core temperature. The convection currents displace the cupula and the person having his ears syringed is likely to feel as if the room is 'swimming'.

The same kind of feeling is often voluntarily induced by children who have discovered that by whirling around very rapidly several times and then stopping, eyes closed and backs pressed safely against a wall, they experience curious feelings of movement. The reason for these feelings is that when you stop abruptly after a period of spinning, the fluid in the ducts continues to flow around for several seconds and the cilia of the cristae are displaced.

Impressions of movement and position are also built up from comparisons, made by the brain, of sensory information from the balance organs on each side of the head. A difference in signal between the sensory receptors on each side is interpreted either as movement (cristae compared) or as a different head position (maculae compared). If there is damage to the vestibular apparatus on one side or impairment of impulse transmission as in *Ménière's disease* then the sufferer will experience feelings of dizziness and apparent movement.

These unpleasant feelings are often complicated by reflex effects triggered by stimulation of the balance organs. These include *nystagmus* (a characteristic pattern of eye movements; see Ch. 29) and postural adjustments (see Ch. 28).

TASTE AND SMELL

The taste of food depends as much on its texture and its smell as it does on chemical stimulation of the taste buds. Think of how food tastes when you have a cold (sense of smell dulled) and how texture (crispness, sliminess, etc.) alters your appreciation of food. Receptors sensitive to the chemicals in food are found in the mucosal lining throughout the digestive tract, but only those in the mouth and nose contribute to the sensation of taste.

MOUTH

Receptors

A variety of different receptors are present in the mouth:

- mechanoreceptors
- thermoreceptors
- nociceptors
- chemoreceptors.

Mechanoreceptors, thermoreceptors and nociceptors
Receptors mediating the sensations of touch, pressure, pain, heat and cold are found in the mucosa lining the oral cavity and the tongue. The mucous membranes towards the back of the mouth are especially sensitive to touch.

> Touching the sensitive mucous membranes towards the back of the mouth and posterior pharyngeal wall elicits the pharyngeal or gag reflex causing constriction of the pharynx. This unpleasant sensation is sometimes experienced when the dentist works on back teeth and droplets from the water jet hit the back of the mouth. In people with extra-sensitive mouths this reflex can be troublesome when cleaning the teeth. Care should be taken when cleaning patients' mouths because eliciting the reflex, apart from being unpleasant, may induce vomiting. This is a method by which vomiting can be induced in an emergency, for example in a conscious child following accidental swallowing of tablets.

Chemoreceptors
The chemosensitive cells are grouped together within *taste buds* (Fig. 24.15) most of which are found on the tongue, but some are also present elsewhere in the mouth and throat (pharynx). These gustatory cells within the taste buds respond to a great variety of chemicals. Tastes have been categorised into at least four types:

- sweet
- sour
- salt
- bitter.

Sour tastes tend to be produced by acids whereas salty tastes are produced by inorganic ions such as sodium and potassium, and their associated anions. Other than this, little correspondence has been found between the chemical structure of a molecule and the taste it produces. Most taste buds tend to be better at mediating one type of taste than another. Consequently, different parts of the mouth are best at detecting different constituents in food (Fig. 24.16).

Sensory neurones, pathways and destinations
Impulses generated by receptors in the mouth are transmitted along cranial nerves V, VII, IX and X to the medulla of the brain to synapse with neurones carrying signals via the thalamus to the somatosensory cortex. Impulses transmitted to the limbic system (see Ch. 31) and the hypothalamus affect appetite (Ch. 14). Stimulation of receptors in the mouth also evokes reflex responses via centres in the medulla, such as the secretion of digestive juices (see Ch. 6) and vomiting (see Ch. 15).

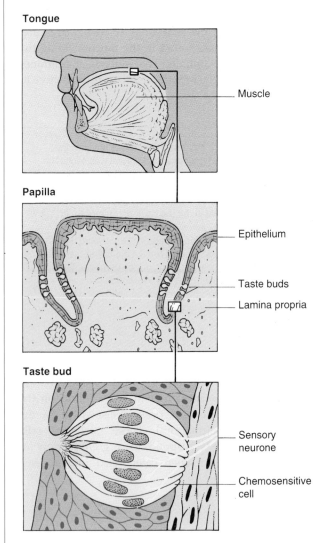

Figure 24.15
Position and structure of the taste buds of the tongue.

Aromatherapy is a branch of alternative medicine practised by qualified therapists that makes use of aromatic essential plant oils in the treatment of some diseases. The oils may also be used by the individual in the following ways: placed directly on a tissue or handkerchief; added to bath water; massaged into the skin; or as a room fragrance added to water and placed on a warm radiator. A few examples: camomile is recommended to calm and sooth; tangerine to refresh and stimulate; sandalwood to relax. Some are reputed to have aphrodisiac qualities, for example nutmeg and sandalwood.

NOSE

The sense of smell (*olfaction*) is not as important to us as humans as it is for some other creatures but its loss temporarily or permanently (*anosmia*) does affect our appreciation of food. The olfactory receptors are tucked away high up in the nasal cavity (Fig. 24.17). Nerve impulses generated by them are transmitted to parts of the brain involved in emotion and motivation, as well as in the control of food intake and its digestion.

Receptors

Structure and location

The olfactory receptors consist of specialised nerve endings embedded in the mucosa of the olfactory cleft (Fig. 24.17). In gentle breathing very little air reaches the receptors whereas, in sniffing, the airflow around the conchae becomes turbulent and more molecules are wafted into the cleft. The receptors possess many

In *coryza* (common cold) the mucous membranes become swollen and the flow of air through the olfactory cleft becomes obstructed. As a result the sense of smell (and taste) is dulled.

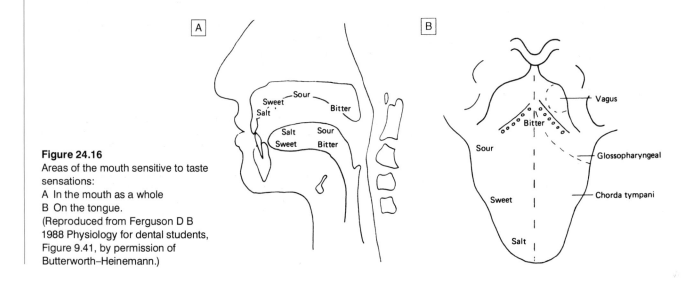

Figure 24.16
Areas of the mouth sensitive to taste sensations:
A In the mouth as a whole
B On the tongue.
(Reproduced from Ferguson D B 1988 Physiology for dental students, Figure 9.41, by permission of Butterworth–Heinemann.)

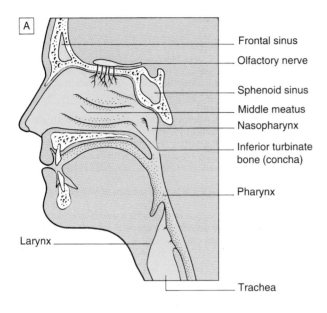

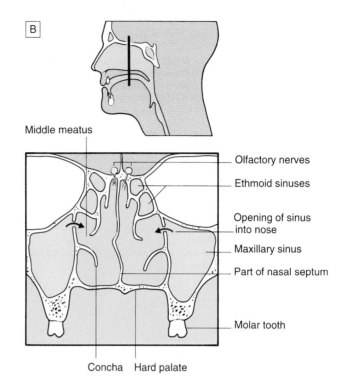

Figure 24.17
Position of the olfactory receptors in the nasal cavity.

cilia presenting a very large surface area for airborne molecules to contact.

Sensitivity
The receptors are amazingly sensitive to airborne molecules. Only a couple of odorous molecules need to be present in a whiff of air for them to be detected. No distinguishing features have yet been found between the receptors, and little is known about the way in which different chemicals give rise to the patterns of information interpreted by the brain as up to 4000 different odours.

Sensory neurones, pathways and destinations
Nerve fibres extend from the receptors, through the *cribriform plate*, and pass to the *olfactory bulb*. Here, the neurones synapse with the next neurones in the system. There is much convergence of information at this level (receptor:neurone ratio of about 250:1) (see Ch. 23) which probably accounts for much of the high sensitivity of the olfactory system.

From the olfactory bulb, nerve fibres pass to the frontal lobes of the brain and to the *prepyriform cortex* of the limbic system. Both of these areas are involved in our emotional and motivational drives (see Ch. 31) and connect with the hypothalamus and the autonomic nervous system, thus affecting appetite and the digestion of food.

KEY POINTS

What you should now know and understand about body senses, proprioception, taste and smell:

- the structure, location and function of sensory receptors in the skin, mucous membranes, muscles, joints, tendons and internal organs
- why some parts of the body, such as the hand, are very sensitive whereas other parts, such as the internal organs, are not
- the nerve pathways through which sensory information travels from the body to the brain
- the significance of different sensory pathways and different destinations for our experience of, and reactions to, various sensations
- the sensory systems contributing to our sense of position and movement (proprioception)
- the structure of the balance organs and how they work
- how and why altered sensation provides clues to the neurologist about the source of an injury or other abnormality
- the basis of some common disturbances of sensory experience such as numbness, tingling and dizziness.

REFERENCES AND FURTHER READING

Ferguson D B 1988 Physiology for dental students. Wright, London
(Clearly written, general physiology text which includes more
information than usual on aspects of oral physiology)

Johansson R S, Vallbo A B 1983 Tactile sensory coding in the
glabrous skin of the human hand. Trends in Neuroscience 6(1):
27–32
(Interesting information about the hand, and how this aspect of
physiology has been investigated)

Junquiera L C, Carneiro J, Kelley R O 1989 Basic histology, 6th edn.
Appleton & Lange, East Norwalk, Connecticut

Mackie R M 1992 Healthy skin: the facts. Oxford University Press,
Oxford
(All aspects of skin and how to keep it healthy. Written for the
general reader)

McMahon S B 1992 Itching for an explanation. Trends in
Neuroscience 15(12): 497–501
(Short specialist review of what is known about itching, and the
theories advanced to explain it)

Penfield W, Rasmussen T 1950 The cerebral cortex of man: a
clinical study of localisation of function. Macmillan, New York
(A now classic book detailing the studies in humans that
revealed so much about the role of different brain areas in
sensation and movement)

Rodnitzky R L 1988 Van Allen's pictorial atlas of neurologic tests,
3rd edn. Year Book Medical Publishers, Chicago
(Useful compact book detailing tests: how they are carried out
and what they mean. Clearly illustrated with line drawings)

Rogers A W 1992 Textbook of anatomy. Churchill Livingstone,
Edinburgh

Wright A 1987 Dizziness: a guide to disorders of balance. Croom
Helm, Beckenham
(Concise clinical text, which begins with a useful overview of
normal balance before delving into medical aspects of signs,
symptoms and physical examination)

Chapter 25
HEARING

Our ears are sensitive to the tiny pressure changes occurring in air when objects vibrate. These pressure changes (*sound waves*) cause the eardrum to vibrate and the vibrations are passed on through the structures in the ear to the auditory receptors (*hair cells*) (Fig. 25.1) which convert the vibratory energy into nerve impulses. Nerve impulses travel along auditory nerve pathways to the auditory areas of the cerebral cortex, giving rise to the sensation of sound.

Deafness occurs if there is either a physical blockage in the transmission of vibrations through the ear or if there is damage to the auditory receptors or pathways. ①

SOUND WAVES

When objects vibrate, they cause the molecules in the air next to the object to be alternately pushed together (*compressed*) and then moved apart (*rarefied*) (Fig. 25.2). This alternating pressure is transmitted to the next layer of air and so on. The alternating wave of pressure in the air caused by a vibrating body is described in terms of its *amplitude* and its *frequency*. The amplitude relates to the loudness of the sound and the frequency to its pitch. Of special importance are the frequencies of sound that are crucial to an understanding of speech.

CHARACTERISTICS

Amplitude and loudness
The *amplitude* of a sound wave refers to the difference in air pressure between the greatest compression and the greatest rarefaction (Fig. 25.3). The bigger the amplitude of the wave, the greater is its intensity in terms of energy and the louder is the sound we perceive. The intensity of a sound is measured in *bels*.

Bels and decibels
The quietest sound that is just audible to a normal ear under ideal conditions is used as a reference level against which the intensity of all other sounds is compared.

$$\text{Intensity (bels)} = \log_{10} \frac{\text{Intensity of the sound}}{\text{Intensity of the reference sound}}$$

As logarithms are used in the calculation (see Ch. 12 and Table 25.1), if the intensity of the sound being measured is exactly the same as the reference sound (0.0002 dynes/cm^2) then:

$$\text{Number of bels} = \log_{10} \frac{0.0002}{0.0002} = \log_{10} 1 = 0$$

The intensity of sound waves in everyday conversation is about 1 000 000 times (10^6) greater than the reference level. As the log of 10^6 is 6, the number of bels is 6 (Table 25.1). As 1 bel = 10 decibels this is 60 decibels (dB).

The intensity of everyday sounds ranges between 0 and about 100 dB (Table 25.2). Sounds of greater intensity may be painful and can cause permanent damage. An increase in decibels from 80 to 100 may not seem very much but it represents a 100-fold increase in sound intensity. An increase to 120 dB at a *very* loud band concert represents an increase of 10 000 times.

①
How important is hearing for the things you do each day?

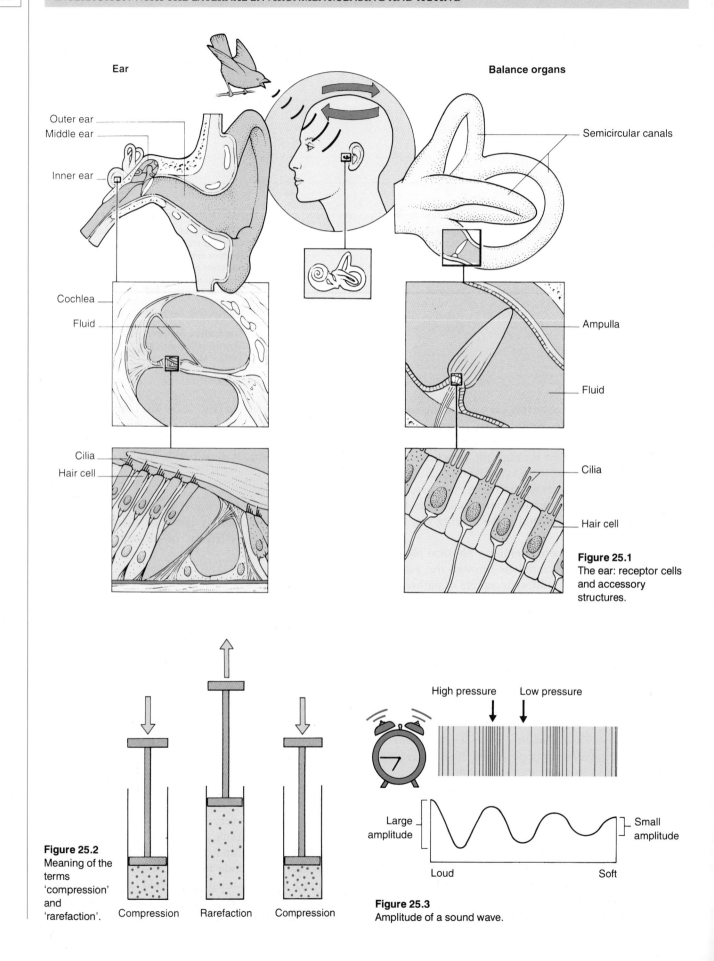

Ear

Balance organs

Outer ear
Middle ear
Inner ear

Semicircular canals

Cochlea

Fluid

Ampulla

Fluid

Cilia
Hair cell

Cilia

Hair cell

Figure 25.1
The ear: receptor cells and accessory structures.

Figure 25.2
Meaning of the terms 'compression' and 'rarefaction'.

Compression   Rarefaction   Compression

High pressure   Low pressure

Large amplitude   Small amplitude

Loud   Soft

Figure 25.3
Amplitude of a sound wave.

Table 25.1 Ways of representing numbers

Number		Power of ten	Logarithm*
10 000	$= 10 \times 10 \times 10 \times 10$	10^4	$\log_{10} 10\,000 = 4$
1000	$= 10 \times 10 \times 10$	10^3	$\log_{10} 1000 = 3$
100	$= 10 \times 10$	10^2	$\log_{10} 100 = 2$
10	$= 10$	10^1	$\log_{10} 10 = 1$
1	$= \dfrac{10}{10}$	10^0	$\log_{10} 1 = 0$
0.1	$= \dfrac{1}{10}$	10^{-1}	$\log_{10} 0.1 = -1$
0.01	$= \dfrac{1}{10 \times 10}$	10^{-2}	$\log_{10} 0.01 = -2$

* To base 10.

AWARENESS OF ENVIRONMENTAL NOISE POLLUTION

Occupational health nurses in industries where there is prolonged intense noise should alert workers to the potential danger of progressive and permanent hearing loss, and encourage the use of special protective earmuffs or earplugs. Where the noise is greater than 90 dB, employers are obliged by law to provide appropriate protection.

Health educators should target groups who may be exposed regularly to loud music in discos or on personal stereos as this causes sensorineural deafness in a significant number of young people. Disco music can be as high as 120 dB.

It is an interesting exercise to compare noise levels in different everyday settings. Why not record noise levels for a 10-minute period in a hospital ward, a college canteen, a city street with road works in progress and your own home, and discuss your findings.

Frequency and pitch

The *frequency* of sound waves is the number of cycles of compression and rarefaction occurring per second.

One cycle per second   = 1 Herz (Hz)
1000 cycles per second = 1000 Hz
                = 1 kiloHerz (kHz)

The frequency of the waves determines the *pitch* we hear (Table 25.3). Waves of low frequency are heard as sounds of low pitch (someone with a deep voice, a motorcycle); waves of high frequency are heard as sounds of high pitch (squeak, dental drill).

Speech sounds

The sounds we hear are usually complex ones made up of a mixture of different frequencies rather than pure notes such as those produced in an audiometer or by a tuning fork. Each sound has a fundamental frequency, but in addition to this there are harmonics and other components that add 'colour' to the sound.

The blend of frequencies in a sound determines

Table 25.2 Intensity of some sounds

Sound	Intensity (decibels)
Very loud band music	120
Heavy traffic	80
Ordinary conversation	60
Whisper	30
Leaves rustling	10
Threshold of hearing	0

Table 25.3 Range of frequencies detected by the human ear

Frequency (Hz)	
20	Lowest detectable sound*
120	Male voice[†]
250	Female voice[†] (about middle C)
4000	Top notes on piano[†]
20 000	Highest detectable sound*

* In young people.
[†] Fundamental frequency.

its quality, whether it sounds harsh or bell-like or shrill for example. It is the differences in harmonics that distinguish one sound from another even though they have the same fundamental frequency. For example, a middle C sounds different sung by the human voice as 'ee' in the word eat as compared with its being played on a clarinet because the blend of frequencies in the two differs (Fig. 25.4). The same is true for different voices.

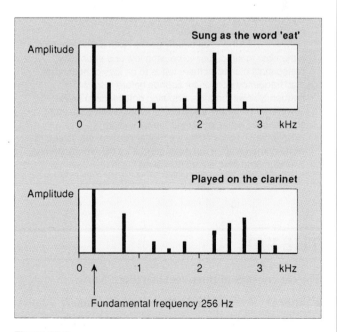

Figure 25.4
Analysis of two sounds of the same pitch (middle C, 256 Hz), one produced by the human voice, the other played on the clarinet. (Adapted from Fletcher 1929.)

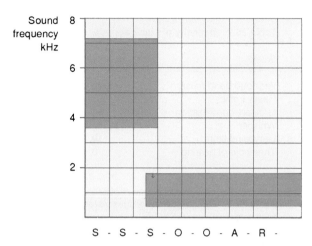

Figure 25.5
Major sound frequencies contributing to the word 'SOAR'. (Data courtesy of D E Evans and H C Richardson.)

No two people sound exactly the same because the blend of frequencies in each voice differs from person to person.

The higher frequency components in human speech are extremely important in enabling us to distinguish one word from another as these are the frequencies used in consonants (see Ch. 29). For example the 's' in the word 'soar' has very high frequency components as compared with the 'oar' sound in the same word (Fig. 25.5).

Presbyacusis – progressive and usually bilateral sensorineural loss of hearing associated with the ageing process – is not necessarily helped by the use of a hearing aid; specialist tests are needed to determine whether residual hearing will benefit.

When speaking to an elderly person with a hearing deficit, remember to keep your voice pitch low and enunciate consonants clearly as there tends to be loss of hearing of high frequency consonant sounds before loss of low frequency vowel sounds. Shouting only tends to make vowel sounds louder and therefore masks the consonant sounds even more, adding to the confusion.

Note that, because they are higher pitched, the voices of women and children are more difficult for the elderly person to understand than are men's voices.

THE EAR

The ear consists of three sections (Fig. 25.6A):

- outer
- middle
- inner.

The outer part funnels sound waves down to the *tympanic membrane* (eardrum) which then vibrates. The vibrations are transmitted through an interconnected set of three small bones (*ossicles*) in the middle ear to the

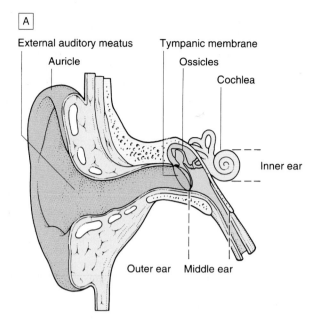

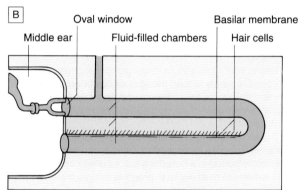

Figure 25.6
Structure of the ear:
A Component parts: outer, middle and inner
B Diagrammatic representation of the cochlea (uncoiled) showing its various parts.

inner ear. The inner ear consists of a small spiral tunnel (*cochlea*) in the bone of the skull, divided internally into three fluid-filled chambers (Fig. 25.6B). Set into the membrane (*basilar membrane*) which divides two of the chambers are the auditory receptors (*hair cells*). When the vibrations are transmitted from the middle ear through the oval window to the fluids of the inner ear, the basilar membrane vibrates, and this excites the hair cells.

OUTER EAR

The *auricle* (*pinna*) of the outer ear (Fig. 25.6A) helps to gather sound waves and direct them along the *external auditory meatus* to the eardrum (*tympanic membrane*). The shape of the auricle causes sound waves coming from in front of us to be picked up better than those from behind. This helps us to locate the source of a sound.

When we turn our heads in response to a sound we are testing out that sound from different directions and in effect taking bearings on it. From this information, derived from both ears, our minds work out the direction from which the sound has come.

The external auditory meatus is the tube leading to the eardrum. The outer third is formed of cartilage and lined by hairy skin possessing sebaceous and wax-secreting glands. The rest is formed of bone and is lined by non-hairy skin. The meatus is not completely straight but is constricted part of the way along. The size and shape of the auditory meatus affects the blend of sounds received by the eardrum. Just as sounds appear different when listened to through a long tube, so the tiny tube of the auditory meatus modifies the blend of sound waves reaching the eardrum.

The eardrum is pearly white in appearance and consists of fibrous tissue. It is covered externally by skin and internally by a mucous membrane.

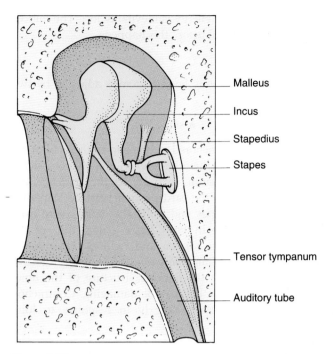

Figure 25.7
Structure of the middle ear.

Awareness of the shape of the external auditory meatus is important when positioning the ear for inspection of the eardrum, instillation of drops and ointment, or for syringing. In order to straighten the meatus it is necessary to pull the auricle up and backwards in the adult and, because of maturational differences, to pull the auricle down and backwards when treating a child.

COMMON PROBLEMS AFFECTING THE EXTERNAL AUDITORY MEATUS

Problems that can disrupt conduction of sound waves and are amenable to treatment, include:

- *otitis externa* (inflammation of the outer ear) – usually associated with infection or trauma, and treated by topical or systemic medication
- *oversecretion of wax* – treated by syringing with warm water to clear the blockage
- *foreign bodies* – treated by either floating out on oily liquid or removing with aural forceps
- *perforated eardrum* – may repair itself if small or can be repaired surgically by grafting a piece of fascia, usually from the temporalis muscle, over the perforation (a procedure called *myringoplasty*).

The eardrum, apart from its mechanical function in conducting sound waves, also closes and protects the air-filled middle ear. A perforated eardrum allows moisture and microorganisms to enter, with the potential to disrupt conduction and cause infection. This is one reason why it is important to ensure that the eardrum is intact before syringing the meatus.

Prompt treatment of respiratory infections and infectious diseases can help prevent ear infection, which may result in some hearing loss. The auditory (eustachian) tube connecting the middle ear and the upper respiratory tract provides easy access for microorganisms.

MIDDLE EAR

The middle ear is a small air-filled cavity which has an opening into the pharynx through the *auditory tube* (*eustachian tube*) (Fig. 25.7). Bridging the gap between the eardrum and the oval window are three tiny bones (*ossicles*). They transmit the vibrations from the eardrum to the inner ear. Vibrations can be damped by the contraction of two tiny muscles, which protect the ear, to some extent, against the damaging effects of loud sounds. Normally the pressure in the middle ear is the same as that in the pharynx, but if the auditory tube is blocked pressures differ and sounds become muffled.

Ossicles

The three bones of the middle ear are the:

- malleus
- incus
- stapes.

These bones act as a lever system so that when the eardrum vibrates the vibrations are transmitted to the *oval window*. In fact the pressures produced are magnified in the process because of the lever action of the bones and because the area of the oval window is much smaller than that of the eardrum. This magnification of the pressure changes is important because at the next stage, when the vibrations are passed on to the fluid of the inner ear, some energy is inevitably lost. The middle ear boosts the signal before this happens.

Muscles

The action of the bony lever system is adjusted by two muscles:

- tensor typanum
- stapedius.

Both muscles are anchored at one end to the wall of the middle ear, and at the other end to one of the ossicles. The tensor tympanum is fixed to the malleus and controls tension in the eardrum whereas the stapedius is fixed to the stapes and pulls this bone away from the oval window. In both cases, contraction of the muscles stiffens the system and reduces transmission of vibrations, muffling the sound. This is a protective response, shielding the delicate structure of the inner ear from vibrations that may be damaging. Contraction of the muscles occurs reflexly in response to loud sounds.

Pressures

Sounds also become muffled when the pressure of air in the middle ear differs from that outside. This can happen when the auditory tubes close or are blocked. The tubes close temporarily when there is an abrupt change in atmospheric pressure (as on take-off or land-

ing of an aircraft). The sweets sometimes offered to airline travellers at the beginning and end of a flight are not just a social gesture. Sucking the sweets increases the flow of saliva, and encourages swallowing. Swallowing (see Ch. 29) opens up the auditory tube. Yawning has a similar effect. Once the pressures are equal again, normal hearing is restored.

INNER EAR

The inner ear consists of a membranous tube (*cochlear duct*) lying in a small coiled tunnel in the bone of the skull (*cochlea*). Within the cochlear duct is the basilar membrane that vibrates when the ear is excited by sound waves.

Cochlea

The cochlea is divided into three chambers (Fig. 25.8A):

- scala vestibuli
- scala media
- scala tympani.

The fluid (*perilymph*) in the outer two chambers differs in composition from the fluid (*endolymph*) in the scala media. The chamber containing perilymph has a small opening linking it with the fluid in the vestibular apparatus (Fig. 25.8A and Ch. 24).

The tissue dividing the scala tympani from the scala media consists of the *basilar membrane* and the *spiral organ (of Corti)*, flanked by supporting cells (Fig. 25.8B & C). The basilar membrane extends from one end of the cochlear duct to the other. If it could be unrolled it would be about 35 mm long.

The auditory receptors (*hair cells*) are in the spiral organ. They are arranged in two sets (Fig. 25.8C):

- inner
- outer.

They are ciliated cells innervated by sensory neurones of the auditory nerve (cranial nerve VIII). The tips of the

---

OTITIS MEDIA (INFLAMMATION OF THE MIDDLE EAR)

Acute otitis media
In infections which involve the upper respiratory tract, the inflammatory response can cause swelling of the mucous membrane lining the middle ear, and exudates may collect in what is normally an air-filled cavity. If untreated, the swelling and fluid will together block conduction, cause severe pain and may eventually rupture the eardrum.

The acute condition is treated with antibiotics and analgesics.

Chronic serous otitis media
This is an accumulation of fluid in the middle ear accompanied by loss of hearing and discomfort, and is common in young children. It is usually a result of blockage of the auditory (eustachian) tube by enlarged adenoids (see Ch. 15) or swollen mucous membrane due to allergy or chronic infection.

The specific cause is identified and treated. The main aim is to ensure that the auditory tube is patent and can fulfil its role of ventilating the middle ear. In addition, it may be necessary to perform a *myringotomy* (opening into the eardrum from the external auditory meatus) to drain the fluid from the middle ear space. A plastic tympanostomy tube (*grommet*) may be inserted into this opening to permit continuous drainage and ventilation of the middle ear. The grommet usually stays in place for 2 or 3 weeks and then dislodges into the external auditory meatus and is discarded. By which time the cause of the original problem should be resolved.

NURSING MEASURES AFTER EAR SURGERY

There are certain specific considerations relating to the care of someone who has undergone ear surgery.

- The patient will need reassurance since, due to dressings blocking the external meatus, his hearing will not improve immediately.
- *Vertigo* (dizziness) is fairly common postoperatively due to disturbances in the balance mechanism of the inner ear, and therefore patients should be mobilised slowly and with full supervision until their stability is established.
- Following reconstructive surgery, patients should be advised against blowing the nose, sneezing with mouth closed, underground or air travel, or using lifts in high buildings, because internal and external pressure changes would dislodge grafts or prostheses. Swimming or getting water in the external meatus should also be avoided, especially where grommets are in situ.

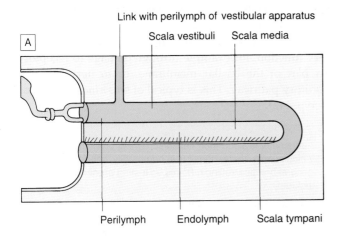

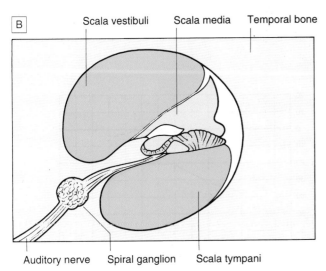

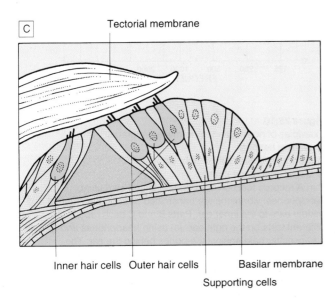

Figure 25.8

The inner ear (cochlea):

A Diagrammatic representation (uncoiled)
B Histological structure in cross-section
C The spiral organ (of Corti).

cilia of the outer hair cells are embedded in another membranous structure, the *tectorial membrane*, lying on top of them. When the basilar membrane vibrates, the cilia are bent first one way and then the other in time with the vibrations. This has the same effect on the auditory receptors as the bending of the cilia has on receptors in the vestibular apparatus. Bending in one direction excites the cells (depolarisation) whereas bending in the opposite direction inhibits them (hyperpolarisation) (see Ch. 24, Fig. 24.12, and Ch. 21).

Basilar membrane

The way in which the basilar membrane vibrates differs according to the frequency and amplitude of the sound waves. If the sound is of low frequency (e.g. 100 Hz), the whole membrane vibrates in time with the alternating pressure wave. Whereas, if the sound is of high frequency (e.g. 2000 Hz), then the part of the basilar membrane furthest away from the oval window does not move at all (Fig. 25.9). The higher the frequency the smaller is the length of membrane that vibrates.

The frequency of a sound wave therefore affects the pattern of impulses in the auditory neurones in two ways:

- by determining the frequency of nerve impulses
- by selecting which neurones are excited.

Both are important in coding the pitch of the sound we hear.

The *frequency code* is best for sound waves of low frequency (<1000 Hz). This is because the theoretical maximum frequency of impulses that neurones can transmit is 1000/second (i.e. 1000 Hz) (see refractory period; Ch. 21).

At frequencies greater than 1000 Hz, it is the *position* of the vibrations on the basilar membrane (Fig. 25.9) that matters most. Because of this, selective degeneration of auditory neurones, as in *presbyacusis*, tends to affect the detection of high frequency sounds more than those of low frequency.

Differences in the amplitude of the sound waves produce corresponding differences in the amplitude of

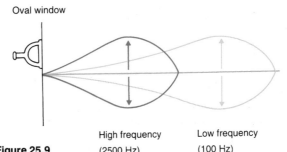

Figure 25.9

Patterns of vibration of the basilar membrane in response to sound waves of high and low frequency.

vibration of the basilar membrane. The larger the amplitude, the greater the number of receptors excited, and the louder is the sound we hear.

SENSITIVITY OF THE EAR

②

What kind of behaviour pattern might lead you to suspect that a person has a hearing deficit?

The human ear is sensitive to frequencies of sound ranging from about 20 to 20 000 Hz (20 kHz), but it is most sensitive between 1000 and 4000 Hz (1–4 kHz).

The sensitivity of the ear to sounds of different frequencies is measured by finding the minimum number of decibels needed for someone to just hear the sound under conditions in which there is very little or no background noise. The results obtained are plotted on a chart to give an *audiogram* (Fig. 25.10).

If the ear is obstructed, for example by wax, or if transmision of sound through the middle ear is impaired, then the intensity of the sounds that can just be heard are all greater than normal (Fig. 25.10B). This is typical of *conductive deafness* (see p. 442). In other cases of deafness only part of the audiogram may be abnormal (Fig. 25.10C). This indicates selective loss of auditory function, for example through damage to receptors on part of the basilar membrane, or to nerves in the auditory pathway. This is typical of *sensorineural deafness* (see p. 442). ②

Audiometry is a common health-screening procedure for which nurses are responsible in community, school and general practice settings. Points on testing procedure include:

- having a soundproof setting
- taking a careful health history
- giving clear instructions to the patient to ensure cooperation and true results (especially important with children and people who have an obvious hearing deficit).

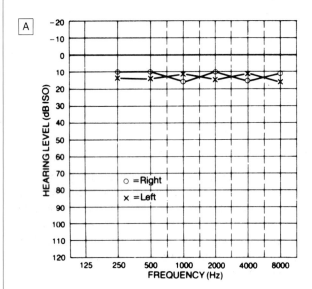

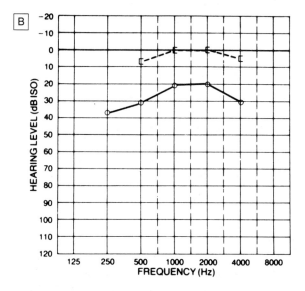

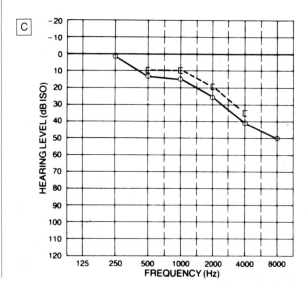

Figure 25.10
Examples of normal and abnormal audiograms:
A Normal hearing
B Conductive deafness in right ear
C Sensorineural deafness.
Part A records tests on right (o) and left (x) ears using headphones: vibrations are transmitted through the external and middle ears to the inner ear. Parts B and C each record two different tests on the right ear: (o) using headphones and ([) using a transmitter held against the bones behind the ear. The transmitter sends vibrations directly to the inner ear via bones in the skull.
In conductive deafness, the two different modes of testing give different results, whereas in sensorineural deafness they do not. (Reproduced from Freeland A P 1989 Deafness: the facts, Figures 4, 6 & 10, by permission of the author and Oxford University Press.)

AUDITORY PATHWAYS

The nerve pathways between the ear and the cerebral cortex (*auditory pathways*) are complex. There are many places at which synapses occur, and therefore at which analysis and modification of the information can occur (see Ch. 23). The main parts of the auditory pathway (Fig. 25.11) include:

- cochlear nucleus
- inferior colliculus
- superior olive
- thalamus.

Each part plays a different role in enabling us to become aware of, analyse and respond to sound waves detected by the ear.

> Excitation of cells of the auditory pathway and auditory cortex in the brain through disease processes or surgical intervention can result in an individual hearing noises that are not there. For example, gross hypertension or ear disease may be accompanied by buzzing noises or *tinnitus* (ringing in the ears).

HAIR CELLS AND SENSORY NEURONES

The majority of neurones in the auditory nerve (about 90%) are associated with the inner row of hair cells. Each of the inner cells is innervated by several sensory neurones, whereas several outer hair cells are all innervated by the same neurone. The cell bodies of all the sensory neurones are gathered together in the *spiral ganglion* (Figs 25.8B and 25.11).

An unusual feature of the auditory system is that the auditory receptors and sensory neurones are innervated by efferent neurones that control their sensitivity. These efferent neurones (*olivocochlear bundle*) originate in the *superior olives*, two nuclei in the medulla oblongata of the brain stem (see Ch. 20). The olivocochlear bundle is believed to play a part in enabling us to tune in to some sounds and to blot out others, for example when listening to conversation at a party.

COCHLEAR NUCLEUS

Nerve axons extend from the spiral ganglion to the *cochlear nucleus* on the same side of the head. The organisation of cells in this nucleus is related to the placing of the receptors along the basilar membrane and to the frequency of the sound (*tonotopic representation*). Cells responding best to a sound of high frequency are situated in one part of the nucleus whereas those responding best to another frequency are at a different place.

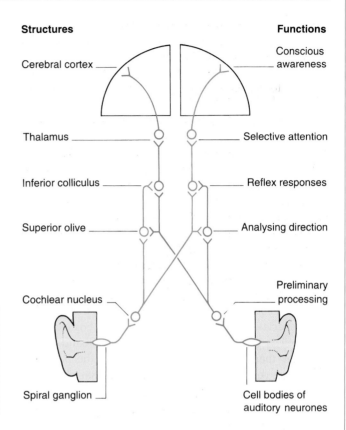

Structures   **Functions**

Cerebral cortex — Conscious awareness

Thalamus — Selective attention

Inferior colliculus — Reflex responses

Superior olive — Analysing direction

Cochlear nucleus — Preliminary processing

Spiral ganglion — Cell bodies of auditory neurones

Figure 25.11
The auditory pathway.

INFERIOR COLLICULUS

From the cochlear nuclei, nerve axons carry the impulses across to the opposite side of the brain either directly or indirectly to the *inferior colliculi*. These two clusters of neurones form part of the system enabling us to turn reflexly in response to a sudden sound. For example if someone cries out, you turn instinctively, to face the source of the sound.

> Someone who has suffered injury to the auditory cortex may still respond to a sudden sound, even though he may be unable to speak or to understand the meaning of the sound. This is because some auditory reflexes are mediated through centres such as the inferior colliculi in the brain stem rather than the higher centres of the cerebral hemispheres.

SUPERIOR OLIVE

One of the indirect pathways between the cochlear nucleus and the inferior colliculus is via the *superior olive*. This group of cells, one on each side of the medulla oblongata, receives an input from both ears. The superior olive probably makes some of the comparisons of sound from each ear that enable us to locate the source of a sound.

THALAMUS

From the inferior colliculi, impulses pass to the *medial geniculate nucleus* of the thalamus. The thalamus is thought to act as a filter for sensory signals and may play a role in selecting the sounds to which we pay attention. Some cells in the medial geniculate nucleus are known to have the property of responding less and less well to a sound that is repeated (*habituation*). In this way we become oblivious to familiar sounds while remaining alert to those that are new.

AUDITORY CORTEX

Nerve impulses reach the auditory areas in the temporal lobes of the cerebral hemispheres (Figs 25.11 and 25.12). The *primary auditory cortex* is the area which first receives the incoming impulses. Here the cells are still organised tonotopically to some extent but they possess more specialised and interesting features. For example, each cell is sensitive to a much narrower band of frequencies than the neurones before it on the pathway, and some cells respond best to sounds that change in pitch, either up or down.

Adjacent to the primary auditory cortex are *secondary auditory areas* in which cells are even more selective in their responsiveness. Some respond best to clicking sounds whereas others even respond selectively to one voice and not to another.

Next to these areas are the *auditory association areas* that play an important role in the understanding and interpretation of sounds (see Ch. 30).

③
What performance outcomes might lead you to suspect that a schoolchild has a hearing deficit?

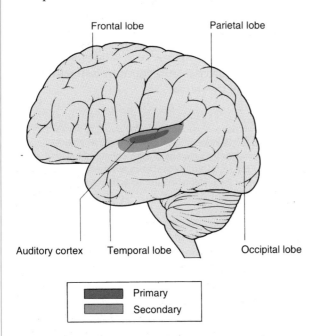

Frontal lobe   Parietal lobe

Auditory cortex   Temporal lobe   Occipital lobe

■ Primary
■ Secondary

Figure 25.12
Position of the auditory cortex in the cerebral hemispheres. (Only the left hemisphere is shown; the right auditory cortex in the right cerebral hemisphere is similar.)

ASSOCIATION AREAS: UNDERSTANDING AND INTERPRETING SOUNDS

Internalisation of familiar sound patterns relating to the context and environment in which we work, and subconscious recognition of changes to the normal pattern, is a phenomenon that is frequently illustrated in nursing. This is particularly true of the expert nurse who has thoroughly internalised the context in which she works. The brain is constantly and subconsciously monitoring sounds in the environment and has the ability to pick out and focus on anything that is different from the expected norm and bring it to conscious recognition.

An example of this is provided by an experienced nurse in a neonatal intensive care nursery where everything was apparently going smoothly as she addressed a group of students. In mid-sentence she stopped and went over to a nearby cot to adjust the control on a chest drain. Her well-attuned ear had picked up an abnormal bubbling pattern in the sound from the drainage bottle and her brain had registered its significance without any apparent conscious effort on her part. Nobody else had 'heard' anything different, nor would they have had the associations with which to interpret that difference had they done so.

DEAFNESS

There are many causes of deafness, some of which are easily treated, and some of which are not. The two main forms are:

- conductive deafness
- sensorineural deafness.

They may be distinguished by simple tests. ③

CONDUCTIVE DEAFNESS

Conductive deafness results when there is obstruction to the transmission of vibrations through the outer and middle parts of the ear. This may be due to a build-up of wax, or it could be due to damage to or disease of the lever system in the middle ear.

SENSORINEURAL DEAFNESS

In *sensorineural deafness*, conduction is normal but the generation and transmission of nerve impulses is impaired. Injury can occur at any level of the auditory pathway. Some common causes of sensorineural deafness are listed in Table 25.4.

The deafness associated with ageing (*presbyacusis*) is due to loss of neurones (see Ch. 36). These losses are greater if there has been repeated exposure to very loud sounds earlier in life (such as using a pneumatic drill, or listening to or playing amplified music at high volume).

Table 25.4 Some causes of sensorineural deafness

Cause	Examples	
	Circumstance	Person(s) affected
Microorganisms	Infection with the rubella virus during early pregnancy	Embryo and fetus
Hypoxia	Asphyxia at birth	Neonate
Antibiotics	Treatment with streptomycin, kanomycin, or quinine	Anyone
Intense sounds	Very loud disco music Personal stereos played at high volume Industrial machinery	Anyone
Uncertain*	Growing older	The elderly

* Cells degenerate and die but why is not known. It may be the result of accumulated exposure to noise throughout life (see Fig. 25.13).

Unfortunately, the serious effects of such exposure are not immediately obvious to the listener. Acute exposure to very loud sounds does cause an immediate decrease in the sensitivity of the ear to sound, but then hearing recovers. However, repeated exposure has cumulative, irreversible effects (Fig. 25.13).

In sensorineural deafness it is often the high frequency components of sound that are lost. This seriously affects the intelligibility of speech because hearing words properly depends crucially upon consonants. Consonants have many high frequency components. For example, the word 'soar' (Fig. 25.5) would be heard as 'oar' if the ear became relatively insensitive to frequencies above about 4 kHz, and would be confused easily with words like it, such as bore, core, door, store etc. ④

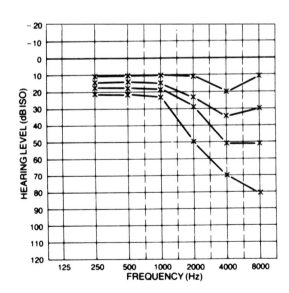

Figure 25.13
Progressive deafness due to years of exposure to dangerous noise. (Reproduced from Freeland A P 1989 Deafness: the facts, Figure 21, by permission of the author and Oxford University Press.)

CHARACTERISTICS OF IMPAIRED HEARING

Many people find hearing impairment embarrassing and are reluctant to admit to deafness, but the following behaviour patterns should alert family or health-care professionals to its presence:

- failure to respond when spoken to and lack of response to sounds that warn of danger in the environment (e.g. approaching traffic)
- straining towards the speaker and turning the better ear to catch what has been said, or requesting that it be repeated
- speaking more softly or more loudly than before
  - a person with conductive deafness will usually speak more softly than normal because he can hear himself through the vibrations from within
  - someone with sensorineural deafness will speak more loudly because damaged nerves cannot transmit sound waves and therefore he cannot hear himself
- developing a flat toneless voice
- a drop in the level of job performance in adults, and social withdrawal.

TESTS

Conductive deafness and sensorineural deafness can be distinguished by simple tests (Fig. 25.14). If the inner ear and the nerve pathways are normal then a person with conductive deafness will be able to hear the sound of a tuning fork if it is placed on the bone just behind the deaf ear. The vibrations bypass the outer and middle ear reaching the inner ear by being conducted through the bone of the skull. If the vibrating tuning fork is then placed on the forehead, assuming the other ear is normal, the sound will surprisingly appear to be loudest in the deaf ear. This is because the vibrations here are not masked by other environmental sounds.

In sensorineural deafness, however, the vibrating tuning fork is not heard either when it is sounded next

④ *An elderly patient complains that her hearing aid is not working, even though it is in good order. What do you think could be the matter?*

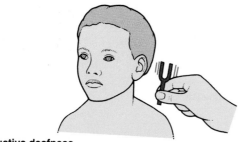

Conductive deafness

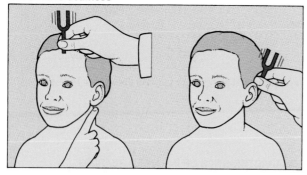

Sensorineural deafness

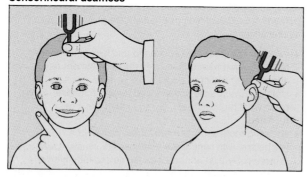

Figure 25.14
Determining the cause of a left ear deafness using simple tests with a tuning fork (usually 512 Hz – one octave above middle C).

to the deaf ear or when it is placed on the bone behind the ear. This is because the receptors and nerves are damaged, and consequently impulses cannot be transmitted properly to the cerebral cortex. If the vibrating tuning fork is placed on the forehead, its sound will be heard best in the ear opposite the deaf one.

KEY POINTS

What you should now know and understand about sound and hearing:

- the structure and function of different parts of the ear
- what sound waves are and how their energy is transformed into nerve impulses
- what a decibel is and the meaning of the decibel scale
- the frequencies of sound commonly present in the human voice and their importance in speech
- how our ability to hear, to listen and to respond to sounds depends on different parts of the brain
- different forms of deafness and how they may arise
- the basis of simple hearing tests.

REFERENCES AND FURTHER READING

Carpenter R H S 1984 Neurophysiology. Edward Arnold, London
Emslie-Smith D, Paterson C R, Scratcherd T, Read N W (eds) 1988 Textbook of physiology, 11th edn. Churchill Livingstone, Edinburgh
Fletcher H 1929 Speech and hearing. Macmillan, London
(An historically interesting book, lucidly describing the wealth of knowledge gained by researchers at the Bell Telephone Laboratories in the early days of telephone and radio)
Freeland A 1989 Deafness: the facts. Oxford University Press, Oxford
(Very readable paperback describing many of the causes of deafness, methods of testing and treatment)
Jahn A F, Santos-Sacchi J 1988 Physiology of the ear. Raven Press, New York
(Specialist book for reference, containing a wealth of information)
Loeb M 1986 Noise and human efficiency. John Wiley, Chichester
(Deals with the effects of noise on human performance. Useful for workplace managers as well as students of human biology)
Pickles J O 1988 An introduction to the physiology of hearing, 2nd edn. Academic Press, London
(Advanced very well referenced student text, describing the auditory system and its experimental investigation in detail)
Royle J A, Walsh M (eds) 1992 Watson's Medical–surgical nursing and related physiology. Baillière Tindall, London
Sataloff R T, Sataloff J 1993 Hearing loss, 3rd edn. Marcel Dekker, New York
(Very useful, clearly written reference book. Includes chapters on dizziness and facial paralysis)

Chapter 26
VISION

Vision is the sensation created in our minds as a result of the stimulation of sensory receptors in our eyes. The stimulus exciting the receptors is electromagnetic radiation.

The quality of the picture formed in our minds depends upon:

- the optics of the eye
- the photoreceptors in the retina
- the processing of information in the nervous system.

These things affect the detail we can see, how much illumination we need to be able to see, and whether the picture in our minds is in colour or in black and white.

In order to appreciate the impact of visual impairment on activities of daily living and develop your sensitivity, try the following exercise with a colleague. Blindfold her and then lead and talk her through all her usual daily activities. Discuss the effects of sensory deprivation and loss of functional and psychosocial independence from her perspective as the affected person, and from your perspective as the helper.

ELECTROMAGNETIC RADIATION

Electromagnetic radiation is the energy given out by excited atoms. The energy released depends on the nature of the atoms and on how excited they are. Often they have been excited by heat.

Forms of electromagnetic radiation range from low energy radio waves (long wavelength and low frequency) to very powerful cosmic rays (very short wavelength and high frequency) (Fig. 26.1). However, our eyes are sensitive only to a narrow band of radiation in the middle of this range (400–700 nm in wavelength). This is the *visible* part of the electromagnetic spectrum.

All forms of electromagnetic radiation travel at the same speed (about 1100 million km per hour), and in straight lines unless they are deflected by a surface (*reflection*) or slowed down by entering a medium that is denser than space or the atmosphere, in which case they bend (*refraction*) (Fig. 26.2). Short wave radiation is refracted more than long wave. This is why sunlight striking raindrops, and being refracted as it passes through them, gives rise to the rainbow. The electromagnetic radiation radiated by the sun contains a mixture of rays including those of the visible spectrum. Each of these is refracted to a different extent.

Radiation can pass straight through tissues or be absorbed by molecules within them. For example, X-rays penetrate soft tissues but are absorbed by bone,

---

Ultraviolet radiation from the sun is absorbed by the corneal epithelium, and overexposure can cause corneal damage. The ozone layer surrounding the earth normally acts as a filter to these harmful rays, but with its continuing depletion there is increasing danger of overexposure.

Additionally, if protective goggles are not worn, radiation damage can occur during sun-lamp treatment and the use of arc-welding equipment.

Examples		Wavelength (metres)	
		10 000	
Long wave (LW)	Radio waves	1000	1 km
Medium wave (MW)		100	
Short wave (SW)		10	
Television			
FM radio		1	1 m
Radar	Microwaves	10^{-1}	
Cooking		10^{-2}	
		10^{-3}	1 mm
Hot machinery	Infra-red rays	10^{-4}	
		10^{-5}	
Sunlight		10^{-6}	1 µm
	Ultraviolet rays	10^{-7}	
		10^{-8}	
	X-rays	10^{-9}	1 nm
Diagnostic imaging		10^{-10}	
		10^{-11}	
	Gamma rays	10^{-12}	1 pm
		10^{-13}	
		10^{-14}	
	Cosmic rays	10^{-15}	1 fm

Figure 26.1
Forms of electromagnetic radiation.

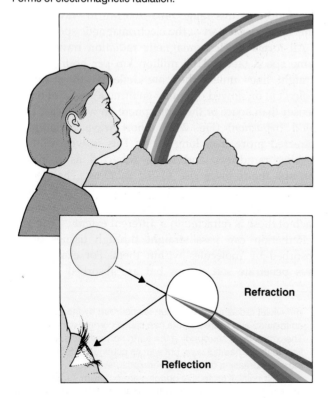

Figure 26.2
Reflection and refraction of electromagnetic radiation.

whereas micro-waves and infra-red rays are easily absorbed by soft tissue and do not penetrate very far (see Ch. 16, Fig. 16.3). The radiation of the visible spectrum is also absorbed by skin and underlying tissues but passes straight through tissues that are crystalline in structure, such as the cornea and lens of the eye.

THE EYE

The eye (Fig. 26.3) is housed within the orbit of the skull, protected by the eyelids, and kept moist by the fluid secreted by several glands, including the *lacrimal glands*. The optical structures of the eye, the *cornea*, the *lens* and the fluid-filled chambers in front of and behind the lens, are all normally transparent. Electromagnetic radiation is refracted as it passes through them to be focused on the light-sensitive surface (*retina*) at the rear of the eyeball.

PROTECTIVE STRUCTURES

Eyelids
The eyelids consist of two folds of tissue which meet at the *medial canthus* and *lateral canthus* (Fig. 26.4A). Each eyelid consists of connective tissue, muscle and small glands, and bears two or three rows of hairs (*eyelashes*). The inner side of each lid is covered by mucous membrane (*conjunctiva*) that extends over part of the eyeball.

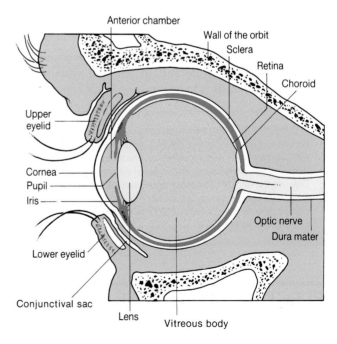

Figure 26.3
Structure of the eyeball and orbit. (Reproduced from Rogers 1992 (Fig. 23.2) by permission of the publishers.)

The space between the eyelids and the eyeball is the *conjunctival sac* (Fig. 26.3).

Lacrimal glands

The lacrimal glands lie under the upper eyelids (Fig. 26.4B) and secrete a watery solution containing anti-bacterial substances, including *lysozyme*. Secretion is increased by irritation of the cornea and conjunctiva, by a parasympathetic reflex. Fluid is swept over the cornea regularly by reflex blinking of the eyelids. Irritation provokes blinking and helps to protect and moisten the delicate tissue of the eyeball.

The fluid swept across the eyeball drains away through two small openings, close to the medial canthus, one in each eyelid (*lacrimal punctum*) (Fig. 26.4A). From the lacrimal punctum the fluid flows through a series of small vessels into the nasal cavity (Fig. 26.4B), which is why you need to blow your nose when you cry.

> The normal protective function of the eyelids may be lost when the eyes do not, or cannot, close and the blink reflex is absent, for example:
>
> - in the unconscious patient
> - in diseases affecting the eyelids, lacrimal system or facial muscles
> - when the corneal reflex is absent.
>
> In such cases, measures must be taken to ensure that the eyes are protected and the conjunctiva does not dry out.

OPTICAL STRUCTURES

Cornea

The cornea (Fig. 26.3) consists almost entirely of orderly layers of collagen fibres. The fibres in one layer run at 90° to those in the next forming a regular structure.

The front of the cornea is covered by a multilayered epithelium containing nerve endings but no blood vessels. The inner corneal surface is lined by a thin endothelium. The requirements of the cells in the epithelium and endothelium for nutrients and oxygen are met simply by the diffusion of these substances from the fluids of the eye or from the atmosphere. ①

The outer corneal surface is kept from drying out by the secretions formed by several glands:

- lacrimal glands – watery secretion
- tarsal glands of the eyelids – sebaceous secretion
- mucous glands of the inner lining of the eyelid – mucus.

This mixture is swept over the corneal surface regularly by the blinking action of the eyelids. ②

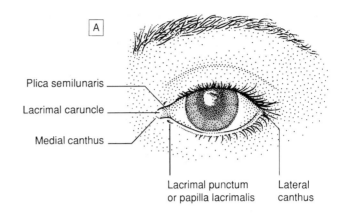

A

Plica semilunaris

Lacrimal caruncle

Medial canthus

Lacrimal punctum or papilla lacrimalis

Lateral canthus

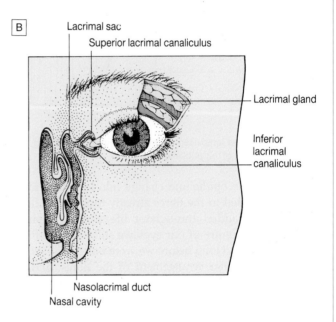

B

Lacrimal sac

Superior lacrimal canaliculus

Lacrimal gland

Inferior lacrimal canaliculus

Nasolacrimal duct

Nasal cavity

Figure 26.4
Protective structures of the eye:
A Eyelids
B Lacrimal glands and drainage system.
(Reproduced from Rogers 1992 (Figs 23.4 & 23.5) by permission of the publishers.)

> The cornea is very sensitive to touch, and it is important to note this especially when performing eye dressings and instilling drops and ointment. A gentle and light touch is essential during all ophthalmic procedures, and drops should be instilled into the outer aspect of the lower conjunctival sac and not dropped directly on to the cornea.

Lens

The lens (Fig. 26.5), unlike the cornea, is composed entirely of cells but the overwhelming majority are dead. They are very long (about 1.0 cm), thin (2 μm) fibres, stacked in an orderly way like very thin wafers in a packet. The fibres are packed full of proteins (*crystallins*). These fibres were formed originally from the living epithelium at the front of the lens. Cells at

① *What characteristic of the cornea enables many ophthalmic drugs to be effective when given as drops or ointment?*

② *Why are protective eye shields sometimes worn by staff in the operating theatre?*

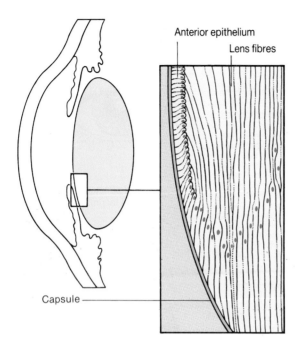

Figure 26.5
The structure of the lens. (Reproduced from Rogers 1992 (Fig. 23. 12) by permission of the publishers.)

the ends of the epithelium change into long thin fibres which are added to the fibres already there. New fibres go on being added throughout life, but increasingly slowly. In the centre of our eyes we still have the fibres that were formed long before we were born.

The very regular arrangement of the fibres, and the nature of the proteins inside them, makes the lens transparent. Opaque patches (*cataracts*) form when the nature and arrangement of the proteins change. Later on, calcium sometimes accumulates in the same area and this increases the opacity. The whole of the lens and the

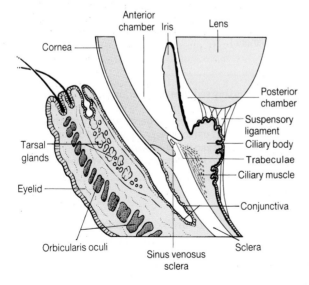

Figure 26.6
The sclerocorneal junction. (Reproduced from Rogers 1992 (Fig. 23.7) by permission of the publishers.)

CATARACTS AND CATARACT EXTRACTION: NURSING RESPONSIBILITIES

Opacity of the lens may be congenital or may develop as a result of the ageing process, injury or disease.

Where a cataract has developed, surgical removal of the opaque lens may be the treatment of choice to restore vision. There are several variations of this procedure, but basically either the whole lens or the contents of the lens capsule are removed. In the majority of cases, an intraocular lens implant (IOL) is used to replace the patient's own lens, but if implantation is not feasible the patient is fitted with aphakic spectacles, which have a thick lens that functions similarly to a normal lens.

Postoperatively, it is essential to observe the basic principles of asepsis, gentle handling and meticulous observation. Infection can result in permanent loss of sight; pressure can damage suture lines or displace IOLs; and meticulous and systematic observation for complications is important because timely intervention is critical in preserving sight.

The patient should be cautioned against rubbing his eyes and told to avoid bending down or lifting heavy objects until healing is complete, as these actions increase intraocular pressure which can cause haemorrhage or glaucoma (see p. 450).

---

epithelium is covered by a thin elastic covering of connective tissue (*capsule*).

The lens is held under tension by the *suspensory ligament* which encircles it and which is anchored to the *ciliary muscle* (Fig. 26.6). When the ciliary muscle contracts, the tension on the lens decreases and the lens *accommodates* by rounding up in shape. This alteration in shape changes the focusing power of the lens (see p. 449). As we get older the lens becomes less flexible and does not round up as much when the tension on the ligament is slackened. Consequently the focusing power cannot be altered to the same extent (see *Presbyopia*, p. 450).

Iris and pupil

Just in front of the lens is the *iris* (Figs 26.6 and 26.3). This is a ring of tissue that includes pigment cells and smooth muscle. The pigment absorbs light rays. The more pigment present, the darker the colour of someone's eyes. Some of the smooth muscle is arranged radially and some encircles the hole in the centre (*pupil*). Contraction of the smooth muscle is controlled by the autonomic nerves (Fig. 26.7):

- parasympathetic fibres constrict the pupil
- sympathetic fibres dilate it.

These autonomic nerves form part of the reflex system controlling the amount of light passing through the pupil to the retina. If the light reaching the retina increases, the pupil reflexly constricts (*pupillary light reflex*); if it decreases, the pupil dilates.

Fluids of the eye

The small spaces between the cornea and the lens (*anterior* and *posterior chambers*) (Fig. 26.6) are filled with a liquid, *aqueous humour*, whereas the the rest of the eyeball is filled with a jelly-like substance, *vitreous body*.

Aqueous humour

The aqueous humour is secreted continuously at the rate of about 2 ml per day by cells of the ciliary body. It flows up out of the posterior chamber, through the pupil into the anterior chamber and is reabsorbed through a meshwork of tiny bands of connective tissue (*trabeculae*), in the angle formed between the cornea and the iris, into a thin-walled vein (*sinus venosus sclera* or *canal of Schlemm*) (Fig. 26.6). If this drainage system is obstructed the fluid pressure (normally 12–20 mmHg) increases. This happens in *glaucoma* (see p. 450).

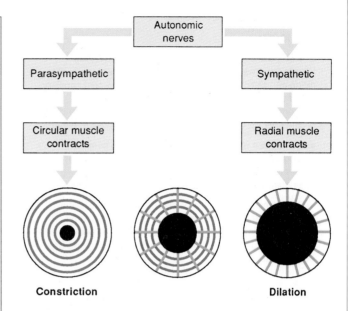

Figure 26.7
Control of pupillary size.

Vitreous body

The vitreous body consists of a jelly-like substance formed largely of hyaluronic acid (see Ch. 2), some collagen fibrils and water. The surface of the jelly is slightly firmer than the rest (rather like skin on custard) and is termed the *vitreous membrane*. This membrane is attached to the inside of the eyeball at two sites. At the front it is stuck to the membrane covering the ciliary body, and at the rear it is bonded to the rim of the optic disc (see p. 452).

FOCUSING THE IMAGE

Normal vision

For a clear image to be formed, the rays of light from an object must be focused on the retina in the same way

③

What immediate problem faces a patient who loses his aphakic glasses after having had a bilateral cataract extraction without lens implants?

GLAUCOMA

Glaucoma is a pathological condition in which raised intraocular pressure can cause irreparable damage to the retina and optic nerve head by restricting essential capillary blood supply. It is a major cause of blindness.

There are several different types of glaucoma depending on the specific cause, but basically they all relate to either:

- an increase in intraocular content, such as over-production of aqueous fluid, bleeding or products of infection; or
- an obstruction in the trabecular drainage mechanism.

Glaucoma may be acute or chronic. An acute onset is accompanied by severe pain, but in chronic glaucoma, where onset is gradual, the condition is initially painless and may be difficult to detect before considerable damage has been done.

Prevention of the effects of glaucoma can best be achieved through:

- regular screening of high-risk individuals and people over the age of 40 years
- meticulous monitoring of postoperative or traumatised patients.

Early detection means that treatment can be started sooner to reduce intraocular pressure.

Treatment depends on the cause, the principle being to reduce the amount of fluid secreted into the eye, or to improve the drainage of fluid out of the eye.

If the cause relates primarily to a defect in the drainage system:

- eyedrops may be used to constrict the pupil and so stretch and open up the trabecular meshwork (e.g. pilocarpine)
- the trabecular meshwork may be opened up by various surgical procedures, creating additional drainage channels (e.g. *trabeculectomy*)
- laser treatment to the trabecular meshwork causes scarring which stretches the tissue between the laser burns and opens the spaces in the trabecular meshwork, thus allowing quicker drainage (*trabeculoplasty*).

If the cause relates primarily to over-production of aqueous humour, the treatment will be medical, using either eyedrops, such as timolol, or oral medication to inhibit production.

If the cause is trauma or surgery, then a combination of measures will be used.

---

that the lens of a camera focuses light rays on to a film. The cornea and the lens are the focusing system of the eye. They refract light rays because of their density and their shapes. The greater their density and their curvature, the greater is their focusing power, measured in *dioptres*.

Cornea

The cornea alone has a focusing power of about 43 dioptres, but this is not enough to focus the light rays sharply on the retina.

Lens

The lens contributes about another 17 to 31 dioptres depending on its shape. At its flattest it contributes an extra 17 dioptres which is sufficient to create a sharp image of a distant object on the retina in a normal eye (*emmetropic eye*). By rounding up, when the ciliary muscle contracts, another 12 to 14 dioptres is added enabling near objects (up to about 10 cm from the eye) to be seen clearly. ③

Myopia and hypermetropia

In some people, the focusing power of the cornea and lens is not well matched to the length of the eyeball. Consequently light rays are brought to a focus either in front of or behind the retina (Fig. 26.8). In either case the image formed is blurred. In *myopia* (short sight) the system is more powerful than normal. Consequently objects can be brought closer to the eye than normal and are seen in more detail but objects at a distance are out of focus. Conversely in *hypermetropia* (long sight), the system is less powerful than normal. As a result distant objects can be seen clearly but close work becomes a problem. Both myopia and hypermetropia can be corrected by lenses of the right optical form and power (Fig. 26.8).

Optical tests

A few simple tests and observations can reveal whether the optical system is normal. These include:

- test charts and objects
- ophthalmoscopy.

Test charts and objects

There are a number of different test charts of which the most common is the *Snellen chart*. This consists of a series of letters of different sizes, which are viewed from a set distance of 6 metres (Fig. 26.9). Each line of letters

PRESBYOPIA

The lens stiffens with age and, as a result, adjusting the focusing power of the eye to the requirements of far and near vision becomes a problem. The nearest point to the eye (near point) that an object can be seen perfectly in focus gets further away. This is termed *presbyopia*. It becomes noticeable after the age of about 40 years. Individuals then find that books and newspapers have to be held further away to be read. Mature students approaching middle years may also find that taking notes in a large lecture theatre becomes a problem because refocusing, from the board to your notebook and back, takes longer than it used to do. Ultimately the lens becomes so stiff that it cannot accommodate at all. It then has a fixed focal power. Some people then need to wear bifocals, or graduated lenses allowing them to focus on distant or near objects according to need.

ASTIGMATISM

In astigmatism, the refraction of light rays by either the cornea or the lens is uneven because of irregularities in the shape of these structures. The consequence is that the image is unevenly focused. Some lines appear sharp whereas others are not. Usually the problem arises because the cornea is not perfectly convex. Instead of being shaped like a section of a ball, it may be slightly more oval (more like a rugby ball than a football). This kind of astigmatism can be corrected by using a lens (cylindrical) that compensates for the unusual dimensions. If astigmatism is mild it can also be corrected by contact lenses as these are perfectly convex in shape.

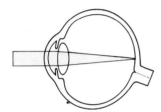

Myopia

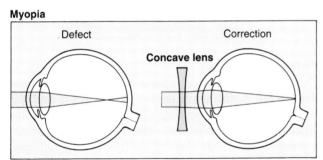

Hypermetropia

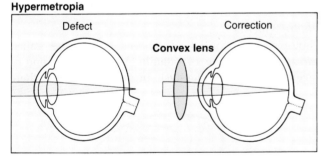

Figure 26.8
Optical problems and their correction.

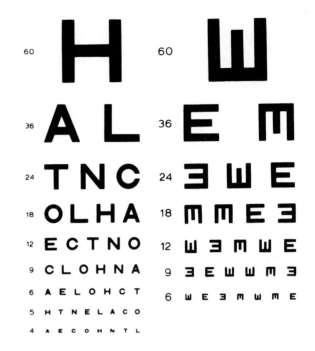

Figure 26.9
Snellen letter and illiterate E test-types. (Reproduced from Parr J 1989 Introduction to ophthalmology, 3rd edn, Figure 3-14, by permission of Oxford University Press.)

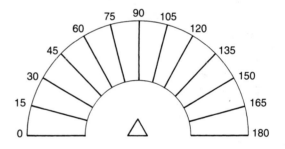

Figure 26.10
Fan of lines used to test for astigmatism.

has a number against it indicating the distance at which someone with normal vision should be able to read those letters. If vision is normal then the line of small letters marked '6' (i.e. 6 metres) should be readable without any mistakes. This is 6/6 vision, meaning that from a distance of 6 metres, the smallest size of lettering that can be seen clearly is the 6-metre line. If, however, only the large letters on the 18-metre line can be read without fault, as may be the case if someone is *myopic*, vision is said to be 6/18. *Acuity* of vision is then said to be less than normal.

Another test object included in the equipment is the *astigmatic* fan (Fig. 26.10). A person with astigmatism will see some lines of this fan as distinctly black, and others as greyish. By noting which appear blackest, an optician can tell how the cylindrical lens should be oriented in order to correct the optical fault.

Ophthalmoscopy

Usually an optometrist or an ophthalmologist will take a look at the structures inside the eyeball using an ophthalmoscope. This instrument enables a small beam of light to be shone into the eye. The rays reflected off the structures inside are focused by a series of lenses in the head of the instrument. By altering the focus, different parts of the eye, including the retina, and the surfaces of the cornea and lens can all be inspected (see p. 452). ④

④
In a slip of the pen a student wrote, 'The eye examination room should be well alight.' Having spotted the obvious, would you still agree with him? What are your reasons?

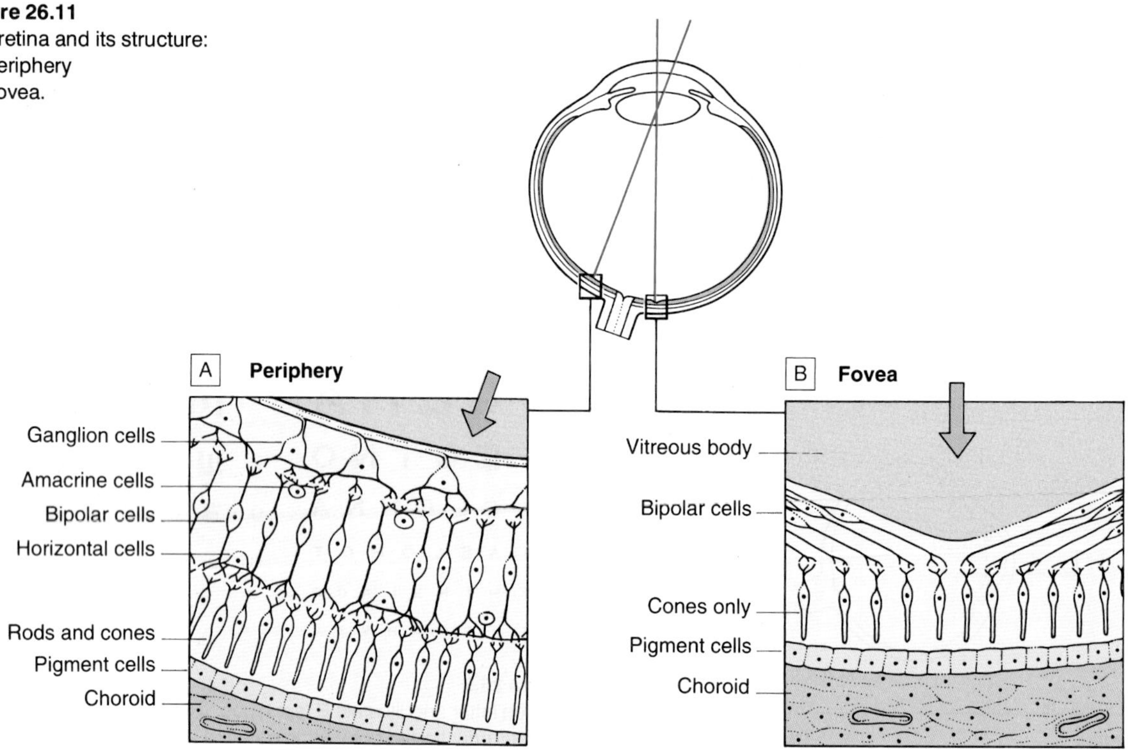

Figure 26.11
The retina and its structure:
A Periphery
B Fovea.

A **Periphery**

Ganglion cells
Amacrine cells
Bipolar cells
Horizontal cells

Rods and cones
Pigment cells
Choroid

B **Fovea**

Vitreous body
Bipolar cells

Cones only
Pigment cells
Choroid

RETINA

The retina (Fig. 26.11) is a thin film of tissue lining most of the inside of the eyeball. It contains:

- blood vessels
- photoreceptors
- nerve cells
- pigment cells.

Viewed through an ophthalmoscope (Fig. 26.12), the retina looks an orangey-red colour. This is because of its blood supply and pigments, together with those of the choroid beneath it. In one part, a whitish patch can be seen (*optic disc*). This consists of axons of the optic nerve, and is the site where these axons leave the eyeball. The disc appears white because the axons here are myelinated (see myelin, Ch. 21).

From the optic disc, blood vessels extend outwards over the surface of the retina. The arteries are narrower than the darker veins. One area does not have any large blood vessels crossing it and appears slightly different in colour (*macula lutea* meaning 'yellow spot'). In its centre is a small depression, the *fovea*.

Patients who have developed acquired immune deficiency syndrome (AIDS) may present with retinitis involving intraretinal haemorrhage and necrosis. The cause is often cytomegalovirus, which may in some cases respond to antiviral agents, for example acyclovir. When AIDS patients present for ophthalmic treatment or for fitting of contact lenses, it is important to note that the human immunodeficiency virus is present in tears, and precautions should be taken as for contact with any other body fluids.

Photoreceptors

There are two types of photoreceptor: *rods* and *cones* (Fig. 26.13). A distinctive feature of both is the multiple layers of membrane stacked closely one on top of the other at one end of the cell. These membranes contain a photopigment that absorbs electromagnetic radiation and activates the receptor.

Photopigments

Photopigments consist of *retinene* (sometimes called *retinal*), a derivative of vitamin A, coupled to one of several lipoproteins (*opsins*). In the human eye there

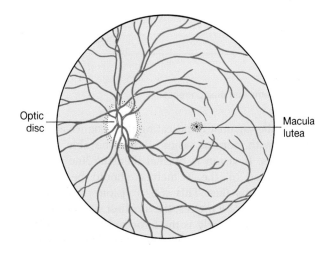

Optic disc

Macula lutea

Figure 26.12
The retina viewed through an ophthalmoscope. (Reproduced from Rogers 1992 (Fig. 23.11) by permission of the publishers.)

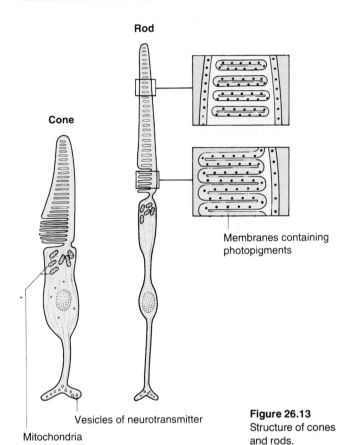

Figure 26.13
Structure of cones and rods.

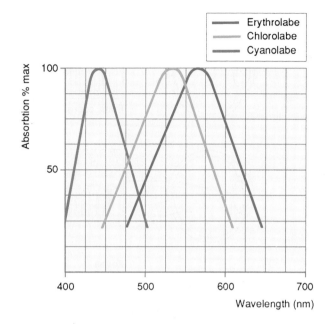

Figure 26.14
Spectral sensitivity of cone pigments. (Based on Marks et al 1964, and Brown & Wald 1964.)

are four different lipoproteins creating four different photopigments:

- *rhodopsin* in the rods
- *erythrolabe, chlorolabe,* and *cyanolabe* in the cones.

Only one type of photopigment is present in each cone.

Each pigment is best at absorbing light rays of a particular range of wavelengths (Fig. 26.14). These ranges overlap. Consequently, rays of one wavelength are absorbed by more than one photopigment, but to differing extents. For example, 580 nm rays are absorbed by both erythrolabe and chlorolabe, but not by cyanolabe.

The sensation of colour is created by the blend of signals generated by the three different types of cone. If one or more types of cone are absent from the retina or lack photopigment then our perception of colour changes (*colour blindness*). Some colours may not be seen at all; others are confused. ⑤

Activation

Absorption of light rays by the photopigment changes the shape of the opsin, which in turn affects ion channels in the membrane, and alters the membrane voltage (see Ch. 21). This triggers the release of neurotransmitter from tiny vesicles in the receptor cells (Fig. 26.13). The neurotransmitter diffuses across the synaptic cleft to activate the adjacent bipolar cell.

COLOUR BLINDNESS

Colour blindness is common among men (8% of the male population; 0.4% of females). It is usually genetic in origin and is carried on the X chromosome (see Ch. 35). The most common form encountered is red–green blindness. Affected individuals confuse greens and reds, but have no difficulty at all with blues and yellows. Usually, red–green blindness is due to a deficiency of chlorolabe (*deuteranomaly*), but it can be due to complete absence of the green or red cones (*deuteranopia* and *protanopia* respectively) or to a deficiency of erythrolabe (*protanomaly*).

Colour vision can be tested very simply. Individuals are asked to match pieces of differently coloured wool from a selection given to them, or are asked to say what numbers or symbols can be seen in pictures composed of a variety of carefully selected coloured spots (Ishihara colour charts). The matches that are made between wools and the numbers and symbols that are seen or not seen in the Ishihara charts reveal any differences from normal.

Innervation

Rods and cones are innervated by bipolar cells but whereas a large number of rods may all be innervated by the same cell, cone cells are sometimes individually innervated (Fig. 26.15). This is characteristic of the cones in the fovea. This difference in innervation is one of the reasons why objects that we look at directly (using the fovea) appear much more detailed than objects seen out of the corner of our eyes (peripheral field of vision).

The bipolar cells pass on the signal to the ganglion cells. These generate action potentials (see Ch. 21) which are transmitted in the nerve fibres of the optic nerve.

⑤
Would colour blindness present any problems in carrying out your nursing duties?

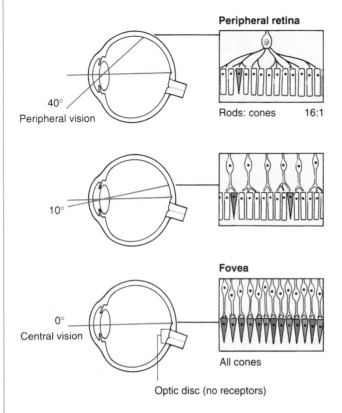

Figure 26.15
Differences in the innervation and distribution of rods and cones at the fovea compared with two peripheral areas of the retina.

Distribution

There is an uneven distribution of rods and cones in the retina (Fig. 26.15). The fovea has cones only, most of which are of the red or green type. Away from the fovea the number of cones decreases dramatically and the number of rods increases. There are no receptors of any type at the optic disc. As explained earlier this part of the eye just contains the axons of the optic nerve. The absence of receptors here creates a small *blind spot* in our field of vision.

You can demonstrate this if you close your right eye and look straight at the patient in Figure 26.16. Now move the book gradually backwards and forwards, whilst still keeping your eye on the patient. You should find a point where the bedpan disappears!

SEEING IN BRIGHT SUNSHINE AND AT NIGHT

The many differences between rods and cones in structure, innervation and distribution, give rise to the different qualities of vision characteristic of vision at night and in daylight. At night, images are not very distinct and lack colour, whereas in bright sunshine objects glow with colour and appear very sharp. At night there is only enough light to excite the rod system, whereas in daylight the cones come into action. The rod system produces an indistinct monochrome image, whereas the cone system, with its three pigments and discrete innervation, creates a colourful, detailed picture.

If we go from bright sunshine into a darkened room, at first all seems black, and we see little, if anything. Gradually, however, our eyes adjust and we begin to make out objects in the room even though the image is indistinct. In bright sunshine the rod vision system, which requires very little light to be activated, has been overwhelmed by the amount of light. So much of the rhodopsin is activated by the bright light that there is very little pigment left in its original state to respond to the small amount of light in a darkened room. Gradually, however, the rhodopsin is regenerated, receptor sensitivity is restored, and we are able to see, albeit indistinctly. The cones adapt as well, so some colour may appear, but this depends on how much light there is in the room.

Nerve cells

The nerve cells in the retina form quite a complex system (Fig. 26.11). At least four different types of cell are present:

- ganglion cells
- bipolar cells
- amacrine cells
- horizontal cells.

The *ganglion* cells are the cells whose axons form the optic nerve (cranial nerve II). The axons lie on the surface of the retina, and are bundled together to form the optic nerve at the optic disc.

The *bipolar cells* are beneath the ganglion cells. They link the ganglion cells with the photoreceptors below. Running horizontally across the retina, the *amacrine cells* and *horizontal cells* allow there to be some communication between adjacent receptors and also between ganglion cells.

Fovea

At the fovea, the structure of the retina looks slightly different (Fig. 26.11B). All the components are present,

Figure 26.16
The blind spot!

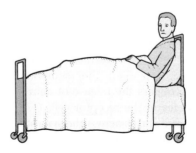

but the bipolar cells and ganglion cells appear to be pushed away from the centre, leaving the photoreceptors more exposed than at any other part of the retina.

Pigment cells and choroid

Beneath all these layers of cells is a *pigment cell layer.* This absorbs electromagnetic radiation that passes through the photoreceptor layer, and limits the amount of radiation that gets through to the *choroid* beneath.

The choroid also contains many pigment cells as well as blood vessels and connective tissue. It performs an important role in nourishing and maintaining the photoreceptors and the pigment cell layer.

The degree of pigmentation of the pigment cell layer and the choroid varies between people and is normally related to skin colour.

Age-related macular degeneration is the major cause of blindness in the elderly in developed countries. Retinal pigment epithelial (RPE) cells wear out with age and are never replaced. Areas where there has been cell loss will eventually shrink and pigment may be dispersed into the macula. This will affect form and colour vision first. With progressive deterioration, abnormal blood vessel membranes may develop from the choroid. These tend to leak fluid behind the central retina and cause distorted and blurred vision.

VISUAL PATHWAYS

The optic nerves from each eye meet up at the *optic chiasma* (Fig. 26.17). Here the nerve fibres carrying signals from the nasal half of the retina cross over to the other side, so that information about objects on the right-hand side of the scene we are looking at (*right visual field*) is carried over to the left side of the brain and vice versa. If injury occurs to the visual pathway on one side of the brain after the chiasma, there will be loss of vision in one half of the visual field of both eyes (Fig. 26.17, B).

From the chiasma, impulses are transmitted to the midbrain to evoke several visual reflexes and to the thalamus and the visual cortex in the cerebral hemispheres to give rise to the sensations of light, colour and movement.

MIDBRAIN

After the optic chiasma, some fibres branch off the optic tract to go to parts of the *pretectal region* and to the *superior colliculi*. These areas are concerned with several visual reflexes including the *pupillary light reflex*, and reflex eye and head movements (see Ch. 29).

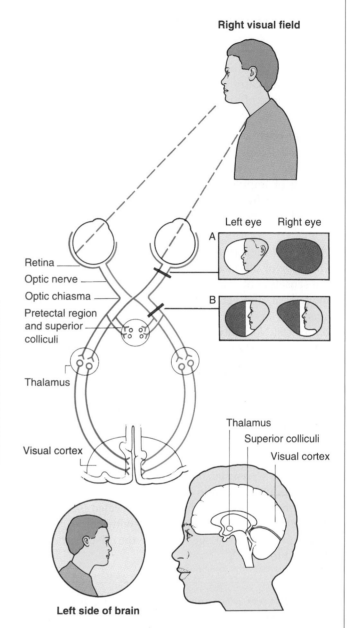

Figure 26.17
Visual pathways showing how the right side of our field of view is represented in the left visual cortex and the resulting effects of lesions of the pathway on vision in each eye: (A) lesion of right optic nerve – loss of vision in right eye; (B) lesion of the right optic tract beyond the chiasma – loss of vision in left visual field of both eyes.

Pupillary light reflex

When light is shone into either or both of the two eyes the pupils normally constrict. Because this reflex is coordinated in the midbrain and not further along the visual pathway it can be evoked in someone who has cortical brain damage. If the visual cortex itself is damaged, someone is unable to see even though the pupillary light reflex is present.

CEREBRAL HEMISPHERES

Axons of the retinal ganglion cells pass to the thalamus in each cerebral hemisphere. From there another set of nerve fibres carry the signals to the visual cortex in the occipital lobe of each hemisphere.

Visual cortex

The visual cortex is made up of a number of different areas, each of which plays a different role in the processing of impulses from the eyes. Each area receives information from both eyes (*binocular vision*) creating a three-dimensional (3D) mental picture of what we see.

Areas and their functions

One area of the visual cortex, referred to as V4, creates the sensation of colour, another creates an awareness of movement, and yet another, the *primary visual cortex* or *striate cortex*, is primarily concerned with the shape of objects. Normally these areas are interlinked, and so the features they represent are fused in our minds. However, if they become disconnected, or if one area is damaged, there can be curious disturbances of perception, such as seeing objects but not properly following their movement.

In each of the different areas, adjacent cells receive signals from adjacent areas of the retina, so that each area of the visual cortex is like a map of the retina (*retinotopic representation*). However, the map is not to scale, because it relates to the number of receptors in the retina and the way they are innervated (see p. 453). As the fovea is richly innervated with nerve fibres, a disproportionately large area of the visual cortex is devoted to it.

> If specific cells in the visual cortex are irritated, perhaps by local spasm of the blood vessels, bright lights are seen in the area of the visual field from which those cortical cells would normally expect to receive impulses.

Binocular vision

When we look at an object close to us, the image of it seen by each eye is not exactly the same. Although the differences are minimised by the way in which our two eyes are caused to swivel inwards, as part of the near response (see Ch. 29) so that the image falls on the fovea in each eye, they are not eliminated because each eye views the object from a slightly different perspective (Fig. 26.18).

We actually see both pictures although we think we are only looking at one, and as a result we gain the impression of depth and perceive three dimensions rather than two.

Controlling the movement of both eyes accurately is

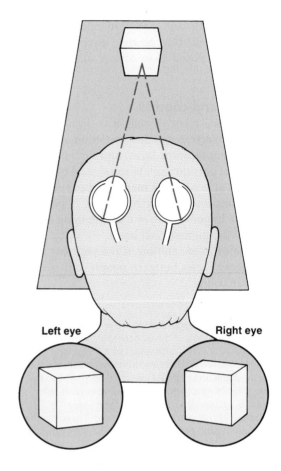

Figure 26.18
Binocular vision.

extremely important for vision. The systems involved and problems that can arise are described in Chapter 29.

> Monocular vision with loss of depth perception may be a result of blindness in one eye, padding occluding an eye, or eyedrops that affect accommodation or the pupillary reflex, and the patient may need to be cautioned about potential hazards. Things will not be exactly where they appear to be and driving especially is contraindicated until adaptation has taken place and the patient has relearned distance perception.

VIEWPOINT

All that has been described begins to reveal how an image is created in our minds, but it does not explain how we know what we are looking at. The black and white picture shown in Figure 26.19 makes this clear. What do you see? Your retina and visual cortex analyse the pattern of light and dark, and create a mental image

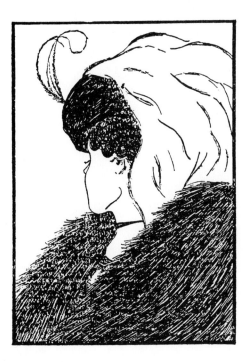

Figure 26.19
Drawing made by the cartoonist A. E. Hill in 1915.

of it. But did you see a young person or an old lady when you first looked at the picture? Your answer will depend on the links (*associations*) formed in your mind between that pattern of black and white and other images remembered from the past (see Chs 30 and 33).

REFERENCES AND FURTHER READING

Boring E G 1930 Apparatus notes: a new ambiguous figure. American Journal of Psychology 42: 444
(The first scientific article to draw attention to Hill's cartoon and its significance for understanding how the mind works)
Brown P K, Wald G 1964 Visual pigments of single primate cones. Science 144: 45–82
Davson H 1990 Physiology of the eye, 5th edn. Macmillan Press, Basingstoke
(Authoritative, clear, magnum text covering all aspects of ophthalmology in detail. Extremely useful for further information)
Elkington A R, Khan P T 1988 ABC of eyes. British Medical Association, London
(Collection of short clinically related articles from the British Medical Journal)
Gaston H, Elkington A 1986 Ophthalmology for nurses. Chapman & Hall, London
(Clearly presented, well-illustrated, concise book)
Hill W E 1915 My wife and mother-in-law. Puck, Week ending November 6
(The original publication of this now very familiar cartoon)
Marks W B, Dobelle W H, MacNichol E F 1964 Visual pigments of single primate cones. Science 143: 1181–1183
Parr J 1989 Introduction to ophthalmology, 3rd edn. Oxford University Press, Oxford
(Clear, concise book covering the anatomy, physiology and optics of vision, as well as the basis of clinical examination and common eye problems)
Perry J P, Tullo A B (eds) 1990 Care of the ophthalmic patient: a guide for nurses and health professionals. Chapman & Hall, London
Rogers A W 1992 Textbook of anatomy. Churchill Livingstone, Edinburgh, p 341, 342, 343, 345, 349

Chapter 27
MOTOR SYSTEMS: AN OVERVIEW

When skeletal muscle contracts it causes movement of parts of the skeleton, for example lifting a leg or bending the neck, or it stiffens and supports different structures, for example tensing the abdominal wall or holding the head up.

Movement usually involves the coordinated activity of different muscles. The simplest form of coordination occurs in reflex movements. These are chiefly mediated via the spinal cord and brain stem. The more complex movements we make when we choose to perform various actions involve other parts of the central nervous system including the motor cortex and basal ganglia of the cerebral hemispheres, and the cerebellum (Fig. 27.1).

REFLEX MOVEMENTS

A reflex is an automatic response triggered by a stimulus. It happens without our thinking about it. It can be simple, like a knee jerk, or more complicated, such as maintaining your balance if you are pushed. Simple reflexes involve just a few sensory receptors and a few muscle groups. Complex reflexes draw upon sensory information from several sources and coordinate activity in many different muscles. A few different reflexes are illustrated in Figure 27.2. ①

ORGANISATION AND TERMINOLOGY

The basic components of a reflex are shown in Figure 27.3. A reflex arc consists of a sensory part and a motor part, linked usually by connecting neurones (*interneurones*). When the sensory receptor is excited,

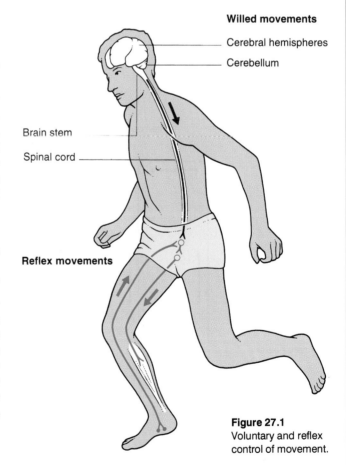

Willed movements
— Cerebral hemispheres
— Cerebellum

Brain stem
Spinal cord

Reflex movements

Figure 27.1
Voluntary and reflex control of movement.

① *What other reflexes can you think of?*

impulses are transmitted to the motoneurones exciting the muscle and causing it to contract.

Muscles that, on contraction, cause extension of a limb are termed *extensors* whereas those that cause flexion are termed *flexors* (Fig. 27.4). Hence some reflexes are

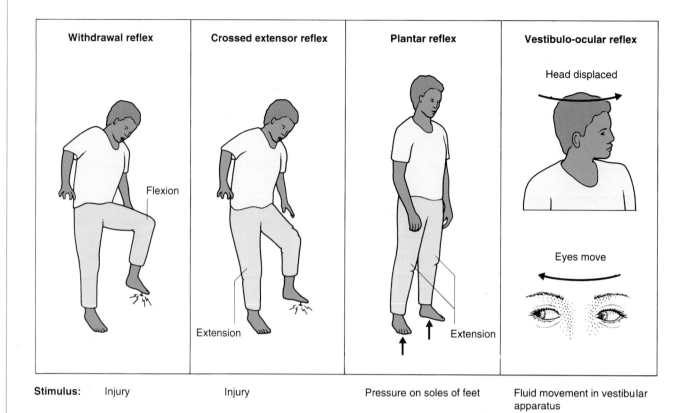

	Withdrawal reflex	Crossed extensor reflex	Plantar reflex	Vestibulo-ocular reflex
	Flexion	Extension	Extension	Head displaced / Eyes move
Stimulus:	Injury	Injury	Pressure on soles of feet	Fluid movement in vestibular apparatus
Function:	Protection	Maintaining balance	Maintaining upright posture	Maintaining observation

Figure 27.2
Examples of reflexes.

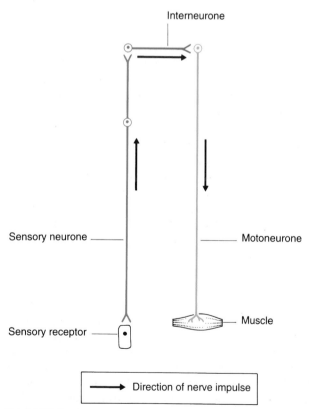

Figure 27.3
Basic components of a reflex arc.

Interneurone

Sensory neurone — Motoneurone

Sensory receptor — Muscle

→ Direction of nerve impulse

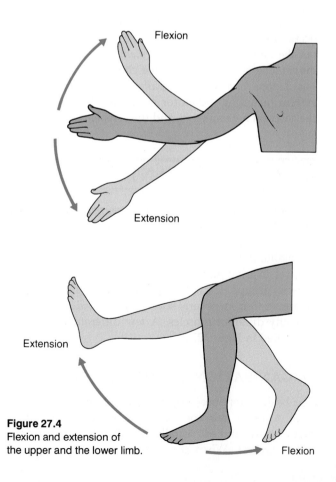

Figure 27.4
Flexion and extension of the upper and the lower limb.

Flexion

Extension

Extension

Flexion

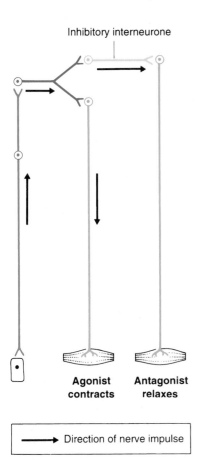

Figure 27.5
Reciprocal innervation of agonist and antagonist muscles.

Inhibitory interneurone

Agonist contracts   **Antagonist relaxes**

→ Direction of nerve impulse

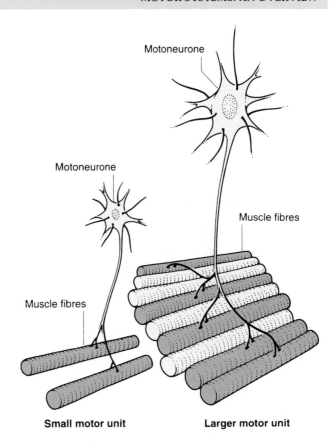

Motoneurone

Motoneurone

Muscle fibres

Muscle fibres

Small motor unit   **Larger motor unit**

Figure 27.6
Motor units of different size (a motor unit is a motoneurone plus all the muscle fibres it innervates).

referred to as 'extensor', for example the plantar reflex, whereas others are termed 'flexor', for example the withdrawal reflex (Fig. 27.2).

Muscles acting in opposite ways at a joint are referred to as the *agonist* and *antagonist* respectively. For example the biceps and triceps muscles of the upper arm operate as an agonist/antagonist pair. Contraction of the biceps flexes the arm; contraction of the triceps extends it (Fig. 27.4). The *agonist* muscle is defined as the one which by contraction causes movement. Thus when the arm is flexed the agonist is the biceps; when the arm is extended the agonist is the triceps.

When the agonist is excited, contraction of *antagonist* muscles is often, but not always, inhibited. The way in which agonist and antagonist muscles are linked into the reflex arc (*reciprocal innervation*) enables them to react in opposite ways to the same stimulus (Fig. 27.5).

SIZE OF THE RESPONSE

Order of recruitment of motor units

When a muscle, such as the biceps, is activated, all its motor units (Fig. 27.6 and Ch. 22) are not usually active at the same time. If the stimulus is small only the smallest motor units are excited. As the stimulus increases in size larger motor units are coopted (*recruited*). Eventually, at maximum contraction, all motor units are participating. This set order of recruitment of the units is determined by how closely packed together the synaptic contacts are on the motoneurones. The smallest motor units are innervated by motoneurones with the smallest cell bodies. In these cells the synapses are very close to one another on the cell body in the central nervous system (Fig. 27.6). This makes it easy for the motoneurones to be excited (see spatial summation, Ch. 21). On the larger cell bodies of the motoneurones of the large motor units the synapses are more spaced out, and many more stimuli are needed to excite the motoneurone.

Spread of excitation

The nerve terminals of the sensory axons and of the interneurones make many synaptic contacts in the brain and in the spinal cord, some of which connect with motoneurones supplying other muscles. If the original stimulus is weak, then only a few muscles are reflexly excited and the movement evoked is small. If the stimulus is stronger, other interneurones and motoneurones are *recruited* and more muscles are activated. This is known as *irradiation* of the stimulus. For example if you

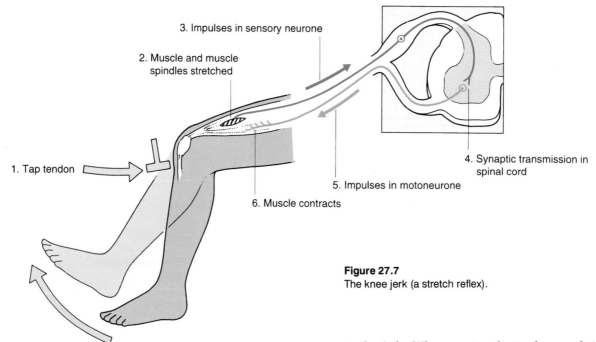

3. Impulses in sensory neurone

2. Muscle and muscle spindles stretched

1. Tap tendon

4. Synaptic transmission in spinal cord

5. Impulses in motoneurone

6. Muscle contracts

7. Leg kicks

Figure 27.7
The knee jerk (a stretch reflex).

touch something hot you may simply withdraw your hand. Only muscles of the arm are excited. But if the stimulus was very large you would probably react by pulling your whole body away. In this case muscles of the trunk and legs would be reflexly excited as well. ②

②
How might an understanding of recruitment and irradiation help the nursing care of a patient with tetanus as the result of an infected wound?

③
What is an ankle jerk? Why might a neurologist want to test this reflex?

> Recruitment of neurones and irradiation of the stimulus are particularly evident in Jacksonian fits. These are focal epileptic seizures which may be caused by cerebral tumours, vascular lesions or an abscess. The 'fit' progresses in a stereotyped manner; for example jerky, spasmodic movements (*clonic spasms*) starting in the thumb and index finger may spread to the hand and arm and perhaps to the rest of the body. The individual may also lose consciousness depending on the extent of the cerebral cortex involved.

MUSCLE TONE AND THE STRETCH REFLEX

Definition and basis

If you lift someone's arm or leg and gently flex and extend it you should feel a very slight resistance. This resistance to movement is termed *muscle tone*. It is due to the reflex contraction of the muscles of the limb you have flexed and extended (*stretch reflex*), in response to the excitation of sensory receptors (*muscle spindles*; see Ch. 24) embedded in the muscle.

You can elicit a stretch reflex too if you tap the patellar tendon just below the kneecap (Fig. 27.7). For this reason stretch reflexes are sometimes referred to as *tendon jerks*. When you tap the tendon you briefly stretch the muscle of the thigh, *quadriceps femoris*, and this stretch excites the muscle spindles. This provokes reflex contraction of the same muscle. Similarly, when you flex someone's leg you stimulate the spindles in the thigh muscles and cause a small reflex contraction of these muscles, which causes the slight resistance to movement that you sense. ③

The degree of resistance felt depends upon the sensitivity of the muscle spindles. If their sensitivity to stretch is high they respond much more vigorously and evoke a much stronger reflex contraction of the muscle. Consequently resistance to passive movement is high (*hypertonia*). Conversely, if the sensitivity of the spindles to stretch is low, very little if any resistance will be felt. As a result the limb will feel limp (*hypotonia*).

> If a nerve supplying muscles of the arm or leg has been severed as a result of an accident, the affected limb will feel very limp in comparison with the uninjured limbs. This is because impulses can no longer pass either to or from the muscles and consequently stretch reflexes cannot occur.

Sensitivity of muscle spindles

The sensitivity of the muscle spindles is controlled by small motoneurones (*gamma motoneurones*) that innervate the muscular part of the intrafusal fibres of the muscle spindle (see Ch. 24). The cell bodies of the gamma motoneurones are intermingled in the anterior (ventral) horn of the spinal cord with the motoneurones supplying the muscle itself. The latter are classified, and often referred to, as *alpha motoneurones* (see Ch. 21).

If the frequency of impulses in the gamma motoneurones increases, the muscle spindle becomes more sensitive to stretch, whereas if the gamma motoneurones fire less frequently the spindles become less sensitive (see Ch. 24).

Changes in tone

If the spindles are more sensitive to stretch, or if alpha motoneurones are more excitable, at least two things occur:

- exaggeration of stretch reflexes
- hypertonia.

This means that when stretch reflexes are elicited by tapping the tendon of a muscle, the muscle jerk is produced much more easily and is bigger, and when the limbs are moved passively, increased resistance to movement is felt by the examiner.

Exaggerated reflexes and hypertonia occur when there is a reduction in impulses from the areas of the cerebral hemispheres involved in the control of movement. This can happen as a result of a spinal injury or a stroke (see p. 466). As the effect of these impulses from the brain is usually inhibitory, their withdrawal makes alpha and gamma motoneurones more excitable. The result is either:

- spasticity, or
- rigidity.

In *spasticity*, reflexes are exaggerated, and there is increased resistance to passive movement of the limbs. In *rigidity*, however, it is noticeable that muscles are tensed even when there is no movement, either active or passive. Also, when an examiner attempts to move the limbs passively, the resistance felt does not feel the same as in spasticity. These differences in tone are related to the specific parts of the brain which are injured or abnormal, and may involve increased sensitivity to stretch of different types of intrafusal fibres (nuclear bag and nuclear chain) (see Ch. 24, Fig. 24.2).

CONTROL OF REFLEXES

Any reflex can be prevented or exaggerated through the influence of impulses from elsewhere in the nervous system. The excitability of interneurones and motoneurones is affected by transmitters released from other nerves making synaptic contact pre- or postsynaptically either with the interneurones or with the motoneurones of the reflex arc (Fig. 27.8). For example, knee jerks are sometimes easier to elicit if someone is feeling tense. This is because the excitability of the motoneurones (alpha and gamma) is increased by a change in the balance of the excitatory and inhibitory inputs. Conversely, if someone is feeling very 'laid back', reflex responses may be smaller because synaptic transmission of impulses is depressed by inhibitory neurotransmitters (see Ch. 21).

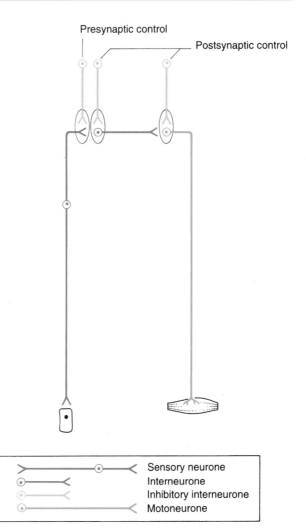

Presynaptic control

Postsynaptic control

>	⊙ <	Sensory neurone
⊙ <		Interneurone
⊙ <		Inhibitory interneurone
⊙ <		Motoneurone

Figure 27.8
Pre- and postsynaptic control of neurones forming a reflex arc.

A characteristic sign of hyperthyroidism is a fine muscle tremor. It has also been found that stretch reflexes occur more swiftly. Thyroxine (see Ch. 10) increases the sensitivity of neuronal synapses to catecholamines, such as noradrenaline and adrenaline. This not only affects the areas of the central nervous system that influence muscle tone but generally makes the patient more excitable or 'jumpy'. Consequently, patients often find it difficult to sleep and are easily awoken by a nurse attempting to record the sleeping pulse rate.

Muscle tension increases in patients who are anxious or nervous. Information can reduce anxiety (Hayward 1976, Boore 1978) so prior to any nursing procedure, particularly invasive procedures such as intramuscular injections or catheterisation, patients should be given both a full, clear explanation of the procedure and the time to ask questions. The consequent reduction in anxiety and muscle tension will make the procedure far less difficult and/or unpleasant for both patient and nurse.

Control by different brain areas

When we choose to move, and/or perform more complex movements (see p. 465), reflexes are allowed or disallowed through the release of neurotransmitters triggered by impulses from several parts of the brain. These areas include:

- cerebral cortex (motor cortex)
- brain stem (reticular formation and vestibular nuclei).

Impulses are transmitted from these areas to the interneurones and motoneurones of the basic reflex loops through several nerve tracts (Fig. 27.9). The tracts are named according to their origin and their destination. Thus the *corticospinal tracts* link the motor cortex with the spinal cord whereas the *vestibulospinal tracts* connect the vestibular nuclei in the brain stem with the neurones in the spinal cord. *Corticobulbar tracts* (not shown in the figure) link the cerebral cortex with the brain stem.

Upper and lower motoneurones

As neurones forming these tracts carry impulses from the brain towards the muscles, they are classified as motoneurones. However, a distinction is made between the motoneurones actually contacting (*innervating*) skeletal muscle (*lower motoneurones*) and those coming from the brain (*upper motoneurones*) that influence the lower motoneurones. Injury to lower and upper motoneurones produces different sorts of disability. Lower motoneurone injury produces:

- paralysis
- flaccidity
- atrophy.

Paralysis occurs because the muscle cannot be excited either reflexly or voluntarily. The muscle feels limp (*flaccid*) because impulses from muscle spindles cannot get through to it and consequently there is no tone. Because the muscle is not used it gradually wastes away (*atrophies*) (see Ch. 22). ④

In contrast, damage to the upper motoneurones alters the ease with which different reflexes are elicited (either increasing or decreasing them) but it does not usually abolish them. What does change is the control that can be exerted over voluntary movements and the way that they are executed (see p. 466).

Spinal shock

If impulses from the brain are cut off completely, because of injury to the spinal cord, the muscles controlled by motoneurones below the level of injury are initially temporarily paralysed (*spinal shock*). Both voluntary and reflex activity is lost. After a time spinal reflexes return, but when they do they are more powerful than normal. This is because many of the reflexes are

④
Damage to the axillary nerve can result from the improper use of crutches when not weight bearing. What consequences might you predict?

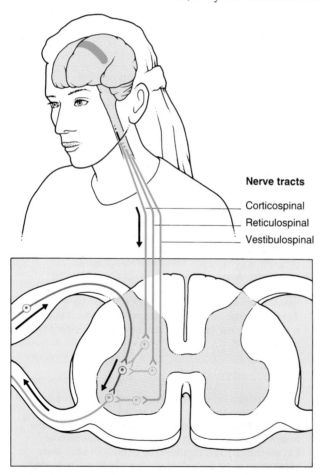

Figure 27.9
Major spinal tracts controlling the movement of the trunk and limbs.

Nerve tracts

Corticospinal
Reticulospinal
Vestibulospinal

SPINAL INJURY

If there is complete transection of the spinal cord causing *paraplegia* (loss of movement and sensation in the lower extremities), the lack of signals to the muscles of the lower limbs results in flaccid paralysis. Once the patient's condition is stable, the flaccid limbs should be put through a full range of movements every day to prevent atrophy and disuse contractures. A *contracture* is a deformity caused by shortening of muscle and an associated thickening of surrounding connective tissue.

The physiotherapy programme will also aim towards building the unaffected parts of the body (i.e. neck, shoulders, arms and trunk) to optimal strength for eventual weight-bearing activities. Such programmes are designed according to each individual's specific neurological deficit.

However, in many patients with paraplegia, spasticity follows the initial flaccidity because the normal balance between excitatory and inhibitory nerve impulses has been upset. Exaggerated reflexes can result in joints becoming flexed and fixed, and painful flexor and extensor spasms occur – often triggered by touch. The position of the limbs is important. The knees must be kept almost straight and the feet supported in dorsiflexion, or standing will become impossible.

normally held in check by the effects of inhibitory neurotransmitters released as a result of activity in the upper motoneurones. If the release of these transmitters is prevented because of injury to the upper motoneurones, reflex responses are unrestrained. ⑤

> Spinal shock is the term given to the loss of all reflex, motor, sensory and autonomic activity below the level of the spinal lesion/injury. It may last several weeks. In addition to being paralysed, patients in spinal shock lack vasomotor tone in their lower extremities and consequently will become hypotensive in an upright position (see Ch. 5). Antiembolic stockings will help prevent pooling of blood in the legs. Whilst positional changes need to be minimised to prevent further trauma, a variety of turning frames can be used to avoid pressure sore formation.

> *Paraplegia* is loss of movement and sensation in the lower extremities.
> *Quadriplegia* (*tetraplegia*) is loss of movement and sensation involving the upper and lower extremities and the trunk.
> *Hemiplegia* is loss of movement and/or sensation on one side of the body.

WILLED MOVEMENTS

When we choose to sit or stand, turn over the pages of a book, look around, run after someone, or perform some other more complicated activity, muscle contraction is coordinated and refined by three parts of the brain:

- motor cortex of the cerebral hemispheres
- basal ganglia
- cerebellum.

Each part differs in its functions. The motor cortex receives impulses from parts of the brain, including the basal ganglia, that link our awareness of ourselves and our environment with appropriate actions. Movements are refined by the cerebellum with the help of sensory feedback from receptors in the muscles and tendons (*proprioceptors*; see Ch. 24) to achieve actions that are as close as possible to those intended. Injury or disease produces different forms of disability depending on the part of the brain affected.

ROLE OF THE MOTOR CORTEX

Specific areas and their functions

The *primary motor area* of the cerebral cortex lies in the frontal lobes of the cerebral hemispheres just in front of the central sulcus (Fig. 27.10). If cells in this area are stimulated, specific movements of different parts of the body occur. A map can be drawn of the parts of the body affected by stimulation of different cells (Fig. 27.11) just as it could for the cells of the somatosensory cortex (see Ch. 23). It can be seen from the diagram (*homunculus* – meaning 'little man') that most of the cells of the primary motor area are concerned with movements of the hands, face and lips.

At least two other areas of the cerebral cortex also have a major role in the control of movement. These are the premotor area and the supplementary motor area (Fig. 27.10). The homunculi in these areas differ from that of the primary motor area. For example most of the cells of the supplementary area are concerned with movements of the limbs, and less are involved with the hands, face and lips.

The cortical cells are normally excited by stimuli transmitted to them from:

- the thalamus (see Ch. 23)
- the somatosensory cortex (see Ch. 23)
- some areas of the association cortex (see Chs 20 and 30).

⑤
How might a knowledge of reflex activity aid you when moving a paraplegic patient from bed to chair?

Figure 27.10
Regions of the cerebral cortex involved in the control of movement.

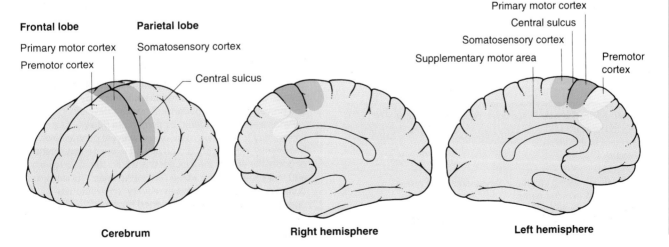

Cerebrum   Right hemisphere   Left hemisphere

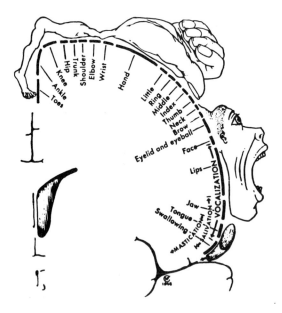

Figure 27.11
Motor homunculus. (Reprinted with the permission of Macmillan Publishing Company from The cerebral cortex of man, by Wilder Penfield and Theodore Rasmussen. Copyright 1950 Macmillan Publishing Company; copyright renewed (c) 1978 Theodore Rasmussen.)

The cells of the motor cortex represent one of the later stages in the process by which our thoughts are translated into actions. Signals from the association areas of the cerebral cortex that are involved in perception and thinking (see Ch. 30) are transmitted to cells of the motor cortex which pass on the information to appropriate upper motoneurones.

Upper motoneurones

Cells of the motor cortex exert control over muscle contraction through two routes:

● direct
● indirect.

The *direct routes* begin in the primary motor area and end on interneurones and/or lower motoneurones in the brain stem (*corticobulbar tracts*) or spinal cord (*corticospinal tracts*). The corticobulbar tracts control muscles of the face and jaws, whereas the corticospinal tracts control muscles of the limbs and trunk.

Table 27.1 General features of disordered function of the motor cortex	
Feature	*Technical term*
Difficulty in making voluntary movements	Paresis
Loss of skill in movements	
Increased muscle tone	
Exaggerated tendon jerks	Spasticity

Many of the lower motoneurones innervating muscles controlling the fingers, lips and tongue are directly innervated by neurones originating in the cerebral cortex. Thus the cerebral cortex is particularly important in the control of activities such as handling objects, writing and speaking (see Chs 28 and 29).

> *Dysarthria* is the collective name given to a number of speech disorders that result from difficulty in controlling the muscles used for speech (see Ch. 29). Impaired control of the muscles of the lips and tongue reduces both the rate of speech and its intelligibility, because consonants become imprecise. Exercise of the affected muscles is important and the nurse will need to encourage patients to practice the exercises taught by the speech therapist. Good results can be expected with patience and repetitious verbal exercises (Myco 1983).

The *indirect routes* pass from the premotor and the supplementary motor areas of the cerebral cortex to the interneurones in the brain stem and the spinal cord, via nuclei in the reticular formation. The nerve tracts originating from the nuclei in the reticular formation that innervate interneurones in the spinal cord are termed the *reticulospinal tracts*. These tracts have a major role in the control of voluntary changes in posture and in moving arms and legs (see Ch. 28).

Effects of injury

Damage to the motor cortex, as for example in a stroke, impairs voluntary movement (Table 27.1). Muscles can still be activated reflexly. In other words, they are not paralysed, but voluntary movements are weak (*paresis*). Some reflexes, for example stretch reflexes such as the knee jerk, are exaggerated. This is because the upper moto-

> **STROKE**
>
> Someone who has suffered a stroke usually experiences a short period of flaccidity followed by the onset of spasticity. The effects are usually most severe in the muscle groups that flex the leg and extend and lift the arm. This is the result of an exaggeration of normal spinal reflexes. The pattern of spasticity is directly related to the reflexes which normally dominate posture. For example, without appropriate care, the shoulder of the affected side will become fixed lower than the unaffected one, with the elbow joint flexed and the fingers clawed. The nurse should therefore ensure proper positioning and support to maintain correct body alignment and prevent abnormal patterns of posture developing.
>
> Passive exercises should be carried out three or four times a day to maintain mobility and prevent contractures. Importantly, nothing should be placed in the patient's hand or under the sole of the foot, for this would stimulate reflexes and make the situation worse. Untreated spasticity leads to contractures, so, to maximise recovery, physiotherapy needs to be complemented by good nursing care and encouragement from relatives.

neurones have a predominantly inhibitory effect on these reflexes (see p. 463), so that, if their influence is withdrawn, reflexes are elicited much more easily. Stretch reflexes are enhanced and muscle tone is increased (*spasticity*). ⑥

ROLE OF THE BASAL GANGLIA (BASAL NUCLEI)

Nature and organisation

The basal ganglia consist of several clusters of cell bodies (*nuclei*) deep within the cerebral hemispheres (see Ch. 20). The nuclei are interconnected, and are linked also to the thalamus (Fig. 27.12).

The basal ganglia receive impulses from different parts of the association areas of the cerebral cortex. They are thus supplied with information about our thoughts. The command signals sent out from the basal ganglia pass first to the thalamus and from there to many different areas of the cerebral cortex including the motor cortex, particularly the premotor and supplementary motor areas.

Effects of disorder

Much of the understanding that has been gained over the years about the role of the basal ganglia in the control of movement has been deduced from studies of patients with movement disorders.

A characteristic feature of all disorders of the basal ganglia is that unsolicited movements occur even when someone is not intending to move. The magnitude and nature of these movements differ according to which group of cells is affected and how their function has become disordered. Some examples are listed in Table 27.2. Information of this kind has led researchers to suggest that the role of the basal ganglia in movement is involved with the initiation, planning and programming of gross movements.

Another characteristic feature of disorders of the basal ganglia is that muscle tone is often increased, but the character of the change (*rigidity*) is different from that characteristic of injury to the motor cortex (*spasticity*). ⑦

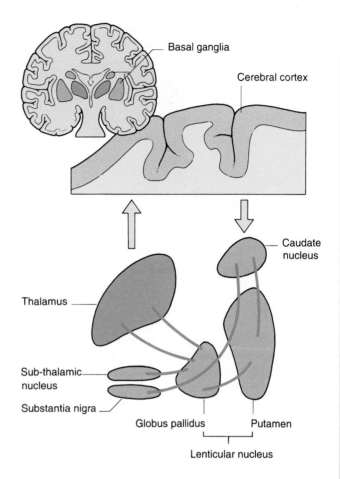

Figure 27.12
The basal ganglia and their relationship to and with the cerebral cortex.

ROLE OF THE CEREBELLUM

Organisation and functions

The cerebellum sits astride the back of the brain stem linked to it by the cerebral peduncles, which consist of afferent and efferent nerve fibres (Ch. 20). There are extensive links between the cerebellum and the balance organs (vestibular system; see Ch. 24), and also with other nuclei in the brain.

One part of the cerebellum (*flocculo-nodular lobe*) (Fig.

⑥
What position is adopted by the legs as the result of spastic paralysis? Why might walking be difficult?

⑦
How would you describe the appearance of a patient with Parkinson's disease?

Table 27.2	Disorders of the basal ganglia	
Disorder	*Characteristic features*	*Site of defect*
Athetosis	Involuntary slow writhing movements (mostly distal muscles)	Lenticular nucleus
Ballismus	Involuntary violent flailing movements	Sub-thalamic nucleus
Chorea	Involuntary rapid jerky movements	Caudate nucleus
Parkinson's disease	Poverty of movement (akinesia) Rigidity Involuntary tremor	Substantia nigra

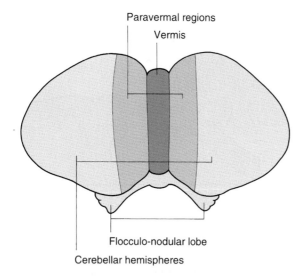

Figure 27.13
Structure of the cerebellum (viewed from the back).

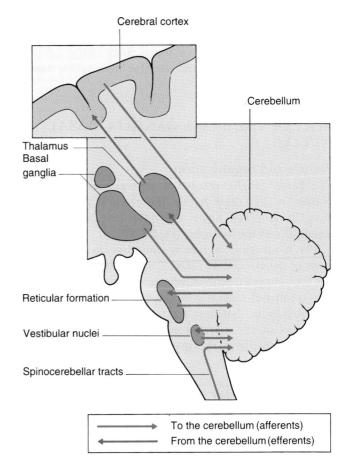

→	To the cerebellum (afferents)
←	From the cerebellum (efferents)

Figure 27.14
Functional connections of the cerebellum with other parts of the motor system.

27.13) is specifically concerned with balance. Other areas (*vermis* and *paravermal regions*) are associated chiefly with walking and gait. The *lateral hemispheres* are involved with the performance of highly skilled movements such as drawing, speaking, and pointing to and placing objects accurately.

The cerebellum receives nerve impulses from all the other areas of the brain involved in the control of movement as well as from sensory receptors including muscle proprioceptors, via the spinocerebellar tracts, and the balance organs, via the vestibular nuclei (Fig. 27.14). It is therefore able to compare information about the movement which is intended with what is actually happening. If there is a difference between intent and performance, corrective adjustments are made by the cerebellum to the movement while it is being performed. Signals from the cerebellum are passed back to the other motor areas with the result that the command signals issued via the upper motoneurones are modified. As a result the movement is made more accurate. In this way the cerebellum controls and coordinates movements that have been initiated elsewhere.

Effects of disorder

Cerebellar disorders are characterised by inaccurate and uncoordinated movements (*ataxia*) (Table 27.3). For example, a person with cerebellar disorder may not be able to reach straight towards an object and pick it up accurately. He will over- or undershoot, then over- or undercorrect and so on until eventually the object is secured. Also, movements that are normally coordinated and performed smoothly may be broken down into their

Table 27.3 General features of cerebellar disorder	
Feature	*Technical term*
Incoordination of movement in general	Ataxia
Drunken gait	Locomotor ataxia
Inaccuracy in positioning hands and feet (as when reaching out to pick up an object)	Dysmetria (past pointing)
Tremor when making a movement	Intention tremor
Inability to perform rapidly alternating movements	Adiadochokinesia

separate parts. The ordinary movement of raising a hand may only be achieved by first moving the shoulder, then the upper arm, and finally the forearm.

As movements in general are less accurate, a different stance may have to be adopted in walking to reduce the likelihood of falling over. Many of the signs of cerebellar impairment, namely unsteadiness in walking, slurred speech and clumsiness are in fact seen in someone who has drunk too much alcohol. All parts of the brain are affected by alcohol but the impairment of skilled activities is easily noticed. Changes in muscle tone are not a prominent feature of cerebellar disorders, but if they do occur the effect is usually a decrease (*hypotonia*).

KEY POINTS

What you should now know and understand about motor systems:

- the meaning of some basic terminology (extensor, flexor, agonist, antagonist, recruitment, motor unit, irradiation)
- what reflexes are and how they work
- how control is exercised over reflexes by other parts of the nervous system
- which parts of the brain are involved in the control of movement and what they do
- what is meant by muscle tone and how it may alter as a result of injury or disease
- the basis of some characteristic features of different types of movement disorder (spasticity, flaccidity, hyper- and hypotonia, rigidity, paralysis, paresis, ataxia)
- what may be the matter if someone cannot move, or moves uncharacteristically clumsily or awkwardly, or makes involuntary movements.

REFERENCES AND FURTHER READING

Boore J 1979 Prescription for recovery. RCN, London
Galley P M, Forster A L 1987 Human movement: an introductory text for physiotherapy students, 2nd edn. Churchill Livingstone, Edinburgh
Goodwill C J, Chamberlain M A 1988 Rehabilitation of the physically disabled adult. Chapman & Hall, London (Excellent reference work covering almost every aspect of care of the patient undergoing rehabilitation)
Hayward J 1976 Information: a prescription against pain. RCN, London
Myco F 1983 Nursing care of the hemiplegic stroke patient. Harper & Row, London
Oliver M, Zarb G, Silver J R, Moore M, Salisbury V 1988 Walking into darkness: the experience of spinal cord injury. Macmillan, New York
Penfield W, Rasmussen T 1950 The cerebral cortex of man: a clinical study of localisation of function. Macmillan, New York (Now classic book describing results of important clinical studies)
Rothwell J C 1987 Control of human movement. Croom Helm, Beckenham (Advanced student text relating basic science to neurological disorders)
Turnbull G I, Bell P A 1985 Maximising mobility after a stroke: the acute patient. Croom Helm, Beckenham

Chapter 28
ACTIONS 1: POSTURE, MOVEMENT AND MANUAL DEXTERITY

Many of the activities filling each day, whether at work or at leisure, such as walking, lifting, digging, cooking and typing, are engineered by movement of the articulated bones of our skeletons. The skeleton gives shape to the body, and supports and protects delicate tissues. The joints between the bones enable us to adopt different postures and to perform many different movements.

Some movements, such as pushing or pulling, are relatively simple but powerful, whereas others such as writing are more intricate. All are powered by the contraction of skeletal muscle and coordinated and controlled by parts of the somatic nervous system.

BONES AND JOINTS

BONE

Bone is a form of connective tissue consisting chiefly of the protein *collagen* liberally impregnated with *hydroxyapatite* (calcium phosphate). This makes bone very hard. Bone is formed by *osteoblasts* and broken down by *osteoclasts*, and once formed is slowly renewed.

Bones come in many different shapes and sizes; some are long, some are flat. Their structures differ according to their function. ①

Formation

Cartilage
Before bone is formed in the body, structural support is provided by *cartilage*. This too consists chiefly of collagen, together with the cells (*chondrocytes* and *fibroblasts*) which form this tissue. Unlike bone, however, collagen is not mineralised. Some bones, such as the long bones of the limbs, are formed by mineralisation of cartilage. The chondrocytes die leaving spaces in the tissue that are invaded by osteoclasts. Other bones, such as those of the skull, develop directly from primitive fetal tissue, without requiring cartilage.

Excavation by osteoclasts
Osteoclasts are a type of macrophage (see Ch. 15). They engulf and digest tissue to which they are attracted, and excavate it leaving tunnel-like spaces. Other cells follow behind them, including endothelial cells of growing blood capillaries, and osteoblasts that line the walls of the tunnel.

① *Can you name three long and three flat bones?*

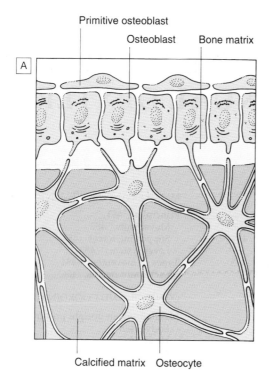

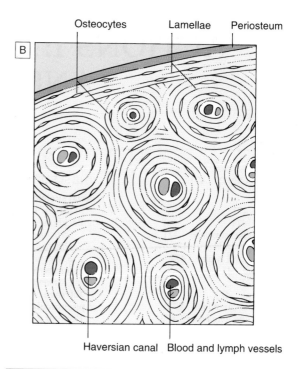

Figure 28.1
Bone:
A Development of bone cells and the interstitial matrix
B Histological appearance of compact bone.
(Part A adapted from Alberts et al 1983.)

Building by osteoblasts

Osteoblasts form bone tissue around themselves, and in so doing become separated from one another and imprisoned within their own handiwork (Fig. 28.1A). However, they communicate with one another through elongated cellular processes extending through tiny spaces in the bone. Imprisoned in the bone they stop forming new tissue but continue as *osteocytes* to be involved in the maintenance of bone and in regulating its replacement.

In this way bone is gradually built up as layers (*lamellae*) of mineralised collagen, that in cross-section often look like sawn across tree trunks (Fig. 28.1B). A space containing blood and lymph vessels (*haversian canal*) remains in the centre of each 'trunk'. The outer surface of bone is covered by a vascular fibrous membrane (*periosteum*).

Remodelling and repair

Remodelling

Once formed, bone is continually overhauled by the excavating activities of the osteoclasts (*resorption of bone*), and the new building works of the osteoblasts (*deposition of bone*). Osteoclasts eat their way through bone at the rate of about 0.05 mm per day with the result that roughly 5 to 10% of the tissue is replaced each year.

BONE WASTING DISORDERS

The term *osteomalacia* means soft bones and is applied to a number of conditions in which the bones of the body are inadequately mineralised, so becoming soft and structurally weak. Bones may bend, deform or fracture on weight bearing. The commonest cause of osteomalacia is vitamin D deficiency. The metabolic pathway of vitamin D is complex and requires normal functioning of the liver and kidneys (see Ch. 13).

Deficiency of vitamin D in the UK occurs where there is poverty, poor diet and lack of exposure to sunlight, and has occurred in Asian immigrants. Milk, liver, eggs and fish are good sources of vitamin D, and milk provides calcium too.

Osteoporosis refers to a group of diseases in which bone resorption outpaces bone deposition, with the result that osteoporotic bones become more porous and lighter. The spinal vertebrae are especially vulnerable to this process, particularly in postmenopausal females (see Ch. 36), as oestrogen affects osteoblast activity. Compression fractures of vertebrae, and fractures of the neck of the femur and the wrist (Colles' fracture) are common. Indeed, osteoporosis is the most important cause of fractures in females over the age of 50 years and is one of the reasons why hormone replacement therapy is currently advocated for postmenopausal women. However, no single deficiency explains all cases of osteoporosis, and an adequate intake of calcium (500–1200 mg/day) and vitamin D, and plenty of exercise are also required.

This process of renewal and remodelling is affected by the stresses acting on the bones. Mechanical stress promotes the formation of bone. If stresses are minimised, as for example in someone who is immobile, then more bone is lost than gained. Conversely, exercise increases the mass of bone tissue. ②

② *What other effects does regular exercise have on the body?*

Despite their strength, bones can be broken (*fractured*). A fracture is treated first by reduction, in which the bone ends are realigned, and then the reduced fracture is immobilised by the application of a cast (e.g. plaster of Paris), or by traction.

Repair

When a bone is broken, the injury activates cells in the tissue that form cartilage. The new cartilage forms a temporary bridge, knitting the fractured ends of the bone together. Subsequently this is broken down by the osteoclasts and replaced by bone through the activities of the osteoblasts. ③

Types of bone

Compact and cancellous

Bone is not uniform in its appearance. *Compact bone* has the characteristic form shown in Figure 28.1B whereas *cancellous bone* looks spongy because there are large spaces filled with *red bone marrow* (Fig. 28.2 and Ch. 4).

Flat bones and long bones

Flat bones, such as the breast bone (*sternum*) and bones

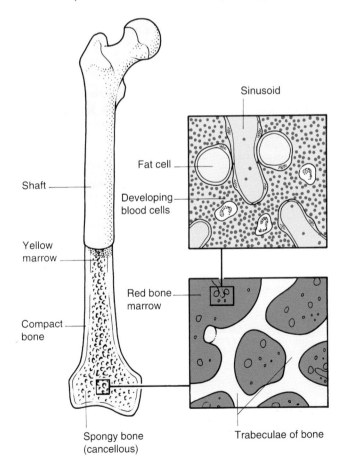

Figure 28.2
Structure of a long bone.

of the skull, consist chiefly of cancellous bone covered by a thin layer of compact bone.

The two ends of a long bone resemble flat bones in consisting of compact bone and cancellous bone, but the shaft is different (Fig. 28.2). It consists solely of a hollow but thick tube of compact bone. The large space in the middle (*medullary canal*) contains *yellow bone marrow* (see Ch. 4).

In long bones that are still growing cartilage is present between the shaft (*diaphysis*) and the secondary centres of ossification at each end of the bone (*epiphyses*). As the bone grows, this cartilage (*epiphysial cartilage*), which is also growing, is gradually mineralised to become bone (see Ch. 35).

JOINTS

Bones are joined to one another by fibrous tissue, forming different types of joint:

- fibrous
- cartilaginous
- synovial.

In a few places, such as the skull, fibrous tissue holds bones together very tightly and rigidly (*fibrous joints*). More often though the jointing allows movement, ranging from the modest flexibility of a vertebral joint (a *cartilaginous joint*) to the free swinging mobility of the shoulder joint (a *synovial joint*). ④

Wherever there is movement, bones are connected to one another by fibrous tissue (*ligaments*) and their contact with one another is cushioned by additional structures. These include the discs between the vertebrae of the spine (see p. 476) and the fluid-filled cavities lying between many of the bones of the arms and legs (see Synovial joints, p. 474). Where there may be friction between the structures surrounding a joint, such as between the ligaments, bone and skin, tissues react by forming their own cushion in the form of a sac of fluid (*bursa*).

A chronic inflammation of a bursa is known as *bursitis* and may be caused by trauma, such as repeated excessive friction. *Bunions* are frequently associated with friction bursitis over the head of the first metatarsal bone (see p. 482) resulting in pain, swelling and limited movement, and often considerable deformity. The prepatellar bursa (see p. 481) may become inflamed in individuals who spend a lot of time kneeling. This bursitis is often referred to as *housemaid's knee*.

Fibrous and cartilaginous joints

Specific features of the fibrous joints in the skull and the cartilaginous joints of the spine will be described later (see Ch. 29 and p. 476 respectively).

③
What factors aid the healing of fractured bones?

④
What other examples of fibrous, cartilaginous and synovial joints can you name?

Synovial joints

Structure

A *synovial joint* consists of a fibrous *capsule*, containing *synovial fluid*, joining the ends of the bones (Fig. 28.3). Synovial fluid is secreted by the cells lining the inner surface of the capsule (*synovial membrane*). The ends of the bones are covered by a smooth layer of cartilage. The capsule may be taut or loose depending on the nature of the joint and its mobility.

Ligaments

Ligaments are fibres formed of collagen that link bones together. Depending on the joint, they may be:

- part of the fibrous capsule
- inside the capsule (intracapsular)
- outside the capsule (extracapsular).

Intracapsular ligaments tether the bones of the joint together, whereas extracapsular ones provide additional support.

Innervation

Sensory nerve endings are embedded in the capsule and the ligaments (*joint receptors*; see Ch. 24). They are excited by the changing tension in these structures as the joint is moved. Impulses from the receptors contribute to the sense of proprioception and pain. The sensory neurones carrying signals to the brain from the joints are bundled together with sensory fibres supplying the skin overlying the same joint.

> *Rheumatoid arthritis* is the most common form of inflammatory arthritis. The inflammation of the synovium produces an increase in synovial fluid and thickening of the synovium. The inflammation, together with the increased amount of synovial fluid which stretches the joint capsule, causes pain.

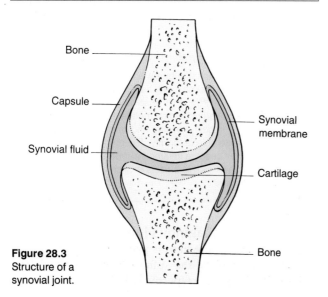

Figure 28.3
Structure of a synovial joint.

THE SKELETON

The skeleton (Fig. 28.4) consists of many different bones jointed together to form a structure which:

- gives support to body tissues
- surrounds delicate tissues such as the brain and lungs
- allows movement.

It can be divided into two parts, *axial* and *appendicular*.

AXIAL SKELETON

The axial skeleton is composed of the skull, spine (*vertebral column*) and rib cage.

Skull

The skull consists mainly of flat bones joined by fibrous joints. There is just one freely movable bone, the *mandible*. Details of the structure of the skull are given in Chapter 29.

Backbone (vertebral column)

The backbone, or spine, consists of 33 vertebral bones stacked neatly one on top of the other (Fig. 28.5). The ones at the bottom are fused together to form the *sacrum* and the *coccyx*, but the remainder are linked by cartilaginous joints.

Structure of a vertebra

All the vertebrae except the *atlas* and *axis* (see Ch. 29) have the same basic structure (Fig. 28.6A & B) although

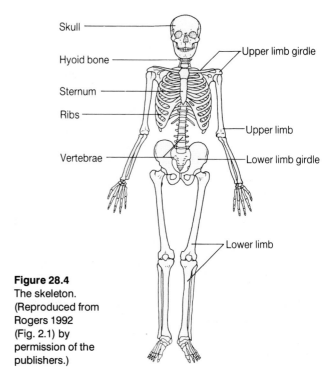

Figure 28.4
The skeleton. (Reproduced from Rogers 1992 (Fig. 2.1) by permission of the publishers.)

Figure 28.5 (*right*)
The skull and vertebral column.
(Reproduced from Rogers 1992
(Fig. 2.8A & B) by permission of
the publishers.)

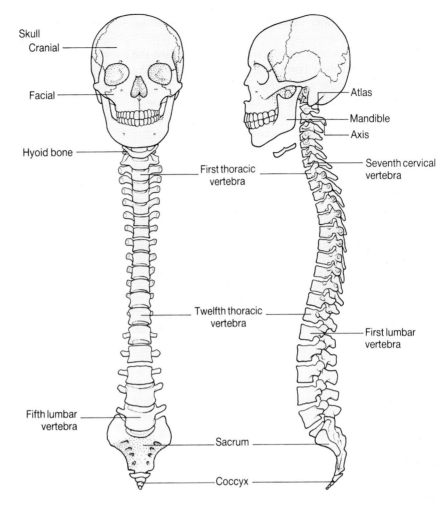

Skull
Cranial

Facial

Hyoid bone

First thoracic
vertebra

Twelfth thoracic
vertebra

Fifth lumbar
vertebra

Atlas
Mandible
Axis
Seventh cervical
vertebra

First lumbar
vertebra

Sacrum

Coccyx

Figure 28.6 (*below*)
Structure of a vertebra:
A Seen from above (superiorly)
B Seen from the side (laterally).
(Reproduced from Rogers 1992
(Fig. 2.9A & B) by permission of
the publishers.)

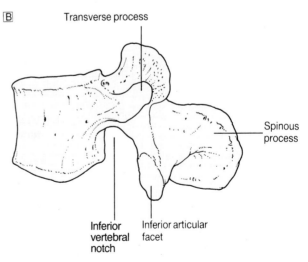

A   Body   Neural arch

Transverse
process

Superior
articular facet

Spinous
process

Lamina

B   Transverse process

Spinous
process

Inferior
vertebral
notch

Inferior articular
facet

they differ in specific features according to their location. Each vertebra has:

- a body – bearing the weight of the column above
- an arch – enclosing the spinal cord
- several processes – attaching to muscles and ligaments.

Some of the processes have smooth regions (*facets*) articulating with vertebrae above or below, and sometimes with other bones.

Differences between vertebrae
The cervical vertebrae are the smallest and differ from the others in having a small hole (*foramen*) in the trans-

verse process on either side, through which the vertebral arteries pass.

The thoracic vertebrae interlock more snugly than the cervical ones, and their laminae and spines overlap like plates on an armadillo's back (Fig. 28.5).

The lumbar vertebrae are the largest, the fifth one at the base being the biggest of all. Here the laminae and spines do not overlap, and because of this it is possible to pass a fine needle between two lumbar vertebrae to perform a *lumbar puncture* when obtaining a sample of cerebrospinal fluid (see Ch. 20).

> The two vertebral arteries run up through channels in the cervical spine in quite close contact to both vertebrae and discs and enter the skull at the foramen magnum (see Ch. 29). Any changes in the vertebrae or discs, for example as a result of arthritis or osteoporosis, may interfere with the flow of blood. Common signs and symptoms include intermittent vertigo – aggravated by movement of the neck, such as tilting the head back – fluctuating weakness of the legs and 'drop attacks', all of which can be attributed to ischaemia of the brain stem.

Spaces for spinal nerves

The shape of the vertebrae, and the way in which they are slotted together, creates small gaps (*intervertebral foramina*) between them, one on either side of each pair of adjacent vertebrae (Fig. 28.7A). These are the holes through which the spinal nerves pass. If these gaps become narrowed, as they may do in *osteoarthritis*, the spinal nerves get pinched. For example, the pain of *sciatica* is caused by pinching of the last two lumbar nerves.

Intervertebral discs

Acting as cushions between the bodies of adjacent vertebrae are the *intervertebral discs* (Fig. 28.7A). They consist of a ring of fibrocartilage (*annulus fibrosus*) surrounding a 'soft centre' of jelly-like material (*nucleus pulposus*). The fibres of the annulus are attached to the vertebrae above and below and to the anterior and posterior ligaments (Fig. 28.7B), which help to keep the disc in place.

The intervertebral discs act as shock absorbers and make the spine more flexible. When the discs degenerate as we grow older (see Ch. 36) the spine loses the cervical and lumbar curves developed in infancy, and takes up a fetal-like curve again.

Although the discs are very strong in children and young people, they deteriorate and can be damaged as we grow older. If for example the ring of fibres weakens, some of the inner soft core may be squeezed out (*prolapsed disc* – known also as a slipped disc) and press on the spinal cord or on the spinal nerves. This excites the nerves and may give rise to the sensation of pain and/or impair movement.

> *Laminectomy* is carried out to remove a ruptured disc when conservative treatment, for example rest, analgesia and/or traction, has failed. There may be varying degrees of pain and sensory manifestations in the initial postoperative period due to temporary inflammatory changes, such as oedema and swelling compressing the nerve roots. It takes some 6 weeks for the ligamentous attachments to heal and thus patients are taught to increase their activity levels cautiously and to avoid putting flexion strain on the spine, (e.g. by stair climbing). However, it is better to avoid back injury, since surgery may lead to a decrease in the flexibility of the spine. Workers should be taught safe lifting techniques in order to reduce the risk of a 'slipped disc', and should never lift with the back in a flexed or rotated position.

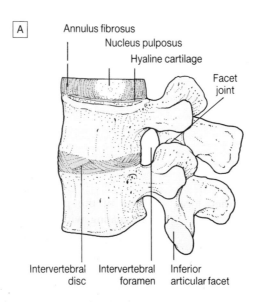
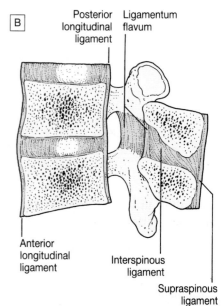

A
Annulus fibrosus
Nucleus pulposus
Hyaline cartilage
Facet joint
Intervertebral disc
Intervertebral foramen
Inferior articular facet

B
Posterior longitudinal ligament
Ligamentum flavum
Anterior longitudinal ligament
Interspinous ligament
Supraspinous ligament

Figure 28.7
Tissues linking the vertebrae:
A Intervertebral discs
B Ligaments.
(Reproduced from Rogers 1992
(Figs 2.10B & 13.7A) by
permission of the publishers.)

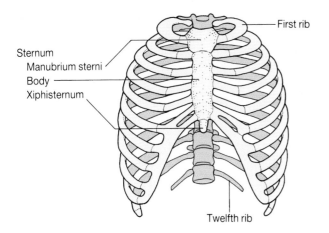

Figure 28.8
Structure of the rib cage. (Reproduced from Rogers 1992 (Fig. 2.11) by permission of the publishers.)

Ligaments

The vertebrae are joined together by several ligaments running between different parts of adjacent vertebrae (Fig. 28.7B):

- body – *anterior* and *posterior longitudinal ligaments* running from end to end of the vertebral column
- laminae – *ligamenta flava* (yellow ligaments) which steady the vertebral column when it flexes
- spines – *supraspinous* and *interspinous ligaments* and their cervical equivalent (*ligamentum nuchae*).

Rib cage

The rib cage (see also Ch. 7) consists of 12 pairs of ribs, each of which articulates with a thoracic vertebra at the back of the thorax. Most of the ribs are joined also at the front, by means of cartilage, to the breastbone (*sternum*) (Fig. 28.8). The sternum consists of three parts:

- manubrium
- body
- xiphoid process (*xiphisternum*).

The xiphoid process varies in shape from person to person.

> If the hands are badly positioned whilst carrying out cardiopulmonary resuscitation, there is a danger of fracturing the xiphoid process and driving it into the liver. It is also possible to fracture ribs, which may subsequently do damage to the lungs or heart.

APPENDICULAR SKELETON

The appendicular skeleton can be divided into four parts (Fig. 28.9):

- pectoral girdle
- pelvic girdle
- upper limb
- lower limb.

Pectoral girdle

Bones

The bones of the pectoral girdle and their relative positions are shown in Figure 28.9. The *clavicle* (collar bone) articulates with the manubrium of the sternum, and with the shoulder blade (*scapula*). These structures support the upper limb enabling it to be moved in many different directions.

> The clavicles are slender bones that extend horizontally across the upper thorax. They provide attachment points for many thoracic and shoulder muscles and act as anterior braces by holding out the scapulae from the upper, narrower part of the rib cage. The clavicles do not resist compression forces well and, if someone falls on to an outstretched hand – put out in an attempt to break the fall – the clavicle may fracture.
> The result is that the entire shoulder region collapses medially as the anterior brace is lost. For this reason a 'collar and cuff' sling is used for support as it holds the shoulder upwards, outwards and backwards from the thorax. However, the patient must be taught how to exercise the elbow, wrist and fingers and undertake regular shoulder exercises in order to retain full movement.

Joints

The joint between the clavicle and the sternum, which takes up the powerful stresses transmitted through the arms to the axial skeleton in pushing, is supported by many strong ligaments and is cushioned by a fibro-cartilaginous disc.

The shoulder joint is a very mobile synovial joint which can be easily dislocated. It is supported more by tendons and muscles than by the interlocking of the head of the humerus into the *glenoid cavity* of the scapula (Fig. 28.10).

Upper limb

The upper limb consists of:

- arm and forearm
- wrist and hand.

Arm and forearm

The end of the humerus fits neatly into a notch in the ulna of the forearm. This joint (*elbow*; Fig. 28.11) operates as a hinge. It is much more limited in its movement than the shoulder joint.

The two bones of the forearm, the radius and the ulna, are linked together practically throughout their length by fibrous tissue (*interosseous ligament*), and articulate with one another at both ends. When muscle contraction pulls the radius around the ulna at the elbow it makes the forearm twist and turns the hand. ⑤

Wrist and hand

There are many bones in the human wrist and hand

⑤
Which bone is broken in a Colles' fracture, and where?

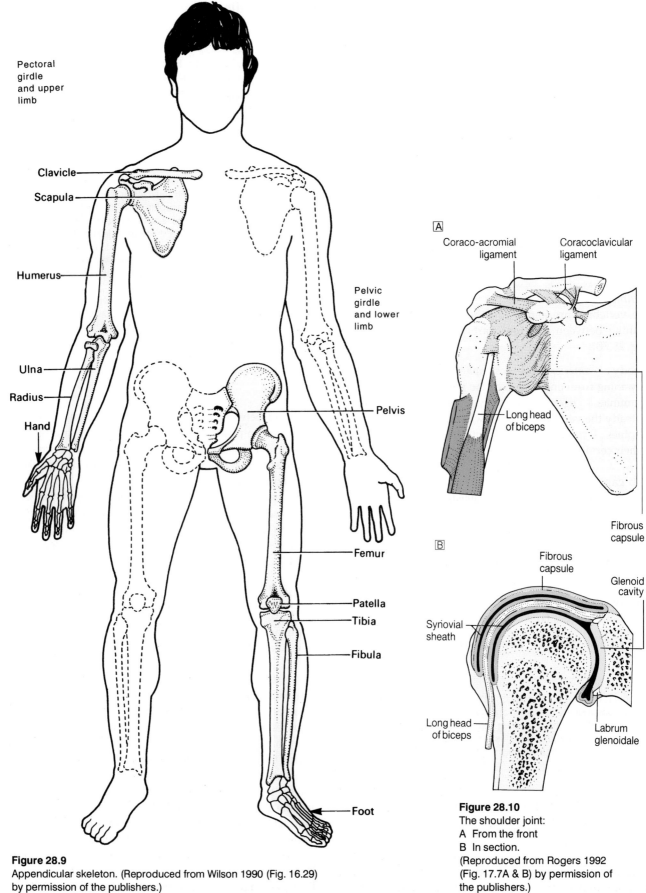

Pectoral girdle and upper limb

Clavicle

Scapula

Humerus

Ulna

Radius

Hand

Pelvic girdle and lower limb

Pelvis

Femur

Patella

Tibia

Fibula

Foot

Figure 28.9
Appendicular skeleton. (Reproduced from Wilson 1990 (Fig. 16.29) by permission of the publishers.)

A

Coraco-acromial ligament

Coracoclavicular ligament

Long head of biceps

Fibrous capsule

B

Fibrous capsule

Glenoid cavity

Synovial sheath

Long head of biceps

Labrum glenoidale

Figure 28.10
The shoulder joint:
A From the front
B In section.
(Reproduced from Rogers 1992 (Fig. 17.7A & B) by permission of the publishers.)

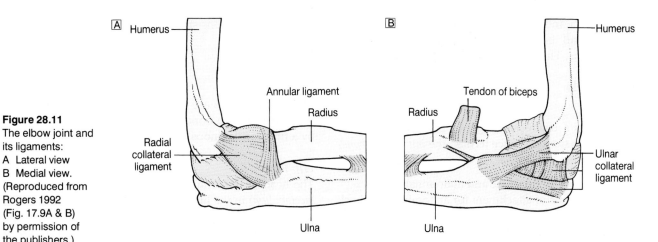

Figure 28.11
The elbow joint and its ligaments:
A Lateral view
B Medial view.
(Reproduced from Rogers 1992 (Fig. 17.9A & B) by permission of the publishers.)

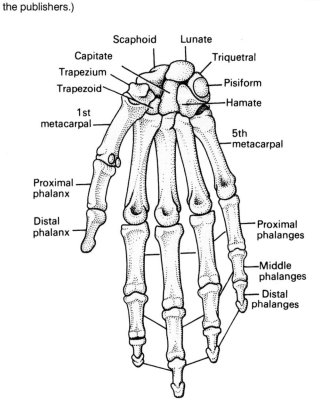

Figure 28.12
Bones of the wrist and hand. (Reproduced from Wilson 1990 (Fig. 16.34) by permission of the publishers.)

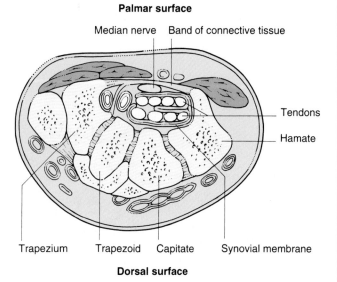

Figure 28.13
Structure and contents of the carpal tunnel.

(Fig. 28.12). They are arranged in a way that gives us an extraordinary dexterity.

The wrist consists of several small *carpal bones*, three of which face the bones of the forearm, and four of which form joints with the bones (*metacarpals*) of the body of the hand. The carpal bones are arranged in a U shape (Fig. 28.13), creating a hollow (*carpal tunnel*) enclosing the tendons linking the muscles in the forearm to the bones of the fingers and thumb. Packed in with the tendons is the *median nerve*, which innervates much of the hand including the muscles at the base of the thumb (*thenar muscles*), and much of the skin covering both the dorsal and palmar surfaces of the hand. If the

space in the carpal tunnel is congested the nerve may be compressed and this may lead to pain (*carpal tunnel syndrome*).

Carpal tunnel compression is particularly common in middle-aged women and may be the result of repetitive strain injury. It causes pain, and burning and tingling sensations in the hand, particularly at night, and may even awake the sufferer. Warmth can aggravate the tingling and housework may exacerbate the condition. Relief may be afforded by resting the affected hand and by the use of a light splint at night. Injections of hydrocortisone may give relief, but in some cases opening the carpal tunnel, a minor surgical procedure which involves division of the anterior carpal ligament, will permanently relieve the symptoms.

The hand itself consists of five rays of jointed bones (*metacarpals* and *phalanges*). The ends of the metacarpals form the knuckles, and articulate with the bones of the digits (fingers and thumb). Each of the fingers consists of three small bones (*phalanges*) hinged together by synovial joints. The thumb has only two phalanges.

Pelvic girdle

Pelvis

The pelvis is a basin-shaped set of bones consisting of the hip bones (*os coxae*, once termed the *innominate bone*) and the sacrum. The pelvis:

- gives support to the pelvic and abdominal organs
- provides points of attachment for abdominal and back muscles
- forms mobile joints with the *femur*s of each thigh.

The shape of the pelvis is shallower and more rounded in women than in men (Fig. 28.14A & B) reflecting modifications necessary for childbearing.

The hip bone consists of three parts:

- ilium
- ischium
- pubis.

These three bones are fused into a single structure. The left and right hip bones are joined together at the front by a fibrocartilaginous joint, the *symphysis pubis*.

Hip joint

The head of the femur fits snugly into a cup-like socket (*acetabulum*) in the hip bone. The opening of the acetabulum is ringed by cartilage (*acetabular labrum*) that helps to hold the head of the femur in the joint. The whole joint is enclosed by a tough fluid-filled capsule and supported by several strong extracapsular ligaments (Fig. 28.15A & B). ⑥

⑥
What types of movement can be achieved by the hip joint?

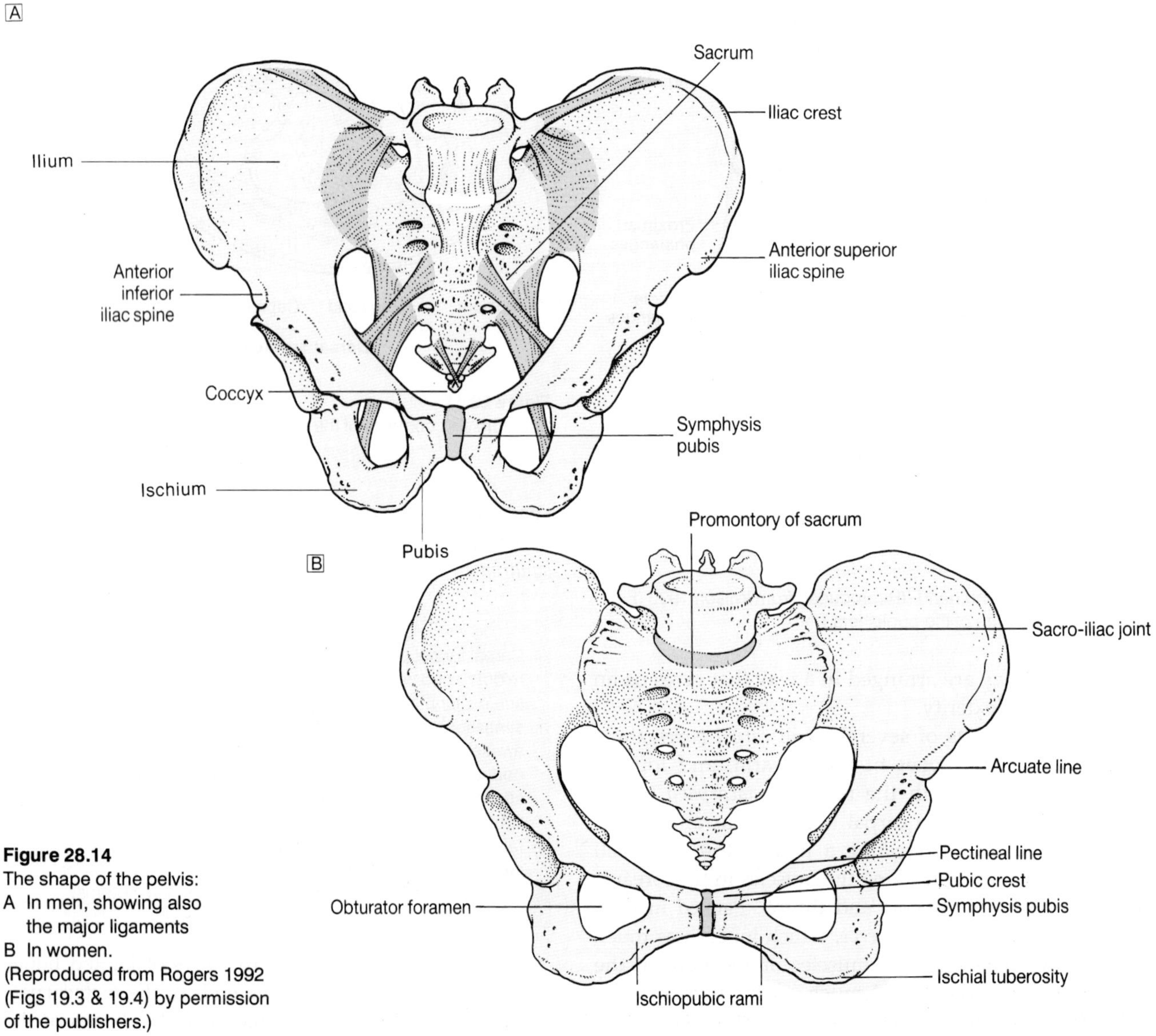

Figure 28.14
The shape of the pelvis:
A In men, showing also the major ligaments
B In women.
(Reproduced from Rogers 1992 (Figs 19.3 & 19.4) by permission of the publishers.)

Figure 28.15
The hip joint:
A With the head of the femur pulled out of its socket
B Showing the ligaments.
(Reproduced from Rogers 1992 (Fig. 19.6A & B) by permission of the publishers.)

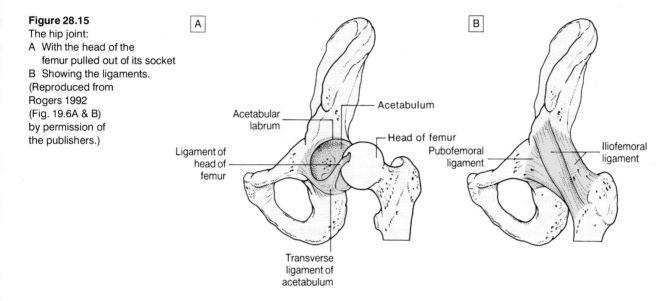

Acetabular labrum
Acetabulum
Ligament of head of femur
Head of femur
Pubofemoral ligament
Iliofemoral ligament
Transverse ligament of acetabulum

During *total hip replacement*, a metal femoral head is fitted into a plastic acetabular socket. The implant is fixed to the surrounding bone with a bone cement.

Following surgery, the leg is usually kept in abduction (see p. 485), to prevent dislocation of the prosthesis, until the soft tissues have healed. There are many ways of positioning the postoperative patient but all have the same objective; to avoid adduction and flexion (see p. 485) of the hip, which may result in dislocation.

Lower limb

The lower limb consists of:

- leg
- ankle and foot.

Leg

The end of the femur articulates with the *tibia* and with the *patella*, a small piece of bone lying just in front of the femur, to form the knee joint (Fig. 28.16A & B). The knee joint is, like the elbow, a hinge joint, but it is more complicated and has several distinctive features. The ends of the femur and the tibia are tethered together by

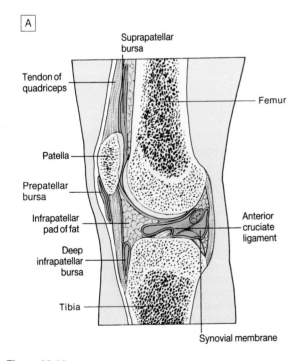

Suprapatellar bursa
Tendon of quadriceps
Femur
Patella
Prepatellar bursa
Infrapatellar pad of fat
Anterior cruciate ligament
Deep infrapatellar bursa
Tibia
Synovial membrane

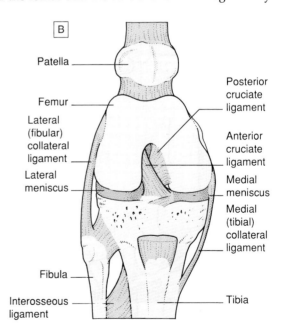

Patella
Femur
Lateral (fibular) collateral ligament
Lateral meniscus
Fibula
Interosseous ligament
Posterior cruciate ligament
Anterior cruciate ligament
Medial meniscus
Medial (tibial) collateral ligament
Tibia

Figure 28.16
The knee joint:
A Front view: patella tendon cut and patella displaced to show the structures underneath
B Section through the left knee joint seen from the side.
(Adapted and reproduced from Rogers 1992 (Figs 19.10 & 19.8) by permission of the publishers.)

two strong intracapsular ligaments (*cruciate ligaments*) within the capsule of the joint, and the whole joint is supported and strengthened by two extracapsular ligaments.

Inside the joint, the tibia, which acts as the weight-bearing bone of the lower limb, is additionally cushioned from the stresses imposed on it from above by two discs of fibrocartilage (*menisci* or *semilunar cartilages*). These lie on top of the smooth cartilage at the end of the bone.

The other bone of the leg is the fibula. It is joined to the tibia along its length by fibrous tissue (*interosseous ligament*) and, with the tibia, articulates with the *talus* to form the ankle joint. The ankle joint is supported by several ligaments.

Ankle and foot

The foot and the ankle, like the hand and the wrist, are composed of a number of bones (Fig. 28.17A & B). The bones of the foot form a sturdy flexible platform enabling us to stay upright as well as walk, run and jump.

There are several ankle (*tarsal*) bones, the largest of which is the *calcaneus*. This bone bears the weight of the body when you are standing upright with your feet flat on the ground. It articulates with the talus above and

with the other tarsal bones in front (*navicular*, *cuboid*, and *cuneiform* bones).

The ankle bones and the bones in front of them (*metatarsals*) are arranged and held in a way that gives the foot an arched shape. Unless you have flat feet, only your toes, the distal ends of your metatarsals and your calcaneous actually press on the ground when you are standing. The metatarsals, cuneiforms, and cuboid bones form arches similar to, but flatter than, the carpal tunnel of the wrist. In addition to this there are two longitudinal arches which raise the central part of the foot off the ground. The arches are supported by the muscles and ligaments of the foot.

The toes are made up of small bones (*phalanges*). The big toe, like the thumb, has only two bones whereas the other toes, like the fingers, have three.

MUSCLES AND MOVEMENT

PRINCIPLES

Movements

When one part of the skeleton is moved by muscle contraction, related parts have to be steadied by other muscles for the movement to be effective. The muscle which pulls on the moving bone (*movable point*) has to

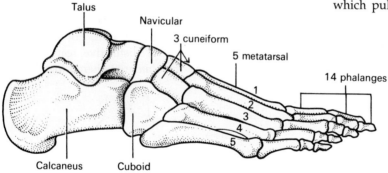

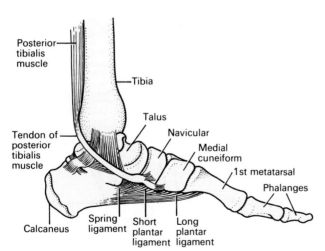

Figure 28.17
Bones and ligaments of the foot. (Reproduced from Wilson 1990 (Figs 16.40 & 16.41) by permission of the publishers.)

ACQUIRED FLATFOOT

Flatfoot occurs when the muscles supporting the arches of the foot are incapable of performing their function fully. Fatigue resulting from many hours of standing or walking may give rise to eversion of the foot (inner border lower than outer border). This will result in the body weight being thrown on to the internal longitudinal arch, which is the weakest. Flattening of the arch may result.

To reduce the risk of acquiring flatfoot, the shoes worn should have an inner border that is straight, with a waist that fits snugly to the arch and a heel that is broad and does not exceed 1 inch in height. Exercises to strengthen the muscles that invert the foot should be performed regularly. These include:

● foot rolling – drawing a circle with the big toe, clockwise for the right foot and anticlockwise for the left
● foot closing -- making a 'fist' of the foot
● placing a tissue on the floor and using the feet to screw the tissue into a ball.

Figure 28.18
Principles of movement:
A Theoretical components
B Relation to movement of the forearm.
(Reproduced from Chilman & Thomas 1987 (Fig. 2.3A & C) by permission of the publishers.)

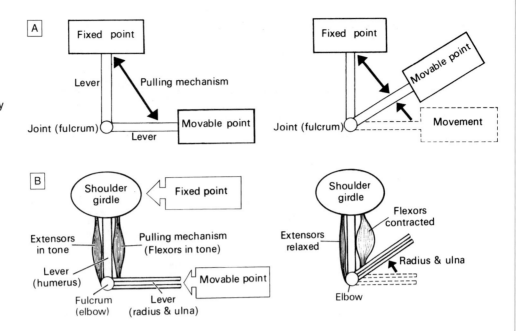

be anchored to another bone which is steadied (*fixed point*). The joint between them acts as the *fulcrum* or pivot of the system (Fig. 28.18A).

Usually there are at least two opposing muscles (*agonist* and *antagonist*) acting on a joint, one causing it to flex (*flexor*), and the other causing it to extend (*extensor*) (Fig. 28.18B and Ch. 27). If the joint allows rotation then there will be other muscles inserted in slightly different places which can twist the bone in one direction or the other when they contract.

Supporting forces

Maintaining an upright posture, whether sitting or standing, requires energy. However, there are efficient and inefficient ways of doing this. If for example someone stands erect, with legs slightly apart, the body is well balanced, and the force of gravity acts straight down the weight-bearing line of the body (Fig. 28.19). Relatively little energy is required to sustain this posture and, if the body sways, only minor additional effort is needed to recentre it. However, if someone slouches, more energy is needed and extra strain is placed on ligaments and joints.

> Poor posture puts a strain on to the muscles of the back, buttocks and legs, increasing fatigue and causing discomfort. It can also lead to deformities of the spine, such as *scoliosis*.

Lever systems

The least stable part of the body is the head, perched on top of the spine. It is balanced on top of the atlas (see Ch. 29) but the weight of the front part, which tends to make the head fall forward, has to be counteracted by a

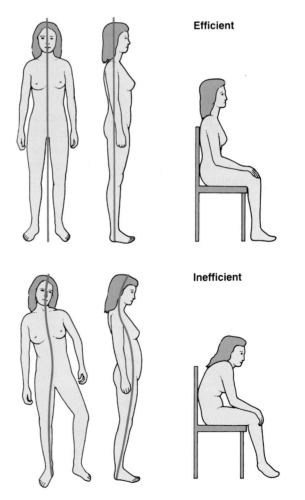

Figure 28.19
Inefficient and efficient postures. (Adapted from Chilman & Thomas 1987.)

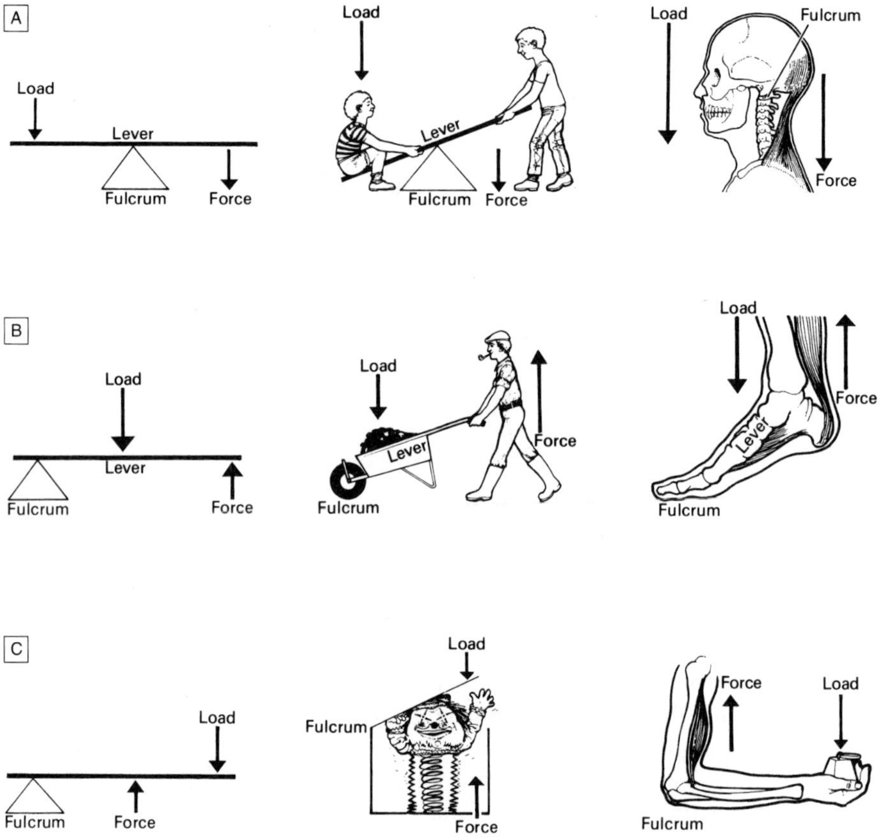

Figure 28.20
Lever systems:
A Head and neck
B Foot
C Arm.
(Reproduced from
Chilman & Thomas
(Fig. 2.4A, B & C) by
permission of the
publishers.)

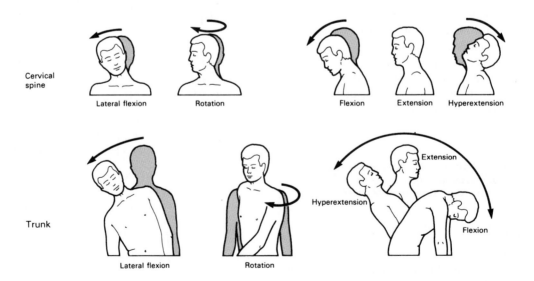

steady downward pull of the neck muscles to the rear (Fig. 28.20A). This is an example of one of several lever systems used in the body that maximise the efficiency of the movements that are made and minimise the energy required to sustain certain postures. Other examples are shown in Figure 28.20B & C.

TYPES OF MOVEMENT

The types of movement, flexion, extension, abduction, adduction and so on, that are possible for different parts of the body are illustrated in Figure 28.21.

Figure 28.21 (*above and right*)
Range of motion exercises for joints: cervical spine, trunk, shoulder, hip, elbow, knee, wrist, ankle, fingers and toes.
(Reproduced from Boore, Champion & Ferguson 1987 (Fig. 13.3A & B, after Henderson & Nite 1978) by permission of the publishers.)

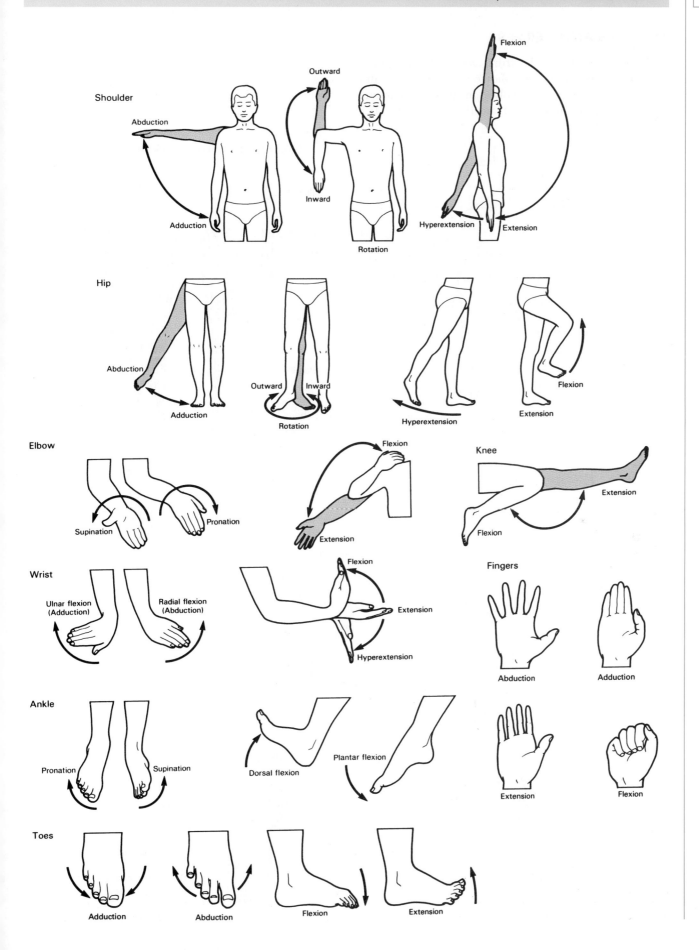

MUSCLES AND NERVES

Superficial muscles of the trunk and limbs, and their relation to major nerves, are shown in Figures 28.22 and 28.23. The major muscles involved in some of the movements shown in Figure 28.21 are listed in Tables 28.1 (p. 487) and 28.2 (p. 488).

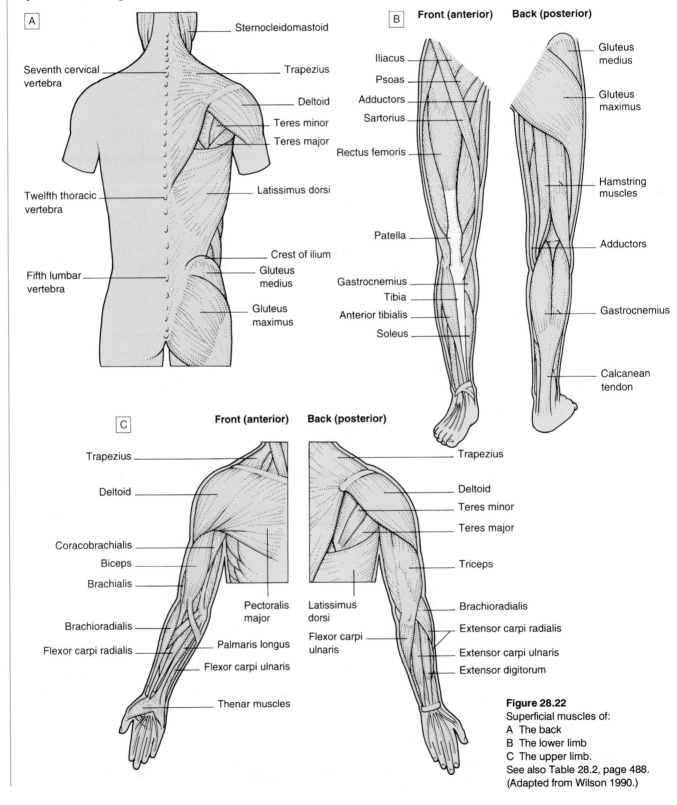

Figure 28.22
Superficial muscles of:
A The back
B The lower limb
C The upper limb.
See also Table 28.2, page 488.
(Adapted from Wilson 1990.)

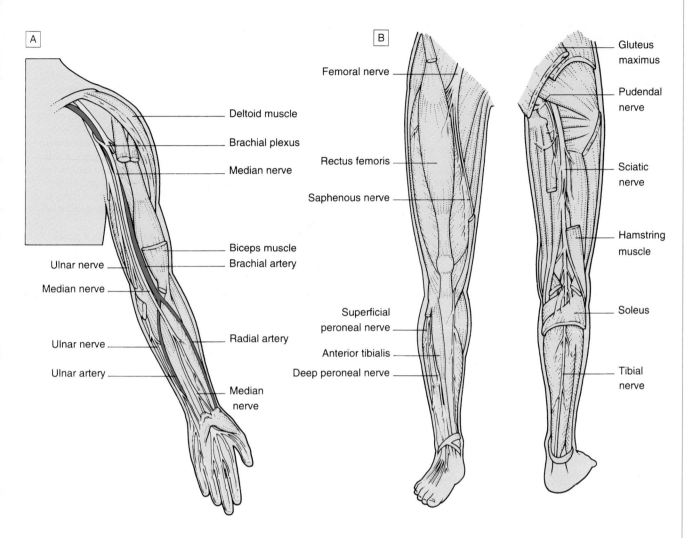

Figure 28.23
Major nerves of (A) the upper and (B) the lower limb and their relation to muscles and blood vessels. (Adapted from Williams et al 1989.)

Table 28.1   Muscles involved in movements of different parts of the body*

| | Movement | | | |
	Flexion	Extension	Abduction	Adduction
Cervical spine	Sternocleidomastoid	Trapezius Sacrospinalis[†]	—	—
Trunk	Abdominal muscles	Sacrospinalis[†]	—	—
Shoulder	Coracobrachialis Deltoid (anterior fibres) Pectoralis major	Teres major Deltoid (posterior fibres) Latissimus dorsi	Deltoid	Pectoralis major Latissimus dorsi
Hip	Psoas, iliacus Rectus femoris Sartorius	Gluteus maximus Hamstrings	Gluteus medius Gluteus minimus	Adductor group

* See Figures 28.21 and 28.22.
[†] These lie underneath the latissimus dorsi and the trapezius muscles and run up the vertebral column from the sacrum.

Table 28.2   Muscles involved in movements of the limbs*

	Movement	
	Flexion	Extension
Elbow	Biceps Brachialis	Triceps
Knee	Hamstrings Gastrocnemius	Quadriceps femoris
Wrist	Flexor carpi radialis Flexor carpi ulnaris	Extensor carpi radialis (longus and brevis) Extensor carpi ulnaris
Ankle	Gastrocnemius Soleus (plantar flexion)	Anterior tibialis Toe extensors (dorsiflexion)

* See Figures 28.21 and 28.22.

CONTROL AND COORDINATION

MAINTAINING AN UPRIGHT POSTURE

Body

Our natural upright posture is maintained by a number of different reflexes (see Ch. 27 and Fig. 27.2) that excite extensor muscles of the lower limbs, trunk and neck.

The *plantar reflex* is evoked by excitation of low threshold mechanoreceptors in the skin of the soles of the feet. When excited these reflexly excite the extensor muscles of the leg.

The balance organs (see Ch. 24) play their part in maintaining balance by detecting movement and reflexly evoking contraction of the extensors through impulses passing along the vestibulospinal tracts (see Ch. 27). If the balance organs are impaired then a person will have difficulty staying upright, particularly with the eyes closed. With eyes open, visual reflexes also help to maintain balance.

Stretch receptors in the muscles (muscle spindles; see Ch. 24) also maintain contraction of the extensor muscles. If you sway slightly to one side, muscles of the leg and trunk of the opposite side are stretched. This reflexly excites their contraction which pulls you back to the centre.

If, in response to a painful stimulus, we reflexly lift one foot off the ground, the *crossed extensor reflex* will at the same time cause increased contraction of the extensor muscles of the other leg to maintain our balance.

Head

Keeping your head up requires strong and maintained contraction of the neck muscles. This is sustained by *tonic neck reflexes* and *righting reflexes* powered by exci-

---

FIRST STEPS

The first years of development of a child (see also Ch. 35) are marked by enormous strides in the development of neuromuscular control. Some simple reflexes are present at birth but these gradually come under the control of other brain areas as the baby gets older. For example, it is well known that babies within a few days of birth can perform walking movements if they are supported by an adult and their feet are allowed to just touch a surface. The stimulus to the skin of the soles of the feet is enough to trigger a spinal locomotor programme that produces alternating contraction and relaxation of the leg muscles. As the baby gets older this activity is inhibited by impulses from other brain areas. Eventually the programme is set into action only when it is actually self-chosen.

The changing pattern of abilities a child has as it grows (see Ch. 35) reveals some of the secrets of motor control that are hidden from us by the sophistications of adulthood. There is a stage, for example, when a child has acquired the ability to pull herself up and can stand unsupported while holding on to a chair or the wall of the cot, but has not yet learned how to sit down gracefully. The grasp reflex of the hands enables the child to hang on firmly to the chair, and extensor reflexes of the legs maintain an upright posture. The problem is how to inhibit these and sit. If someone then reaches down to the child, the touch of their hands on the child's body excites opposing reflexes which make the child release its grip, and its legs go from under it. In time, aided by a variety of learning experiences, motor skills develop and movements become more sophisticated and controlled.

---

tation of receptors in the muscles and joints of the neck, and by the *vestibulocollic reflex* excited by stimulation of the balance organs (see pp. 499 and 500).

MOVING: ROLE OF DIFFERENT BRAIN AREAS

Moving from one posture to the next requires some reflexes to be inhibited while others are facilitated. Some complex patterns of movement, such as those involved in walking, are pre-programmed in the nervous system. Others are acquired only by experience. Brain areas involved include:

- motor cortex of the cerebral hemispheres
- basal ganglia
- cerebellum.

Motor cortex

Cells in the motor cortex of the cerebral hemispheres exert direct control over the interneurones and motoneurones of the reflex arcs in the brain stem and the spinal cord via the corticobulbar and corticospinal tracts (see Ch. 27). The cells in the motor cortex receive impulses from the association areas of the cerebral cortex and from the basal ganglia via the thalamus. They are also influenced by impulses coming from the cerebellum.

Basal ganglia

The role of the basal ganglia in movement control is still not well understood but evidence suggests that these brain areas play a role in allowing or disallowing different patterns of movement (see Ch. 27).

For example, in Parkinson's disease, the commonest disorder of the basal ganglia (Table 28.3), patients may have difficulty in starting and stopping chosen sequences of activity. Walking is no problem once the individual has got going, but making the initial moves is difficult. Likewise, stopping this activity may be a problem. Consequently, a person may find little difficulty in walking outdoors where movement is relatively unobstructed, whereas moving around the house, where continual adjustments need to be made to avoid obstructions, is much more difficult. ⑦

One of the other features of this and other disorders of the basal ganglia is that the patient may have unwanted movements while at rest (see Ch. 27). This suggests that programmes of activity are being allowed that have not been chosen.

Another observation that points to the function of the basal ganglia in posture and movement is that the spontaneous movements that are made usually relate more to the muscles involved in posture and limb movement than those which are concerned with the intricate movements of the fingers (see below). This suggests that the basal ganglia may have a key role in determining the postures we adopt and how we move between them and less to do with the intricate movements of our hands.

Cerebellum

This part of the brain is involved in the development of skilled programmes of activity for rapid targeted movements (see Ch. 27). As the cerebellum coordinates a mass of information from both sensory and motor areas of the nervous system it is able to refine movements so that they are performed efficiently and accurately. Without this function, movements of all kinds become much more clumsy. For example an upright posture can still be maintained but with more difficulty and only by adopting a physically more stable stance: legs placed wide apart to widen the base. Walking is still possible but in a staggering fashion and not in a straight line. ⑧

USING OUR HANDS: ROLE OF DIFFERENT BRAIN AREAS

We use our hands to pick up and hold objects, to feel their shape and explore their texture, and to perform skilled actions such as writing and drawing. All these actions require considerable coordination of visual, somatosensory and motor activity.

Table 28.3   Clinical features of Parkinson's disease

Clinical term	Observations
Tremor	Alternate contraction of agonist and antagonist muscles (e.g. 'pill rolling' movement of thumb and fingers)
Rigidity	Increased muscle tone in both extensor and flexor muscles
Akinesia	Relative lack of voluntary movement Expressionless face Loss of arm swinging while walking

DRUG TREATMENT OF PARKINSON'S DISEASE

The principal features of Parkinson's disease are tremor, rigidity and akinesia (see Table 28.3). It is thought that these signs and symptoms are the result of an imbalance between two neurotransmitters, acetylcholine and dopamine, and that improvement might be expected if the effects of the neurotransmitters could be modified. Currently, drug treatment is aimed at either decreasing cholinergic excitatory activity or increasing dopaminergic inhibitory activity.

Cholinergic activity in the basal ganglia can be blocked by atropine, and the synthetic anticholinergic drugs have a similar action. Such drugs include benzhexol, orphenadrine and procyclidine. They reduce rigidity but do not improve tremor or akinesia. The drug dose is increased gradually until optimum benefit is achieved or toxic effects occur. Toxicity is indicated by the atropine-like effects of dry mouth, blurred vision, constipation and urinary retention.

Dopaminergic activity can be enhanced by the administration of levodopa. Maximum improvement may take up to 6 months, but some 75 to 80% of patients obtain some benefit. Adverse effects include postural hypotension, nausea and vomiting, and involuntary movements, such as jerking of limbs (*myoclonus*), abnormal restlessness (*akathisia*) and facial grimacing. However, in the long term, the benefits of the drug often disappear and, after 5 years, only one-third of the patients prescribed levodopa still show improved function (Gillies et al 1986).

Primary motor and sensory cortex

The primary motor area of the cerebral cortex has a dominant role in the control of these highly skilled activities. The corticospinal tracts directly innervate many of the lower motoneurones supplying the muscles that control the movements of the hands and fingers.

Several cortical reflexes are involved in allowing us to do things like grasp and hold on to an object. For example if the object begins to slip through our hands this is detected by mechanoreceptors in the skin of the palm and our grasp of the object is reflexly strengthened. Similarly when we feel and explore the surface of an object that we are touching, the exploratory movements of our fingers are guided partly by the sensory information detected by cutaneous receptors

⑦
What is the name given to the type of gait that is characteristic of a person suffering from Parkinson's disease?

⑧
What is the general term used to describe unsteadiness in movement?

and transmitted to the somatosensory cortex which lies right next to the motor cortex (see Fig. 27.10).

The hands and the muscles that control them are extremely well represented in both the primary motor cortex and the adjacent somatosensory cortex (see Figs 24.8 and 27.11). The two areas are linked by interconnecting nerve fibres, so that the neurones in the motor cortex can be controlled by the sensory information arriving at the adjacent sensory area.

If there is damage to these parts of the brain it is possible for someone to experience difficulty in handling objects and in writing, without necessarily having difficulty in walking or other movements.

Other areas

The kind of tasks that require a considerable degree of hand–eye coordination involve other parts of the brain too, including the visual cortex. Picking up a small object between finger and thumb, or placing the correct finger on the right place on a keyboard requires knowledge of the position of the target, calculation of the amount of movement required, as well as selection of an appropriate course of action to achieve the task. Feedback of information from sensory receptors may also be used to refine the movement as it is being performed so that it is achieved with the highest degree of accuracy. Here again the cerebellum, particularly the *neocerebellum*, plays its part. If function is disordered, movements are performed with much less accuracy.

Highly skilled learned activities such as writing and drawing, through which we express our thoughts and communicate with others, depend not only on the skill with which we can actually execute the individual movements involved but also on our ability to string together a whole series of different movements in a meaningful and purposeful way. These activities rely on the function of the association areas of the brain in the parietal and frontal lobes of the cerebral hemispheres. This will be described in a later chapter (see Ch. 30).

KEY POINTS

What you should now know and understand about posture, movement and manual dexterity:

- how posture is determined by the bones of the skeleton, the joints between them and muscle contraction
- the main parts of the skeleton and its major bones
- what bone is, how it is made, maintained and mended
- different types of joints and their structure and function
- major muscles of the trunk and limbs and what they do
- how posture and movement of the trunk and limbs is controlled by the nervous system
- how the skilfulness of the hand is created by its structure, the muscles moving its parts, and their control by the nervous system
- the anatomical and physiological basis of some common musculoskeletal problems and their management.

REFERENCES AND FURTHER READING

Alberts B, Bray D, Lewis J, Raff M, Roberts K, Watson J D 1983 Molecular biology of the cell. Garland Publishing, New York, p 935

Boore J R P, Champion R, Ferguson M C 1987 Nursing the physically ill adult. Churchill Livingstone, Edinburgh, p 282, 283

Chaffin D B, Anderson G B J 1991 Occupational biomechanics, 2nd edn. John Wiley, Chichester (Specialist reference work explaining methods of working and the design of work tools and workplaces that help to prevent musculoskeletal disorders)

Chilman A M, Thomas M 1987 Understanding nursing care, 3rd edn. Churchill Livingstone, Edinburgh, p 33, 34

Ger R, Abrahams P 1989 Essentials of clinical anatomy. Churchill Livingstone, Edinburgh

Gillies H C, Roger H J, Spector R G, Trounce J R 1986 A textbook of clinical pharmacology, 2nd edn. Edward Arnold, London

Goodwill C J, Chamberlain M A (eds) 1988 Rehabilitation of the physically disabled adult. Chapman & Hall, London (Excellent reference covering almost every aspect of care of the patient undergoing rehabilitation)

Gunn C 1992 Bones and joints: a guide for students. Churchill Livingstone, Edinburgh (Covers all the bones and joints – including teeth – concisely and clearly, using simple line drawings)

Henderson V, Nite G 1978 Principles and practice of nursing, 6th edn. Macmillan, New York

Jenkins D B 1991 Hollinhead's Functional anatomy of the limbs and back, 6th edn. W B Saunders, Philadelphia (Not just bones and muscles but what moves what and how)

Lumley J S P 1990 Surface anatomy: the anatomical basis of the clinical examination. Churchill Livingstone, Edinburgh (Clearly presented book. Photographs plus line drawings indicating position of structures beneath)

Murray P D F 1985 Bones: a study of the development and structure of the vertebrate skeleton. Cambridge University Press, Cambridge (Classic book describing the experimental basis of fundamental knowledge about the development and growth of bones)

Oliver J 1993 Back care: a teaching manual. Butterworth–Heinemann, London (Practical manual for those providing information and advice to patients with back problems. Explains what happens to discs, joints and ligaments when we move)

Rogers A W 1992 Textbook of anatomy. Churchill Livingstone, Edinburgh, p 14, 21, 22, 23, 168, 239, 242, 278, 282

Rothwell J C 1987 Control of human movement. Croom Helm, Beckenham (Advanced student text relating basic science to neurology)

Williams P L, Warwick R, Dyson M, Bannister L 1989 Gray's Anatomy, 37th edn. Churchill Livingstone, Edinburgh

Wilson K J W 1990 Ross & Wilson Anatomy and physiology in health and illness, 7th edn. Churchill Livingstone, Edinburgh, p 366, 369, 371, 372, 381, 386, 394

Chapter 29
ACTIONS 2: LOOKING, COMMUNICATING AND EATING

A welcoming smile, a word, or taking a mouthful of food are different actions with different purposes but all involve activity of muscles of the face and jaws. Several different parts of the brain, including the brain stem, the limbic system, the cerebral hemispheres and cerebellum, are involved in controlling the muscles, according to the specific movements performed and their role.

This chapter outlines the structure of the head and neck and describes how a variety of different actions such as looking, speaking and eating are performed and controlled. This will provide a basis for understanding some of the problems that arise as a result of injury, disability or disease.

ANATOMY OF THE HEAD AND NECK

BONES

Skull

The skull (Fig. 29.1) is composed of several bones, all but one of which, the *mandible*, are fixed together to form a rigid structure. In the fetus and in young babies, the joints between the bones (*sutures*) are flexible, but they gradually become calcified with age forming immovable joints.

The skull consists of two parts:

● cranium   ● bones of the face.

Cranium

The cranium forms a protective case around the brain. The top part (*vault*) arches over the cerebral hemispheres. The lower part (*base*) (Fig. 29.2) lies under the cerebellum and brain stem and is pierced by a number of holes (*foramina*) of different sizes through which nerves and blood vessels pass. The largest of these (*foramen magnum*) surrounds the lowest part of the medulla oblongata which merges into the spinal cord.

The vault and the base are each composed of several bones (Figs 29.1 and 29.2):

Vault	*Base*
frontal	temporal
occipital	occipital
parietal	ethmoid
	sphenoid

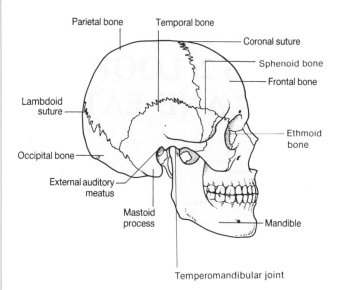

Figure 29.1
Structure of the skull. (Reproduced from Rogers 1992 (Fig. 14.2) by permission of the publishers.)

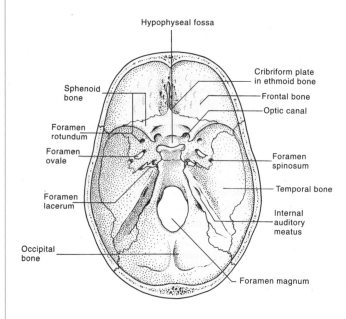

Figure 29.2
Bones of the base of the skull from the inside. (Reproduced from Rogers 1992 (Fig. 14.6) by permission of the publishers.)

The *occipital* bone, forming part of the vault as well as the base, is the one perched on top of the neck bones (see p. 475). The *ethmoid* bone forms part of the structure of the nose (see Ch. 15 and Fig. 29.9). The *sphenoid* bone has a number of extensions connecting with other bones and tissues and includes a small cavity (*hypophyseal fossa*) enclosing the pituitary gland (see Ch. 10). The *temporal* bone houses the auditory apparatus (see Ch. 25).

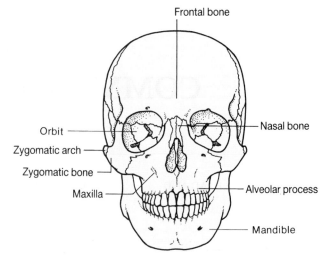

Figure 29.3
Bones of the face. (Reproduced from Rogers 1992 (Fig. 14.3) by permission of the publishers.)

Bones of the face

The framework of the face is created by several bones (Fig. 29.3). Several interlock with the anterior part of the cranium, including:

● cheek bone (*zygomatic bone*)
● upper jaw bone (*maxilla*)
● bones forming the walls of the nasal cavity (*nasal bones, vomer, palatine bones, inferior concha*).

The *maxilla* consists of two bones that become fused during development. It bears the upper teeth and forms:

● the roof of the oral cavity (*hard palate*)
● part of the lateral walls of the nasal cavities
● the floor of the socket of the eyeball (*orbit*).

CLEFT LIP OR PALATE

During the tenth week of fetal life, the maxillary bones and the palatal processes fuse as the beginning of human face construction. Sheets of skin and muscle start to organise themselves around the landmarks of the mouth, nose and eyes. A single flap grows symmetrically down the middle to form the forehead, the upper eyelids, the front of the nose and the web that links the inside of the upper lip and the gum. If the bones fuse normally, but the overlying skin does not close, the result is a *cleft lip*, sometimes called a 'harelip' because it looks like the lip of a hare. This abnormality may appear on either the right or left side of the lip, the cleft running down from the nostril.

Sometimes, there is imperfect fusion of the underlying bones leaving a large gap in the hard palate, in which case the nasal cavity opens into the mouth and the nasal septum and vomer bone are often absent. Such an abnormality is called *cleft palate* and often, but not always, occurs in conjunction with cleft lip.

In infancy, cleft palate and cleft lip both limit the child's ability to suck and may lead to malnutrition. Cleft palate may later lead to the development of speech difficulties. Both abnormalities can be corrected by surgery.

Figure 29.4
View of a section through the skull, showing the air-filled sinuses. (Reproduced from Rogers 1992 (Fig. 14.5) by permission of the publishers.)

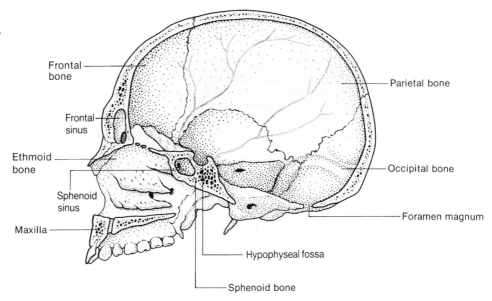

The only freely mobile bone of the skull is the *mandible*. Like the maxilla it bears teeth and forms early in development from the fusion of two bones. It articulates with the temporal bone of the cranium via the *temporomandibular joint* (Fig. 29.1). This hinged joint also allows the mandible to slide forwards and backwards.

Air-filled sinuses
Several of the bones, the frontal, sphenoid, ethmoid and maxilla, contain hollow air-filled spaces (*sinuses*) (Fig. 29.4). These sinuses are lined by a ciliated mucous epithelium. Secretions formed by the epithelium drain through several openings into the nasal cavity (see Ch. 15). ①

SINUSITIS

Normally the mucous membrane of the paranasal sinuses responds to environmental stress by flushing the surface with mucus, but as the lining becomes inflamed, the communicating passages narrow. With the accumulation of mucus in the sinuses, the drainage slows down and congestion occurs. The condition is known as *sinusitis*. The victim experiences headaches and a feeling of pressure and heaviness within the facial bones. Sinusitis is accompanied by *rhinitis* (an acute or chronic inflammation of the nasal mucous membrane caused by infection or an allergic reaction) because the mucous membranes of the sinuses are continuous with those of the nose. General malaise and fever accompany the local symptoms when an infection is present.

Chronic sinusitis may occur as a result of a deviated nasal septum. The most common location of deviation is the junction between the bony and cartilaginous portions of the septum (Fig. 29.9). If the deviation prevents drainage of one or more of the sinuses, chronic infection and inflammation may occur. Deviated septa may result from the development of abnormalities, such as polyps, or injuries to the nose.

Q: The maxillary sinus is most prone to infection. Can you think why this might be?

Neck bones

There are seven *cervical vertebrae* (see Ch. 28). Joints between the vertebrae allow bending of the neck forwards and backwards. Turning of the head to the left and to the right is enabled mainly through rotation of the first cervical vertebra (*atlas*) upon the peg-like vertebra below (*axis*) (Fig. 29.5). The peg (*odontoid process*)

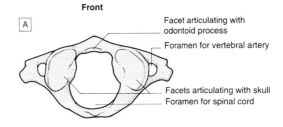

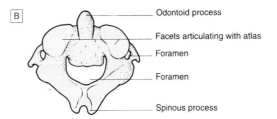

① *What do you think is the function of these sinuses?*

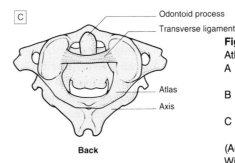

Figure 29.5
Atlas and axis:
A Atlas from above
B Axis from above and behind
C Atlas in position on top of axis.
(Adapted from Wilson 1990.)

is held in position by the *transverse ligament*. The atlas supports the skull above.

Whiplash is a nonspecific term applied to injury to the spinal cord and spine due to sudden extension of the neck, as in sudden stopping or starting of a vehicle. It is a common injury sustained in car accidents.

TEETH AND PERIODONTAL TISSUES

Teeth

Two sets of teeth, *deciduous* and *permanent*, develop during life within the maxilla and mandible (Fig. 29.6). The deciduous or *milk* teeth (20 in total) begin to erupt from around 6 months of age but are gradually pushed out later, from the age of 6 years, by the permanent teeth (see Ch. 35). Both sets include:

- incisors (8)
- canines (4)
- premolars (or deciduous molars) (8).

The permanent teeth also include a maximum of 12 more, the *molar* teeth. Incisors, canines, premolars and molars differ in their structure and function. Incisors cut food into pieces, whereas the premolars and molars crush and grind it.

Structure of a tooth

Each tooth consists of two parts (Fig. 29.7):

- an outer calcified part (*dentine, enamel* and *cement*)
- an inner region of connective tissue (*pulp*).

Most of the outer part consists of *dentine*. This is harder than bone and consists of a framework of collagen fibres impregnated with inorganic materials. Although hard, the dentine is not impenetrable, as there are many minute tubules extending through it to the pulp in the centre. Dentine is formed throughout life by cells lining its inner surface.

The part of the tooth embedded in the jaw bone (*root*) is covered by a thin layer of *cement*, a substance similar to dentine but less hard and not containing any tubules. Like dentine it is continually formed throughout life.

The other part of the tooth (*crown*) is covered by a thin layer of *enamel*, the hardest tissue in the body. Once formed, enamel cannot be renewed or extended. ②

② *What is the role of the enamel?*

The pulp in the interior of the tooth consists of a number of different cells, including *odontoblasts*, *fibroblasts* and *macrophages*, lodged in an intercellular matrix consisting of collagen and glycoproteins (see Ch. 2). The pulp contains blood vessels and lymph capillaries, and is innervated by autonomic and somatic nerve fibres. Some nerve endings extend a short distance into the dentine. Excitation of these nerves gives rise to pain (see Ch. 32).

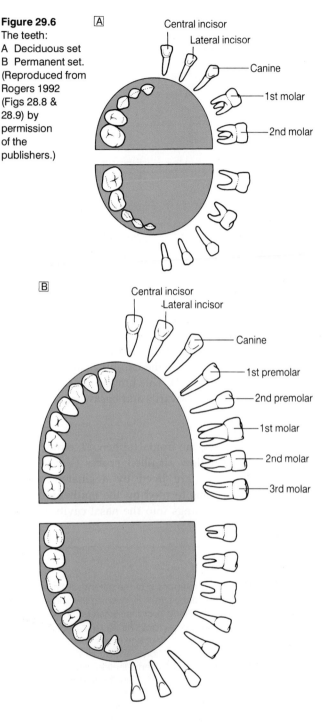

Figure 29.6
The teeth:
A Deciduous set
B Permanent set.
(Reproduced from Rogers 1992 (Figs 28.8 & 28.9) by permission of the publishers.)

Periodontal tissues

Periodontal membrane

The root of each tooth is attached to the surrounding bone by the *periodontal membrane* (or *ligament*) (Fig. 29.7). This consists of bundles of collagen fibres anchored at one end to the bone of the jaw, and at the other end to the cement covering the tooth. This strong fibrous tissue holds the tooth firmly but not rigidly. The periodontal membrane is well supplied with nerves. These detect the pressures developed during chewing and biting (see p. 506).

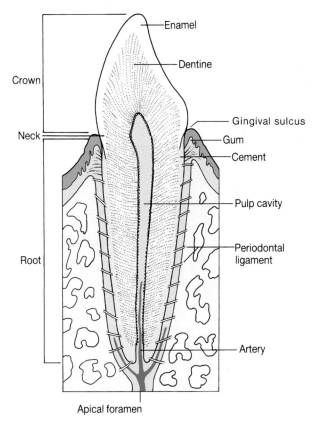

Figure 29.7
Structure of a tooth. (Reproduced from Rogers 1992 (Fig. 28.7) by permission of the publishers.)

TOOTH DECAY

Our teeth play an essential role in breaking down food into smaller particles. Unfortunately, some of these food particles, especially the refined carbohydrates (sugar), remain in the mouth after meals and provide nourishment for oral bacteria, which are responsible for most common teeth problems but are harmless until sugar enters the mouth.

One would expect all the food we eat to leave the mouth with the action of saliva and the tongue and, even if some particles were left behind, that the antibacterial constituents of saliva would kill these bacteria. Their survival on the surfaces of the teeth depends on the sticky matrix they produce, which traps food particles and creates plaque deposits that start to ferment. The fermentation produces acids that remove calcium and phosphate from the surface enamel of the teeth. The plaque deposit provides food for bacteria, as well as protecting them from saliva. Once the acids have eaten away a crevice in the tooth, the destructive process accelerates, because the bacteria are most active when hidden away from the air. The result is cavity formation in the tooth, known as 'dental caries'.

If nothing is done to prevent further bacterial activity within the gingival sulcus (Fig. 29.7), the acids produced begin to erode the connection between the neck of the tooth and the gingiva. The gums appear to recede from the tooth and a periodontal disorder develops, the invading bacteria progressively destroying the periodontal ligament and eroding the alveolar bone. This loosens the tooth and eventually causes it to be lost.

Gingiva

Extending from the periodontal membrane over the jaw bones is a mucous membrane (*gingiva* or *gum*) consisting of squamous epithelium and connective tissue. The gingiva is firmly bound to the outer covering of the bone (*periosteum*) and contains many sensory receptors. Normally the gingiva covers the junction between the enamel and the cement (*cervical margin*) but recession of the gum occurs as we grow older, exposing the junction. This process is accelerated by gum disease, such as gingivitis.

ORAL CAVITY, NOSE AND PHARYNX

Oral cavity

When you look into your oral cavity through the mouth you will see a number of different structures (Fig. 29.8). The most prominent, which gets in the way of seeing much else if it is not pressed down, is the *tongue*. The tongue consists almost entirely of muscle fibres. Some are anchored to the *mandible*, the *hyoid* bone (see p. 507, Fig. 29.20), and the *styloid process* of the temporal bone.

The upper surface of the tongue is richly supplied with a variety of sensory receptors including taste buds (see Ch. 24) and touch, pressure and temperature receptors.

The roof of the oral cavity is formed by the *hard palate* which merges into the *soft palate* at the back of the mouth. The exit from the oral cavity into the pharynx is framed by two arches, formed of folds of mucous membrane. Associated with these are the *palatoglossal* and *palatopharyngeal muscles*. Lying between the arches are clumps of lymphoid tissue (*palatine tonsils*) (see Ch. 15).

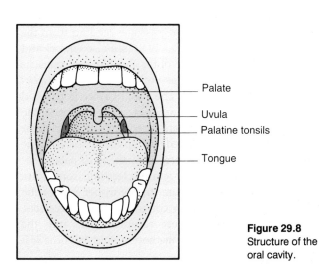

Figure 29.8
Structure of the oral cavity.

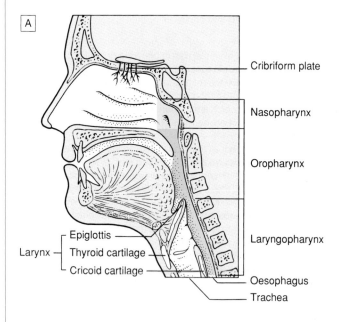

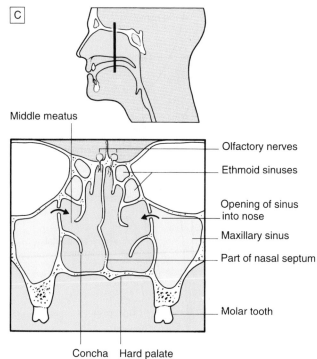

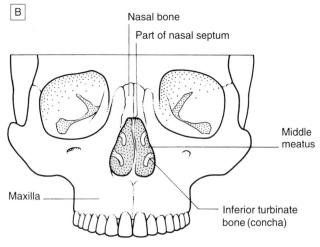

Figure 29.9
Section through the head showing nasal, pharyngeal and laryngeal structures.

Nose

The nose consists of sculpted passages leading from the nostrils into the pharynx (Fig. 29.9) (see also Chs 15 and 24). The framework of the outer flexible part consists of cartilage, whereas that of the inner passages (*nasal cavity*) is formed by bone. The nasal cavity is divided into two by the *nasal septum*. On walls opposite the septum (*lateral walls*) there are three projections (*conchae* or *turbinate bones*) separated by spaces (*meatus*). The floor of the nasal cavity is formed by the hard palate.

The nasal cavity and the sinuses leading from it are lined by a mucous epithelium. In the upper part of the nasal cavity the epithelium contains *olfactory receptors*. The nerves innervating these receptors pass into the brain through perforations in the ethmoid bone (*cribriform plate*).

BLEEDING FROM THE NOSE

Nosebleed or *epistaxis* is a common condition involving the vessels of the mucosa covering the cartilaginous portion of the septum. Bleeding results from any factor affecting the integrity of the epithelium or the underlying vessels after a blow to the nose, or it may be the result of sneezing, picking the dry nostrils or blowing the nose. Other contributing factors are infections, allergies, blood clotting disorders or high blood pressure (hypertension), which may provoke nosebleed by rupturing small vessels.

Following traffic accidents, a watery, blood-stained fluid issuing from the nose may be a sign of escaping cerebrospinal fluid (CSF) from a fractured skull. Such 'bleeding' can cause a considerable loss of blood and CSF, and the casualty may swallow or inhale much of it, resulting in vomiting and affecting breathing. In such a situation, the main aim of care is to prevent further complications by safeguarding breathing and preventing inhalation of vomit.

The nose is supplied with blood by branches of both the maxillary and facial arteries. There are anastomoses (see Ch. 5, p. 100) between these two supplies. One site of anastomosis near the entrance to the nostrils is the most common site of spontaneous nosebleeds.

Pharynx

The *pharynx* is a tube consisting chiefly of muscle covered inside and out by fibrous tissue, and lined by epithelium. When the muscles contract, as they do during swallowing (see p. 506), the tube is narrowed and shortened.

The pharynx leads from the oral cavity and nose to the *larynx* and *oesophagus*. It consists of three parts (Fig. 29.9):

- nasopharynx   • oropharynx   • laryngopharynx.

Nasopharynx

The nasopharynx extends from the base of the skull to the soft palate. Like parts of the nose and the respiratory tract, it is lined by a ciliated mucous epithelium. There are several clumps of lymphoid tissue. Some (the *tubal tonsil*) is near the opening of the *auditory (eustachian) tube*. Swelling of this clump of lymphoid tissue as a result of an infection can block the tube and cause temporary deafness (see Ch. 25). Other clumps of lymphoid tissue (*adenoids*) are present on the roof and upper back wall of the nasopharynx. They are most prominent in children and decrease during adolescence (see Chs 15 and 35).

Oropharynx

The oropharynx is the part between the soft palate and the epiglottis that looks red with inflammation when you have a sore throat. It is framed by the *palatoglossal* and *palatopharyngeal arches* and is lined by squamous epithelium.

Laryngopharynx

The laryngopharynx extends from the epiglottis to the oesophagus (Fig. 29.9). The laryngeal opening faces the back wall of the pharynx. There is a small recess (*piriform fossa*) on either side of the larynx in which small food items such as fish bones sometimes get stuck. In addition to the constrictor muscles, the pharynx also has three longitudinal muscles. When these contract, as they do in swallowing (see p. 507), they raise the larynx.

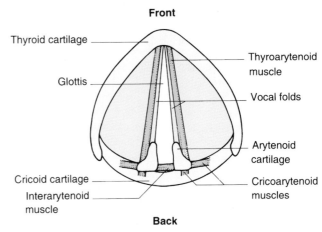

Figure 29.10
Position of the vocal folds in relation to other laryngeal structures.

Larynx

The larynx is a box-like structure formed from several pieces of cartilage (Fig. 29.9):

- epiglottis
- thyroid cartilage (part of which forms the 'Adam's apple')
- cricoid cartilage
- arytenoids (two small movable pieces).

Stretched between the arytenoids and the thyroid cartilage are the vocal cords (Fig. 29.10).

MUSCLES AND NERVES

Some of the many muscles of the head and neck, their innervation and actions are shown in Figures 29.11 and 29.12.

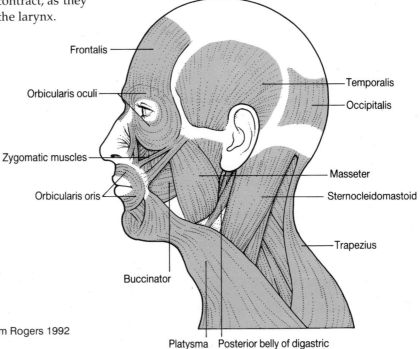

Figure 29.11
Muscles of the head and neck. (Reproduced from Rogers 1992 (Fig. 15.1) by permission of the publishers.)

Figure 29.12
Innervation and functions of
muscles of the head and neck.

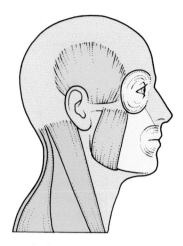
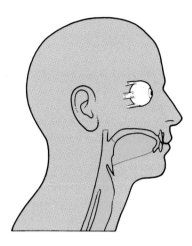

Nerves		Muscles	Functions	
Cranial	Spinal			
III, IV, VI		Eyeball		Looking
VII		Face, lips, brow	Facial expression	
(a) V		Jaw (masseter, temporalis)		
(b) IX		Pharynx	Eating	Vocal communication
(c) X		Pharynx, larynx		
XII		Tongue		
	Phrenic nerve Intercostal nerves	Diaphragm Intercostal	Breathing	
XI		Neck (trapezius sternocleidomastoid)		Head turning
(a), (b), (c), includes sensory innervation of naso-, oro- and laryngopharynx respectively				

LOOKING

Our ability to see depends on the motor systems controlling the movement of our eyes and of our heads, as well as on our sense of vision. These motor systems enable us to look around and to fix our eyes rapidly and accurately on any objects of interest. They also enable us to keep track of what we are looking at, even if we or it is moving.

EYE MOVEMENTS

Movement of each eyeball is controlled by three pairs of muscles (Fig. 29.13), innervated by cranial nerves III, IV and VI:

- superior and inferior rectus
- superior and inferior oblique
- lateral and medial rectus.

These muscles enable us to look around as well as swivel our eyes inwards in order to view a near object (*convergence*). ③

There are two kinds of movement:

- pursuit
- saccadic.

In a *pursuit movement* the eyeballs turn slowly and steadily in one direction, keeping track of the object in view, until the eyeballs have turned as far as they can. At this point the pursuit movement stops and the eyeball flicks back to its centre position. This rapid flick is a ballistic

③
Can you explain why virtually any movement of the eyes requires the joint action of several muscles, albeit to different degrees?

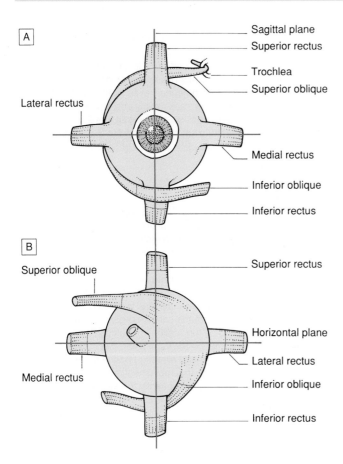

Figure 29.13
Muscles of the eyeball seen from in front and from behind.

Labels (A, top): Sagittal plane, Superior rectus, Trochlea, Superior oblique, Lateral rectus, Medial rectus, Inferior oblique, Inferior rectus

Labels (B, bottom): Superior oblique, Superior rectus, Horizontal plane, Medial rectus, Lateral rectus, Inferior oblique, Inferior rectus

movement (*saccade*). The combination of movements, pursuit followed by saccade, is seen in rail travellers as they view the passing scenery.

When we are not looking at anything in particular but just looking around, we use saccadic movements too, to fix our eyes first on one point and then on another. From these several snapshots we build up in our minds a full picture of the scene.

CONTROL

The movement of our eyes is controlled:

- reflexly
- voluntarily.

Reflexes make us look at a new object of interest and keep it in view regardless of whether we or it is moving. Voluntary control enables us to look around or deliberately focus on an object of our choice, as in reading this book for example.

Reflex control

Noticing a new object
When a novel object suddenly appears in our field of view we usually feel impelled to turn and look at it.

Depending on where it is, we may simply turn our eyes, or we may turn our heads and bodies too. These movements are entirely reflex. They are triggered by the novelty of the stimulus, and their purpose is to enable us to bring the image of the novel stimulus on to the foveal part of the retina, which provides us with the clearest and most detailed vision (see Ch. 26). ④

We do not have to be conscious of the stimulus to react to it. We respond automatically because the parts of the brain that coordinate these responses are in the brain stem (see Ch. 20) and not the thalamus and cerebral cortex, which are involved in consciousness (see Ch. 31). Consequently, a person who has sustained cerebral injury involving the visual cortex, may still respond to an abrupt change in his surroundings, such as a flash of lightning, even though he cannot actually see it (see Chs 23 and 27).

Similar reflexes enable us to turn our heads and bodies to face a new stimulus when we are startled by a sound, such as breaking glass, or by an unexpected tap on the shoulder. Again, the purpose of the reflex movement is to enable us to face and look at the novel stimulus.

Fixing on an object while you move
When walking down the road looking at the scenery, although your body goes up and down at each step, the picture in your mind's eye of the buildings or trees and bushes does not. However, if you attempt to take a photograph while walking the resulting picture is usually blurred (unless you use a very fast shutter speed).

The picture we see with our eyes is not blurred but remains steady chiefly because reflex movements of our eyes and head compensate for the movement of the body. The displacement of our bodies is rapidly detected by sensory receptors in the vestibular apparatus (see Ch. 24), and this sensory information reflexly triggers contraction of the appropriate muscles of the eyeball (*vestibulo-ocular reflex*) and of the neck (*vestibulocollic reflex*) (Fig. 29.14). As a result, the image of the object we are looking at is kept centred on the foveal part of the retina.

Tracking a moving object
Keeping our eyes fixed on a moving object, such as a bird or a car, depends upon a different reflex (*optokinetic reflex*). The movement of the object of interest is registered by cells in the visual areas of the cerebral cortex (see Ch. 26). Impulses from these cells are used to power a pursuit movement of the eye which is used to track the moving object and keep the image of it on the foveal region of the retina for as long as possible.

Viewing a near object
When we glance from a distant object to a near object,

④ *How does the foveal part of the retina provide us with the clearest and most detailed vision?*

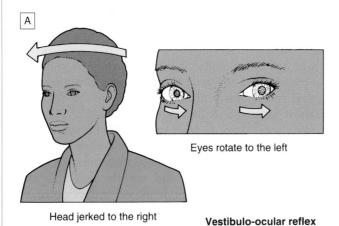

Head jerked to the right

Eyes rotate to the left

Vestibulo-ocular reflex

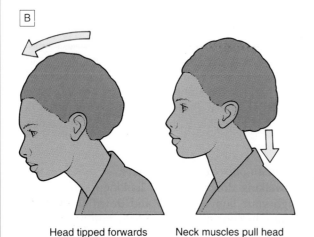

Head tipped forwards

Neck muscles pull head back

Vestibulocollic reflex

Figure 29.14
Reflexes stabilising eye position.

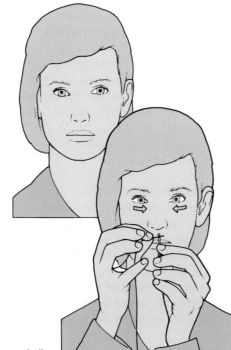

Figure 29.15
Movement of the eyeballs for near vision.

Convergence

NYSTAGMUS

Nystagmus is a distinctive pattern of involuntary eye movement occurring sometimes in neurological disorders. An observer looking at someone's eyes would see that they do not remain steady but track rapidly and repeatedly in one direction. The pattern consists of a pursuit movement followed by a recentring saccade. There are two main sources of nystagmus:

- vestibular
- cerebellar

Vestibular nystagmus
Vestibular nystagmus is provoked by signals originating from the vestibular system. Normally, movements of the eyes are reflexly triggered when movement of the body is sensed by the balance organs (*vestibulo-ocular reflex*) (Fig. 29.14). This reflex depends partly on a comparison, made by cells of the vestibular nuclei, of the signals received from the balance organs on each side of the head.

If the vestibular system on one side is defective, the difference in signals from the balance organs on each side of the head is noted by the vestibular nucleus. This difference gives someone the impression that movement is occurring when it is not, and also triggers the reflexes normally associated with that movement, such as the vestibulo-ocular reflex. Consequently the eyes move as if pursuing an object and then recentre and begin the pursuit again, and keep on doing this.

Vestibular nystagmus is often accompanied by vertigo and nausea (Bouchier & Morris 1976). Nurses can help the afflicted persons by advising rest in a quiet darkened room because the condition can be very frightening for the patient. The nurse will need to stay with him to provide reassurance and protection from physical harm during the worst stages of an attack.

Vestibular nystagmus can be evoked temporarily in healthy people by the simple manoeuvre of spinning someone around in a rotating chair, and then stopping the chair abruptly. The fluid in the subject's semicircular canals continues to spin for several seconds and, while it does, the vestibular receptors are stimulated, the impression of movement is created, and the vestibulo-ocular reflex is triggered giving rise to nystagmus.

Cerebellar nystagmus
Nystagmus of cerebellar origin differs from vestibular nystagmus in that it happens only when movement is attempted (see p. 501). It is a form of *intention tremor* (see Ch. 27) occurring when the gaze is shifted from one object to another. It disappears once the new object has been fixated.

our eyeballs turn towards one another (*converge*) so that both point directly at the new object of interest (Fig. 29.15). This binocular movement is powered by a cortical reflex, which forms part of the *near response* (see Ch. 26).

Convergence is guided by the difference in the images of the object viewed through each eye. Convergence stops when the two images (formed by right eye and left eye) fit together best in the 'mind's eye'. These two images of a near object can never be exactly the same, but they are near enough for our minds to form an apparently single image.

The slight differences that continue to exist produce the three-dimensional view of objects (*stereoscopic view*) that we normally enjoy. This three-dimensional view helps us to form an impression of the relative distance of objects from us.

If there is weakness in one or more of the ocular muscles of either eye, it may become impossible for the two eyes to work together. Because they no longer point at the same object (*strabismus* or *squint*) the result is double vision (*diplopia*). If this occurs in young children, one of the two images may be suppressed. This can lead to irreversible changes in the visual cortex so that sight from one eye is permanently impaired.

Voluntary control

Voluntary control of eye movements, for example in looking around or reading, depends upon normal function of regions of the motor cortex and the cerebellum (see Ch. 27).

Looking around

When we look around, we scan the scene around us and fix our eyes briefly on different objects. This provides us with a number of snapshots of the scene from which we may choose one to inspect. Once something has caught our attention, the vestibulo-ocular, vestibulocollic, and optokinetic reflexes maintain the position of the object of interest on the fovea, until we are distracted by something else or choose voluntarily to look at a different object.

Reading

When we read a book or a letter, our eyes do not move steadily across the page but jump from one point to the next in a series of saccades. Some techniques designed to improve reading speed do so by reducing the number of saccades necessary to read a page of text. Reading difficulties may sometimes be caused by disordered control of eye movements.

COMMUNICATING

We communicate with one another in many different ways by vocal and non-vocal means. We use sounds to express our thoughts in words, and the intonation of our voices to express how we feel. We use facial expression and body language as well to convey messages and display our moods and attitudes.

VOCAL COMMUNICATION

We produce sounds using the vocal apparatus of the

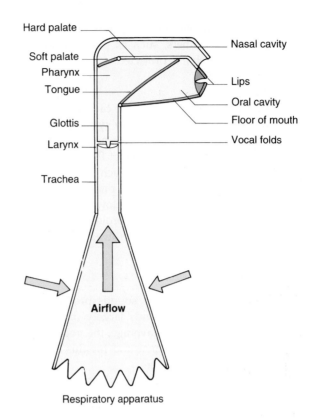

Figure 29.16
The vocal instrument.

Legend: Moving parts in the supraglottal chambers

larynx and associated structures of the oral cavity, throat and pharynx. Many different muscles are involved. Their activity is controlled by cells in several parts of the brain, including the brain stem and limbic system as well as the cerebral cortex, cerebellum and basal ganglia. The production of clear speech involves many brain areas. If the function of any part is disturbed, speech is impaired (*dysarthria*).

> A local paralysis of the laryngeal muscles may render someone completely silent although his mastery of language remains unimpaired; he can still convey his thoughts in writing and make graceful and eloquent use of language.

Mechanics of sound production

Sounds are produced by the vibration of parts of the vocal apparatus, shown diagrammatically in the form of a musical instrument in Figure 29.16. The vocal folds in the larynx vibrate when air is forced past them through the glottis (the gap between the folds). Other vibrations are added by structures such as the lips, tongue and soft palate often when airflow is abruptly altered. The pitch of a sound (high or low) depends upon the length and tension of the vibrating structures whereas the form of the sound (e.g. aaah, eee, ooo) depends upon the shape and size of the chambers, such as pharynx, nose and oral cavity into which it is projected.

Vibration

The normal sounds of breathing are caused by vibration of structures within the respiratory system as air flows in and out of the lungs through the airways. If there is narrowing of airways or presence of fluid, other abnormal sounds may be produced such as wheezing in asthma, or the crepitations heard in pneumonia.

In speaking and singing (see below) the respiratory muscles are used to produce a prolonged expiration, and air is forced through the narrowed glottis causing the vocal folds to vibrate.

Pitch and form

The fundamental pitch of the sounds produced when the vocal folds vibrate depends largely on the length and tension of the folds. On average, the vocal folds are longer in men than in women and for this reason the pitch of a man's voice is lower.

The shape of the cavity into which the sound is projected determines which harmonic frequencies will resonate best. This alters the blend of frequencies in the sound and determines its form and character (see Ch. 25). As the relative dimensions of the structures of the pharynx, nose and oral cavity differ slightly from person to person, voices sound different too.

> The action of the resonating cavities in the head is illustrated by the change in quality of the voice when a person has a severe cold and the nose and sinuses are congested.

Neural control of sound production

We use our voices to cry out when we are hurt, to laugh when we are amused, and to sing and speak. The neural control mechanisms range from the simple reflex of the cry of alarm, to the complexity of cerebral and cerebellar control of speech.

The cry of alarm

The cry or scream of alarm is the most primitive of sounds we make. It is basically the result of a simple brain stem reflex triggered by pain or danger. Neurones in the vicinity of brain areas associated with pain pathways, such as the peri-aqueductal grey matter (see Ch. 32), are involved.

Crying and laughing

The more complicated patterns of sound characteristic of crying, moaning, and laughing etc. involve the limbic system and the hypothalamus (see Ch. 31). The motor cortex, cerebellum and thalamus exert relatively little control over the production of these sounds. Thus,

patients who have suffered injury to the cerebral cortex leaving them unable to speak (see Ch. 30) may still be able to laugh and cry.

Speaking and singing

Speaking and singing involve the coordinated contraction of over 100 different muscles controlled by the motor areas of the cerebral cortex, the basal ganglia and the cerebellum, acting through the lower motoneurones of the pons, medulla and spinal cord in the cranial and spinal nerves (Ch. 27).

Speaking

The processes involved in speaking and singing can be divided into several components:

- producing an airstream
- producing sounds
- modifying sounds by *resonance*
- smooth transitions between one sound and the next (*articulation*).

Producing an airstream

The pattern of breathing is altered when we speak or sing. Instead of the usual regular pattern of inspiration and expiration (see Ch. 7), sharp inspirations are interspersed with periods of steady expiration. In speech and singing, expiration is not a passive process but is controlled by muscle contraction. Both internal and external intercostal muscles are involved, acting to brake the usual recoil-powered expiration, and to maintain airflow at an appropriate rate when the recoil force lessens or would have ceased.

When we speak, the automatic inspiratory–expiratory cycle, set by the respiratory centres in the pons and medulla (see Ch. 7), is overruled by impulses from the motor cortex. The intercostal nerves are controlled directly by impulses in the corticospinal tracts rather than by impulses originating from the brain stem.

Producing sounds

When breathing without speaking, the glottis is open. When we speak, the glottis is narrowed by the contraction of several laryngeal muscles including the cricoarytenoid and interarytenoid muscles (Fig. 29.10). Air forced out through this narrow opening causes the cricovocal ligaments (vocal folds) to vibrate. This vibration compresses and rarefies the air and produces sound waves (see Ch. 25). Contraction of the muscles sets the length and tension in the folds and thus determines the pitch of the sound. Muscle spindles (see Ch. 24) monitor the length of the muscle fibres, helping to maintain them at the length required. The motoneurones innervating the laryngeal muscles form part of the laryngeal nerves, which are branches of cranial nerve X (vagus).

The consonants of speech, such as 't', 'p', 'k' and 'd', are produced by briefly closing off the oral cavity in a variety of different ways using the muscles of the jaws, lips and tongue. The sudden release of air causes other structures, such as lips, to vibrate, adding further frequencies of vibration to those originating from the vocal folds.

The sounds we produce as 'p', 'b' and 'd' consist of vibrations produced by the vocal folds, as well as vibrations produced by other structures. In sounds like 'sss' and 't', however, the vocal folds are not used at all. The vibrations are created by air flowing through the narrow openings formed by the lips and tongue. When we whisper, we hardly use the vocal cords at all.

Resonance

The primary sound formed by the vocal folds is modified by the shape of the chambers within which it resonates. For the human voice, the chambers include the pharynx, the oral and nasal cavities, and the air-filled sinuses. We change the shape of several of the chambers by opening and closing our mouths, including or excluding the nasal cavity by elevating the soft palate, and altering the relative positions of lips, tongue, teeth and cheeks (Fig. 29.16). This is how we produce different vowel sounds.

To produce 'a', 'e', 'i', 'o', and 'u', we normally use the oral cavity alone and block off the nasal cavity with the soft palate. If the nasal cavity is used as well, nasal vowel sounds are formed. These are used a lot in some languages, such as French. If the nasal cavity is open when the oral cavity is closed, then nasal consonants like 'm', 'n', and 'ng' are produced.

Articulation

Speech consists of a series of different sounds linked together to form words, and words linked together to form phrases. It is a highly skilled motor activity requiring smooth transitions, in a short space of time, from one pattern of muscle activity to the next. The movements required have to be exceedingly precise. Very small differences in the position of the lips and teeth alter the sounds produced. The differences made to speech by the loss of teeth or the acquisition of dentures are well known. Considerable coordination of activity is required to ensure that the correct sequencing of sounds is achieved easily and crisply. Without this, speech

becomes slurred or laboured. This precision is achieved by the control exercised by the motor cortex and the cerebellum.

Dysarthria

Defects in the motor control of speech lead to characteristic speech impairments (*dysarthrias*). Speech is disordered if there is impairment of (Fig. 29.17):

- the muscles of speech: respiratory, pharyngeal, facial etc.
- lower motoneurones: cranial nerves – V, VII, IX, and XII; spinal nerves – phrenic, intercostal
- upper motoneurones: e.g. corticospinal and bulbar tracts
- brain areas: motor cortex, basal ganglia and cerebellum.

There are four main types of dysarthria:

- flaccid
- spastic
- ataxic
- hypokinetic.

Flaccid dysarthria

Flaccid dysarthria results from injury to one or more lower motoneurones. The effects on speech depend

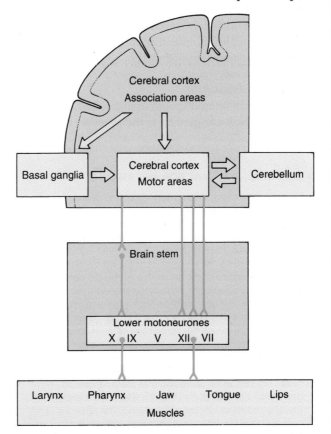

Figure 29.17
Neural control of the muscles involved in speech.

The lips, tongue and the soft palate play an important role in articulation. However, if damage occurs at higher levels, as it does in strokes, the patient may suffer from one of the various forms of *aphasia* (Ch. 30), which means the inability to express oneself linguistically. The neuromuscular apparatus of the voice and tongue may be intact, but the patient cannot put his thoughts into words.

upon which lower motoneurones are affected. The effects may include breathiness in phonation, nasal emission of air, and audible inspiration.

The tone of the affected muscles is reduced, as in any lower motoneurone lesion (see Ch. 27), which is why this form of speech disorder is termed a *flaccid dysarthria*.

> A temporary dysarthria can result from dental anaesthesia.

Spastic dysarthria

The lower motoneurones of the lips, tongue and cheeks are directly innervated by neurones from the motor cortex (*corticobulbar tracts*) (Fig. 29.17). If there are lesions of these tracts, or of the cerebral cortex, speech becomes slow and words are articulated imprecisely and with difficulty. If there is extensive cortical damage then speech becomes impossible, as will any voluntary movement of the mouth, face and tongue. In addition, muscle tone (see Ch. 27) is increased, which is why the disorder is termed *spastic*.

Ataxic dysarthria

Speech is also imprecise and not well articulated if there is damage to the cerebellum. Words can still be formed but with much less precision, and they are not as smoothly articulated in sentences. The slurred speech resulting from alcohol intoxication is a good example of the results of cerebellar dysfunction.

Hypokinetic dysarthria

One example of altered speech associated with defective function of the basal ganglia is the *hypokinetic dysarthria* that may appear in Parkinson's disease. The articulation of speech is normal and words are properly formed, but there is a monotony of pitch and loudness. This makes speech seem dull because many of the usual stresses that we add in saying words and sentences are absent. Another feature sometimes present is difficulty in actually beginning to speak. These features parallel the difficulties that people with Parkinson's disease tend to have in making other movements (*akinesia*) (see Ch. 28).

NON-VOCAL COMMUNICATION

Much communication occurs without a single word being spoken. The way we look at another person, and the way he or she looks at us, conveys a lot of information as does the body language of posture and gesture. We convey feelings and attitudes such as those of happiness, expectancy and welcome, or of hostility, anger and withdrawal. We study one another's faces and read facial expressions. ⑤

Facial expression

The facial expressions adopted in emotions such as fear, anger, disgust, sadness, surprise and happiness are similar in different cultures and countries, suggesting that they are pre-programmed reflex patterns of muscle contraction triggered by our emotional state (see Ch. 31).

When we are surprised we raise our eyebrows; when we are angry we lower them. When we are happy we pull up the corners of our lips by contracting the zygomatic muscles in order to smile and we screw up our eyes by contracting the outer part of the orbicularis oculi (see Fig. 29.11). We can pretend various emotions by voluntarily contracting the same muscles but it is interesting that most people do not seem to be able to

⑤
What means of non-vocal communication have you used when nursing patients?

HAPPINESS, SATISFACTION AND SMILING

The concept of happiness is very difficult to define. Aristotle, one of the great Greek philosophers, described it as 'an activity of the soul in accordance with moral and intellectual virtues'. From the viewpoint of physiology, it might be useful to use the description of Joseph Butler (1692–1752), who saw happiness as 'the by-product of the satisfaction of desires for things'. If satisfaction that meets the person's genuine needs (including physiological needs, such as for food to satisfy hunger) might be the key to genuine happiness, one may speculate that it is this 'genuineness', felt internally, to which the contraction of the outer part of the orbicularis oculi responds in those who cannot contract it voluntarily.

This notion can be very helpful for nurses and other health workers when assessing and planning care of depressed patients, some of whom may force a smile (usually known as 'smiling depression'). The absence of contraction of the orbicularis oculi may indicate the lack of genuine happiness even though the patient says that he or she is happy.

FACIAL PARALYSIS

Paralysis or *paresis* of the facial muscle served by the seventh cranial nerve (Fig. 29.12) is called Bell's palsy. It is most common in persons between 20 and 40 years of age. The condition is characterised by a vague sensation of muscle tension on the affected side, in which there is flaccidity, and drooping of the mouth. There may also be watering of the eye. The paralysis is conspicuous in that the person fails to smile, whistle or grimace.

Nursing principles focus on keeping the patient comfortable, helping him to cope with a changed body image and preventing complications. Since patients are self-conscious about their appearance, their desire for privacy should be respected, especially during meals. Families are warned not to show surprise at the patient's appearance or make comments that may embarrass him or remind him of the change. The condition may sometimes be relieved within a week or a month without treatment other than rest, a nutritious diet and vitamins. In other cases, the disorder may persist for months or years.

contract the outer part of the orbicularis oculi voluntarily. Only genuine happiness seems to act as the trigger. ⑥

If there is impairment of motor function, some of these natural forms of expression may be affected too, and the cues that tell us how that person is feeling may be lacking. A face may be expressionless but that does not necessarily mean that the person behind the face has no feelings. In Parkinson's disease, for example, a patient may have an expressionless ('*dead-pan*') face. This is because of the patient's difficulty in putting motor programmes into action (see Ch. 28).

EATING

By biting and chewing we reduce food to manageable well-lubricated lumps that are easy to swallow. Whether the food that is swallowed has been well chewed or not seems not to matter much for digestion. However, someone's ability to chew does affect choice of foods, and may therefore influence nutritional state indirectly.

Biting and chewing are voluntarily initiated as is the first stage of swallowing, but thereafter reflexes take over, propelling the swallowed food along the oesophagus into the stomach (see Ch. 6).

BITING AND CHEWING

Mouth closure and mouth opening involve contraction of different groups of muscles (Figs 29.11 and 29.18):

Mouth closure	*Mouth opening*
masseter	digastric
temporalis	infrahyoid group
medial pterygoid	lateral pterygoid

When someone is sitting upright, mouth opening is helped by gravity. In chewing and grinding movements, the jaw is also swung from side to side by alternating contraction of the muscles on either side.

In chewing, a very important role is played by the tongue. It pushes the food between the teeth, crushes some of it against the hard palate, and selects and forms the well-chewed portions into a conveniently sized portion (*bolus*) for swallowing. Because the tongue is very sensitive to chemical and mechanical stimuli (see Ch. 24), it detects particles of food lingering in the mouth and sweeps them up for swallowing. Tension of the muscles in the cheeks (*buccinator*; Fig. 29.11) helps to keep food between the biting surfaces. ⑦

> **DRY MOUTH**
>
> An impairment of salivation (Ch. 6) resulting in a dry mouth and coated secretions can have detrimental effects on an individual. Any disorder that affects the mouth and associated structures can impair the ingestion, mastication and swallowing of food, affect the sense of taste, and interfere with speech. The physical appearance is also affected and respiratory disorders can occur.
>
> Removing coated secretions and encouraging frequent and thorough mouth washes and copious small drinks can help to freshen the mouth and stimulate salivation. Such measures will make the mouth feel comfortable and the patient will be able to speak and masticate food with ease.

Chewing patterns

The exact pattern of biting and chewing depends on the food ingested, the shape of a person's mouth and on dentition. Europeans commonly shuttle food from one side of the mouth to the other and thus chew food alternately on either side, whereas others, such as the Aboriginal people of Australasia, chew food simultaneously on both sides.

⑥
As an exercise at home, stand before a mirror and try to force a smile. Can you observe the outer parts of your orbicularis oculi muscles contract?

⑦
What other functions does chewing have besides breaking food into small pieces?

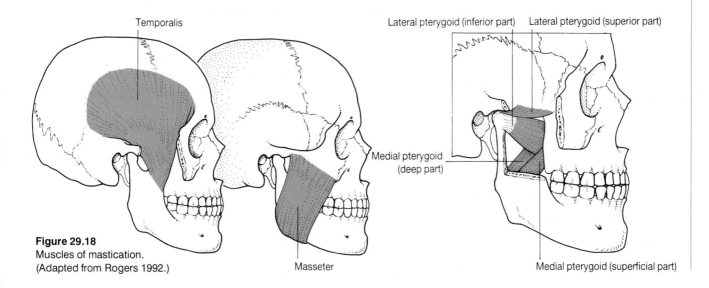

Figure 29.18
Muscles of mastication.
(Adapted from Rogers 1992.)

Temporalis

Masseter

Lateral pterygoid (inferior part)   Lateral pterygoid (superior part)

Medial pterygoid (deep part)

Medial pterygoid (superficial part)

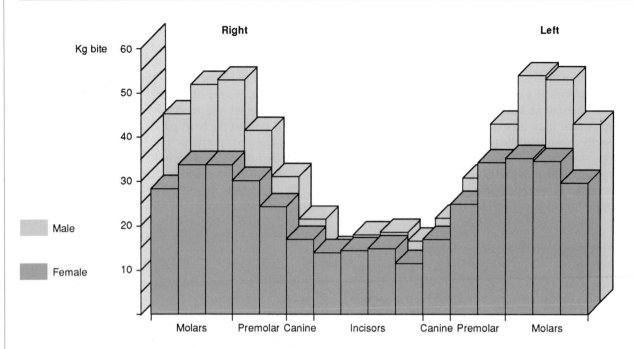

Figure 29.19
Typical biting forces for different teeth in young adults. (Adapted from Worner 1939.)

Forces

Considerable forces can be developed in biting. The maximum forces developed between the molar teeth by the action of the jaw muscles are 40 to 60 kg in people of European origin (Fig. 29.19), though smaller forces (about 30%) are normally used in chewing. The maximum force is limited by the sensitivity of the teeth and gums rather than by the power of the muscles. When wearing dentures maximum forces developed are smaller (15–20 kg). Some peoples, such as the Inuit people of the Arctic, who regularly chew seal skin, can achieve much greater forces (up to 160 kg).

Neural control

Chewing is basically an automatic process initiated by the presence of food in the mouth. Careful control has to be exercised over the powerful forces produced in biting and chewing to avoid injury to the delicate structures of the oral cavity. ⑧

Sensory receptors in the oral cavity excite cells in the medulla oblongata (*masticatory centre*) that set the basic programme of chewing movements. The masticatory centre is influenced by activity in the feeding and satiety centres of the hypothalamus (see Chs 14 and 31). The basic process of chewing and biting is refined by control

⑧
Fortunately for us, tongues heal very quickly. Have you ever bitten your tongue or inner lip whilst chewing food? If so, can you suggest how this happened?

In *bruxism*, also called *bruxomania*, a person unknowingly tightens the jaw and grinds the teeth, usually in sleep. Repeated and continuous grinding of the teeth over a long period of time can wear down or loosen teeth and cause bone loss.

from higher centres including the basal ganglia, thalamus and cortex, and is influenced by sensory feedback from the teeth and gums. There is, for example, very rapid inhibition of muscle contraction on biting as soon as food has been broken, protecting the teeth and gums against injury.

SWALLOWING

Swallowing is an almost completely reflex process. It has three stages:

- oral
- pharyngeal
- oesophageal.

Several muscles are involved and their contraction is coordinated by a cluster of cells (*swallowing centre*) close to the respiratory centres in the medulla oblongata of the brain stem. When swallowing occurs, breathing is normally interrupted. The motoneurones controlling the muscles involved in swallowing form part of cranial nerves IX, X and XII.

Oral stage

The oral stage is usually initiated voluntarily but may be a reflex triggered by the presence of substances in the mouth. The masticated food is formed into a bolus by the lips, cheek muscles and tongue and positioned on the back of the tongue. Contraction of several muscles including those of the tongue forces the bolus back into the oropharynx. The pressure developed in the process can be as great as 75 mmHg (10 kPa).

Pharyngeal stage

From the pharyngeal stage onwards, swallowing is entirely reflex. Once the process has been triggered it cannot be interrupted voluntarily. The reflex is triggered by irritation of receptors at the back of the oral cavity and involves propulsive movements as well as those that seal off all exits other than the oesophagus. ⑨

Reflex excitation

The presence of food at the back of the mouth excites sensory receptors around the entrance to the pharynx, on the soft palate, tonsils, epiglottis, base of the tongue and the posterior wall of the pharynx. These receptors excite the cells in the swallowing centre of the medulla oblongata. The swallowing centre controls the con-

---

A LUMP IN THE THROAT

A sense of food sticking in the throat or of pain causing difficulty in swallowing (*dysphagia*) may signal the presence of an organic disorder, such as oesophageal cancer, peptic oesphagus or stricture. The sensation may be felt in the throat or upper sternum, even when the obstruction is in fact at the lower end of the oesophagus. Dysphagia that is physiological requires treatment, for example surgery.

Sometimes, under emotional tension (such as in grief) the cricopharyngeus muscle may go into spasm, although coordination during swallowing is normal (Rees & Trounce 1988). This spasm leads to a painful sensation of tightening in the throat and is usually described as a 'lump in the throat'. Dysphagia of this sort is referred to as *globus hystericus*. It has no organic cause and the treatment is reassurance (Kumar & Clark 1990).

---

traction of several pharyngeal muscles and inhibits the cricopharyngeus muscle, which forms part of the upper oesophageal sphincter. A stimulus of some kind is needed to evoke these responses, even if it is only the presence of saliva at the back of the mouth. Without this, swallowing is very difficult, if not impossible.

Sealing off other exits

The bolus of food is propelled through the pharynx into the oesophagus with some force and speed (up to 20 m.p.h.). As there are two other exits from the pharynx, there is a risk of food being forced either up into the nose or down into the larynx (Fig. 29.20A). Normally, this does not happen. The exit into the nose is sealed off by the elevation of the soft palate, caused by contraction of the levator and tensor palati muscles. Contraction of these muscles also opens the auditory tubes (eustachian tubes) which is why swallowing helps to relieve the discomfort felt in the ears by air travellers on landing and take-off (see Ch. 25).

The laryngeal exit is avoided (Fig. 29.20) by:

- pulling the larynx upwards and forwards under cover of the tongue
- diversion of the bolus away from the laryngeal opening by the epiglottis
- bringing together of the vocal folds (closure of the glottis).

Oesophageal stage

Once the bolus has entered the oesophagus it is carried along by a wave of peristalsis (see Ch. 6) controlled

⑨
Is it possible to swallow food whilst standing on one's head? If so, how?

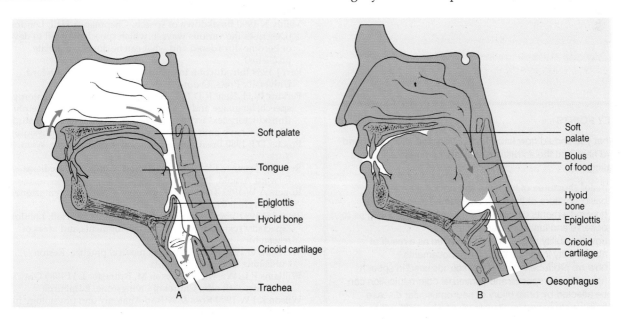

Figure 29.20
Position of structures in the mouth and throat during:
A Breathing
B Swallowing.
(Reproduced from Rogers 1992 (Fig. 5.11) by permission of the publishers.)

by the 'swallowing centre' in the medulla oblongata. Secondary waves of peristalsis are triggered by irritation of the oesophagus by any food particles left behind. A food bolus takes several seconds to reach the stomach, whereas liquids travel much more quickly, aided by the effect of gravity if someone is sitting upright.

IMPAIRMENT OF SWALLOWING

Swallowing may be impaired for a number of different reasons. For example, damage to the swallowing centre may cause partial or complete paralysis, resulting in an inability to swallow. If paralysis occurs in the pharyngeal area, food may pass into the trachea and nasal cavities. If the sphincter at the oesophageal opening remains relaxed during breathing, air is drawn into the oesophagus during inspiration. If the swallowing reflex is absent (e.g. in an unconscious patient or during general anaesthesia) food or water may be inhaled into the lungs, resulting in choking and possible airway obstruction, lung collapse and pneumonia.

Nursing care in a patient with swallowing impairment includes:

- observing him/her constantly while eating
- providing meals in liquid, semi-liquid or soft form
- ensuring that soft food is divided into small pieces and eaten slowly
- avoiding hot or iced foods
- taking care not to distract the patient while he/she is swallowing.

Where appropriate, sitting the patient up facilitates feeding.

KEY POINTS

What you should now know and understand about the head and neck and the activities of looking, communicating and eating:

- major structures of the head and neck
- basic structure of the teeth and gums
- how movements of the eyes are controlled, enabling us to observe and inspect objects of interest
- how the ability to see may be impaired as a result of abnormality in the control of eye movements
- how we produce the variety of sounds used in speech
- how and why speech and nonverbal communication can be affected by brain injury or neuromuscular disease
- how we chew and swallow food, and how difficulties may arise with these activities.

REFERENCES AND FURTHER READING

Anderson D J 1956 Measurement of stress in mastication I. Journal of Dental Research 35: 664–670
Besford J 1984 Good mouthkeeping. Oxford University Press, Oxford
(Written for parents but useful to all involved in dental health education. Lucid and comprehensive explanation of problems and their prevention)
Bouchier I A D, Morris J S 1976 Clinical skills. W B Saunders, London, p 314
Carpenter R H S 1988 Movements of the eyes, 2nd edn. Pion, London
(Advanced text lucidly presenting and discussing the experimental basis of knowledge)
Darley F L, Aronson A E, Brown J R 1975 Motor speech disorders. W B Saunders, Philadelphia
Dutia M B 1989 Mechanisms of head stabilisation. News in Physiological Sciences 4: 101–104
Fawcus M 1991 Voice disorders and their management. Chapman & Hall, London
(Text for speech therapy students. Useful for reference)
Ferguson D B 1988 Physiology for dental students. Wright, London
(Lucid text, containing more detail than other basic texts of physiology on oral physiology and speech)
Fletcher H 1929 Speech and hearing. Macmillan, London
(Classic, and now historically fascinating, book describing fundamental research work collated and carried out by the Bell Telephone Company in the early days of telephone and radio)
Garner R 1989 Acute head injury. Chapman & Hall, London
(Very useful, concise, readable book, covering all aspects of rehabilitation)
Hardcastle W J 1976 Physiology of speech production. Academic Press, London
Jenkins G N 1978 The physiology and biochemistry of the mouth. Blackwell, Oxford
Jurgens U, Ploog D 1981 On the neural control of mammalian vocalisation. Trends in Neuroscience 4: 135–137
Kumar P J, Clark M L 1990 Clinical medicine. Baillière Tindall, London
Martini F 1989 Fundamentals of anatomy and physiology. Simon & Schuster, Anglewood Cliff, New Jersey
Milloy N 1990 Breakdown of speech. Chapman & Hall, London
(Describes the various ways in which speech may fail to develop or become disordered and what can be done to alleviate problems)
Parr J 1989 Introduction to ophthalmology, 3rd edn. Oxford University Press, Oxford
Perkins W H, Kent R D 1985 A textbook of functional anatomy of speech, language and hearing. Taylor & Francis, Philadelphia
(Introductory text written in self-instructional mode for students who may have limited knowledge of anatomy and physiology)
Procter D F 1980 Breathing, speech and song. Springer, Wien, New York
Rees P J, Trounce J R 1988 A new short textbook of medicine. Edward Arnold, London
Rogers A W 1992 Textbook of anatomy. Churchill Livingstone, Edinburgh, p 69, 180, 182, 183, 203, 429, 430
Titze I R 1992 Vocal fold physiology. Chapman & Hall, London
(Specialist text addressing new developments and areas of research)
Wensel L O 1980 Acupuncture in medical practice. Reston Publishing Company, Virginia
Williams P L, Warwick R, Dyson M, Bannister L H 1989 Gray's Anatomy, 37th edn. Churchill Livingstone, Edinburgh
Wilson K J W 1990 Ross & Wilson Anatomy and physiology in health and illness, 7th edn. Churchill Livingstone, Edinburgh
Worner H K 1939 'Gnathodynamics' The measurement of biting forces. The Australian Journal of Dentistry 43: 381–393

Part C
ASPECTS OF EXPERIENCE

We think, plan and remember; we acquire new knowledge and use written and spoken language to communicate with others. We practise new skills and devise new activities. We feel joy and sadness. We feel agitated or relaxed. We spend most of our life awake but for about a third of it we sleep.

The chapters in this part:

- identify the areas of the nervous system that are specifically involved in these aspects of experience and behaviour
- show how mental phenomena, such as consciousness and memory, relate to the organisation and functioning of nerve cells
- explain the basis of some examples of altered experience and behaviour caused by injury, drugs or disease
- describe and explain the biological basis of pain and pain relief.

Chapter 30
THE MIND: KNOWING AND DOING

Through our minds we:

- make sense of our surroundings and experiences
- share our perceptions with others
- engage in the varied activities of each day.

The process of understanding what we see, hear, feel, etc. involves attaching meaning to sensory experience. To do this we link sounds with sights and feelings and associate them with other information stored already in our brains.

Sharing our understanding with others involves translating our thoughts into a form that others can recognise and interpret. We communicate by producing a sophisticated set of sounds (speech), by drawing and using symbols (writing, typing) and by the picture language of facial expression, gestures and posture.

In work and play our mental plans are translated into ordered patterns of behaviour. The tasks we perform may be routine or may require us to devise new sequences of activity.

All these faculties of the mind are the result of the functioning of the *association areas* of the two cerebral hemispheres, each of which contributes different but interrelated capabilities.

MENTAL ABILITIES

KNOWING

Understanding what our senses tell us depends on the linking together of separate pieces of sensory information. Understanding even the most ordinary of daily activities involves the *association* of a surprisingly large number of bits of information. Consider, for example, the many separate sensations experienced by a child

Table 30.1 Some of the sensory experiences contributing to a child's understanding of washing up
What am I doing?
I can feel a liquid It feels warm I can feel bubbles They 'pop' on my hands They tickle my nose There is a smell of water/soap/soapy liquid I bend and stretch my arm to make the water move My fingers close and open to catch bubbles
I can feel the edge of a bowl It feels round It is bigger than my hand The water in it comes up to my elbow It makes a swishy noise It makes a gurgly noise It tastes soapy I don't like the taste and pull a face I can make the water move I can see coloured patterns in the water
In the water I can see an object It fills with water It pours out the water It is slippery
Answer: I am washing the dishes
Reproduced from Longhorn F 1988 A sensory curriculum for very special people, by permission of the author.

who is washing up (Table 30.1). Each sentence in the table identifies a different sensory feature of the activity. All these features linked together create the mental concept of what is going on. When that concept is then linked to the words 'washing up', the sounds made by those words are given meaning. For whenever they are heard, they conjure up the memory of that rich pattern of sensory experience.

Role of parietal and temporal lobes

The main areas of the brain concerned with the association of different sensations are found in the *parietal* and *temporal* lobes of the cerebral hemispheres, between the primary sensory areas for vision, hearing and somatic sensation (Fig. 30.1). Damage to the parietal and temporal lobes gives rise to difficulties in comprehension.

Lesions close to the visual areas may result in someone being unable to recognise an object from its appearance although it can be identified from its feel. This disturbance of understanding is termed *visual agnosia*. Conversely, lesions closer to the somatosensory areas result in *astereognosis*, the inability to identify an object from its feel although it can be recognised by sight.

Injury to the parietal lobe may also be revealed in someone's drawings (Fig. 30.2). The problem does not lie in performing the necessary movements but in understanding how component parts of an object fit together (*spatial agnosia*).

Damage to areas of the association cortex nearer to the temporal lobe and the auditory areas usually gives rise to difficulties in understanding sounds, and in interpreting the meaning of words (see p. 516).

Caring for patients with communication difficulties requires special skills to find a satisfactory means by which the person can converse. Help and advice for nurses and relatives is usually provided by hospital and/or community speech therapists.

VISUAL AGNOSIA

Can you imagine how you would feel if you awoke one morning and could not recognise some common objects? You are looking for your toothbrush; it is there in front of you, but until you chance to pick it up it is unrecognisable. Perhaps the nearest one can get to experiencing visual agnosia is to take part in one of those competitions which require one to identify a strange object from the past or a highly specialised tool. To be told to use the object would be a waste of time; even handling it would not help, although that is usually the first thing one does on being shown something new, and a feeling of puzzlement would ensue.

Visual agnosia is not common and for that reason it is easily overlooked, the affected person being termed 'difficult' or 'not interested'. The person will often begin to ask where things are: 'Where are my glasses?'

'Right in front of you.'

'Oh, are these my glasses?'

Relatives soon find this sort of dialogue frustrating, especially when repeated dozens of times a day.

Some people are able to make the connection between feeling and recognising and will automatically handle objects. Those who have a failing memory, for example, may not make this connection. In hospital, a patient may ask for a cup of tea, then leave the tea untouched simply because he does not recognise the cup. When such a person is required, or wishes, to use an object it is necessary to place it in his hands so that he can use tactile sensations for recognition.

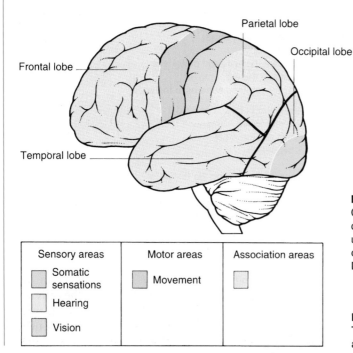

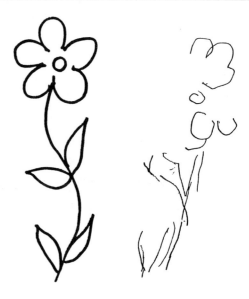

Figure 30.2 (*above*)
Copy (right) made by a patient with bilateral parietal lobe dysfunction of a drawing of a flower (left). The loss of understanding in the patient's mind of the relationship between component parts is evident. (Courtesy of Dr J S Snowden, Department of Neurology, University of Manchester.)

Figure 30.1 (*left*)
The lobes of the cerebral hemispheres showing the position of the association areas of the cerebral cortex.

DOING

Performing a task such as washing up, and being able to talk about it, depends on being able to translate the concept of it into action. This depends on normal function of the muscles involved and on the correct control of their activity by the nervous system. It is thus possible for someone to understand what is going on around them but not be able to express themselves fully in their speech and by their actions. Links have to be made between those parts of the nervous system that detect and analyse sensory experience and those parts that use that information to power muscle activity. ①

Role of parietal and frontal lobes

Areas of the association cortex involved in translating thoughts into action include parts of the parietal cortex as well as regions of the frontal lobes close to the motor areas (Fig. 30.1). Injury to these areas may result in someone being unable to perform tasks with which they were previously familiar, and which are still understood. This form of disability is termed *apraxia*. There may also be difficulties in assembling words in an appropriate order in speech (*motor aphasia*; see p. 517).

Injury to other parts of the frontal lobes gives rise to more subtle changes in behaviour related to planning for, and worrying about, the future. In humans, the frontal lobes are exceptionally large. They are linked with:

- the parietal and temporal association areas
- the limbic system
- the basal ganglia. ②

Information passes between the parietal and temporal association areas and the frontal lobes by means of large intracortical tracts of nerve fibres. The limbic system is involved in emotion (see Ch. 31), and the basal ganglia are involved in the planning and programming of movement (see Chs 27 and 28).

The functions of much of the frontal lobes were a puzzle for many years, for it was known that, even if this part of the brain was injured or it was cut off from the rest, as in a frontal leucotomy (see below), there appeared to be little impairment of intelligence. However, it is now known that the frontal lobes are involved in the elaboration of more complex behaviours, and in the expression of emotion.

Effects of injury to the frontal lobes

In the 19th century a mining engineer, by the name of Phineas Gage, sustained enormous damage to his left frontal lobe. He had an accident with some dynamite, which drove a rod of iron through his face and out through the top of his skull. Amazingly, he survived and, despite the extensive damage to his left frontal lobe, he suffered very little physical or mental disability.

What did change, however, was his personality. Before the accident he had been of a fairly sober disposition. After it, he was temperamental, used foul language, and cared little about what other people thought.

Studies many years later in the 20th century demonstrated that, if the frontal lobes were cut off from the rest of the brain (*frontal leucotomy*), anxiety was considerably reduced, without grossly affecting intellectual functions. Before the advent of tranquillisers and antidepressants, frontal leucotomy was used with some success to bring relief to those suffering from chronic depression and anxiety. ③

Closer study of people who have undergone surgery or who have suffered injury to this area of the brain has revealed that one of the resulting changes in behaviour is difficulty in planning and organising activities. There is difficulty in retaining the knowledge necessary to be able to proceed from one task to another. This includes knowledge of what has just been done (so that the action is not repeated), as well as a knowledge of what should happen if a particular course of action is, or is not, pursued. If there is difficulty in predicting what the consequences of a particular action are, this may be why injury to the frontal lobes is associated with a reduction in anxiety. As far as the individual is concerned there may seem to be little to worry about.

Another characteristic feature of frontal lobe injury is often some change in emotional expression, for example loss of facial expressiveness.

FRONTAL LOBE LESIONS

A person with a frontal lobe lesion (tumour, haematoma) may well be dismissed as suffering from senile dementia or, if younger, from pre-senile dementia. Initially the affected person fails to grasp whole situations, perhaps seeming to act impulsively having previously been thoughtful. The powers of reasoning disintegrate and he becomes careless about his appearance, often neglecting to wash and change clothes. Normal social inhibitions are lost. The person is often incontinent of urine and faeces but this is not due to any lack of function of the bladder and bowel; he no longer understands the impropriety of relieving himself instantly. He may also indulge in simple jokes and puns, giving the impression of cheerfulness, though the jokes are often not appropriate to the situation. It is difficult to know which is the more distressing for the carer to cope with, continual jokes or bouts of temper and depression.

ASYMMETRY OF CEREBRAL FUNCTION

The two cerebral hemispheres are linked together by a very large bundle of nerve fibres (*corpus callosum*) (Fig. 30.3). This allows cross-talk between the two

① *Where is voluntary muscle activity initiated?*

② *Can you name the basal ganglia?*

③ *What does the word 'leucotomy' actually mean?*

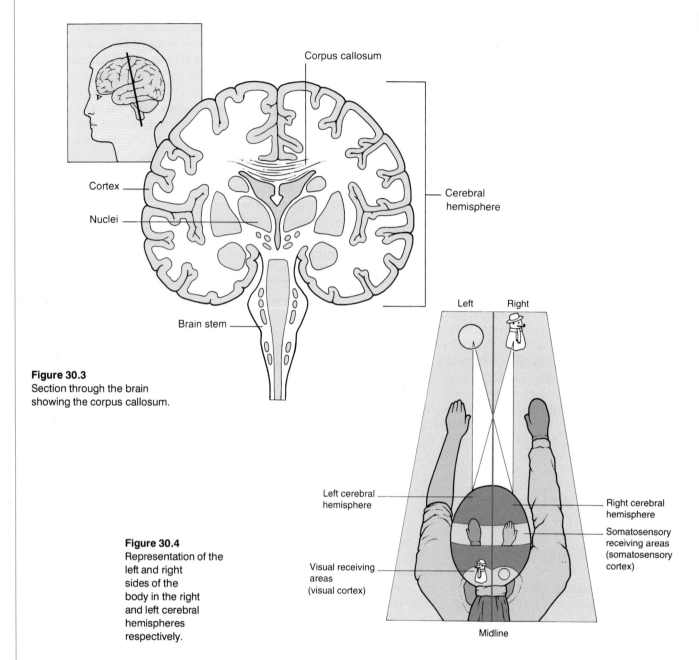

Figure 30.3
Section through the brain showing the corpus callosum.

Figure 30.4
Representation of the left and right sides of the body in the right and left cerebral hemispheres respectively.

hemispheres. Normally our thoughts and actions are influenced by activity in both hemispheres. As explained in earlier chapters (see Chs 23 and 27), sensory and motor systems are usually ordered in such a way that the left-hand side of the body is represented in the right cerebral hemisphere and vice versa (Fig. 30.4). Were it not for the corpus callosum it would indeed be the case that the 'left hand would not know what the right hand was doing'.

Some very interesting facts about the function of the cerebral hemispheres in humans were discovered a number of years ago in a group of patients who were treated for intractable epilepsy by cutting the corpus callosum. The purpose of this apparently rather radical operation was to limit the very severe epileptic seizures from which these people suffered.

STUDIES IN 'SPLIT-BRAIN' PATIENTS

After the operation in which the corpus callosum had been cut across it was possible to direct sensory signals selectively either to the left or to the right hemisphere (Fig. 30.4). It was found that, if a picture of an object was displayed in the *left* visual field, the subject could select the correct object from a number of objects hidden from view behind a screen, but only by using the *left* hand. If selection was attempted with the right hand instead, the number of times that the correct object was chosen was no better than by chance. Intriguingly, when the investigator then asked the subject what the object was that had been displayed in the left visual field and handled by the left hand, the subject could not say. Yet if the same object was now displayed in the *right* visual field

Table 30.2 Cerebral specialisation in most people (>90%)	
Left hemisphere	Right hemisphere
Verbal	Nonverbal
– speech	– visuospatial awareness
– writing	drawing
– use of symbols	route finding
	recognising faces
	– musical ability
	– expressing and understanding emotion

	Left hand	Right hand
Preoperative		
Postoperative		

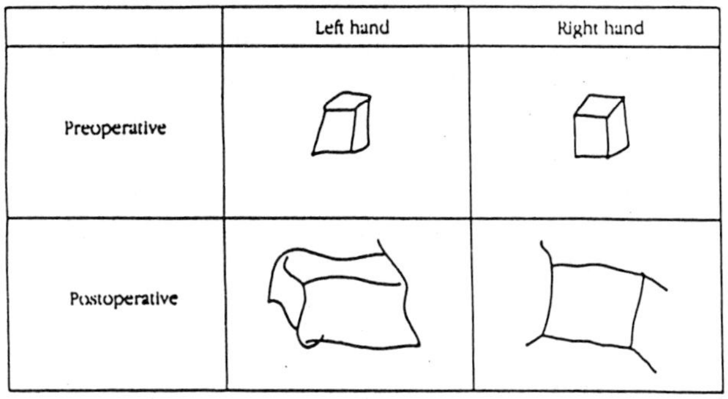

Figure 30.5
Drawings of a cube made by a right-handed person before and after an operation in which the corpus callosum was transected. Preoperatively, the patient could draw the cube with either hand. Postoperatively the patient drew a better picture of the cube using the left hand. Movement of the left hand is controlled by the right cerebral hemisphere. (Reproduced from Gazzaniga M S, LeDoux J E 1978 The integrated mind, Figure 18, by permission of the authors and Plenum Publishing Corporation.)

and handled by the *right* hand, no difficulty was experienced in naming it.

These and many other experiments have revealed that the left and the right cerebral hemispheres do not have exactly the same functions. In the majority of people, the associations that enable us to speak are developed largely in the left hemisphere whereas the right hemisphere specialises in nonverbal associations (Table 30.2).

ROLE OF EACH CEREBRAL HEMISPHERE

The left hemisphere

The hemisphere that enables us to speak has been termed the *dominant hemisphere*. It was originally believed that this hemisphere literally dominated our minds, and that the other hemisphere was of minor importance. This view is no longer held (see below).

In about 93% of people, the left hemisphere is the major controller of speech. If there is damage to it, as a result of a stroke, for example, the power of speech is often lost. ④

In a small percentage of people (5%) the speech centres are located in the right hemisphere. In the remaining 2% language functions are more or less equally represented on both sides.

The right hemisphere

In function, the right hemisphere has many capabilities that may be labelled intuitive: the ability to know that you know someone because you recognise facial

---

THE SODIUM AMYTAL TEST

Sometimes before major brain surgery, a simple test is performed to determine which of the two hemispheres houses the language centres. A small quantity of sodium amytal (an anaesthetic) is injected into either the left or the right carotid artery. Each of these vessels supplies the corresponding half of the brain and so each hemisphere can be temporarily sedated. The patient is asked to read or count, and speech will be interrupted or disorganised for several minutes if the injection is made on the side which is dominant for speech.

---

features even though you may not be able to 'put a name to the face'; the appreciation of music; an awareness of how things fit together (Fig. 30.5).

The right hemisphere also appears to be more closely involved with the recognition and expression of emotions. In the split-brain experiments described above it was found that a person could react with laughter or embarrassment to a picture presented to the right hemisphere, without being able to say what had been seen. Intuitive knowledge and emotions do not require words. The right hemisphere enables us to know, understand and express some things in a nonverbal way.

DOMINANCE AND NON-DOMINANCE

As the left and the right hemispheres normally do communicate with one another, intuitive knowledge does express itself in words and, conversely, words can be transformed into other actions and feelings. Now that the functions of both hemispheres are being better understood the terms dominant and non-dominant hemispheres become less suitable. It is truer to say that the two hemispheres specialise in different activities rather than that one is dominant for our understanding and actions. It is now usual to refer to one or other hemisphere as dominant for a given activity, such as speech, rather than being dominant overall.

HANDEDNESS AND SPEECH

Asymmetry of cerebral function is evident too in the preferences we have in using either the right or the left hand. 90% of people are right handed and in the overwhelming majority of these (95–99%) the left hemisphere controls speech. In the remaining 10%, who are

④
What is a stroke?

left handed, the control of speech is not necessarily centred in the right hemisphere. Indeed in the majority (60–70% of left-handers) speech is localised to the left hemisphere too. Interestingly in most left-handers *both* hemispheres have some speech function. The fact that stuttering is more common amongst left-handers than in right-handers has led some to speculate that in left-handed people who have a stutter, centres in both hemispheres may be involved in controlling speech.

LANGUAGE

The spoken and written word is very important to us as humans. Without it, our ability to communicate with one another would be much more limited. ⑤

⑤
What other methods of communication are there?

At its simplest, language involves associating a symbol or sound with an object or activity (Fig. 30.6). But in addition to this we communicate a much richer understanding of our experience by the way in which we bring those symbols together to form sentences. In order to communicate fully we need to be able to do both those things. The first concerns our vocabulary (chiefly nouns and verbs); the second relates to syntax (the construction of sentences).

The spoken word

Two areas of the cerebral cortex that have a major role in vocabulary and in syntax are:

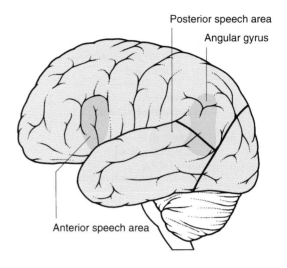

Figure 30.7
Major language areas of the left cerebral hemisphere.

- the posterior speech area (Wernicke's area)
- the anterior speech area (Broca's area).

The posterior speech area lies at the junction of the temporal and parietal lobes of the cerebral cortex whereas the anterior area lies just in front of the primary motor cortex (Figs 30.7 and 30.1). These areas were identified many years ago by two doctors (Wernicke

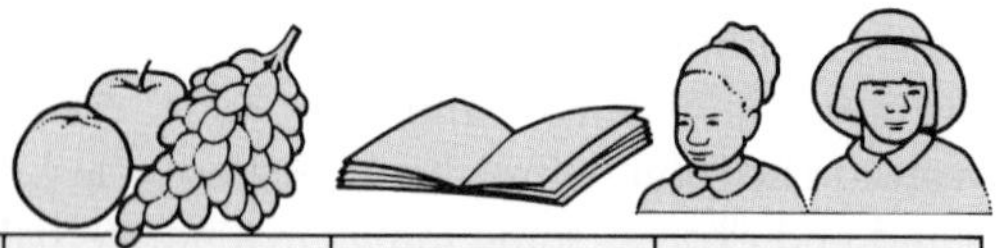

German	*Obst*	*Buch*	*Kinder*
Swahili	*Matunda*	*Kitabu*	*Watoto*
Arabic	فُوكّه	كِتَاب	أطْفَال
Hindi	फल	किताब	बच्चे
Japanese (Chinese)	くだもの （果物）	ほん （本）	こども （子供）
Korean	과 일	책	아이들

Figure 30.6
A few words in a few languages. (Courtesy of staff and students of the School of Biological Sciences, University of Manchester.)

LEFT OR RIGHT HANDED?

An old lady who had broken her right wrist and was normally right handed said, 'Isn't it silly, we have two perfectly good hands and spend our lives concentrating on the use of one. Why can't we use both equally well?'

There are probably a few who are completely ambidextrous, others who are normally right handed use the left for some activities, while others are definitely right or left handed. There are others still who are not quite sure of the difference between right and left, and will have to think before obeying instructions.

What about footedness? Does right footedness go with right handedness? Not necessarily. Some people are born with *crossed lateralisation*; they are right handed and left footed or vice versa. Some older people are naturally left handed and left footed but, as children, were forced to use the right hand for writing etc.

These may seem relatively unimportant points but, apart from the connection with certain learning difficulties, this confusion with right and left has significance when nursing patients. The obvious is making sure that bedside lockers are placed on the patient's preferred side, unless of course that arm or hand cannot be used. Less obvious is the problem of the right-handed/left-footed person who requires assistance with walking. It is so easy to assume that the patient 'leads' with the right foot, either when walking or climbing stairs. Try starting up stairs with your non-dominant foot; it is likely that you will not feel so well balanced and your other foot will not follow so readily. Under these circumstances the patient may need extra support and reassurance.

Table 30.3 Several different forms of aphasia and their key features

Type of aphasia	Fluency of speech	Comprehension	Ability to name objects	Ability to repeat spoken words
Broca's	*	*****	*	***
Wernicke's	*****	***	***	***
Global	*	*	*	*
Conductive	*****	*****	***	***
Anomic	*****	*****	***	*****

Key: ***** = moderate to good; *** = impaired to a greater or lesser degree; * = severely impaired

and Broca) who noticed that specific disorders of spoken language (*aphasias*) exhibited by some of their patients were associated with damage to these two parts of the brain.

Damage to the posterior area chiefly created problems with vocabulary and comprehension of the spoken word (*Wernicke's aphasia*) whereas damage to the anterior area resulted mainly in difficulty in constructing sentences and in actually speaking (*Broca's aphasia*). Other types of aphasia, including global, conductive and anomic, have since been described (Table 30.3). *Global aphasia* usually results from extensive damage to both speech areas, whereas *conductive aphasia* is thought to be due to impaired impulse transmission between the two areas. *Anomic aphasia* is a more selective language impairment often seen in patients who have recovered from other, more severe, forms of aphasia.

Vocabulary and comprehension

In *Wernicke's aphasia*, which is sometimes referred to as a form of *sensory* or *receptive* aphasia, an individual has difficulty in selecting the correct word for different objects and activities. This is one form of *anomia* (difficulty in naming objects). Words do come to mind and are used but they are the wrong ones. Sentences are formed from the words found and are articulated and spoken, often very fluently, but what is said may make little sense. Not surprisingly, there is also poor understanding of what other people say.

> *Wernicke's aphasia* is a very distressing disorder causing frustration, anxiety and anger. Imagine trying to converse with someone who only speaks an obscure language, without being able to share words for objects and activities because they change frequently! Extreme patience and understanding are required from all who care for the patient.

Forming sentences and speaking

Conversely, in *Broca's aphasia*, which is sometimes referred to as a *motor* or *expressive* aphasia, understanding of speech is much better. The correct nouns and verbs are chosen to describe objects, but there is difficulty in saying them and in forming sentences. Prepositions and conjunctions tend to get left out, so that sentences are often reduced to a bare minimum. A sentence such as, 'I am feeling very tired and I would be glad if I could go home soon,' might be reduced to 'tired . . . go home'. People who display Broca's aphasia can have difficulty in understanding sentences whose meaning crucially depends on the order of words. A sentence such as, 'The patient that the nurse was helping was tired,' could leave them wondering who was helping whom, and whether the patient or the nurse was tired!

As the anterior speech area is close to the primary motor cortex, injury to this general area usually also results in features characteristic of damage to the motor cortex such as slowness of speech and difficulty in articulation (*dysarthria*) (see Ch. 29). ⑥

The written word

Other areas of the cerebral cortex are specifically involved in creating the associations enabling us to read and write. Adjacent to the posterior speech area is the *angular gyrus* (Fig. 30.7). The angular gyrus performs the same sorts of function as the posterior speech area but is concerned more with the written rather than the spoken word. Injury to this area leads to an inability to read (*alexia*) or to difficulties in reading (*dyslexia*).

Translating thoughts into written symbols is different from translating them into spoken words. Writing depends on a slightly different set of associations involving control of finger and hand movements. It can be impaired (*agraphia*) independently of other aspects of language. ⑦

INDIVIDUAL DIFFERENCES

So much of what we say and do each day depends upon the normal functioning of all these areas of the cerebral cortex. Each of us will have known times when we have not been able to find the right word, or have surprised ourselves by coming up with things we had not thought

⑥
What is the difference between aphasia, aphonia and dysarthria?

⑦
What do the suffixes -lexia and -graphia mean?

of before, or have been totally disorganised in our planning. All these experiences are features of the links that are, or are not, normally being made within our brains.

We differ as people, in intellectual ability and in practical expertise. This too is a consequence of the different links existing within the neural networks of the brain, and of the associations that have been forged in the course of development, and learned through experience (see Ch. 33). Our abilities change as we grow, and as we age (see Chs 35 and 36). In the elderly, damage to small areas of the cerebral cortex as a result of minor cerebral haemorrhages can lead to impairment of understanding, communication and behaviour.

It is vitally important for anyone working with people to understand that loss or absence of one intellectual or practical ability does not mean that a person is completely stupid, devoid of understanding, or incapable. It is especially easy to make that mistake if people cannot express themselves in speech, for it is then much more difficult for us to know what they are thinking. People like Christopher Nolan, the writer, who developed cerebral palsy through brain damage at birth, have opened a window of understanding for many of us on the life of those with physical and mental disabilities. Similarly the work of the artist Stephen Wiltshire (Fig. 30.8), and others like him, has revealed the skill and ability that can lie within the mind of someone who in other ways may appear to be unintelligent. The challenge to us all is to seek out the keys that will unlock the hidden potentials lying within the minds of others, and to enable each one to use that potential to the full. Our fast increasing knowledge of the workings of the human brain is likely to help us to do just that.

DYSLEXIA

In medical terminology, dyslexia means difficulty with reading or word blindness, but it has been used as a blanket term to cover several learning difficulties including problems with reading, writing and counting. If a person cannot properly recognise letters and words, it follows that he will not be able to write them recognisably. The motor activity of writing is often adequate but the ability to arrange letters to form recognisable words is lacking to various degrees.

Letters and numbers are symbols and for some people the brain is unable to make sense of these symbols, especially when letters are combined to form words. It is not known how a child is perceiving words and letters until an attempt is made to write them down; then, for example, letters are often written back to front, particularly b, d, p and q. Reversing letters in this way is, however, fairly common in children when they first begin to write and is not of itself indicative of dyslexia. This is a complex disorder with many individual variations; for example one young girl said that she found great difficulty in reading upper case letters. While at school, children are helped by educational psychologists, and support for both adults and children is provided by the Dyslexia Institute.

Case history
A student nurse gaining community nursing experience was alone in the health visitors' office. She took a telephone message and wrote it down for the appropriate health visitor. The message was difficult to interpret. One health visitor said, 'She can't spell, can she?'

Another recognised something more than bad spelling. Words badly spelled are usually more or less phonetically correct, for example 'delited' and 'scervy' for delighted and scurvy. Dyslexic words, however, may be recognisable because the right letters are in the wrong order, for example suptum for sputum, and not phonetically correct.

The student admitted to being dyslexic and was willing to explain how she managed to hide her difficulties. For example, she asked someone else to write down her letter of application so that she could copy it – which took several attempts.

In nursing, the main concern is whether the person will be a safe practitioner, i.e. is able to understand written instructions, provide legible written information and interpret drug prescriptions correctly. With professional help, this student passed her final examination at the third attempt.

A MISUNDERSTANDING

(The story is true: names and places have been changed.) 'People don't seem to understand you round here,' said Mrs Phillips as we walked slowly to the front door of the elderly people's home. Our friend seemed a little more confused than usual. We said goodbye and promised to visit again soon. When we did, a few days later, we chatted briefly with the staff on duty, mentioning that our friend was going to have her eightieth birthday soon. 'Eightieth?' said the staff member. 'She's long past that you know. Close on 90 she is!'

Now there were many things that we did not know about Mrs Phillips, but of this we were sure. She was shortly to be 80 and was looking forward to it. 'It's on her records . . . I'll show you the file,' said the staff member opening the drawer of the filing cabinet and thumbing through the folders, 'Here it is. Mrs Phillips from Normanton. Born 23rd April 19. . .'

'Normanton?' we exclaimed, 'Mrs Phillips has lived all her life in *this* town. She doesn't come from Normanton!' There was a pause.

'Oh Lord!' said the staff member pulling out a second file marked 'Mrs Phillips'. Her face fell as she glanced through both of them. 'Oh! The drugs . . .' she groaned.

There were two Mrs Phillips in residence in that home for the elderly, and for several days they had been given one another's medication. Maybe that was the reason why our friend had seemed confused on our previous visit. But then we remembered the comment she had made then: 'People don't seem to understand you around here.' She was right. She had been misunderstood, and *knew* it.

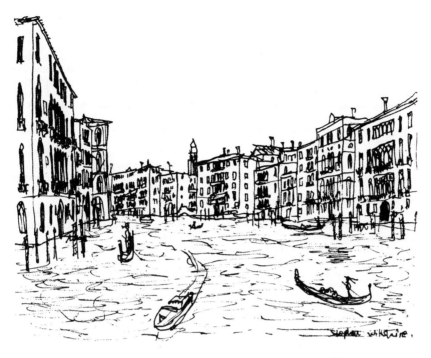

Figure 30.8
'Imaginary Venice'. One of innumerable drawings by the artist Stephen Wiltshire, who has autism. The picture was drawn from his imagination after a 5-day stay in Venice and took him just 5 minutes. (From: Floating cities, by Stephen Wiltshire (Michael Joseph, 1991) copyright (c) Stephen Wiltshire, 1991. Reproduced by permission of Penguin Books Ltd.)

KEY POINTS

What you should now know and understand about the mind and its capabilities:

- which parts of the brain are involved in enabling you to read and to understand this and other books
- which parts of the brain are involved in enabling you to speak and to write about what you know
- what is meant by the association areas of the cerebral cortex and what they do
- differences in function between the left and the right cerebral hemispheres
- how brain injury may affect someone's ability to understand, to communicate and to act
- why a stroke may or may not affect someone's ability to speak
- why someone's intelligence and capabilities should never be underestimated.

REFERENCES AND FURTHER READING

Blakemore C 1990 The mind machine. BBC Books, London
(A fascinating book for the general reader as well as the student)
Bradshaw J L 1989 Hemispheric specialisation and psychological function. John Wiley & Sons, Chichester
(Specialist text reviewing the experimental basis of current understanding)
Carpenter R H S 1984 Neurophysiology. Edward Arnold, London
Critchley M 1971 The parietal lobes. Hafner, London
Gazzaniga M S, LeDoux J E 1978 The integrated mind. Plenum Press, New York, p 52
Graham R B 1990 Physiological psychology. Wadsworth Publishing, Belmont, California
(An interesting student text stressing concepts and providing useful background to current theories)
Hewson L 1986 When half is whole: my recovery from stroke. Colling Dove, Blackburn, Victoria, Australia
(Illuminating personal account of one woman's recovery from stroke)
Kertesz A 1979 Aphasia and associated disorders: taxonomy, localisation and recovery. Grune & Stratton, New York
Kleinke C L 1986 Meeting and understanding people. W H Freeman, Oxford
(Useful book, describing how we form impressions of others from their physical appearance, verbal and nonverbal behaviour)
Longhorn F 1988 A sensory curriculum for very special people. Souvenir Press (E & A), London
(Written for those working with children and adults with profound learning disabilities. Full of practical and imaginative ideas for developing sensory awareness)
Murdoch B E 1990 Acquired speech and language disorders. Chapman & Hall, London
(Textbook providing more detail on the neuroanatomical and neurophysiological basis of language, and its disorders)

Nolan C 1981 Damburst of dreams. Pan Books, London
(Poems, stories and autobiographical writings of a young man, with cerebral palsy, whose exceptional literary talent was revealed when a combination of new drugs and new technology allowed him to express his thoughts in written form for the first time)
Plum F (ed) 1988 Language, communication and the brain. Raven Press, New York
(Collection of interesting specialist articles reviewing different aspects of language, its development and its disorders)
Prigatano G P, Schacter D L 1991 Awareness of deficit after brain injury: clinical and theoretical issues. Oxford University Press, New York/Oxford
(Collection of articles, written by specialists. First book since 1955 devoted to altered self awareness. Interesting; useful for reference)
Reinvang I 1985 Aphasia and brain organisation. Plenum Press, New York & London
Springer S P, Deutsch G 1989 Left brian, right brain, 3rd edn. W H Freeman, New York
(Very readable, fascinating account of the development of understanding of the activities of the two hemispheres. Extremely well referenced)
Wiltshire S 1991 Floating cities. Michael Joseph, London
(An amazing book, one of several by this extremely talented autistic artist, containing many intricate drawings of buildings and places. A delight to own and a revelation to read)

Chapter 31
SLEEP, EMOTION AND BEHAVIOUR

Sleep is important. Without it we become irritable and concentration suffers. When awake, we may feel alert or drowsy, responsive to events or sluggish. These different levels of consciousness are set by neural systems that influence the cerebral cortex. Their activity can be modified by drugs.

Closely linked to our level of arousal, but different from it, is the experience of how we feel. We talk about being happy, or sad, angry or afraid. Emotional experiences are complex. They draw together many different aspects of brain function: a specific sensory experience, for example passing an examination, triggers distinctive patterns of behaviour, such as surprise, and laughter; and this includes both somatic control (e.g. of facial expression) as well as autonomic responses (e.g. increased heart rate through excitement).

Many different parts of the brain are involved in our emotions but a central role is played by the limbic system which acts as an interface between the somatic and visceral components of the nervous system. The somatic components include the association areas of the cerebral cortex, whereas the visceral control areas comprise the hypothalamus, the pituitary gland and the autonomic nervous system.

Brain injury can result in changes of mood. Conversely, our moods can affect our bodies and our state of health.

SLEEPING AND WAKING

We become drowsy and go to sleep when activity in cells of the cerebral cortex becomes synchronous. Synchrony is achieved by regular pulsing of the cortex by impulses from particular groups of cells in the thalamus (*nonspecific nuclei*). The result of this pulsing is that impulses reaching the brain from sensory receptors are no longer registered properly in the cerebral cortex, and as a result we are unaware of them.

When we are awake, pulsing of the cerebral cortex by the thalamus is prevented by excitatory activity reaching the thalamus from groups of cells within the reticular formation of the brain stem (Fig. 31.1 and Ch. 23). These cells form part of the system that produces the regular sleep/wake cycle and determines the characteristics of sleep, such as its depth and episodes of dreaming. The neurotransmitters involved include serotonin, noradrenaline and acetylcholine.

SLEEP/WAKE CYCLE

The activity of groups of cells within the reticular formation of the brain stem, such as the *raphe nuclei* and the *nucleus locus coeruleus* (Fig. 31.1), waxes and wanes daily, driven by a 'biological clock' in the hypothalamus. Activity is also affected by impulses in sensory systems, allowing us to be aroused from sleep, or conversely prevented from sleeping.

Biological clock
The cells in the hypothalamus acting as a clock are those in the *suprachiasmatic nucleus* (Fig. 31.1 and Ch. 18). The

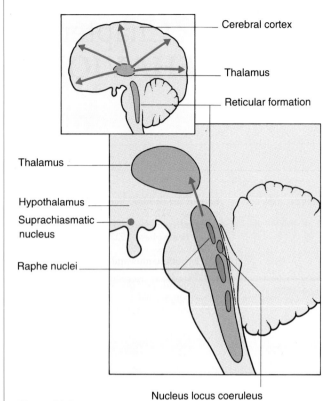

Figure 31.1
Parts of the brain involved in determining the level of consciousness.

circadian rhythm set by this clock causes most of us to be awake for about 16 hours and asleep for about 8 hours each day, though the pattern changes from birth to old age (see Ch. 36) and there are individual variations particularly in the duration of sleep. If someone is allowed to go to sleep and get up when he or she wishes, in an environment which provides no clues as to time of day, a regular cycle of sleeping and waking occurs with a period of about 25 hours. The cycle is normally entrained to the 24-hour day by cues, *zeitgeber*, such as light, the ringing of an alarm, and social habits. Any routine events can function in this way, and therefore cue us into sleeping and waking. ①

Arousal

The activity of cells in the reticular formation is also affected by impulses in the sensory systems. Signals from almost all our senses enter the reticular formation along fibres that are branches (*collaterals*) of the main sensory pathways. These impulses raise the level of excitation in the reticular formation and disrupt the regular bursts of impulses generated by the thalamus. As a result we wake up. This is why it is difficult to get to sleep when we are awake and wanting to sleep but are being bombarded with information from our senses about sounds and lights around us. Conversely, when stimulation is lacking, perhaps in a darkened, warm classroom or lecture theatre, when listening to a very

SLEEP AND THE NURSE

Most people consider sleep to be very important. There are a few who get by with a succession of catnaps, their longest period of sleep being about 4 hours. Others are not happy unless they achieve 8 hours or more. Like the weather, sleep often provides a major topic of conversation, how late one went to bed, what disturbed one's sleep, how early one had to get up, and so on. As one gets older, sleep tends to become less important and the period of sleep required shorter (see Ch. 36). Helping a ward of patients to achieve what they consider to be the right quantity and quality of sleep often requires much ingenuity on the part of the nurse. Much may depend on what has happened to the individual patients during the day; some may be night-shift workers and find it extremely difficult to sleep at night while in hospital (see Ch. 18). Sleeping tablets are not always the answer.

Case history

A male nurse found that an elderly gentleman stayed awake all night and disturbed other patients. The nurse noticed that as soon as he put the patient's light on in the morning and gave him a wash and a cup of tea he went to sleep! The day staff did not report the patient as being difficult during the day. The nurse decided to carry out the morning routine of a wash and cup of tea at around 11 p.m. The elderly gentleman slept soundly all night and the day staff reported him as requiring more attention because he no longer slept all day.

Most people develop a bedtime routine. These routines are as varied as the people using them, a hot drink, a shower, reading, exercise, listening to music, yoga, and so on. Without these routines, sleep is often difficult to capture. Once a person is hospitalised it can be extremely difficult to follow any sort of pre-sleep routine, and, in addition, there are a variety of stimulants with which the sensory receptors have to cope. The people who can sleep soundly under any circumstance or after taking a couple of paracetamol tablets are to be envied. 'Nurse can't you give me something to help me sleep?' is a frequent question.

The reasons for not sleeping need to be explored before resorting to sleeping tablets; they might, for example, include pain, anxiety, noise, light, or an uncomfortable bed. If it is not possible to resolve the problem with simple remedies then short-term night sedation might be prescribed. Alternatives, such as relaxation, massage therapy and aromatherapy are sometimes used with effect. Whenever possible, anxiolytics (e.g. diazepam, lorazepam) and hypnotics (e.g. nitrazepam and the barbiturates) should be avoided and, if prescribed, should be short term.

monotonous voice, there is less to disturb the regular activity of the thalamic cells and we may easily drift off to sleep.

CHARACTERISTICS OF SLEEP

When we fall asleep and stay asleep for a while, our level of consciousness alters, and the state of mind and body alternates regularly between two types of sleep:

- non-REM
- REM.

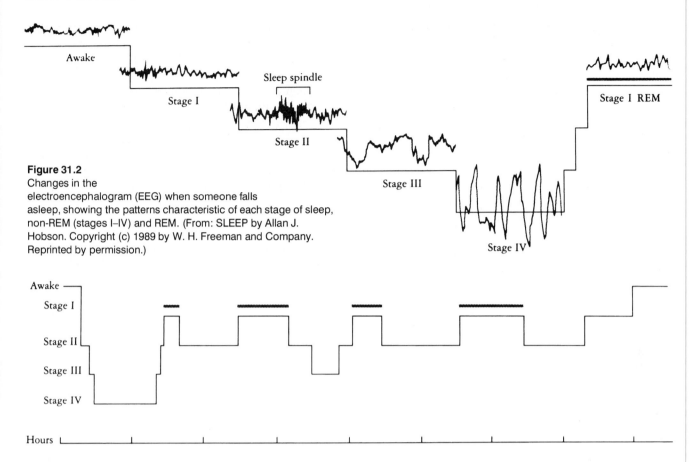

Figure 31.2
Changes in the
electroencephalogram (EEG) when someone falls
asleep, showing the patterns characteristic of each stage of sleep,
non-REM (stages I–IV) and REM. (From: SLEEP by Allan J.
Hobson. Copyright (c) 1989 by W. H. Freeman and Company.
Reprinted by permission.)

Figure 31.3
Pattern of sleep stages during a night's sleep. Episodes of REM sleep are indicated by the horizontal bars (From: SLEEP by Allan J.
Hobson. Copyright (c) 1989 by W. H. Freeman and Company. Reprinted by permission.)

Each form of sleep is marked by characteristic patterns of the EEG, and distinctive changes in muscle tone, mental activity, heart rate and breathing.

Non-REM sleep

When we fall asleep the pattern of electrical activity recorded in the EEG changes (Fig. 31.2 and Ch. 23), and heart rate and blood pressure fall. Four stages (I–IV) of non-REM sleep have been distinguished by EEG. The last of these, stage IV, is sometimes referred to as deep sleep or slow wave sleep. It is more difficult to arouse someone from this level of sleep than from the other three. Stage IV sleep is also the one in which sleepwalking and talking, nightmares and tooth grinding may occur in some people, particularly when someone is young. The amount of stage IV sleep tends to diminish as we grow older, with the benefit that these phenomena tend to disappear.

When we first fall asleep, we progress rapidly through the four stages of sleep, spend a short while at the lowest level reached and then return through them. This cycle recurs at about 90- to 100-minute intervals throughout the night, but with the depth of sleep becoming less as the night progresses (Fig. 31.3).

During stage IV sleep, the blood pressure and pulse rate fall. If it is essential to record blood pressure and pulse during the night and this is carried out without rousing the patient, then the chart should be marked 'sleeping'. This will account for a, possibly, marked difference from the previous and subsequent recordings.

REM sleep

A different form of sleep, REM sleep, occurs at regular intervals during a period of sleep (Fig. 31.3). It is associated with a number of distinctive features, including:

- rapid eye movements (REM)
- dreaming
- profound muscle relaxation
- increase in blood pressure, pulse and breathing.

When the changeover occurs between non-REM sleep and REM sleep, the EEG pattern alters abruptly to one resembling the awake state (Fig. 31.2). Yet, paradoxically the sleeper is very deeply asleep. For this reason REM sleep has been termed '*paradoxical sleep*'. If the sleeper is aroused from REM sleep he will often report that he has been dreaming. This is why there is movement of the eyeballs, as in his mind he is visualising and following the events of his dream. There may be occasional twitches of the body, but overall, muscle tone and activity is profoundly reduced. The mind, especially the imagination, is active but the body is relaxed. Blood pressure, pulse and rate of breathing, however, increase and vary much more than during non-REM sleep.

The first episode of REM sleep lasts for only a few minutes, but as the night progresses the episodes gradually lengthen. The transition from REM sleep to non-REM sleep and vice versa is marked by an increase in body movement, and a change in body position. The rest of the sleeping time, whether REM or non-REM, is generally associated with muscle relaxation.

②
How many drugs can you name that affect the level of consciousness?

> Sleep research has not shown that any serious, long-term ill effects are produced by sleep deprivation. Tiredness, irritability and impaired judgement are the most usual effects. REM sleep is the most important part of the sleep cycle and is needed to refresh cognitive ability. Too many very late nights combined with early shifts may well affect a nurse's ability to function efficiently – to the detriment of patient care.

NEUROTRANSMITTERS

The cells of the *raphe nuclei* in the brain stem secrete *serotonin* (5-HT or *5-hydroxytryptamine*), whereas the cells of the *nucleus locus coeruleus* secrete *noradrenaline*. Both these amines are associated with states of arousal and their secretion falls during sleep. Other cells in the brain stem secrete *acetylcholine*. Its secretion increases in REM sleep.

These different groups of cells in the brain stem, each secreting different substances, form part of much bigger systems of neurones innervating many areas of the brain. These systems modify (*modulate*) the process of synaptic transmission throughout the brain and therefore change the general level of activity within the nervous system.

Changing levels of these substances are responsible for the alteration in levels of consciousness and behaviour characteristic of different periods of sleep, as well as for the differing levels of arousal in the awake state (see p. 522). Many drugs affecting the central nervous system interfere with the release and action of these substances and therefore alter levels of consciousness and affect sleep. ②

EMOTION AND MOTIVATION

DEFINITION AND BASIS

Emotion and motivation are familiar terms, yet it is not easy to define exactly what each consists of and how each is produced by our nervous systems.

Emotion

We know what we mean when we say that we feel emotional, or when we describe someone else as acting emotionally. But emotion is difficult to describe and explain biologically because it includes so many different aspects of our experience and behaviour, all of which are bundled together to produce the states of mind and body that we call happiness, sadness, anger, fear etc. Any emotion includes:

- particular patterns of behaviour (smiling, shaking fist etc.)
- autonomic effects (racing heart, sweaty hands etc.)
- our conscious perception of these responses (feelings)
- the description we give to our feelings (happy, angry etc.)
- the stimuli acting as triggers (success, a missed bus).

Each of these involves the activity of different parts of the nervous system and the effects produced on the tissues and organs that are controlled by them. Thus emotional experience and behaviour involve many parts of the brain including:

- cerebral cortex and basal ganglia
- limbic system
- hypothalamus
- autonomic nervous system and pituitary gland.

In our emotions, activity in the parts of the brain which are chiefly concerned with the control of the internal environment (hypothalamus, pituitary gland and autonomic nervous system) is closely associated with activity in the somatic nervous system (cerebral cortex

> **SLEEPING PILLS**
>
> Drugs used as sleeping pills include the barbiturates and the benzodiazepines. Barbiturates depress nervous activity in general, rather like general anaesthetics (see Ch. 23) whereas benzodiazepines promote the inhibitory effects of the neurotransmitter GABA (*gamma aminobutyric acid*). One of the actions of GABA is to depress the secretion of serotonin which is one of the substances associated with states of arousal (see p. 000). This may be one way in which the benzodiazepines exert their sedative effect.
>
> The term 'sleeping pill' is a misnomer in that these pills do not produce the regular cycles of activity characteristic of a good night's sleep. At best, they merely depress activity, and quieten the nervous system, making it more likely that sleep will occur. At worst, they disrupt normal mechanisms, induce tolerance and create dependence (see Ch. 19), and result in even worse insomnia when they are withdrawn. Benzodiazepines actually suppress stages III and IV of non-REM sleep, and barbiturates suppress REM sleep. Neither therefore actually produces a normal night's rest.

and basal ganglia). The limbic system acts as the interface between these two.

Motivation

Motivation springs from our need to satisfy basic drives for:

- food
- warmth
- water
- survival (through sex and reproduction).

Satisfaction of these needs depends upon our ability to behave appropriately (go shopping, turn on a tap, put on clothes, date a boyfriend/girlfriend etc.) as well as upon the internal controls of blood sugar, osmolality and temperature, and gonadal function described in Chapters 13, 14, 16 and 34. We have to work to buy food; we have to consider how best to clothe and house ourselves and our families. To do these things we need to know and understand about shops, materials, and money etc., as well as be motivated to make use of them.

Motivation couples the need to satisfy our basic drives, with our perception of the likely results of different courses of action. If a strategy (for example going for a hot drink) appears to fulfil a basic need (for water, for example) it will be attractive to us, whereas if it appears to be harmful (raising body temperature) we will be inclined to avoid it. If there is danger but the possibility of reward (for example standing one's ground in a crowd of people all trying to buy a hot drink during the interval at a show), we may react aggressively. These behaviours are intimately interwoven with our different emotions. Things that are attractive and rewarding usually bring pleasure; those that appear harmful make us feel afraid; if our actions are frustrated we may feel anger.

All of this involves a detailed assessment both of our internal bodily state and of our surroundings, and the selection of a pattern of behaviour appropriate to our needs. The limbic system has a central role in this overall process of assessment and decision and therefore plays a key role in motivation as well as in our emotions.

> Patients who are confined to bed are unable to satisfy all of their basic drives. Needing a drink of water, or to empty the bladder, becomes a problem for such patients. When planning care the nurse must be aware of the basic drives so that she can meet patients' needs before they become problems. Thus, emotions such as anxiety ('I might lose control and wet the bed') and anger ('they've forgotten my drink again') are reduced.

LIMBIC SYSTEM

The limbic system is a complex system, which is very important in determining our behaviour. It has links with other parts of the nervous system including:

- neocortex of the cerebrum
- hypothalamus
- olfactory system.

Structure

The main parts of the limbic system and their situation in the brain are shown in Figure 31.4A & B. The limbic system consists of a number of clusters of cell bodies (*nuclei*) linked together with neural tissue in which the cells are arranged in layers (*cortex*). The overall appearance is of a ring of neural tissue bordering on the neocortex surrounding it (*limbus* means border).

The limbic system represents the highest level of brain activity in some animals. In humans, the limbic system has been swamped by the development of the neocortex (see Ch. 20 and Fig. 31.4A) functionally as well as structurally (the limbic system is buried underneath the cerebrocortical mantle). Consequently our behaviour is much more complex than that of other intelligent creatures.

Functions

It has been difficult to obtain information about the functions of the limbic system in humans, because the various structures are buried deep within the cerebral hemispheres. Some functions have therefore been inferred from the results of studies of animal behaviour. In experimental studies in the 1950s, it was found that rats appeared to enjoy having parts of their limbic system stimulated electrically. If they were enabled to deliver their own stimuli by means of a lever they would go on doing so for hours! It was concluded that in some way stimulation was experienced by the animals as rewarding. Conversely, stimulation of other areas led to avoidance of the lever, suggesting that in some way the stimulus was unpleasant.

There have been some studies in humans of the effects of stimulation of parts of the limbic system. Subjects have reported stimulation as evoking feelings of pleasure, relaxation, anger, fear, and even terror. Other information in humans has been derived from the effects of lesions or injury to the limbic system. Damage to the amygdala, for example, has been shown to produce a loss of aggression in men as well as feelings of hypersexuality.

Links with other brain areas

Neocortex of the cerebrum

Links between the limbic system and the neocortex enable information, gleaned from our senses about the outer world, to be received and logged. One region of the limbic system, the *hippocampus*, appears to play a crucial role in our memory of sensory experiences (see

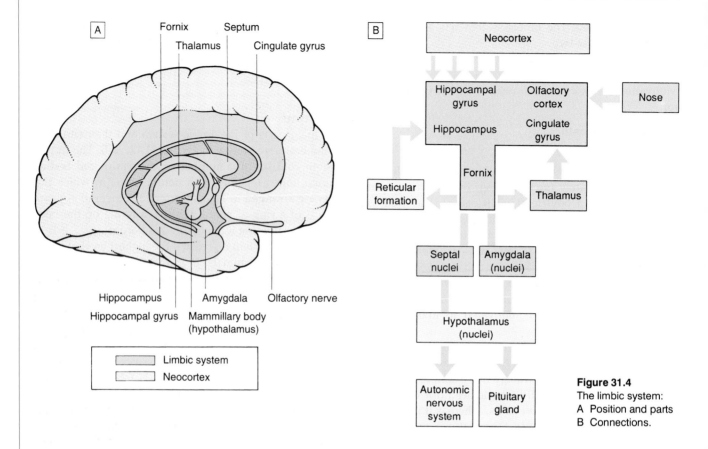

Figure 31.4
The limbic system:
A Position and parts
B Connections.

Ch. 33). This is probably of importance in determining our learned emotional responses to different situations. If an event in the past was associated with unpleasant consequences (maybe a destructive response of a teacher or parent to our failure in an examination), when we encounter a similar situation again we will remember the previous experience, and 'relive' its unpleasant associations. Consequently we may react as we did before even if this time the consequences are quite different (for example tutors being helpful and constructive). ③

③
What other common examples of learned emotional responses can you think of?

> It is important for the nurse to understand learned emotional responses because, by helping to prevent unpleasant associations for patients, she can lessen anxiety related to future admissions to hospital. A painful injection may make a patient become very tense prior to subsequent injections, thus increasing the possibility of pain. Painful experiences in hospital, both physical and emotional (e.g. seeing another patient die), are likely to be remembered more readily than happier ones (e.g. the staff being kind and approachable).

Hypothalamus

The links between the limbic system and the hypothalamus enable our behaviour to be controlled in a way that serves the needs of the internal environment. For example, the control of body temperature (see Ch. 16) involves the choices we make about what clothes to wear, and whether or not to turn up the central heating, as well as autonomic responses such as vasodilation and vasoconstriction of cutaneous blood vessels. Choosing to turn up the central heating requires that we have learnt some basic information about heating systems and how to work them. We have to access that information, logged in the neocortex and hippocampus, in order to create a comfortable environment and maintain body temperature.

Another example is the control of the desire to eat. There are two areas in the hypothalamus concerned with feeding and fullness (*satiety*) (see Ch. 14). These areas are linked with specific regions of the amygdala (Fig. 31.5). It has been shown in animal studies that stimulation or lesions in these areas of the amygdala can either cause an animal to overeat or not to eat at all. Interestingly these changes in feeding behaviour are associated with changes in emotional behaviour too. The combination of going off one's food and feeling tired and depressed is familiar to most people. Here we see some of the complex links that may be involved in certain behaviours, and the associations between one's state of mind and activities such as eating.

Olfactory system

Part of the limbic system is linked directly to the olfactory system (Fig. 31.4; see also Ch. 15). This sensory

ANOREXIA NERVOSA

Anorexia nervosa has been recognised as an illness for over 100 years, being first described as 'the want of appetite due to a morbid mental state'. The cause is unknown and has been attributed to either psychological factors, arising from conflicts during puberty and adolescence, or disordered functioning of the hypothalamus in relation to the control of eating and some endocrine production. Rarely, a tumour of the hypothalamus causes the same symptoms.

The mechanisms involved are complex, as is the human brain, and the disorder has been widely researched. Sufferers are now treated sympathetically, which has not always been the case. Those affected are usually young girls in their teens, although boys and older people of both sexes are sometimes also affected. It is not possible to be specific about the circumstances surrounding the onset of the disorder but, for some, it may be associated with the inability to accept sexual development, a desire to retain a childlike figure; others start dieting and find that they get such a lift from the initial starvation that they continually strive to maintain the sensation; for others the causative mechanism may not be established.

The anorexic person is liable to become so emaciated that life is threatened; food is refused and, if eaten, is usually voluntarily vomited by a finger down the throat. There is a distorted image of body size (even when thin the person still feels fat), personality changes occur and there may not be insight, causing denial of illness. In girls, ovulation and consequently menstruation cease (see Chs 34 and 35). In severe cases, the effects of malnutrition are obvious, loss of hair, swollen gums, skin disorders.

Treatment, which may be prolonged, is usually carried out in a psychiatric unit where sympathetic and consistent care can be provided. Sufferers are no longer subjected to traumatic treatment, such as insulin coma therapy, high doses of largactil and electroconvulsive therapy, as they once were.

system is unique in our bodies in that sensory signals do not pass via the thalamus to the cerebral cortex but go instead straight to the limbic cortex. The sense of smell is a powerful regulator of behaviour in animals. It is less obviously important in us, but even so smells are probably more powerful in evoking emotional feelings, whether of pleasure or disgust, than any other sensation. ④

ROLE OF THE CEREBRAL HEMISPHERES IN EMOTION

Right hemisphere

In the previous chapter we saw that, in the majority of people, the right hemisphere specialises in such things as the recognition of faces, in musical appreciation, and in nonverbal forms of expression such as laughter and facial expression. These facts and the results of a variety of studies have revealed that the right hemisphere plays an important role both in our expression of emotion and in our recognition and understanding of the emotions expressed by others. For example in patients with 'split brains' (see Ch. 30), funny pictures presented to the left visual field (evoking activity in the right hemisphere) are more likely to evoke laughter than if they are presented to the right visual field (therefore to the left hemisphere). Studies of normal subjects reveal that our facial expressions are more intense on the left side of our faces (that is the side controlled by the right hemisphere). Also damage to the right hemisphere can reduce the emotional intonation of speech and our ability to understand the emotional cues given in the speech of others.

Left hemisphere

However, the left hemisphere also appears to contribute to emotion. Study of the consequences of injury to the right or left hemisphere in patients who have had a stroke has revealed that changes in mood can occur in either case. Injury to the left hemisphere is associated with a higher incidence of negative emotions, such as feeling depressed. Conversely, injury to the right hemisphere more often produces the opposite effect. For

④ *Appetising food stimulates secretion of digestive juices. How do you think this is brought about?*

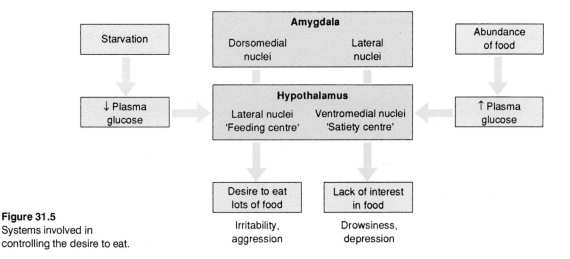

Figure 31.5
Systems involved in controlling the desire to eat.

example, there may be an inappropriate indifference to a situation, or there may be optimism or even joviality. Other evidence of an opposite emotional bias between right and left hemispheres has come also from observations made in psychiatric patients who have received unilateral electroconvulsive therapy (ECT) and in people suffering from temporal lobe epilepsy.

> Electroconvulsive therapy was used extensively between 1940 and 1960 before antidepressant (e.g. amytriptyline) and antipsychotic (e.g. chlorpromazine) drugs became available. It was primarily used to relieve depression and the disordered mental states associated with schizophrenia. Today it is less commonly used but may be effective in bringing a person out of severe, immobilising depression more quickly than drug therapy. A weak electric current passed between the temples, or one temple and the frontal region on the same side, produces the effects of an epileptic seizure. However, muscular spasms do not occur because the patient is anaesthetised and given a muscle relaxant. The improvement in depressive states may be due to the release of noradrenaline and serotonin by such seizures.

Frontal lobes

As mentioned in Chapter 30, the frontal lobes of the cerebral hemispheres seem to be involved in allowing or disallowing certain behaviours. After injury to this part of the brain a person may become less anxious and more carefree. This occurs most often if the damage is to the right frontal cortex. Damage to the left frontal cortex in contrast can result in depression.

THE HYPOTHALAMUS AND VISCERAL CONTROL

The hypothalamus consists of several clusters of neurones (*nuclei*) (Fig. 31.6) that are concerned with the control of different aspects of the internal environment (Table 31.1). These cells are linked with the somatic nervous system through the limbic system. They control the activity of our internal organs (viscera) through the autonomic nervous system and the hormones of the pituitary gland (Table 31.2).

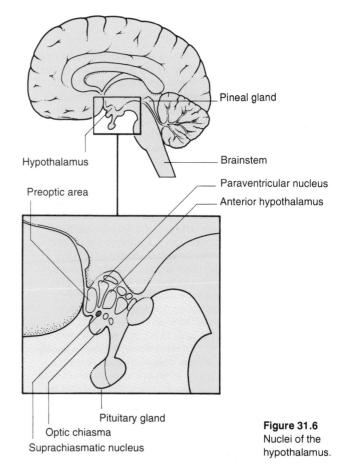

Pineal gland

Hypothalamus

Brainstem

Preoptic area

Paraventricular nucleus

Anterior hypothalamus

Pituitary gland

Optic chiasma

Suprachiasmatic nucleus

Figure 31.6 Nuclei of the hypothalamus.

Autonomic nervous system and hormones

When we feel excited, whether angry or desperate to run away from a threatening situation, or buoyed up with eager anticipation, the sympathetic nervous system is activated producing many changes in the activity of the viscera (see Ch. 19 and Fig. 19.5). We are conscious of many of these changes, for example the pounding heart is sensed in our chest, our hands feel damp from the sweat, and the changed tone of the gastric and intestinal muscle makes us feel queasy. All these things contribute to the emotional experience we have of excitement, anger or fear. ⑤

Different emotions are thought to be associated with slightly different patterns of activation of the autonomic

⑤ *Can you think of any other feelings you have experienced that result from changes in visceral activity?*

Table 31.1 Functions of nuclei and/or areas in the hypothalamus		
Nuclei/area	Functions	Chapter reference
Lateral and ventromedial	Feeding/fasting	14
Supraoptic and paraventricular	Water balance	13
Anterior/posterior	Temperature regulation	16
Preoptic area	Reproduction	34, 35
Suprachiasmatic	Circadian rhythms	18

Table 31.2 Hormones of the pituitary gland

Hormone	Abbreviation	Target gland
Adrenocorticotrophic hormone	ACTH	Adrenal cortex → corticosteroids
Antidiuretic hormone	ADH	
Follicle stimulating hormone	FSH	Gonads → oestrogens
Growth hormone		
Luteinising hormone	LH	Gonads → oestrogens / progesterone / testosterone
Oxytocin		
Prolactin		
Thyroid stimulating hormone	TSH	Thyroid → thyroxine

nervous system and different balances of hormones. Whereas the secretion of adrenaline and noradrenaline is linked with anger and fear, anxiety is associated with raised levels of ACTH and corticosteroids, and aggres-sion can be correlated with the levels of androgens, particularly testosterone in males. Other hormones that have been implicated in changes in mood and behaviour include insulin, thyroid hormones, gonadal hormones in women and endogenous opioids. ⑥

Psychosomatic phenomena

It is clear that extensive links exist between the mind and the body through the systems described above. Our state of mind can clearly influence activity in our viscera through the autonomic nervous system and through the hormones released from the pituitary gland. Increased secretion of catecholamines (adrenaline and noradren-aline) is implicated in coronary heart disease, whereas catecholamines and cortisol have both been linked with the development of diseases that may be associated with suppression of the immune system (such as duodenal ulcer and cancer). Conversely, strategies such as relax-ation therapy and meditation lower the secretion of these stress hormones and have a beneficial effect.

⑥
What are the endogenous opioids? When and where are they produced?

STRESS AS AN EMOTION

Long-term emotional stress sometimes produces physical symptoms that are distressing for the individual, or collections of signs and symptoms that form a specific disease. Diseases which are entirely or partly manifestations of severe emotional stress are termed psychosomatic, a word which once suggested that the illness was 'all in the mind' and that those affected should 'pull themselves together'. More recently, the term stress-related illness or disease has been used.

Today most people are aware that stress plays a significant part in our lives. Some seem to thrive on stress, while others begin to suffer physical symptoms in the presence of fairly low levels of stress. Stress as an emotion is liable to alter normal levels of hormones and enzymes, for example the production of excess catecholamines, which in turn may affect the function of an organ or system. Alterations in the immune system may increase susceptibility to infection and the development of cancerous tissue. Even many accidents can be directly attributed to stress.

Nurses, whether in hospital or the community, are in an ideal position to discover evidence of stress. For example, is the stress of being in hospital and/or ill impeding recovery? Is there a long-term worry which the patient has considered too trivial to mention?

Most people are aware of the illnesses and conditions that are made worse by emotional stress: high blood pressure; asthma; skin diseases such as eczema and psoriasis; digestive disorders from flatulence to ulcerative colitis. But what about the colds, headaches, aches and pains from tense muscles, rashes and various types of indigestion that occur on starting a new job or school? Nurses are encouraged to recognise stress in themselves and engage in relaxing pursuits, such as exercise or listening to music. Research into the part played by stress in disease is ongoing and more definite links may be discovered.

KEY POINTS

What you should now understand about sleep, emotion and behaviour:

- why we go to sleep and what happens when we do
- factors that help or hinder sleep and how they work
- differences between natural sleep and the effects of sleeping pills
- neural systems involved in determining our moods, feelings and desires
- biological basis of some common emotional experiences such as excitement, euphoria and anxiety
- basic drives influencing our behaviour and how they may alter in health and disease
- how states of mind can affect bodily function.

REFERENCES AND FURTHER READING

Agras W S 1985 Panic: facing fears, phobias and anxiety. W H Freeman, Oxford
(Discusses basis of various disorders and their treatments as well as what friends and family can do)

Bloch G 1985 Body and self: elements of human biology, behaviour, and health. William Kaufmann, Los Altos, California
(Lucid student text setting physiology and psychology firmly within everyday experience)

Donovan B T 1985 Hormones and human behaviour. Cambridge University Press, Cambridge
(Overview of research findings concerning the relationship between the nervous system, hormones and behaviour)

Feuerstein M, Labbé E E, Kuczmierczyk A R 1986 Health psychology: a psychobiological perspective. Plenum Publishing Company, New York
(Wide ranging book addressing the relationship between a person's physical condition and their psychological state)

Graham R B 1990 Physiological psychology. Wadsworth Publishing Company, Belmont, California
(Student text providing more information about sleep, mood and behaviour, and the experimental basis of current knowledge)

Hobson J A 1989 Sleep. W H Freeman, New York
(An interesting book, including experimental background to current knowledge, written for the general reader as well as the student)

Hughes J 1987 Cancer and emotion: psychological preludes and reactions to cancer. John Wiley & Sons, Chichester
(Examines links between psychology and cancer and vice versa, in a clear non-technical way for patients, their families and professional carers)

Logue A W 1986 The psychology of eating and drinking. W H Freeman, Oxford
(Overview providing interesting and useful insights into many different normal and abnormal behaviours, even including wine tasting)

Mendelson W B 1987 Human sleep: research and clinical care. Plenum Publishing Company, New York
(The physiology, pharmacology and pathology of sleep. Practical guidelines for the management of sleep disorders)

Strongman K T International review of emotion. John Wiley & Sons, Chichester
(Biannual volumes containing specialist reviews)

Chapter 32
PAIN

Like vision, hearing, touch, smell and taste, pain is a sensation evoked by the excitation of nerve cells in the brain. It usually occurs when specific sensory receptors are excited, but, like other sensations, it can be experienced whenever and however pain pathways are stimulated. The character (sharp or burning) and perceived location of a pain (discrete or vague) depend on:

● the types and situations of the receptors excited
● the pathways through which the impulses are transmitted
● the ultimate destinations of the signals within the brain.

Pain alerts us to damaging forces in or around our bodies and triggers a variety of protective responses and behaviours. Some of these provide important clues to the health worker about the source of the injury.

Pain differs from other sensations in the degree to which it is associated with emotional reactions, such as anxiety, fear and alarm, and with their accompanying

autonomic reflex responses. It is these reactions and responses that give pain much of its distinctive and unpleasant character. Fortunately, pain can often be controlled by appropriate therapy or drug treatment.①

THE SENSATION OF PAIN

Damage to tissues is not invariably felt as pain. For example, the small intestine can be cut and cauterised without pain being felt. Likewise, in brain surgery, once a hole has been made in the skull under local anaesthesia, brain tissue can be cut without the patient feeling anything. However, at the other extreme, even slight injury to tissues such as the skin and the peritoneum (see Ch. 6) can produce very sharp and discomforting pain. This shows that receptors sensitive to tissue damage, which mediate the sensation of pain, are not uniformly distributed throughout the body. Lining layers, such as the skin (see Chs 15 and 24) and peritoneum, tend to be more richly supplied with receptors than internal structures, such as the liver (see Ch. 9) and the intestines (see Ch. 6).

THE EXTERNAL SURFACE: SKIN

Types of sensation

The skin is abundantly supplied with receptors excited by noxious stimuli (*nociceptors*), most of which are

① *Think of a pain that you have experienced. What did you think about at the time? How did it make you feel? What did you do? Did you notice it disappear?*

In some conditions, such as rheumatoid arthritis, chronic pain may serve a protective function. In others, like back pain, it may have outlived its usefulness as a warning. The back pain sufferer commonly believes that painful movements will lead to further injury. However, after the initial acute phase, lack of exercise leads to muscle wastage and further pain. Back pain patients commonly require education and physical retraining to overcome this.

unspecialised nerve endings (see Chs 15 and 24). When the skin is damaged, two recognisably different qualities of pain can be distinguished. There is the sharp, well-localised pain felt at the time of injury, and the longer-lasting, more diffuse discomfort experienced shortly afterwards. These two types of sensation are sometimes referred to as 'fast' and 'slow' pain. The differences between them are due to differences in the receptors stimulated and in the routes and destinations of the impulses within the nervous system.

Fast pain

The receptors activated include mechanosensitive nociceptors responding to the forces producing the injury. They are innervated by small diameter myelinated nerve fibres (Aδ) (see Ch. 21) that synapse in the spinal cord and brain stem with tracts carrying these signals directly to the thalamus (*spinothalamic* and *trigeminothalamic tracts* respectively) and from there to the somatosensory cortex (Fig. 32.1). Because of this direct and fairly discrete routing, the pain felt is relatively sharp and well localised (see Ch. 23).

Slow pain

When tissues are damaged, a variety of cellular products are released, including bradykinin and prostaglandins (see Chs 10 and 15), some of which stimulate a different class of pain receptors, the *polymodal nociceptors*. These are so called because of the range of stimuli to which they will respond. They are innervated by unmyelinated nerve fibres (C fibres; see Ch. 21) that synapse, within the spinal cord and the brain stem, with tracts carrying the signals first into the *reticular formation*

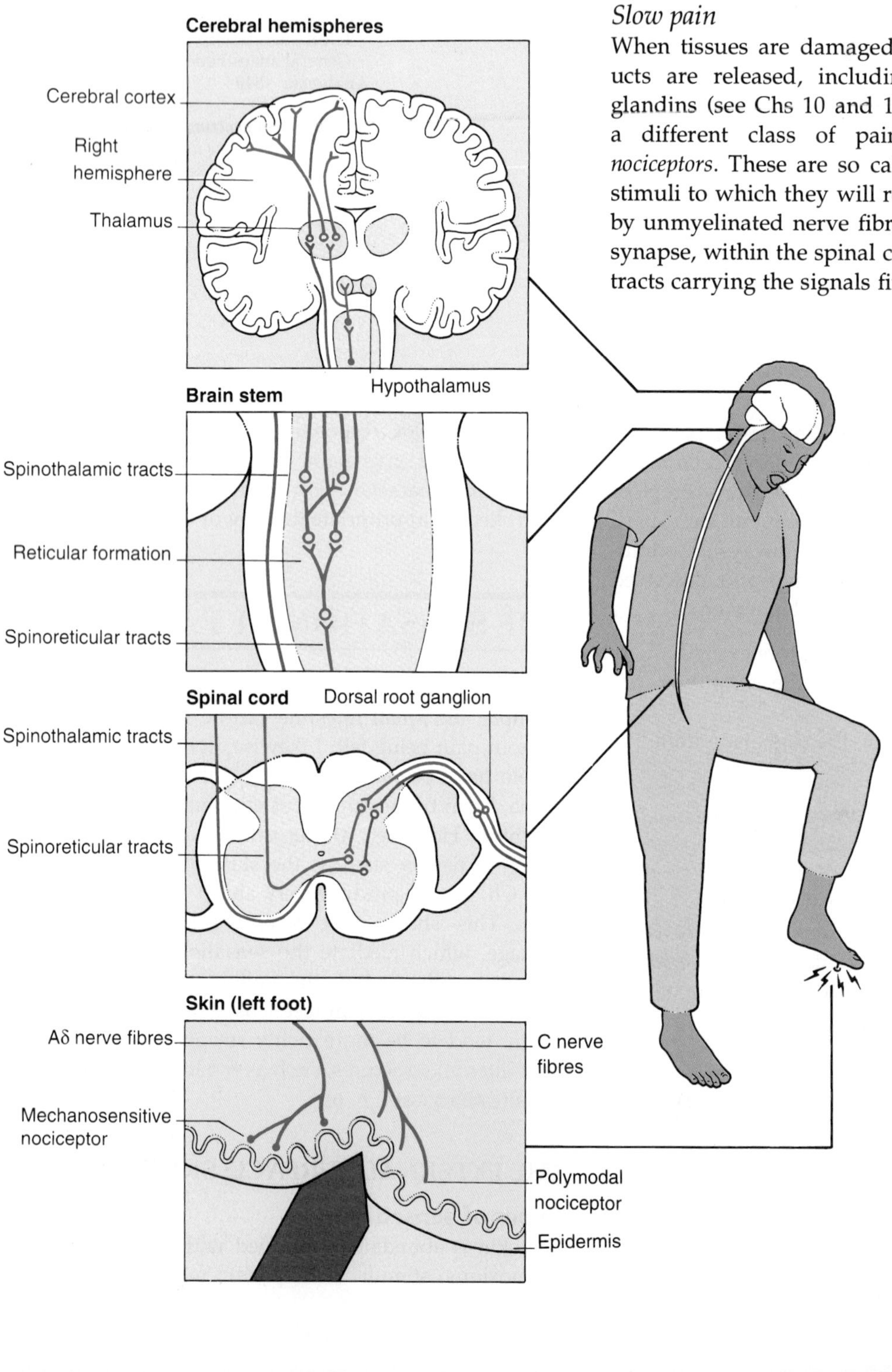

Figure 32.1
Routes through which impulses from nociceptors in the skin are transmitted to the brain, giving rise to the sensations of 'fast' pain (red lines) and 'slow' pain (blue lines). (Note that the skin receptors being excited are on the left side of the body whereas the destination of the nerve impulses in the brain is on the opposite side.)

of the brain stem (see Ch. 23), via the *spinoreticular tracts*, and thence to the thalamus and the cerebral cortex (Fig. 32.1). Within the reticular formation, the excitation does not remain discretely localised but spreads out to activate adjacent nerve cells so that the excitation becomes more diffuse and more areas of the brain are activated including parts involved in our emotional responses, such as the hypothalamus (see Ch. 31). Consequently our perception of the site of injury is vaguer and we experience more distress.②

Physiological pain control: the pain gate

It is well known that the discomfort experienced when we injure ourselves can be made to feel different: just rubbing the injured part has a soothing effect; courageous rescuers are sometimes unaware of serious injures they have sustained until after an emergency is over; 'positive thinking' can influence what we feel. None of this is in any way mysterious. The transmission of any signals within the nervous system can be inhibited at synapses. The first place this occurs in pain pathways is within the spinal cord or brain stem.③

Melzack & Wall (1965) coined the word 'gating' to describe the way that signals from nociceptors arriving at the spinal cord could be prevented from being transmitted further, thus reducing the sensation of pain and producing *physiological analgesia*. Disturbances and diseases affecting this pain control system give rise to a variety of abnormal sensations including 'pins and needles' (*paraesthesia*) and supersensitivity to painful stimuli (*hyperalgesia*).

Physiological analgesia

The crucial feature in the body's system of pain control is the presence of inhibitory interneurones, which synapse with neurones in the pain pathway (Fig. 32.2). These inhibitory interneurones are activated by:

- simultaneous activity in other sensory neurones (usually large diameter myelinated fibres (Aβ) carrying information about touch and pressure from the skin)
- nerve fibres carrying signals down from the brain.

② Describe and compare your feelings when you last experienced: (a) a burn; (b) a cut; (c) toothache; (d) a headache.

③ Next time you hurt yourself, notice the difference in quality between the immediate sensation and delayed pain. How do you instinctively try to alleviate this?

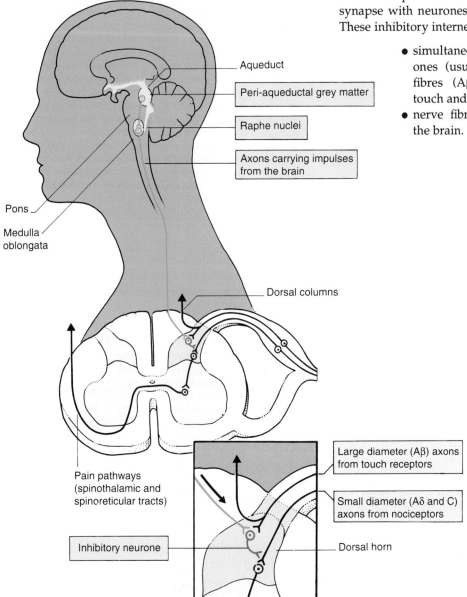

Figure 32.2
Component parts of the body's system of pain control. The transmission of signals in the 'pain pathway' can be inhibited by simultaneous activity in (1) other sensory neurones conducting impulses from the skin and (2) axons conducting impulses from the brain, both of which excite inhibitory interneurones.

The axons of sensory neurones conveying signals about touch and pressure from the trunk and limbs become the dorsal columns of the spinal cord (see Ch. 24). Just before they do, these axons branch in the dorsal horn forming collaterals that synapse with the inhibitory interneurones. Consequently, when the skin in the vicinity of the injured area is gently rubbed (which excites the large diameter fibres), these inhibitory interneurones are activated and this reduces the transmission of signals in the 'pain pathways'.

The nerve fibres coming down from the brain, that have similar effects, include some which originate in two areas of the brain stem (Fig. 32.2):

- peri-aqueductal grey matter
- raphe nuclei.

Some of the nerve cells involved in influencing (*modulating*) the transmission of pain are cells secreting a different class of neurotransmitters, the *endogenous opioids*, which include peptides such as:

- endorphins
- enkephalins
- dynorphin.

> The gate control theory highlights the presence of ascending and descending influences on pain perception. Pain is never solely physical or purely psychological. The relative influence of these factors will vary according to the extent of tissue damage, the context in which the pain occurs and individual interpretation.

Paraesthesia and hyperalgesia

The discomfort experienced a short while after a leg or an arm has gone numb when you have been lying on it awkwardly is very familiar. When the limb comes 'back to life' again, a mixture of sensations are felt (*paraesthesia*) and the pain can be excruciating.

When tissue is compressed and becomes ischaemic the nerve axons stop transmitting nerve impulses, and sensation is lost (see Ch. 21). As blood flow recovers, the axons recover too but this takes longer for the large diameter fibres than the smaller ones. Consequently, after a period of numbness, the small diameter unmyelinated nerve fibres, some of which transmit signals from nociceptors in deeper tissues of the limb, begin transmitting signals before the large diameter fibres involved in the gating of pain have recovered. Briefly, activity in the small diameter fibres is uninhibited by gating mechanisms and the affected individual experiences the result! As activity returns to normal in the larger fibres the transmission of signals from the small diameter fibres is gated again and the discomfort fades.

Other examples of imbalance in transmission giving rise to abnormal sensations include the *hyperalgesia* that may be experienced for a short time when a severed nerve regrows, and *postherpetic neuralgia*.

STRATEGIES FOR CONTROLLING PAIN

Recent research into the transmission of pain has enhanced our understanding of therapies that are known to be effective in reducing acute or chronic pain. Acupuncture and transcutaneous electrical nerve stimulation (TENS) are both thought to stimulate the release of endogenous opioids. TENS appears to activate the large fibre sensory neurones. It is administered via a small portable apparatus with two electrodes which are attached to the skin close to the painful area. Once switched on, a small electrical current is released which has a physiological effect similar to rubbing the painful area. TENS can be administered in short bursts or may be used continuously throughout the day for people with persistent pain. Although it is not effective for everyone, it can provide substantial relief and has no side effects. It has the advantage that patients can apply it themselves to suit their own needs.

Personal control is known to be associated with success in coping with pain, and patients gain much benefit from learning ways in which they can help themselves to avoid or reduce pain. Strategies depend upon the type of painful condition but may include appropriate exercises, relaxation, imagery, distraction and, more recently, the introduction of patient controlled analgesia (PCA). PCA allows patients with acute pain or chronic malignant pain to deliver their own doses of analgesic whenever they feel they need it, up to a predetermined limit. Patients using PCA postoperatively have been shown to achieve better pain control while using less analgesia, although not all patients will feel confident enough to use it. Psychological control is now known to be intimately related to physiological pain control through the involvement of descending as well as ascending neuronal pathways. Hence, the manner in which care is delivered is now recognised to be as important as the treatment being administered.

The hyperalgesia occurring some while after a nerve has been severed is caused by the smaller fibres growing fastest and re-innervating their sensory receptors first (see Ch. 21). As a result, the area of the skin innervated by the regenerating fibres will, for a time, be hypersensitive to painful stimuli. In postherpetic neuralgia, a common sequel to shingles (*herpes zoster*), prolonged excruciating pain results from the damage caused to large diameter myelinated fibres by viruses.

INTERNAL STRUCTURES

Pain is felt when some but not all internal tissues are damaged or stressed. Tissues and organs are innervated by autonomic and somatic nerve fibres. The quality of the sensations felt and the stimuli that evoke pain differ according to the type of innervation.

Sources of pain

Pain arises if there is:

- local ischaemia (e.g. inadequate skeletal muscle or coronary blood flow)

- chemical damage (e.g. leakage of enzymes in the pancreas)
- spasm of smooth muscle (e.g. of the intestines)
- overdistension of a hollow organ (e.g. bladder)
- irritation of the peritoneum, pleurae or pericardium.

Some tissues, such as the alveoli of the lungs and the liver acini, are insensitive to injury whereas neighbouring structures, such as the bronchi, the capsule of the liver and the bile ducts, are very sensitive.

Innervation

The sensory nerve axons mediating pain run in:

- autonomic nerves
- somatic nerves.

Autonomic nerves

Many of the axons transmitting signals from nociceptors are unmyelinated C fibres running in the sympathetic nerves. They transmit signals from many internal organs and from tissues, such as skeletal muscle, and include axons innervating the walls of blood vessels.

Somatic nerves

The axons mediating the sensation of pain are small diameter fibres (Aδ and C). They innervate:

- the parietal peritoneum (see Ch. 6)
- the pleurae (see Ch. 7)
- the pericardium (see Ch. 5)
- the connective tissue associated with some organs (e.g. mesentery of the intestines – see Ch. 6; capsule of the kidney – see Ch. 8).

Qualities of sensation

The sensations experienced are broadly of two kinds:

- localised and acute
- diffuse and debilitating.

In some cases the pain is actually felt at a different site (*referred pain*) to that from which it originates.

> Pain in children is particularly difficult to assess. Many find it difficult to describe the location or intensity of the pain. Parents will know how their child usually responds when ill and they should be consulted when nurses assess and monitor a child's pain.

Localised and acute

The character of the painful sensations arising from excitation of axons in the somatic spinal nerves is similar in some respects to that of cutaneous pain. It can be sharp in character, and is usually localised to the injured area. For example the sharp stabbing pain of an inflamed appendix, that is felt in the lower right hand part of the abdomen, is a result of irritation of the overlying parietal peritoneum.

Diffuse and debilitating

The character of the pain felt when sensory axons in the autonomic nerves are stimulated is quite different. It is usually more diffuse, long-lasting and debilitating. For example, the burning pain of gastritis or pancreatitis is of this kind, as is the intense pain of intermittent claudication caused by muscle ischaemia. The cramping quality (*colic*) of abdominal pain such as 'stomachache' and period pains (*dysmenorrhoea*) is due to periodic contraction of the smooth muscle in the affected tissue.

> In the case of a *phantom limb* (see Ch. 23, p. 411), the pain apparently has no identifiable source. When a limb has been removed, the pain and sensory pathways above the level of amputation remain intact and may persist in transmitting signals that reflect the state of the limb prior to amputation. This type of pain can be very difficult to treat.

Referred pain

If pain originates from the viscera, it may be felt as coming from the surface of the body at a site distant from the injured organ. The axons running in the autonomic nerves innervating the internal organs are believed to converge in the spinal cord with somatic sensory nerve fibres coming from a particular part of the body surface (Fig. 32.3). This convergence arises from the fact that embryologically both parts (viscera and skin) developed from the same primitive tissue. As the brain does not have a 'picture' of the internal organs as it does of the body surface (see sensory homunculus, Chs 23 and 24), signals from internal organs are interpreted as having come from the body surface. They are said to be *referred* to that surface. Consequently, appendicitis gives rise to a cramping pain around the umbilicus, at a distance from the appendix, as well as the stabbing pain felt in the vicinity of the inflamed tissue itself. Other parts of the body to which pain may be referred as a result of injury to various thoracic and abdominal organs are shown in Figure 32.4. ④

Effective stimuli

The kinds of stimuli that are effective in evoking pain also differ according to whether autonomic or somatic nerves are involved. Surgeons can make an incision in the intestines (autonomic innervation) without pain being felt whereas a similar cut in the parietal peritoneum (somatic innervation), stimulating the mechanosensitive receptors of the Aδ system, is very painful. Conversely, local ischaemia of the intestines caused by muscular spasm or overdistension, that excites polymodal nociceptors and the C fibre system running in the sympathetic nerves, produces great discomfort.

④ Where would the referred pain of (a) cholecystitis, (b) angina, be felt? What other conditions may give rise to referred pain?

Figure 32.3
The basis of referred pain using the pain of appendicitis as an example: when the appendix is inflamed, some pain is experienced in the region of the umbilicus, although the source of the nerve impulses giving rise to the pain is actually the appendix.

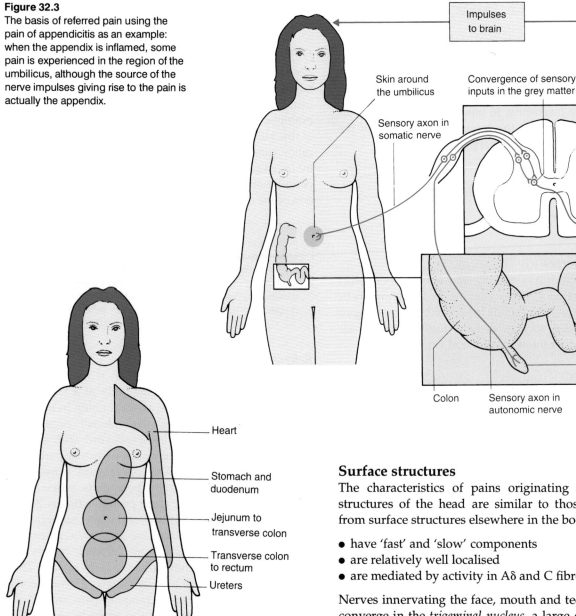

Figure 32.4
Parts of the body to which pain may be referred as a result of injury to various organs.

PAIN IN THE HEAD

The principles described so far apply also to the different kinds of pain felt in the head. Damage to surface structures (such as skin of the face and scalp, and mucous membranes of the mouth and teeth) is usually associated with sharp focused pain, whereas stimuli affecting internal structures (such as sinuses, muscles and intracranial structures) tend to produce more diffuse pain that is often referred to other parts of the head.

Surface structures

The characteristics of pains originating from surface structures of the head are similar to those originating from surface structures elsewhere in the body. They:

- have 'fast' and 'slow' components
- are relatively well localised
- are mediated by activity in Aδ and C fibres.

Nerves innervating the face, mouth and teeth (Fig. 32.5) converge in the *trigeminal nucleus,* a large group of cells within the brain stem and top two segments of the spinal cord. The organisation of cells within this nucleus resembles that in the dorsal horn of the spinal cord (see Ch. 20 and Fig. 32.2). Signals arising from nociceptors of the surface structures may be 'gated' in this nucleus by activity in large diameter fibres.

In *trigeminal neuralgia* there is hypersensitivity to stimuli delivered to discrete areas of the skin, giving rise to excruciating pain. One theory is that there is an imbalance of signals between the large and small diameter cutaneous afferents as a result of damage to the larger afferents.

Toothache

Teeth (see Ch. 29) are richly innervated by myelinated and unmyelinated sensory nerve fibres (including Aδ

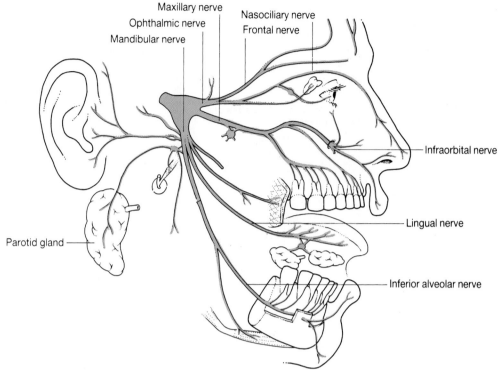

Figure 32.5
Nerves innervating the face, mouth and teeth. The trigeminal nerve (cranial nerve V) contains sensory fibres carrying impulses to the trigeminal nucleus in the brain stem. (Reproduced from Rogers 1992 (Fig. 25.8) by permission of the publishers.)

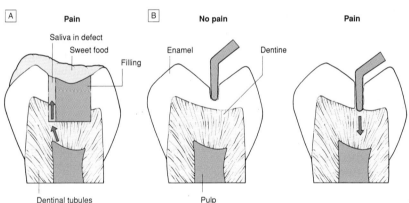

and C). Each tooth is innervated by over 2000 nerve fibres. Most fibres are located in the dentine and in the outer parts of the pulp. The nerves can be stimulated by a change in temperature or by factors which cause movement of fluid in the dentine tubules (Fig. 32.6). Sugary solutions for example draw fluid by osmosis out of the tubules, stimulating receptors. Likewise, if a dentist presses with a dental probe into a bit of exposed dentine, fluid is forced through the tubules. The effect can be excruciating.

Pain may also occur if the pulp is inflamed due to infection (*pulpitis*). In this case, vasodilation increases pressure within the pulp and excites the receptors. The tooth may throb with pain because of the arterial pulsations.

Internal structures
Irritation of internal structures gives rise to various

Figure 32.6
Ways of getting toothache:
A Sugar from the food seeps into a hole in the enamel and draws fluid by osmosis through the dentinal tubules exciting nerves in the pulp
B Pressure on the dentinal tubules (in this case from a dental probe) forces fluid through them.
(Adapted from Mumford J M 1984 Causes and alleviation of dental pain, Figures 5.3 & 5.4. In: Holden A V, Winlow W (eds) The neurobiology of pain, by permission of the author and the Manchester University Press.)

forms of headache. Some headaches are a result of damage and stresses to tissues of the brain whereas others originate from other structures of the head (Fig. 32.7).

Brain tissue
As in other parts of the body, it is the membranes wrapped around the brain (meninges; see Ch. 20), and

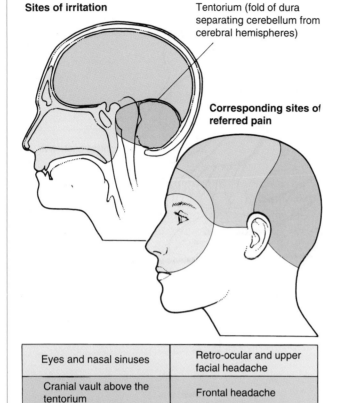

Sites of irritation

Tentorium (fold of dura separating cerebellum from cerebral hemispheres)

Corresponding sites of referred pain

Eyes and nasal sinuses	Retro-ocular and upper facial headache
Cranial vault above the tentorium	Frontal headache
Cranial vault below the tentorium	Occipital headache

Figure 32.7
Headaches: where they originate and where they are felt.

⑤
A patient complains of headache and asks for paracetamol. What precautionary assessment and observations would you make?

the walls of blood vessels, that are richly innervated with sensory nerve fibres, whereas brain tissue itself is largely insensitive to injury. Pain occurs therefore when there is:

● any tugging on the venous sinuses
● stretching of the dura
● damage to the blood vessels of the dura.

The pain of *migraine* headaches, for example, is associated with vascular changes. As a result of an abnormal burst of impulses, a short period of local vasoconstriction occurs followed by a prolonged period of vasodilation. The timing of the intense pain tends to coincide with the vasodilation.

Other structures
Headaches may also be caused by stimuli arising in:

● muscles of the neck and temple
● nose and sinuses
● eyes.

In each case the sensory signals are referred to various parts of the head.

Most people have experienced *tension headache* at

> *Migraine headache* is often preceded by visual disturbances and accompanied by nausea or vomiting. The headache is often unilateral and highly localised. Drug and biofeedback therapies may be effective in avoiding or ameliorating attacks. *Tension headaches* are common among people, such as typists, who adopt unnatural arm and head postures for long periods. A workplace assessment may assist many sufferers to resolve the problem.

some time. In an anxiety state there is a general increase in muscle tension throughout the body, including muscles in the neck and temple. Increased tension in these muscles probably causes local ischaemia which excites receptors in the blood vessels. The impulses arriving in the sensory cortex from the muscles are interpreted as coming from surface structures of the head with the result that pain is not felt in the tensed muscles but in the head in a vague and discomforting way. ⑤

REACTIONS TO PAIN

As well as creating the sensation of pain, activation of nociceptors elicits a variety of reflex responses. Many of these are protective, although they may add to our discomfort. Some contribute to the emotions we feel as a result of injury.

REFLEXES

The reflexes elicited by excitation of nociceptors may be divided into two groups:

● somatic   ● autonomic.

Somatic reflexes
The simple reflex response to the excitation of nociceptors in the skin is the *withdrawal reflex* (see Ch. 27), which pulls the injured part of the body away from the source of damage. Excitation of receptors inside the body also evokes characteristic responses. Irritation of the peritoneum for example reflexly causes contraction of abdominal muscles overlying the injured area. This is the so-called *guarding response*.

Impulses giving rise to referred pain can also evoke reflex contraction of the muscles that would ordinarily be stimulated by injury to the skin.

Secondary muscle pain
If the reflex contraction of muscles is prolonged, the muscle tissue itself may become ischaemic. As a result nociceptors within the muscle are excited leading to further pain. Consequently muscle pain (*myalgia*) may be added to the original pain and discomfort increases.

Autonomic reflexes

Activation of pain receptors also excites several autonomic reflexes producing effects that contribute to a general feeling of malaise and weakness. When you stub your toe on a piece of furniture or suffer from griping pain (*colic*) due to a stomach upset or painful periods you may well feel weak at the knees and light headed. This is a result of sympathetic and parasympthetic reflex effects on the circulatory system altering the distribution of blood flow between tissues and lowering blood pressure.

EMOTIONS

Our emotions are complex in that they consist of a blend of feelings, thoughts and behaviour (see Ch. 31). When

Acute pain is commonly associated with anxiety and fear, while chronic pain may be associated with anxiety, depression, anger or acceptance. Terminally ill patients may experience a wide range of emotions. Some patients express their emotions while others conceal them; a quiet patient may be suffering just as much as one who complains.

we feel pain we also tend to react emotionally with anxiety, alarm or fear. Each of these states is associated with activation of the sympathetic nervous system (see Ch. 19).

These emotional reactions to injury can be dissociated from somatic reflex responses and the specific sensation of pain. Damage to the frontal lobes of the brain, or the now infrequently performed operation of *frontal leucotomy* or *lobotomy* (see Ch. 31 and Fig. 32.8) can result in someone feeling less troubled by pain even though it is still sensed.

PAIN CONTROL

Pain can be controlled by interfering with the transmission of impulses in the nervous system, often with drugs but sometimes by other techniques such as TENS (see p. 534), or even surgery.⑥

Methods that block the transmission of impulses in general within the nervous system reduce our awareness of all sensations (*anaesthesia*), including pain, whereas those that act more selectively on pain pathways diminish pain sensation (*analgesia*) without having much effect on other sensations.

ANAESTHESIA

Drugs that produce anaesthesia do so either by blocking the transmission of action potentials along nerve axons (*local anaesthetics*) or by reducing activity within the reticular activating system (*general anaesthetics*).

Local anaesthetics

Local anaesthetics, such as lignocaine, work by blocking sodium channels in nerve axons thus preventing the transmission of action potentials along nerve fibres (see Ch. 21). When injected locally, all nerves in the area tend to be affected, including other sensory axons (e.g. for touch) as well as motoneurones. However, the smaller diameter fibres mediating pain are generally blocked more easily than the large diameter ones involved in touch and movement. Anaesthetic injected *epidurally* locally anaesthetises the spinal cord and blocks transmission of impulses through that section of the cord.

PAIN AS A PERCEIVED THREAT

The onset of pain is usually worrying or alarming. The way in which we interpret and experience pain is influenced not only by the extent of tissue damage but by our expectations of pain. These are based upon our culture, knowledge and past experiences, belief in our own ability (or that of others) to control the pain and the circumstances in which pain occurs. Uncertainty about what is causing the pain and what may happen as a consequence generates anxiety and fear, which intensify the pain. These emotions can be reduced or allayed by giving patients information about what is happening, explaining procedures, and helping patients to learn strategies for coping. This is particularly relevant where a painful process, such as childbirth or surgery, is anticipated or planned. However, many people with chronic pain experience fear and poor pain control because no one has taken the time to explain the likely causes or consequences of the pain nor the rationale for the treatments offered.

Lack of information is a significant cause of worry and even anger for some patients, and most benefit from information which enables them to feel more in control. On the other hand, some become more distressed when confronted with details and prefer not to know. Denial is a way of coping that should be respected but it should never be assumed that those who do not ask do not wish to know. Therefore it is important to assess each patient's needs on an individual basis. The nurse may then negotiate a plan of care with the patient to suit those needs.

The main difference between acute pain, chronic pain and pain in terminal illness is the degree of uncertainty or hopelessness (loss of control) associated with the condition. This affects doctors and nurses as well as patients, their relatives and friends. Nurses can help those with intractable benign or malignant pain by encouraging them to express their feelings and needs in an atmosphere of empathy and encouragement. Nurses working with terminally or chronically ill patients require support networks and stress management skills that enable them to deal with the demands made upon them. Only by confronting our own beliefs and feelings can we help others to face up positively to theirs.

⑥ How many ways can you identify that lay people use to control (or cope with) their own pain? Do people in different cultures deal with pain in different ways?

General anaesthetics

General anaesthetics, such as thiopentone, and halothane, have a nonspecific effect on all nerve membranes making them less excitable, but the part of the brain whose function is affected first is the reticular activating system (RAS) (see Chs 23 and 31). This system sensitises much of the cerebral cortex to incoming sensory signals, so that when activity in the RAS is reduced impulses arriving in the primary sensory areas of the cerebral cortex fail to excite other cortical areas. Consequently during surgery under anaesthesia no pain or other sensations are usually experienced even though the surgeon's knife is causing injuries that excite many receptors. Later on, as the effects of the anaesthetic wear off, the usual sensitivity of the cortical cells is restored, consciousness returns and pain is felt.

ANALGESIA

A variety of different strategies of specific pain relief are available, including:

- drug therapy
- physiologically based methods
- surgery.

> Nurses and doctors commonly underestimate patients' pain. They may still adhere rigidly to a 4-hourly drug administration regime, hold the mistaken belief that opioid analgesia for acute or malignant pain will cause addiction, or think that a quiet adult or child is pain free. These attitudes lead to undermedication and unnecessary suffering. Good communication between doctors, nurses and patients (or parents) and regular assessment should reduce the problem.

Drugs

Drugs having an analgesic effect generally work in one of two ways:

- peripherally   • centrally.

Peripherally acting analgesics work by altering the conditions around the nociceptors thereby reducing their level of excitation, whereas centrally acting analgesics interfere with the transmission of impulses at synapses within the brain and spinal cord.

Peripherally acting analgesics

These include the *non-steroidal anti-inflammatory drugs (NSAIDs)* (e.g. aspirin and paracetamol). NSAIDs inhibit an enzyme, *cyclo-oxygenase*, involved in the production of prostaglandins (see Ch. 10). Prostaglandins sensitise nociceptors to the effects of bradykinin, one of a number of substances, including prostaglandins, released by tissue injury. Bradykinin is a potent stimulant of the nociceptors.

Centrally acting drugs

Some drugs, such as the *opioids* (e.g. morphine), mimic the action of endogenous neurotransmitters, such as the endorphins, at 'pain gates' in the spinal cord and in the brain. Others, such as the *antidepressants* (e.g. amitriptyline), interfere with neurotransmission involving neurotransmitters like noradrenaline and act by influencing emotional reactions to pain as well as the sensation of pain itself.

Some pain however can be intractable and very large doses of drugs may be needed to bring any kind of relief. Unfortunately drugs have their side effects (see Ch. 19) as they act on similar membrane receptors throughout the body, many of which are not involved in pain transmission. In pain control, therefore, the benefits of intensive drug therapy have to be weighed against its complications. In terminal illness there is likely to be much to gain, but in an otherwise healthy person other methods of pain relief may be sought. ⑦

Physiologically based methods

The variety of methods of making use of the body's own system of pain control range from the psychology of positive thinking to the physical effects of TENS (see p. 534).

Psychology

It well known that even a glucose tablet can affect a patient's awareness of pain provided he believes it will do so. This is the *placebo effect*. It is thought that the positive encouragement given to the individual convincing him that he *will* feel better when he has swallowed the tablet activates his own physiological mechanisms of pain control (see p. 533 and Fig. 32.2). Endorphins are released and anxiety is reduced, both of which lessen the discomfort. Encouragement and distraction *do* help whereas a dispiriting environment makes matters worse. ⑧

> Pain clinics are available in most health districts to help patients with all types of intractable benign pain (including back pain). In addition to a range of medical and surgical treatment, some offer programmes designed to increase patients' knowledge of their condition, improve levels of exercise and activity, teach relaxation and reduce both dependence on drugs and reliance upon other people.

Surgery

If all other means of pain control have been tried and failed, surgical procedures may be adopted as a last resort (Fig. 32.8). For example in *dorsal rhizotomy* one or more dorsal roots are severed, preventing sensory signals from entering the spinal cord, without affecting outgoing motor impulses. The problem with these procedures is that unfortunately they rarely give perman-

⑦
What steps should nurses working with terminally ill patients take to ensure that pain is kept well under control?

⑧
What ethical problems are associated with giving a patient a placebo drug that is known to have no therapeutic value?

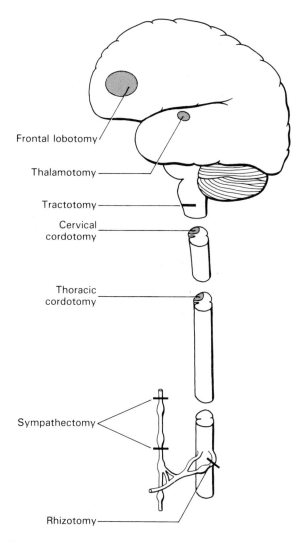

Frontal lobotomy

Thalamotomy

Tractotomy

Cervical cordotomy

Thoracic cordotomy

Sympathectomy

Rhizotomy

Figure 32.8
Sites of some of the surgical operations used in the relief of pain. (Reproduced from Allan 1988 (Fig. 21.7) by permission of the publishers.)

ent pain relief. Often the pain returns over a period of months, and may then be even worse than before.

However, chronic pain is not necessarily the end of the world. People can and do learn to live with it, or rather in spite of it.

PAIN ASSESSMENT

Assessment is a key aspect of the nursing management of pain. It enhances communication between patient, nurse and doctor. Regular assessment of acute or malignant pain provides a basis for the provision of optimum levels of analgesia. Pain intensity, together with the dosage, frequency and effectiveness of analgesia should be individually assessed and monitored to ensure that pain relief is adequate and sustained. Pain measures for all age groups are available, for example numerical scales (0 to 10), word scales (no pain to worst pain imaginable), descriptive scales (physical qualities like burning or aching, emotional qualities like frightful or punishing or evaluative qualities such as miserable or unbearable), colour intensity scales or happy/sad faces. It is necessary to select the method preferred by the particular patient group. Body charts may be used to locate the sources of pain. Assessment frequently reveals discrepancies between the assumptions of health professionals about the patient's pain and the patient's own reports. For patients with chronic pain, the use of a diary may help to identify triggering factors that could be avoided or pain relieving factors that could be better utilised. The patient's own observations provide valuable diagnostic information and help nurses and doctors to understand their feelings.

'Pain is what the patient says it is.' Affective words like 'cruel', 'fearful' or 'vicious' indicate that the patient cannot tolerate the pain. This may be due, in part, to a range of factors which need to be considered in an assessment of the 'whole person'. Unresolved past experiences, family problems, bereavement, employment difficulties, inability to meet commitments or lack of information may all influence someone's ability to tolerate physical pain. The nurse will not necessarily be able to resolve these issues but patients will benefit from knowing that they can, if they wish, share their feelings with someone who understands. The nurse and patient can then plan together a realistic and optimistic strategy for pain control in an atmosphere of mutual trust.

KEY POINTS

What you should now understand about pain:

- why some pain feels sharp whereas other forms feel more diffuse
- why some forms of pain are more bearable than others
- why pain is sometimes felt at a site in the body distant from the injury causing it
- what is meant by the 'pain gate' and how it is believed to work
- why pain is not always felt when tissues are damaged
- some of the reflex responses associated with pain and how they are produced
- some of the causes of common aches and pains such as toothache, headache and stomachache
- the differences between anaesthesia and analgesia
- the basis of some of the methods used in the management of pain, including drugs, TENS, counselling and surgery.

REFERENCES AND FURTHER READING

Allen D (ed) 1988 Nursing and the neurosciences. Churchill Livingstone, Edinburgh, p 308

British Medical Bulletin 1991 Pain: mechanisms and management. British Medical Bulletin 47(3) (Collection of specialist reviews)

Cailliet R 1992 Head and face pain syndromes. F A Davies, Philadelphia (One of a useful series of paperbacks on pain in different parts of the body. Other titles include: Low back pain; Shoulder pain; Neck and arm pain; Foot and ankle pain; Hand pain and impairment; Soft tissue pain and disability; Understanding your backache)

Campbell A 1987 Acupuncture: the modern scientific approach. Faber & Faber, London (Paperback)

de Dombal F T 1991 Diagnosis of acute abdominal pain, 2nd edn. Churchill Livingstone, Edinburgh (Lucidly written book providing useful insights into how the physician works out what the cause of pain may be)

Guyton A C 1986 Textbook of medical physiology. W B Saunders, Philadelphia, ch 50

Latham J 1991 Pain control, 2nd edn. Austen Cornish Publishers, London (Short paperback guide to the clinical and theoretical background to the nature of pain, written for health professionals)

Melzack R, Wall P D 1965 Pain mechanisms: a new theory. Science 150: 971–979

Melzack R, Wall P D 1991 The challenge of pain. Penguin, London (Authoritative paperback for the general reader describing and explaining all aspects of pain, and pain control in some detail. Includes short glossary of terms)

Mumford J M 1983 Toothache and related pain. Churchill Livingstone, Edinburgh

Mumford J M 1984 Causes and alleviation of dental pain. In: Holden A V, Winlow W (eds) The neurobiology of pain. Manchester University Press, Manchester, p 87, 89

Rang H P, Dale M M 1991 Pharmacology, 2nd edn. Churchill Livingstone, Edinburgh (Useful reference for drugs)

Rogers A W 1992 Textbook of anatomy. Churchill Livingstone, Edinburgh

Sofaer B 1992 Pain: a handbook for nurses. Chapman & Hall, London (An introduction to the physical, psychological, spiritual and cultural factors influencing pain, together with methods of pain assessment and appropriate therapies)

Wall P D, Melzack R 1989 Textbook of pain, 2nd edn. Churchill Livingstone, Edinburgh (Huge book. Useful for reference)

Chapter 33
LEARNING AND MEMORY

The physiological basis of learning is the formation and modification of synaptic contacts between neurones. The physiological basis of memory is the connections existing between neurones. While these persist we retain the ability to perform learned tasks and to 'relive' past experiences in our imagination.

Brain areas having a key role in learning and memory include the hippocampus of the limbic system, the cerebral cortex and the cerebellum. Neurones in these areas have the potential to form an amazing number of synaptic contacts. The greatest changes in synaptic contact occur in the early years of life but some flexibility of contact is retained throughout our adult years.

Motor skills, once learned, are largely automatic. We do them 'without thinking'. However, remembering things that we have heard or seen or felt depends upon forming an imprint of the experience in our minds and on bringing that imprint from our subconscious minds to consciousness. If we cannot remember, it may be because long-lasting contacts have not been formed, or because contacts have been lost, or because we cannot gain access to the relevant neural circuits.

DEFINITIONS

LEARNING

When we *learn*, changes are occurring in the connections between neurones in the nervous system. Some of these changes, such as those in infancy and childhood involved in learning to sit, stand and walk, are genetically pre-programmed. Others, such as learning to speak Japanese, or how to play the clarinet, depend on our specific experiences as individuals. Experience affects the chemistry of our brains through specific changes occurring at well-used and at under-used synapses as well as through the excitatory and inhibitory effects associated with different states of arousal and emotion (see Ch. 31).

Thus, we learn as we grow and as our nervous systems develop in utero, through infancy and in childhood (see Ch. 35), and we go on learning as we continue to be exposed to new stimuli, experiences and circumstances throughout our lives. The potential for learning is greatest while our nervous systems are still developing but considerable scope still exists after the nervous system has reached developmental maturity. ①

MEMORY

If learning is defined as the process of forming or modifying contacts between neurones, memory can be defined as the changes in synaptic contact that outlast the period of learning. The new pattern of synaptic contact may consist of links involving our motor systems

①
When does the nervous system reach developmental maturity?

allowing us to exercise a new skill, such as riding a bicycle, or they may be links between sensory experiences enabling us to remember the word for an object, or recall a past event, such as what happened last Thursday.

Skills

It is said that once you have learned to ride a bicycle you never forget. After a long spell of not riding, your first attempts may be a little inexpert but you instinctively remember what to do. You don't have to think about it – you just ride. Motor memories (skills) differ from thought memories in that we can make use of them without conscious thought. A skilled pianist can play a complex piece of music 'from memory' without actually having to *think* about how to play. ②

Thoughts

Memory of past experiences, however, can be both conscious as well as unconscious. We carry in our minds a complex record of all that has happened to us in our lives, though for most of the time we are unaware of it. When fragments of this record are brought to consciousness we actually remember. When we cannot bring the record to consciousness, the memory is still there in the connections between neurones, but our recollection of it is impaired.

Having a 'poor' memory

In everyday conversation we talk of having a poor memory, meaning that we have forgotten the name of a new friend or that we find difficulty in remembering what we have done recently or read for example (how much can you remember now of the chapter you read before this one?). Some people, through injury or disease, experience loss of memory (*amnesia*). Although in conversation we seem to be talking about the same thing, namely a difficulty with memory, the causes of that problem vary. Memory may be poor because:

- synaptic contacts do not form very easily (really a difficulty in learning)
- contacts between cells have not been maintained (actual loss of memories)
- recall of the stored memory is impaired (memory intact but not brought to consciousness).

To understand how learning takes place and memories are formed we need to begin by looking first at the factors that influence the formation of synaptic contacts, and how, once such contacts are formed, they are maintained.

② *What nursing skills can you think of that, once learnt, might be performed without thinking?*

③ *How are impulses transmitted through the neurones?*

DEVELOPMENT AND MAINTENANCE OF CONTACTS BETWEEN NEURONES

The number of nerve cells in the brain reaches a maximum early in life. After this no *new* nerve cells are formed. However, like all nucleated cells, neurones have the ability to grow and develop (see Chs 2 and 21). Provided the cell body of a neurone is intact there can be:

- growth of axons and dendrites
- formation of new synapses between neurones
- modification of existing synapses.

All these processes are influenced by the chemical environment of the cells as well as by the internal activity of the cells themselves. Both vary as impulses are transmitted through the neurones, and as neurotransmitters and other agents are released and recycled. By these means new links can be forged between neurones, and the effectiveness of existing synapses can be altered. This ongoing flexibility in connections between neurones is termed *plasticity*. It is greatest in the early years of life but is retained in adulthood. In contrast to many other cells, however, mature nerve cells cannot reproduce. When nerve cell bodies are injured and die they cannot be replaced. ③

PLASTICITY

Developmental

The total number of synapses in the brain reaches a peak around the age of 5 years and then decreases to a plateau in the adult years (Fig. 33.1). The number of

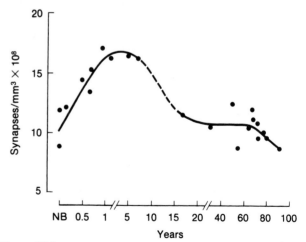

Figure 33.1
Number of synapses per mm³ at different ages in part of the cortex of the frontal lobe of the cerebral hemispheres. (Reproduced from Huttenlocher P R 1979 Synaptic density in human frontal cortex: developmental changes and effects of ageing, Figure 3, by permission of the author and Elsevier Science Publishers.)

cells and synapses in the brain is affected by our experience. If our senses receive plenty of stimulation in early life many synaptic contacts are established and maintained. But if relevant experiences are lacking, synapses are less profuse. For example, early visual deprivation leads to permanent visual disability. In humans the key period for visual development lasts up to 5 to 10 years of age.

During development, synapses that are used are strengthened and retained, whereas those that are inactive deteriorate and are eventually lost. In this way each of us develops a unique pattern of contacts shaped by our unique experience as individuals. No two brains can be exactly alike because no two lives are ever exactly the same.

EARLY DEVELOPMENT

All aspects of child development have been studied to a greater or lesser degree; some activities lend themselves more readily to investigation than others. The sequence of developmental steps is the same for all infants because it depends on the maturation of motor and visual skills, and the ability to coordinate those skills. Those professionals whose job it is to assess the development of infants use a series of milestones (or stepping stones), which are more detailed than when the infant smiles, sits or crawls, as criteria for normal progress (see Ch. 35). Consider, for example, the ability to reach for and grasp an object. A month-old baby will stare fixedly at an interesting object – grasping with the eyes! By about 2 months the baby will start swiping at objects with a closed fist. By 4 months the baby will be using an open hand and judging the distance by glancing from hand to object. By 5 months the object is reached for and grasped accurately.

It has been found that in families where the infant is given frequent stimulation and encouraged to reach for interesting objects, the developmental milestones for reaching and grasping will be arrived at earlier than the normal age. When a baby is fed, changed and returned to his cot without time being given for 'play' the milestones will be achieved at the normal age. Frequent, appropriate stimulation throughout childhood encourages the formation and maintenance of synaptic contacts and the child tends to progress more rapidly. Health visitors advise mothers and other carers on providing appropriate stimulation during the early years. Not all mothers find it easy to play with babies and young children and so need extra help.

In adulthood

Plasticity still exists in the adult brain but to a lesser extent. We continue to be able to learn new things, though not with the same facility as in our younger years.

If there is injury to the brain, for example through a cerebral haemorrhage, it is possible for nearby uninjured neurones to sprout and form new contacts replacing ones that have been lost (*reactive synaptogenesis*). The extent to which this occurs depends on age, the extent to which the neurones are used, and the degree of injury.

In old age, the number of cells and synapses may decrease. In senility there is a big reduction in the number of cells and synaptic contacts in several parts of the brain including the cerebral cortex and the hippocampus.

THE CHEMISTRY OF SYNAPTIC CONTACT

Making contact

Nerve cells are stimulated to grow by *trophic factors* that promote growth and guide its direction (see Ch. 21). These factors may be chemicals released from adjacent nerve cells or by glial cells nearby. The trophic factors attract the growing nerve endings. Sometimes cells, such as astrocytes in the brain, act as a framework guiding the direction in which growth occurs (see Ch. 20). ④

One of the fascinating things revealed in recent years by sophisticated filming techniques is the dynamic nature of these events. Speeded up film of nerve cells in culture reveals just how active cells really are and how much exploratory activity goes on. Dendrites are seen to move around, extend and retract, contacting other cells and surfaces in the vicinity as they do so (see Ch. 21). If the chemistry is right when contact is made, a closer association is formed, and synapses develop; if it is not, the dendrite retracts and tests other sites.

The chemistry that matters includes the chemistry of recognition between molecules on the membranes of the cells in contact as well as the chemistry of the local environment. Influential substances include neurotransmitters such as noradrenaline, acetylcholine, dopamine and serotonin. Noradrenaline, for example, fosters the development of synapses.

Some substances are influential during a specific period of development. For example, the hormone thyroxine is necessary for normal brain development in the first few years of life. If this hormone is deficient at that time, profound mental retardation results that cannot be reversed by giving thyroxine later on (*cretinism*).

Most babies in the UK are screened for thyroxine deficiency at the same time as screening for phenylketonuria is carried out – 5 to 7 days after birth. Approximately 1 in 3000 babies is unable to produce thyroxine, sometimes due to the absence or underdevelopment of the thyroid gland. Replacement therapy is commenced immediately, thus preventing the development of cretinism.

Keeping contact

Once contact has been established the maintenance of the synapse depends on its usage. Inactivity and activity produce different local chemical states that, in turn, affect cell function. Modifications in the junction can occur both pre- and postsynaptically.

The neurotransmitter released by the presynaptic

④
What are the glial cells and where are they found?

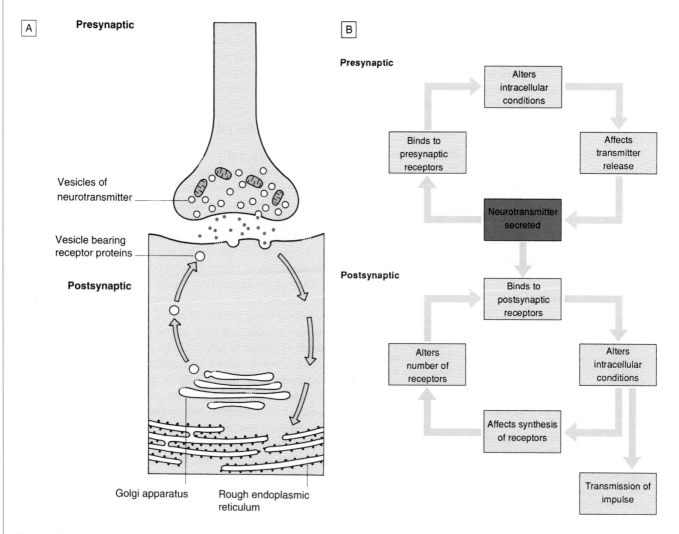

Figure 33.2
Regulatory effects of neurotransmitters at pre- and postsynaptic components of a synapse.

terminal is picked up by receptors on the presynaptic membrane as well as binding to receptors on the postsynaptic membrane (Fig. 33.2). These presynaptic receptors regulate the functioning of the nerve ending, and the amount of transmitter released.

At the postsynaptic membrane, long-term changes in the number of receptors inserted into the membrane affect the responsiveness of the cell to the transmitter released by the presynaptic ending. The sensitivity of the receptors is also influenced by regulatory proteins in the membrane adjacent to the receptors, which are themselves affected by local conditions.

Some of the changes occurring at synapses, such as the changes in concentrations of intracellular ions and second messengers (see Chs 2 and 21), will be short-lived. But those that involve restructuring of the membranes and organelles of the synapse, through the control of protein synthesis, will result in long-lasting changes.

ASSOCIATIVE LEARNING

INSTINCT AND INTELLECT

The links developing between neurones during growth and development, as a result of genetic pre-programming, create instinctive patterns of behaviour. You touch something hot and instinctively pull your hand away, not because you have learned by experience to do so, but because of the pattern of neural connections between nociceptors and muscles (see Ch. 27) determined by your genes. What we learn with experience is to recognise hot objects before we touch them. We can then intelligently choose either not to pick them up or, alternatively, aim to do so with great care.

CONDITIONING

It was shown by the Russian scientist Pavlov that responses to certain stimuli could be *conditioned*. If a bell

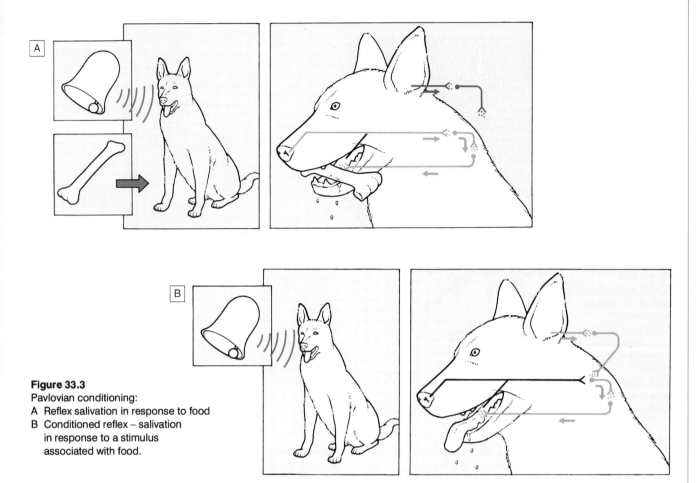

Figure 33.3
Pavlovian conditioning:
A Reflex salivation in response to food
B Conditioned reflex – salivation
in response to a stimulus
associated with food.

was regularly sounded at the same time that food was presented to one of his dogs, after a while the dog would salivate in anticipation of the arrival of food whenever the bell was rung, even though there was not a whiff or sight of food anywhere.

The way in which this association of sensory signals and responses may develop is shown in Figure 33.3. Simultaneous activity in salivatory and auditory pathways is believed to create the right chemical conditions for the development of synaptic contacts forging links between the auditory system and the salivary glands. This may occur by the strengthening of existing contacts or by the establishment and growth of new ones.

The association created externally by ringing the bell at the same time as presenting food is thus transformed into actual physical connections made between the nerve fibres. Once this has happened our brains have a *long-term memory* of that association recorded in the connections developed between the neurones. If association is not renewed from time to time the connections may weaken and eventually be lost.

KEY BRAIN AREAS

The parts of the brain that are believed to have a key role in learning (cerebral cortex, hippocampus and cerebellar cortex) contain cells that have two distinctive features:

- huge dendritic trees
- dendritic spines.

The pyramidal cells of the cerebral cortex and hippocampus and the Purkinje cells of the cerebellar cortex all possess huge dendritic trees (Fig. 33.4A). The dendrites possess tiny spurs, not commonly seen on other nerve cells. Synaptic contacts are made with these spurs (Fig. 33.4B). The number of dendritic spines and synapses is affected by experience. For example, visual deprivation in the early years of life decreases the numbers of spines formed on cells of the visual cortex.

DEVELOPING SKILLS AND KNOWLEDGE

Although the principles of associative learning are the same regardless of the nature of what is being learned, there are some differences between the learning of motor skills and the development of intelligence.

Motor skills
The learning of new motor skills is an important function of the cerebellum. This part of the brain has a major role in enabling us to coordinate and refine our

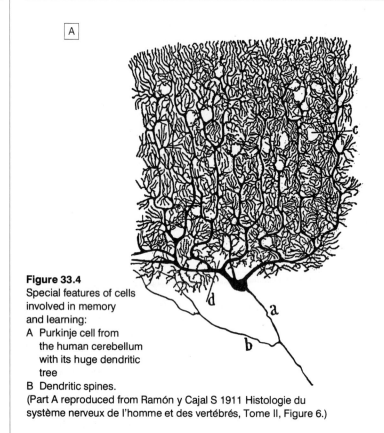

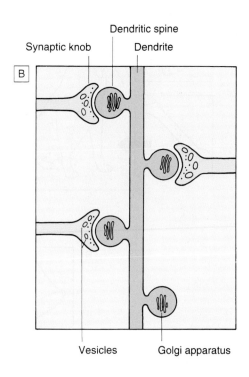

Figure 33.4
Special features of cells involved in memory and learning:
A Purkinje cell from the human cerebellum with its huge dendritic tree
B Dendritic spines.
(Part A reproduced from Ramón y Cajal S 1911 Histologie du système nerveux de l'homme et des vertébrés, Tome II, Figure 6.)

movements (see Chs 27–29). It also has extensive connections with many other parts of the brain that are concerned with movement, and receives information from proprioceptors (see Ch. 24) about how the movement is actually being performed. This feedback is important in learning. If the action is successful, associations are strengthened.

The learning of a new motor skill has been divided into three phases:

- cognitive
- associative
- automatic.

Cognitive phase

In the cognitive phase you concentrate on how to perform the task in hand. This involves knowing the actions needed, the sequence in which they should occur and how quickly they should be performed. In your mind you consciously and deliberately link together all the elements of the task.

Associative phase

In the associative phase these links are strengthened. You then concentrate not so much on *how* to perform the task, but on refining and improving it, so that it is performed with increasing ease and minimum effort. It is thought that the brain builds up a pattern of associations between the command signals and their outcome, rather in the way that you may plot a graph

between two variables (Fig. 33.5). In this way we do not have to learn every possible movement but instead we build up a set of rules (*schema*) that can be used to determine the command needed for a 'new' task of a similar kind. It may be for this reason that the development of motor skills is often best achieved by practicing different but related movements, rather than by repeating exactly the same movement over and over again.

Learner nurses sometimes find difficulty in refining and improving specific movements. Sometimes, as in pouring a dose of medicine from a bottle to a measure, the basic movements are already learned. The schema has been formed by actions such as pouring a precise amount of milk into a cup or pouring beer carefully into a glass so as to avoid the development of too much froth. Other movements, such as the controlled wrist action required to shake down the mercury in a clinical thermometer, do not always have a comparable set of rules or schema. Hammer and peg toys help children develop the wrist movement needed; similar activities in adults are chopping vegetables, hammering tacks and playing darts. But not everyone has acquired these skills, which may account for the difficulty experienced by some learner nurses in shaking down the mercury in a thermometer.

Automatic phase

Ultimately the action being learned becomes automatic. It can be performed without conscious control. A skilled pianist for example can play a piece of music without

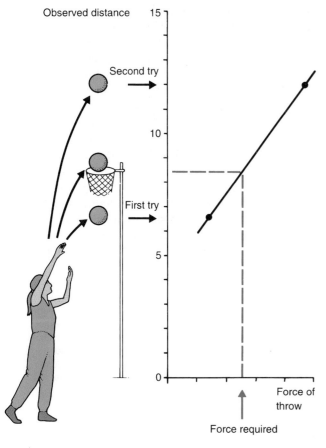

Figure 33.5
Development of rules in our minds (schema) linking actions with outcomes.

TEACHING MOTOR SKILLS

The ability to analyse skills when teaching junior colleagues and patients is very important; miss a crucial point in the cognitive phase of learning and the teaching will probably fail. Most of us, especially now that various sports' shoes are so popular, gain much experience in tying bows. Can you remember when you couldn't tie a bow? The actions have been rehearsed (*associative phase*) so often that they are memorised and recalled when needed without conscious thought – it is possible to chat about last night's party while tying your trainer laces (*automatic phase*).

Try writing down step-by-step instructions for tying a bow or doing up a button; this is the *cognitive phase* of the task. Then ask a friend to follow your instructions; she must try not to use her previous knowledge. When she has tried this, ask her whether your instructions were adequate. Finding out how to break down a complex procedure into a series of steps that can be followed successfully by another person is the first step in learning to teach motor skills.

It may be necessary to teach a mentally handicapped child to pull up her pants. She may not be able to understand verbal instructions and just tugs at her pants ineffectually. Then you think, 'Why is it so easy for me?' You analyse your own actions only to be told by the child's mother, 'I don't do it that way'. With physical guidance, the child will reach the associative phase – possibly forming her own rules, which might be different from both yours and her mother's.

Many nursing skills also become internalised, and careful analysis is required prior to teaching. Some skills, for the sake of safety, are bound by strict rules (administration of drugs) and principles (asepsis). These major skills have been partially analysed, but other commonplace actions, such as pouring medicine into a measure or handling forceps skilfully, need further analysis by the teachers so that they may be well taught.

---

looking at the scripted music or thinking about when, where and how to move his fingers. Most of our day-to-day activity consists of automatic programmes triggered by the routine events of the day. ⑤

Skills do not develop overnight. They take time. In the early stages recognisable gains in skill occur quite quickly. But refinement of movement and the establishment of those patterns takes longer. It is said that complex patterns of behaviour, such as personal habits, take about 2 years to become properly established.

Learned motor activities, once established, are not easily forgotten. If practice does not continue, performance may deteriorate but the memory remains. Why learned movements should be retained so well is not clear. It may be that some basic components of the activity are common to other tasks so that 'practice' continues though in a different guise. It may also be that movements learned subsequently interfere less with what has already been learned than is the case for 'thinking' memory.

Knowledge

At its simplest, knowledge is the linking together of inputs from several senses (see Ch. 30). Learning the meaning of words, for example, involves associating either the sound of a word or its appearance in print with the characteristics of the thing that the word describes. In most people these linguistic associations develop chiefly in the parieto-occipital and temporal areas of the left hemisphere of the cerebral cortex, whereas visuospatial associations, such as the shape and form of objects, form in the right hemisphere (see Ch. 30).

Once links have been established, the presentation of one stimulus, such as the spoken word, will be sufficient to call up the associated sensory experiences in our imagination. So having said the word 'apple', in the mind's eye we imagine an apple: we recall something of its appearance, its flavour, its smell and how it feels, even though the relevant sensory receptors are not activated. We *know* what an apple is like because the memories of its features are fixed in our minds in the pattern of synaptic connections between neurones. This is an example of *semantic* memory. Another form of memory is termed *episodic* and relates to the memory of more complex experiences such as events.

⑤
Apply these phases to your learning of a nursing skill – what procedures are you now performing automatically?

THAT IS NOT AN ORANGE

Very few adults, if any, can remember learning to associate the word 'apple' with the roundish, edible, green/red object found on trees, in shops and at home in the fruit bowl. Small children often spend much time presenting an apple, for example, to an adult and saying 'orange' or 'ball'. There may be several reasons for this: it may be a game; the child – knowing that an apple is neither an orange nor a ball – may want to learn a new word; but more importantly he may be confused by previous responses. Confusion arises like this:

   Child: 'Orange?' (offering an apple).
   Adult: 'No, it's not an orange. It's an apple.'

This method of attempted teaching reinforces the child's initial idea that the object is an orange. He hears 'orange' and does not recognise or understand the negative, so the new word 'apple' does not become associated with the object. This is particularly important when teaching mentally handicapped children. The correct response is to point to the apple and say clearly 'apple', repeating the word as necessary. It may be possible also to demonstrate its sensory aspects of smell, taste, texture and shape. Eventually the memory links will be established.

When teaching patients and colleagues, it is useful to refer always to the positive aspects of the concept to be learned. For example, anxious patients and the elderly, in particular, may find difficulty in remembering how to use an aerosol inhaler if only an explanation is given. If the patient is given supervised 'hands-on' experience, then the links are likely to be stronger and longer lasting. This is because the sensory attributes of the inhaler (shape, feel, movement of parts) become fixed in the pattern of synaptic connections between neurones in the patient's brain. If the manufacturer decides to change the name of a specific inhaler, the patient will still be able to use it. Similarly, if the patient becomes unable to remember the name of the inhaler, or even recognise it, then sensory information gained from handling it will convey its use.

Intellectual learning, unlike motor learning, is known to be particularly sensitive to:

- our level of arousal
- our degree of motivation.

Arousal

Moderate levels of arousal are necessary for optimum learning. If someone is either overexcited or drowsy, learning is not as good. The level of activity in the reticular activating system (RAS) (see Chs 23 and 31) creates background conditions that facilitate or depress learning. Raised levels of activity in the reticular formation are associated with the release of noradrenaline which is known to have a widespread influence on neurones in the brain (see Ch. 31). It raises the level of excitability and facilitates learning.

Motivation

Things that are well remembered are usually those that arouse our emotions, whether pleasantly or unpleasantly.

Activity in the limbic system, part of the brain involved in the elaboration of emotion (see Ch. 31), is involved in learning. Hippocampal neurones are believed to control the ease with which synaptic contacts are formed in other parts of the brain. Also, the limbic system is known to be involved in determining our choice of behaviour. Stimulation of certain areas of the limbic system has been shown to evoke feelings of either pleasure or displeasure, and behaviour that either seeks to repeat the experience or to avoid it at all costs. As synaptic changes are consolidated by repetition, any system encouraging the repetition of specific actions will play a significant role in learning. As the psychologist Thorndike stated from his studies in animals, 'of several responses made to the same situation, those which are accompanied or closely followed by satisfaction (*re-inforcement*) will be more likely to recur'.

Thorndike's findings from his animal studies usually work equally well with human beings. When teaching, whether children, learner nurses, junior colleagues or patients, positive reinforcement is more likely to achieve good results. Constant criticism and 'putting down' is liable to cause despondency and lack of interest in all but the strongest personalities.

REMEMBERING AND FORGETTING

The development of synaptic contacts can explain how associations between sensory signals become literally fixed in our minds as memories, but it does not readily explain how we remember things from moment to moment, such as the number that we have just found in the telephone book, the name of someone to whom we have just been introduced, or what we have just read. This *short-term memory* (or *working memory*) differs from long-term memory. Each is the result of different processes and can be disrupted in different ways.

We are unconscious of most of what we have learned. The memories are there in the patterns of synaptic contact that develop over our lives, but we are not conscious of all that is stored in our minds. Most of what we know intellectually is kept below the level of consciousness until such times when it is recalled or 'brought to mind'.

SHORT-TERM MEMORY

It is believed that sensory information is, for a short while, passed around neuronal circuits repetitively so that the experience lingers in our minds (Fig. 33.6). Neuronal circuits of this kind are termed *reverberating*

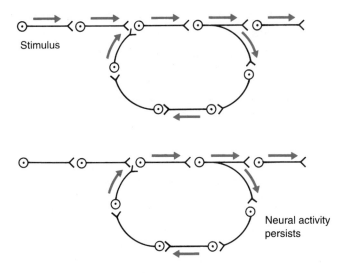

Figure 33.6
A reverberating circuit of neurones and how it works.

circuits. It may be that if neural activity persists for long enough, under the right circumstances it is then converted into physical changes in synaptic contacts so that the memory becomes long term.

> When listening to a lecture, a great deal of information is received in a relatively short space of time. It is possible that only a proportion (often small!) of the lecture content produces sufficiently sustained neural activity for the concepts to enter long-term memory. The making of notes to aid the memory and for later study will assist the processing of important information, which will be retained for future recall.

If short-term memory processes are disrupted acutely, long-term memories are not formed. For example, an individual who is knocked out by a blow to the head may not remember the events around the time of the injury at all well. The same kind of memory loss is experienced by those who are given ECT (electro-convulsive therapy). Events immediately preceding the shock treatment are not remembered. This is termed *retrograde amnesia*. However, the remembrance of earlier events is unaffected as is the formation of new memories subsequently.

LONG-TERM MEMORY

The ability to form new long-term memories is affected if there is damage to parts of the temporal cerebral cortex and the limbic system, especially the hippocampus. Damage to the temporal cerebral cortex is associated with loss of semantic memory whereas injury to the hippocampus gives rise to loss of episodic memory. ⑥

When there is damage to the hippocampus, new information is retained only for a very short space of time before it is lost completely. Thus no new long-term memories of events are formed (*anterograde amnesia*). The person affected remains locked in the past and has great difficulty learning and remembering new experiences. Interestingly, some tasks can be learned but the individual cannot *remember* having learned them.

> **MEMORY LOSS AND THE ELDERLY PERSON**
>
> The elderly person who suffers from memory loss usually becomes very irritating to all but the very placid and patient. The type of memory loss varies from individual to individual. It is not like just having a poor memory where retrieval is possible given the right cues. The total blankness and the knowledge that retrieval is impossible, when faced frequently with something that one knows one must have done, is quite unnerving and has to be experienced to be understood fully.
>
> Many elderly people are able to give detailed descriptions of events which occurred decades earlier, but cannot remember what they were told 5 minutes ago. This is why some elderly people manage better in their own homes, with help, than in, say, a home for the elderly. Once moved from the environment that is familiar, the details of which are stored in long-term memory and can still be retrieved, it is difficult either for the features of the new accommodation to be processed and stored or for the information to be retrieved. The elderly person may well wander about trying to find familiar surroundings and the whereabouts of certain people. The label 'confused and disoriented' is often applied. Attempts to sedate the person, frequently make matters worse whereas appropriate stimulation and individual attention may help to relieve the anxiety. For some there is no alternative to 'living in the past'.

RETRIEVING INFORMATION

Remembering involves retrieving information that has been stored and bringing it to consciousness. This process is distinct from those that form memories in the first place. All are needed for us to have a 'good memory' (Fig. 33.7).

Figure 33.7
Learning and remembering.

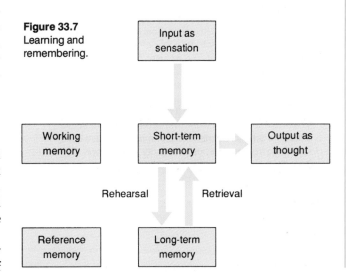

⑥
What can you do to aid development of long-term memory?

We will all have had the experience of trying desperately hard to remember something important and then finding that when we turn to something else, suddenly the answer comes 'out of the blue'. Our conscious minds are oblivious to the 'computer search' in progress until the answer is found. The retrieval of information is assisted by association. It is often the case that a related though different fact will act as the trigger. It helps the search to take place in the relevant 'files' in our minds.

The recall of information is influenced by brain chemistry. The concentration of acetylcholine appears to be of especial significance but noradrenaline and adrenaline also affect the process. There is evidence to suggest that the memory loss associated with ageing and senility is caused by a deficiency of acetylcholine within the hippocampus. This part of the limbic system seems to be involved both in the establishment of long-term memories and in their retrieval into consciousness.

THE UNCONSCIOUS

More goes on in our minds below the level of conscious awareness than we ever imagine. We can absorb information subconsciously, process it, store it and make use of it often all without conscious thought.

This buried information influences and directs our behaviour without our knowing. For example some people suffer from unaccountable *phobias* in which a particular object, circumstance or set of events produces immediate fear and panic. Some may feel afraid of going out; others may have a fear of lifts; others still may feel panicky at the sight of a feather. These reactions may be inexplicable to the person concerned. It may be that inappropriate associations have been formed early in development. If these reactions seriously hamper a person's life then attempts may be made to decondition inappropriate responses and build more helpful associations. ⑦

⑦
What are the words used to describe 'fear of going out' and 'fear of being shut in'?

Community nurses may be the first to recognise the so-called 'school phobia' in a child. This is not usually a fear of school; it is more likely to be a fear of being separated from the security of a parent. The excuses for non-attendance at school are rewarded by the parent – the child is allowed to stay at home and receives extra attention – and are therefore likely to persist. If early separation phobia is not recognised and treated then it may well return in adulthood as a result of stress at work. The separation phobia then manifests itself as agoraphobia. The sufferer fears being separated from the source of security and support – often the wife or husband.

KEY POINTS

What you should now know and understand about learning and memory:

- parts of the brain having a key role in memory and learning, and their distinctive features
- what is happening to neurones in childhood and in adulthood when we are learning
- some of the factors that promote or hinder learning and how they may act
- reasons why someone may have a poor memory
- types of memory loss and how they may be caused.

REFERENCES AND FURTHER READING

Agras W S 1985 Panic: facing fears, phobias and anxiety. W H Freeman, Oxford
(Discusses basis of disorders and their treatments; uses case histories and gives advice to friends and families)
Boakes R A 1987 Food, physiology and learned behaviour. John Wiley & Sons, Chichester
(Specialist reviews of the ways in which people acquire food preferences and eating habits)
Brown M C, Hopkins W G, Keynes R J 1991 Essentials of neural development. Cambridge University Press, Cambridge
(Excellent resource for background to nerve cell growth, contact, plasticity, injury, basis of learning etc.)
Cottam P, Sutton A 1985 Conductive education: a system for overcoming motor disorder. Croom Helm, Beckenham
(First comprehensive overview in English of this novel system of education developed in Hungary)
Davey G 1987 Cognitive processes and Pavlovian conditioning in humans. John Wiley, Chichester.
(Collection of specialist reviews)
Freeman Somers M 1991 Spinal cord injury. Appleton & Lange, East Norwalk, Connecticut
(Book written for physiotherapists involved in rehabilitation following spinal cord injury. Basic understanding of spinal cord injuries)
Hoyenga K B, Hoyenga K T 1988 Psychobiology: the neurone and behaviour. Brooks/Cole Publishing Company, Pacific Grove, California
(Advanced well-referenced student text)
Huttenlocher P R 1979 Synaptic density in human frontal cortex: developmental changes and effects of ageing. Brain Research 163: 195–205
Kidd G, Lawes N, Musa I 1992 Understanding neuromuscular plasticity: a basis for clinical rehabilitation. Edward Arnold, London
(Engaging book written for therapists, teachers of the handicapped and others. Explains scientific basis of rehabilitation)
Ramón y Cajal S 1911 Histologie du système nerveux de l'homme et des vertébrés, Tome II. A Maloine, Paris (Reprinted CSIC, Madrid, 1972)
(Classic book by a great histologist)
Schmidt R 1982 The schema concept. In: Kelso J A S (ed) Human motor behaviour: an introduction. Erlbaum, Hillsdale, New Jersey, p 219–235
Schmidt R 1989 Motor control and learning – a behavioural emphasis. Human Kinetics Publishers, Champaign, Illinois
(Student text providing more information about movement and learning)
Winlow W, McCrohan C R (eds) 1987 Growth and plasticity of neural connections. Manchester University Press, Manchester
(Collection of specialist reviews by researchers)

Section 4
VARIATIONS IN FORM AND FUNCTION

Section Contents

We begin life as a single cell and grow to form a body consisting of millions of cells. As we grow to maturity, age and then die, systems change, and form and function alter.

The chapters in this part describe and explain:

- how human life begins and ends
- the structure of the male and female reproductive systems and the process of reproduction
- how pregnancy affects a woman's body
- the main changes in form and function occurring throughout life.

Chapter 34
SEX, REPRODUCTION AND PREGNANCY

Although a few people began their lives in the clinical environment of a test tube, the overwhelming majority of us were conceived through the sexual union of a man and a woman. The male and female reproductive organs have the functions of:

- producing the germinal cells (*ova* and *sperm*) from which a new individual is created
- providing a means for sperm and ova to meet through sexual union (*coitus*)
- creating the right environment for the development of ova and sperm, and later for the fertilised cell as it grows into a baby.

If conception occurs, and a woman becomes pregnant, profound changes occur throughout her body. These changes are designed to enable her to nourish and maintain the growing fetus whilst maintaining her own inner equilibrium (homeostasis). A vital role is played by the placenta, a structure which develops from the fertilised cell. When the baby is born (*parturition*) the mother's organs and tissues revert to the non-pregnant state over a period of several weeks (the *puerperium*), but milk production (*lactation*) continues for many months for the nourishment of the new-born child.

REPRODUCTIVE ORGANS AND TISSUES

MALE

The male reproductive organs and their situation in the adult are shown in Figure 34.1. The main structures are:

- the testes (housed within the scrotum)
- the penis
- several glands.

Sperm cells and exocrine secretions produced by the testes flow through tubules in the *epididymis*, along the

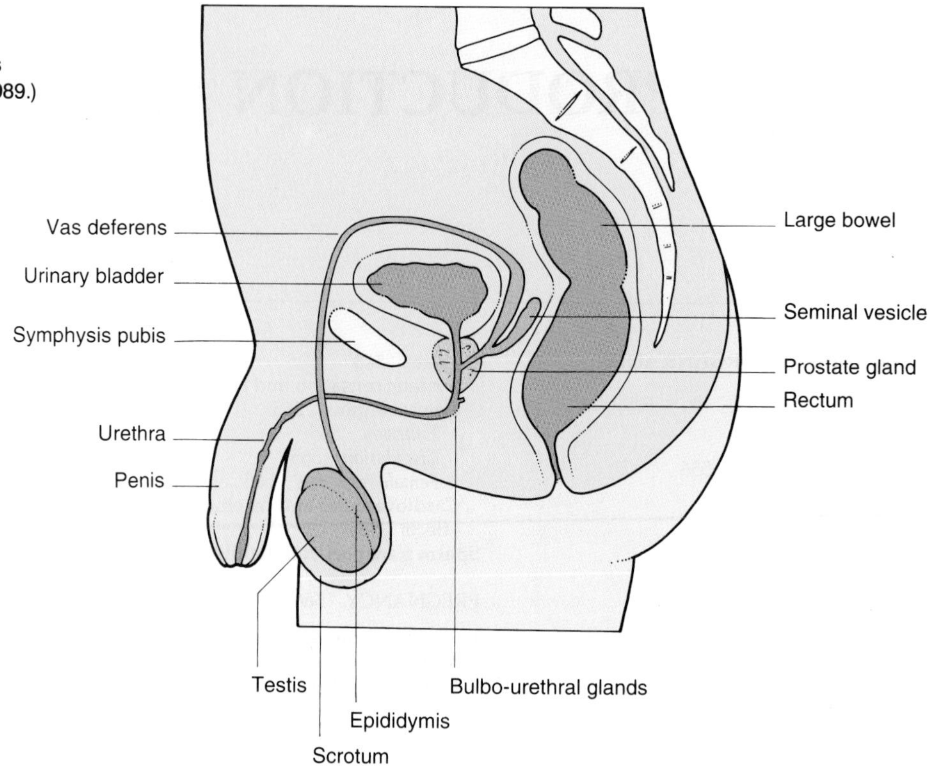

Figure 34.1
The male reproductive organs and
their relation to neighbouring structures
in the pelvis. (Adapted from Bancroft 1989.)

Vas deferens

Urinary bladder

Symphysis pubis

Urethra

Penis

Large bowel

Seminal vesicle

Prostate gland

Rectum

Testis

Epididymis

Scrotum

Bulbo-urethral glands

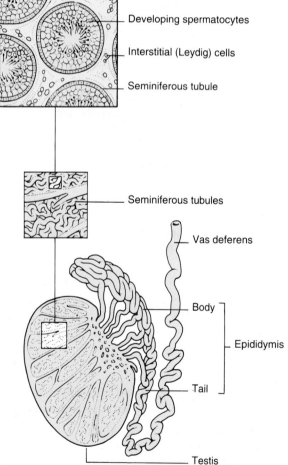

Developing spermatocytes

Interstitial (Leydig) cells

Seminiferous tubule

Seminiferous tubules

Vas deferens

Body

Epididymis

Tail

Testis

Figure 34.2
Structure of the testis. (Adapted from Rogers 1992.)

vas deferens and ultimately the *urethra*. En route, secretions are added to the testicular fluid by several glands, including the *prostate*, and the *seminal vesicles*, forming *semen*. The penis consists largely of spongy tissue which becomes engorged with blood during sexual excitement and consequently enlarges and stiffens. This renders it firm enough to be pushed into the vagina so that sperm, ejaculated from the urethra, can be deposited in the female reproductive tract.

Testes

There are two testes, one usually slightly larger than the other. Each consists of many *seminiferous tubules*, the site of sperm production, and *interstitial cells of Leydig* producing the hormone *testosterone* (Fig. 34.2).

Sperm production

Sperm cells (*spermatocytes*) are produced continuously throughout adult life, from puberty (see Ch. 36) onwards. Primitive cells in the wall of the seminiferous tubules (*spermatogonia*) divide mitotically (see Ch. 2) and then meiotically (only half the number of chromosomes in each cell; see Ch. 35) to form millions of mature *spermatozoa* (Fig. 34.3). The entire maturation process takes about 2 to 3 months.

The *Sertoli cells* forming the bulk of the tissue of each seminiferous tubule support the development of spermatozoa and also secrete some fluid. Mature spermatozoa become detached and move along the tubules to the *epididymis*. The epididymis consists largely of an excep-

Seminiferous tubule

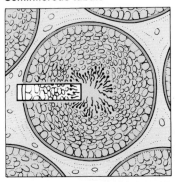

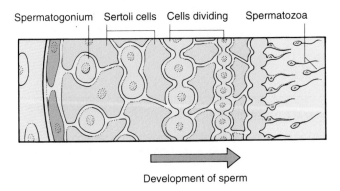

Figure 34.3
Development of sperm within a seminiferous tubule.

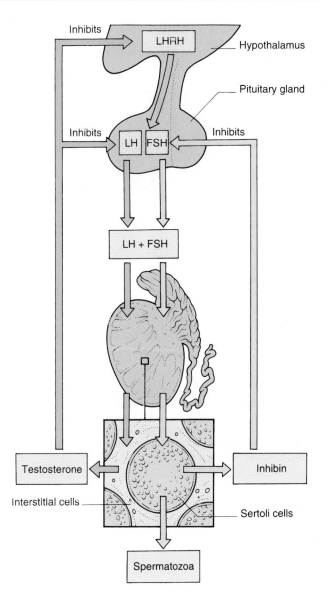

Figure 34.4
Hormonal control of testicular function.

tionally long coiled tube. It takes 2 to 4 weeks for sperm to pass along the tube to the end of the epididymis (*tail*) where sperm are stored until they are ejaculated, leak out in the urine or die and are phagocytosed. Movement is aided by waves of peristalsis.

Sperm production is promoted by:

● follicle stimulating hormone (FSH)
● testosterone.

FSH is secreted by the anterior pituitary. Its secretion is stimulated by luteinising hormone releasing hormone (LHRH) from the hypothalamus and inhibited by *inhibin* formed by Sertoli cells of the testes.

Testosterone
Testosterone is a steroid hormone (see Ch. 3). It:

● supports the production of sperm
● develops and maintains the male secondary sex characteristics (androgenic action; see Ch. 35)
● has growth-promoting (anabolic) effects.

Production of testosterone by the interstitial (Leydig) cells is stimulated by luteinising hormone (LH) from the anterior pituitary (see Ch. 10). LH secretion is promoted by LHRH and inhibited by testosterone (Fig. 34.4). ①

Penis

Penises vary considerably in length, being between 5 and 10 cm long when flaccid, and extending to about 15 cm when erect. The penis consists mainly of blood vessels and supporting connective tissue, covered by skin (Fig. 34.5).

The arteries supplying the penis empty into three distensible rods of tissue (*corpora cavernosa* and *corpus spongiosum*) which expand and fill with blood in an erection. Each rod of tissue is surrounded by connective tissue supporting the engorged vessels. Running through the centre of the corpus spongiosum is the urethra. At its tip, the corpus spongiosum forms the *glans penis* which is encircled by a flap of skin (*prepuce* or *foreskin*).

The skin of the penis is hairless but contains many sensory nerve endings which are important in sexual

① *What do you understand by 'steroid hormone'? Can you name some other examples?*

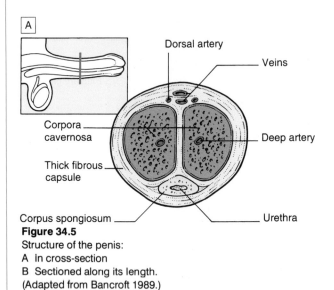

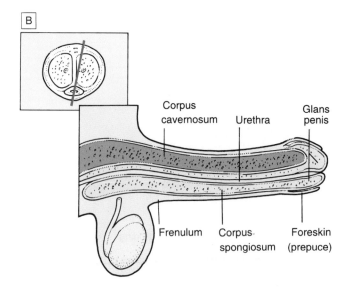

Figure 34.5
Structure of the penis:
A In cross-section
B Sectioned along its length.
(Adapted from Bancroft 1989.)

arousal. The most sensitive areas are the glans penis and the *frenulum* on the underside of the penis.

> The double fold of skin which forms the prepuce or foreskin is usually mobile and can easily be retracted over the glans. To avoid infection, the area beneath the foreskin should be kept clean and free from accumulated secretions. Some consider that removal of the foreskin (*circumcision*) is more hygienic than leaving it in place.

Glands

There are several different glands in the male reproductive tract (Fig. 34.1), the chief of these being:

- seminal vesicles
- prostate gland
- bulbo-urethral glands (Cowper's glands).

The secretions formed by these glands mix with testicular secretions to form *semen*.

The *prostate gland* consists of a collection of tubulo-alveolar glands enclosed by a capsule containing smooth muscle. The gland completely encircles the urethra.

> Enlargement of the prostate gland can cause obstruction to urine flow. This condition is not uncommon in older men.

Semen

Semen consists of a mixture of secretions (Fig. 34.6); 60 to 70% is contributed by the seminal vesicles, which secrete a sticky yellowish secretion, and about 20% by the prostate gland. Substances secreted by the seminal vesicles are important in activating and nourishing the sperm.

About 3 ml of semen are produced at an ejaculation, only 2% of which is sperm. This tiny volume, however,

> **MALE INFERTILITY**
>
> The most obvious question to answer when seeking the cause of male infertility is, 'can the semen be ejaculated?' If there are no obstructions of the seminal ducts, either congenital or acquired by injury, infection or tumour, and semen is being produced, then the next question to consider is, 'are sufficient live, normal sperm being produced?' There may be abnormalities of the testes, either congenital (e.g. undescended testes) or aquired (e.g. bilateral inflammation of the testes (*orchitis*) caused by the mumps virus, which, though rare, causes sterility). Working in excessive heat or wearing tight clothing may affect sperm production. General diseases, such as diabetes mellitus, coeliac disease and endocrine disorders may lead to defective spermatogenesis. More specifically, dysfunction of the anterior pituitary gland or the hypothalamus may prevent production of FSH, LH and LHRH, thus affecting testicular function and the formation of healthy sperm.

contains about 300 million sperm cells (100 million/ml of semen). If the cell count is less than 20 to 40 million/ml the chances of conception are slim.

FEMALE

The structures of the female reproductive tract and their positions within the pelvic cavity are shown in Figures 34.7 and 34.8. The main structures are:

- ovaries
- uterus (womb)
- uterine tubes (fallopian tubes)
- vagina
- vulva (external genitalia).

The other part of a woman's body that is specifically adapted to support reproduction is breast tissue (*mammary glands*).

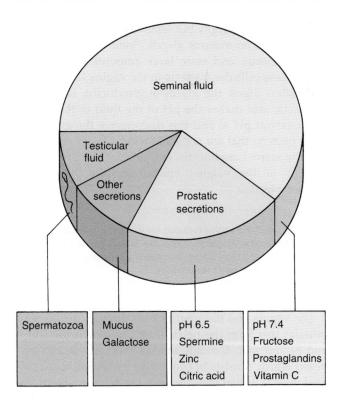

Figure 34.6
Composition of semen.

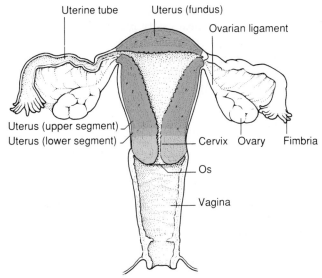

Figure 34.7
Female reproductive organs. (Reproduced and adapted from Rogers 1992 (Fig. 9.5) by permission of the publishers.)

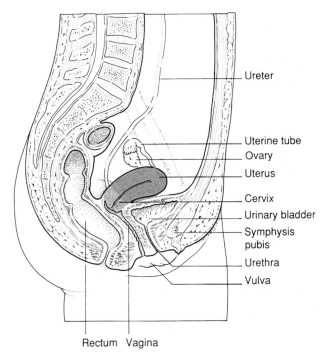

Figure 34.8
Position of the reproductive organs in the female pelvis. (Reproduced and adapted from Rogers 1992 (Fig. 9.6) by permission of the publishers.)

From puberty until the menopause (see Ch. 36), reproductive organs and associated tissues undergo cyclical monthly changes (*menstrual cycle*) resulting in the release of an egg (*ovum*) and the preparation of the woman's body for the implantation and growth of an embryo. Usually one ovum is released each month, wafted into a uterine tube and then propelled through it to the uterus. If sperm have been deposited in the vagina, some will swim up into the uterus and one may fertilise the ovum. If fertilisation does not occur the prepared richly vascularised lining of the uterus breaks down, and blood and cell debris (*menstrual fluid*) drains out of the uterus for a few days, leaking out of the body through the cervix and vagina. The whole cycle then begins again.

Ovaries

There are two ovaries. Each lies within the peritoneal cavity (Fig. 34.8) up against the wall of the pelvis, one on either side. The ovaries are supplied with blood by the ovarian arteries (branches of the abdominal aorta) and are anchored to the uterus by connective tissue (*ovarian ligaments*) and by a layer of peritoneum forming part of the *broad ligament*. The ovaries house the ova and manufacture and secrete *oestrogens*.

The ova are formed during fetal life. At birth a female child possesses about 1 to 2 million ova. By the time she reaches reproductive years at adolescence, numbers have fallen to about half a million, and go on decreasing during adulthood until, by the age of about 50 years, there are none left (see Ch. 36, Fig. 36.13).

Uterine tubes

Each uterine tube is about 12 cm long, extending from the uterus towards the ovary. The end next to the ovary is fringed with finger-like projections (*fimbriae*) wafting fluid from the peritoneal cavity into the tube. The wall of the tube consists of muscle and is lined internally by a ciliated secretory epithelium. Contractions of the muscle and beating of the cilia help to propel the fluid in the tube towards the uterus.

Uterus

The uterus is a small hollow pear-shaped organ lying just behind the urinary bladder (Fig. 34.8). The bulbous part is the body and the narrower part is the cervix, part of which protrudes into the vagina (Fig. 34.7). The uterus is normally in an *antiverted* position meaning that it is at an angle in the pelvis, leaning forward with the cervix pointing backwards.

Body

The body of the uterus consists largely of muscle (*myometrium*) lined internally by a glandular layer (*endometrium*). Part of this layer is shed at menstruation. New cells grow from the remaining tissue to replace those that are lost.

Cervix

The cervix consists mostly of connective tissue (see Ch. 2) and has few muscle cells. It too is lined by a secretory epithelium which includes many glands (*cervical glands*). However, unlike the endometrial layer, this secretory epithelium is not shed during menstruation although its secretory activity changes during the menstrual cycle.

Vagina

The vagina is an expandable muscular tube consisting mostly of longitudinally arranged bundles of smooth muscle cells. The vagina is lined internally by tissue that

② What does pH stand for?

CERVICAL SMEAR TEST (PAPANICOLAOU OR PAP TEST)

Early malignant disease of the cervix can be detected by the examination of cells obtained directly from the cervix. Carcinoma of the cervix is the second commonest cancer in women worldwide. Current research interest is in the relationship between the presence of the human papillomavirus on the cervix and cervical cancer (Wilkinson 1992). The cervical smear test is available for all women and is generally painless. It should be repeated at regular intervals depending on age, health and the results of previous tests. The cells are obtained by gently scraping the cervix with a specially shaped cervical spatula. Microscopic examination will show whether any malignant cells are present. Management may consist of:

- punch biopsies which, if positive, are followed by laser ablation
- a diathermy loop excision biopsy following a positive smear test
- hysterectomy (removal of the uterus) if the malignancy is extensive.

---

has a rich blood supply but relatively few sensory nerve endings, and no mucous glands. Some of the epithelial cells synthesise and store large amounts of glycogen. When these cells die, bacteria in the vagina (*Lactobacillus acidophilus*) digest the glycogen, producing lactic acid. The lactic acid makes the pH of the fluid in the vagina acidic (about pH 4) and this discourages the growth of other bacteria that are not acid loving. This environment and the many lymphocytes and neutrophils (see Ch. 15) present in the vaginal epithelium provide defence against infection. ②

Douching of the vagina reduces the numbers of lactobacilli present and consequently raises the vaginal pH. Contrary to popular expectation therefore, douching may promote infection rather than prevent it.

The vagina and the urethra pass through the layer of muscles that form the pelvic floor (*levator ani*; see Chs 6 and 8) and then through another layer of tissues (*perineum*) which consists of connective tissue and more striated muscle. When they contract, the pelvic and perineal muscles act like a sphincter around the opening of the vagina (Fig. 34.9A & B).

In the perineum to either side of the vaginal opening are two small masses of erectile tissue (*bulb of the vestibule*) similar in origin and tissue structure to the corpus spongiosum of the penis. The external opening of the vagina may be partially covered by a thin flap of connective tissue (*hymen*).

An intact hymen was considered to be a sign of virginity, and its tearing, with associated bleeding, at intercourse was believed to be confirmation of virginity. The now common use of tampons results in the hymen being stretched, so that it is no longer torn during the first sexual intercourse. Gentle stretching, with the fingers, of a tight hymen is recommended if this is the cause of painful intercourse (*dyspareunia*). Rarely, the hymen completely closes the vagina. This condition (*imperforate hymen*) is usually discovered when menstruation begins. The hymen is then opened surgically.

Vulva

The external genitalia (*vulva*) (Fig. 34.10) consist of several folds of tissue (*labia majora and minora*) surrounding the vaginal and urethral openings together with more erectile tissue equivalent to that of the penis in the male (see Fig. 34.5). The corpora cavernosa and corpus spongiosum together form the *clitoris*, the glans of which (just above the urethral opening) is the most sensitive part erotically. The vulva has both sebaceous and sweat glands and a number of mucus-secreting glands around the urethral and vaginal openings. It is also well supplied with sensory nerve endings.

GENITAL INFECTIONS

When sexually transmitted diseases are mentioned, most people think of diseases given frequent media coverage, such as AIDS, gonorrhoea, syphilis and herpes, but there are other infections of the genital tract, such as candidiasis and trichomoniasis, that can be transmitted by sexual intercourse.

Candidiasis (thrush)

Candida albicans is a widespread yeast-like organism which is normally present in nose, mouth, bowel and on the skin. If conditions in the vagina predispose to the organism becoming *pathogenic* (disease producing), for example loss of normal vaginal bacteria during antibiotic therapy, reduced resistance to infection, increased humidity (wearing tights with closed gusset or tight jeans), then uncomfortable symptoms arise. There is usually *pruritus* (itching), watery or thick and cottage-cheese-like discharge and discomfort when passing urine (*dysuria*). When the condition occurs in the male, there are small curd-like plaques or red spots on the glans penis and sometimes dysuria. Both men and women may be asymptomatic but still pass on the organism to partners.

Vaginal thrush is fairly common during pregnancy because the urine often contains some sugar which encourages the growth of *Candida albicans* in the vulval area.

Trichomoniasis (trike)

Trichomonas vaginalis is a *protozoon* (unicellular animal) possessing flagellae. It is capable of surviving for short periods outside the body in moist conditions and therefore can be transmitted on shared towels, after swimming for example. Infection results in an unpleasant discharge that is often profuse and fishy smelling, and may be yellow/green, frothy and watery. It is usually accompanied by pruritus and inflammation. In the male there is a similar discharge from the urethra, and dysuria. The condition may be asymptomatic.

Because these infections can be asymptomatic, it is important for both partners to be treated; otherwise there is always the possibility of one re-infecting the other. The regular and correct use of condoms helps to prevent the spread of such infections.

Breasts

The breasts consist of glandular tissue. Each mammary gland consists of about 20 separate tubulo-alveolar glands each of which possesses a separate duct opening out at the nipple (Fig. 34.11). In the female the glandular tissue undergoes further development at puberty (see p. 605), whereas in the male it normally remains immature.

Enlargement of the breasts can occur in men as a result of endocrine disorder (*gynaecomastia*).

The individual glands of the breast are separated from one another by connective tissue and fat. The glands are supported by ligaments (*Cooper's ligaments*)

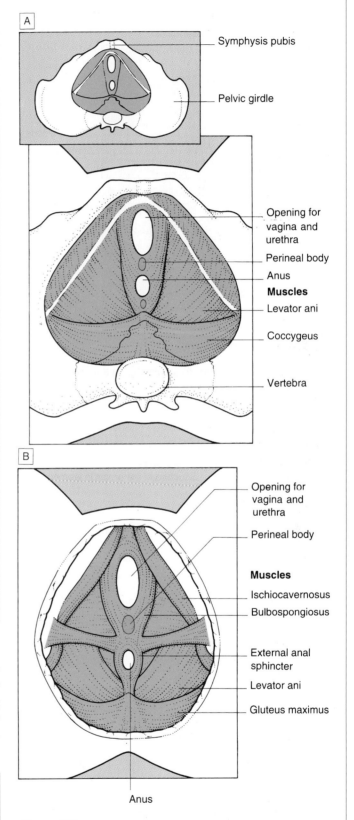

Figure 34.9
Muscles of the pelvic floor and perineum in women.
A Pelvic floor viewed from above
B Muscles of the perineum viewed from below.
(Part A adapted from Chamberlain & Dewhurst 1986; part B adapted from Williams et al 1989.)

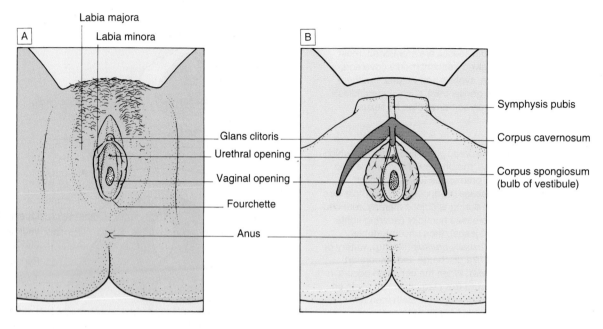

Labia majora
Labia minora

A

Glans clitoris
Urethral opening
Vaginal opening
Fourchette
Anus

B

Symphysis pubis
Corpus cavernosum
Corpus spongiosum (bulb of vestibule)

Figure 34.10
Female external genitalia (vulva):
A External features
B Internal features (compare these with Fig. 34.5 which shows equivalent tissue in the male).
(Adapted from Bancroft 1989.)

③
What do you think 'ampulla' means.

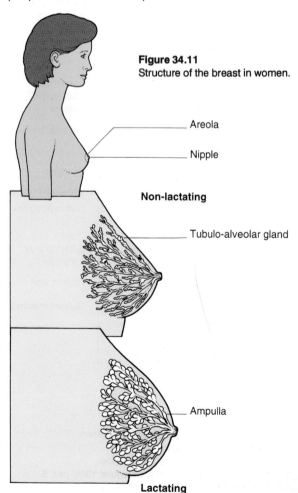

Figure 34.11
Structure of the breast in women.

Areola
Nipple

Non-lactating

Tubulo-alveolar gland

Ampulla

Lactating

anchoring them to the skin and to the underlying covering (*fascia*) of the muscles of the chest wall.

There is an enlargement of each duct (*ampulla* or *sinus*) just before it passes through the nipple. These sinuses are surrounded by smooth muscle fibres. The ducts too have contractile cells (*myoepithelial cells*) in their walls which contract reflexly in response to suckling (see p. 580) expelling the milk contained within them. ③

The skin around the nipple is the *areola*. It darkens during pregnancy due to the production of extra melanin. The areola has many glands, including tiny mammary-type glands (*Montgomery's tubercles*), and sebaceous glands secreting an oily substance that creams and protects the nipple during suckling.

About 75% of the lymph draining from the tissues of the breast drains through the lymph nodes of the armpit (*axilla*).

In a *radical mastectomy* the axillary lymph nodes are removed in an attempt to eradicate cancerous cells that may have spread to the nodes from the primary tumour in the breast.

SEXUAL ACTIVITY

Human sexual experience is complex. It involves minds and emotions as well as genitalia. In a sexual response there are:

- changes in the reproductive organs
- experiences of pleasurable erotic sensations
- an altered state of arousal.

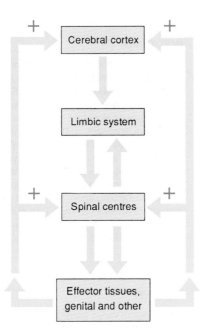

Figure 34.12
Neural control of the sexual response.

At its most basic level, stimulation of sensory receptors in the genital region evokes spinal reflexes which cause changes in male and female genitalia, including vasocongestion and increased secretion. The vasocongestion of erectile tissue firms up the genitalia in both sexes, enlarging the penis in the male and the coital canal in the female ready for sexual union. The experience of pleasurable sensations together with associated attractive stimuli provides the motivation for the sexual behaviour which brings two people together. The sensations evoked by sexual intercourse have a positive feedback effect in this system (Fig. 34.12) leading ultimately to a climax (*orgasm*) in which there is a sudden increase in the intensity of erotic sensations coupled with muscular contractions and, in men, the ejaculation of sperm. This intense but pleasurable experience is rapidly followed by a period of profound relaxation.

When a woman fails to conceive and the couple seek advice, the initial counselling must establish that sexual intercourse is taking place. Occasionally marriages are not consummated and, even with increased emphasis on sex education, some couples remain ignorant of what sexual intercourse entails.

SEXUAL AROUSAL

Sexual arousal may be provoked by stimulation of receptors locally in the genitalia, as well as by psychic factors, some conditioned by experience. These stimuli evoke many changes in the genitalia and increase the general state of arousal.

Local stimuli and reflex effects

The skin covering the glans penis and the glans clitoris is richly supplied with sensory receptors. There are also other receptors close by especially at the back of the penis and in the vulva. Stimulation of these receptors evokes spinal reflexes (sacral spinal cord) causing several effects including:

- vasocongestion in reproductive organs
- fluid secretion
- muscle contraction.

Vasocongestion

Vasocongestion occurs in the penis and in the equivalent vessels of the clitoris caused by dilation of blood vessels. The penis and the clitoris become engorged with blood and therefore expand. The increasing tissue pressure increases stimulation of the cutaneous receptors, thus increasing the intensity of sensation and the reflex responses. Vasodilation may be due to decreased afferent activity in the sympathetic nerves.

In men, the swelling compresses the penal veins, thus reducing the outflow of blood from the penis. As a result pressure increases within the organ and it lengthens and becomes hard. At full erection the pressure of blood within the penis is only just below systolic arterial blood pressure (see Ch. 5). The throbbing sensed is due to arterial pulsations. Additional stiffening is due to reflex contraction of the *ischiocavernosus* and *bulbospongiosus* muscles (striated muscles at the base of the penis; Fig. 34.13).

Erections also occur in men and boys in the absence of sexual stimulation, for example during sleep and on waking, and in arousing but non-sexual situations.

In women, expansion of the vulva creates a firmer cuff of tissue at the opening to the vagina and lengthens the coital canal. Vasocongestion also occurs in the

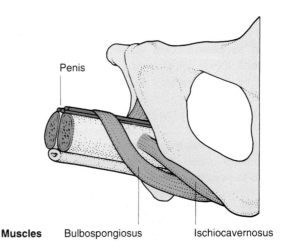

Muscles   Bulbospongiosus   Ischiocavernosus

Figure 34.13
Muscles of the penis. (Adapted from Bancroft 1989.)

uterus. Contraction of smooth muscle in the tissues supporting the uterus and the vagina causes the upper part of the vagina to elongate and enlarge.

Fluid secretion

In women, as sexual arousal proceeds, fluid is secreted by the walls of the vagina, and there is secretion of mucus by the vestibular glands (Bartholin's) at the vaginal opening. Both fluids help to lubricate the movement of the penis within the vagina. The vaginal fluid may also provide a more favourable environment for the survival of ejaculated sperm.

In men too, there is increased glandular secretion during sexual arousal. The amount varies between men but can be great enough to drip from the penis.

Muscle contraction

In men contraction of muscles in the genitalia also causes elevation of the testes and contraction of the scrotum. In women there may be erection of the nipples. ④

Psychic factors

The spinal reflexes producing these various genital effects are influenced by impulses from the brain such that the sight of a person or an object, or internal imagery in fantasy, also excites or inhibits sexual responses. These responses are mediated by the limbic system which plays a central part in determining mood and emotion (see Ch. 31). Specific areas of the hypothalamus (*medial, preoptic/anterior*) may be involved. The effectiveness of stimuli in evoking responses depends also on the pre-existing general level of arousal (see Ch. 31).

> Alcohol depresses activity in the central nervous system. Although at low doses this may reduce inhibitory effects and increase responsiveness, at higher doses sexual responses are progressively reduced.

The stimuli which are sexually arousing differ from person to person. One person may be attracted by another's looks; another may be influenced more by touch or even possibly by smell (*pheromones*). Some people, mostly men, develop particular sexual responsiveness to parts of the body or objects associated with the body, such as clothes or materials (e.g. rubber or leather). This *fetishism* can become a problem in a sexual relationship when it becomes more important than person-to-person encounter.

How these various responses are established is still uncertain. Many are thought to be learned by association (see Ch. 33) as a result of good and bad experiences in infancy, childhood and adolescence, but some, such as sexual responsiveness to persons of the same sex (*homosexuality*), may in some people be determined

④
At what other time might nipples be erect?

IMPOTENCE

Primary impotence is rare – that is for a man never to have attained and maintained an erection for sufficient time to perform normal sexual intercourse. Secondary impotence may have organic causes or may result from taking certain medications or alcohol. Psychological factors are important too; stress, tiredness, guilt and depression are all possible causes. A man may worry so much about his failure that he is liable to fail again – and again. Adverse comments from his partner about his performance may bring about impotence or prolong it if it has already occurred. There may be something about his current partner that acts as a 'turn-off' (this does not imply lack of love) and, should he be able to perform satisfactorily with someone else, the original problem can be exacerbated by guilt.

FRIGIDITY

Sexual desire varies considerably from person to person. Some women are not particularly interested in sexual activity. If such a woman's partner makes more demands on her than she feels able to enjoy then she will probably label him 'oversexed' and he will label her 'frigid'.

Frigidity suggests unbending coldness and has been used to cover many aspects of female psychosexual problems. Sexual activity is not absolutely essential to a happy and loving relationship. Like any other activity it is fine if it is enjoyed, but it should not become so important that emotional distress results for either or both partners. There may, however, be physical causes for lack of enjoyment of the sexual act, such as pain due to infection or following suturing of the perineum.

Other causes of frigidity may be fear of pregnancy or of contracting a disease, a recent stressful life event or tiredness. Some women with a new baby find that the mother/baby relationship is totally satisfying. For others, there may be something about their partner's behaviour or demands which act as a 'turn-off', for example boredom with the same ritual foreplay. Deep feelings about sex are sometimes instilled during childhood (e.g. sex is dirty), which prevents enjoyment later in life. Some women never experience an orgasm, approximately 10% of women are physically incapable of orgasm (Edwards & Bouchier 1991). Concern about this may cause physical or mental ill-health, the woman thinking that she is frigid. It does not matter what labels are used, if emotional distress is present in either partner then counselling is required.

---

also by genetically and hormonally controlled events prior to birth.

General arousal

The effects of sexual arousal on the rest of the body are similar to those produced by other forms of excitement and activity, and reflect a general increase in activity within the sympathetic nervous system. Thus there are increases in:

- blood pressure
- heart rate
- rate of breathing.

The pupils dilate, and there are changes in blood flow and secretory activity in the skin.

ORGASM

This intensely pleasurable experience is one of the least well understood aspects of sexual physiology. It is characterised in both sexes by a peaking of sexual tension followed by a rapid release. In men, this climax is marked by emission and ejaculation of semen, whereas in women there are rhythmic contractions of muscles in and around the vagina.

Somatic sensation and responses

Orgasm is characterised by an explosion of sensory feeling that may simply be localised to the perineal region or may spread out from there to other parts or even the whole of the body. The experience differs from person to person, the only common features seeming to be the mounting intensity, and peaking of feeling which suddenly dies away. In some instances the extreme change in feeling suggests an altered level of consciousness, bordering even on loss of consciousness.

The sensations of orgasm are accompanied by involuntary contractions of many muscles of the body which can include those of the limbs, abdomen, neck and face. In extreme instances these contractions may resemble convulsions. Very quickly this brief period of muscular spasms is followed by profound muscular relaxation coupled with a sense of calm.

Genital organs

Propulsion of semen from the male reproductive tract occurs in two stages:

- emission
- ejaculation.

Emission

In emission, contraction of the smooth muscle in the vas deferens, seminal vesicles and prostate gland causes the secretions there to be expelled into the urethra. Muscle contraction is evoked by a sympathetic reflex mediated via nerves leading to (*pudendal*) and from (*hypogastric*) the upper lumbar parts of the spinal cord.

Ejaculation

The semen within the urethra is then expelled from it by contractions of the striated muscle at the base of the penis (*bulbospongiosus* and *bulbocavernosus muscles*). Simultaneously there is contraction of the internal sphincter of the bladder coupled with relaxation of the external sphincter. The whole process is quite complicated and involves several different reflexes coordinated in the sacral part of the spinal cord.

If all goes to plan, the events of emission and ejaculation occur at the climax of sexual excitement. In men,

especially those who are older, it can take a little while for the whole system to recover. Consequently another erection cannot be produced immediately after orgasm.

Female responses

In women the climax of sexual excitement is usually marked genitally by repeated contraction of the ring of muscles at the opening of the vagina and the muscle of the vaginal walls. Contractions of the muscle in the uterus is believed to occur too. In contrast to men, once orgasm has occurred re-excitement can be achieved in women quite quickly.

Cardiovascular and respiratory effects

Just before orgasm there is a sharp increase in respiratory rate, and often in women and in some men a flushing of the skin overlying the trunk. At orgasm, heart rate and blood pressure both increase sharply and then fall. Heart rate increases by between 20 and 80 beats per minute, the size of the increase depending on the level of anxiety, as well as the sexual response and physical activity. The same applies to blood pressure. Increases range from 25 to 120 mmHg for systolic pressure and 25 to 50 mmHg for diastolic pressure. In non-stressful situations the demands placed on the cardiovascular system by sexual activity have been estimated to be similar to modest physical exercise.

SPERM TRANSPORT AND VIABILITY

Sperm deposited in a woman's vagina move through the genital tract quite rapidly and reach the uterine tubes within an hour. The spermatozoa have to negotiate the mucus of the cervix before swimming through the fluids in the uterus. At the time of ovulation, when the mucus is thin (see p. 567), penetration by sperm is easier than at other times. ⑤

Sperm survive for up to 2 days in a woman's reproductive tract. During this time they change (*capacitation*) in ways that enable them to adhere better to an ovum. Of the millions of sperm deposited in the vagina less than 100 actually reach the ovum. Of these, normally only one will penetrate the membrane to fertilise the egg (see p. 568).

Sperm cells are foreign to a woman's body and therefore should be recognised and attacked by her immune system just like any other foreign body. However, they are protected by substances secreted in semen that inhibit local immune responses.

⑤ *What other name is commonly used for the uterine tubes?*

> The immunosuppressive effect of substances in semen is believed to contribute to the increased incidence of cervical cancer in sexually active women. Cancerous cells are not destroyed as readily because immune mechanisms locally are suppressed.

CONTRACEPTION

Contraception or family planning is the means by which conception may be prevented. The only 100% effective contraceptive is abstention from sexual intercourse (even sterilisation has a failure rate). Failure rates for other methods are calculated per 100 women years of use (HWY) – this is the number of women who would become pregnant if 100 women used the same method for 1 year. There are five groups of contraceptive methods.

Natural methods

- *Coitus interruptus* involves withdrawing the penis before ejaculation takes place. The failure rate is high (17 per HWY) because semen leakage often occurs before ejaculation.
- Abstaining from sex during the time of ovulation is a method that involves establishing, by various means, when ovulation is taking place. Changes in early morning body temperature (see p. 568) and the consistency of cervical mucus are two indicators of ovulation. The failure rate for these methods varies from 1 to 11 per HWY.
- Breast feeding in developing countries provides effective contraception because ovulation does not occur while the baby is suckling regularly (see p. 580). If supplementary bottle feeds are given instead of suckling the baby, or the night feed is missed, ovulation is likely to recommence.
- *Vaginal douching* is used by some women, but as the very motile sperm can reach the internal cervical os within 90 seconds the method is ineffective. There is also the added risk of increasing susceptibility to vaginal infection (see p. 560).

Barrier methods

These methods provide a physical barrier between the semen and the cervix. Spermicides give additional protection. For men, there is the *sheath* or *condom*, and for women, the *diaphragm*. The failure rate for both is 2 to 15 per HWY.

Vaginal sponges are gaining popularity for older women or those who are breast feeding, and at other times when fertility may be reduced. There has been controversy about the failure rate – it may be as high as 25 per HWY.

Intrauterine contraceptive devices (IUCDs)

These devices (there are several types) are inserted into the uterine cavity by a doctor using a special applicator. The IUCD is thought to act in three ways:

- the endometrium is rendered less suitable for implantation
- prostaglandin production may be increased, causing expulsion of the fertilised ovum
- uterine tubal motility may be increased, again causing expulsion of the ovum.

The failure rate is 0.3 to 4 per HWY.

Hormonal methods

These are known collectively as 'the pill'. The combined pill contains oestrogen and a synthetic form of progesterone – progestogen; there is also a progestogen-only pill. They act by suppressing the production of FSH and LH. Consequently, the ovarian follicles do not mature and ovulation does not take place (see p. 568). The failure rate for the combined pill is 0.1 to 1 per HWY, and for the progestogen-only pill, 0.3 to 5 per HWY.

Sterilisation

In women, the uterine tubes are divided and clipped to obstruct the passage of the ovum to the uterus. The effect is immediate and reversal is possible. There is an increased risk of ectopic pregnancy following reversal (see p. 570). The failure rate for clips is 2 per 1000 cases.

In men, each vas deferens is divided (*vasectomy*) and sutured. The effect is not immediate because sperm remain viable in the vas deferens distal to the occlusion for up to 4 months. Other contraceptive methods should be used until two consecutive sperm counts have been negative. Reversal is possible but fertility does not always return. The failure rate is 0 to 0.2 per HWY. Further information about contraceptive methods can be found in Bennett & Brown 1989.

PREGNANCY

During her reproductive years a woman's body goes through a series of changes each month preparing her to conceive and bear a child. If conception does not occur, preparations are abandoned, the materials produced are scrapped and a fresh cycle begins. This regular sequence of changes is termed the *menstrual cycle* because of the discharge of fluid (*menses*) occurring via the vagina at regular intervals.

If, however, the ovum is fertilised, many tissues swing into action driven by hormonal signals gearing the woman's body, as well as her womb, to house, nourish and protect the developing new individual. A key structure which forms from the conceptus, not the mother, is the *placenta*, the lifeline between her and her offspring. Through this organ the fetus gains all it needs and disposes of its waste. Extensive changes occur in almost all systems in a woman's body in pregnancy. Some developments such as *lactation* support the baby after its birth but all are designed to nourish and protect the new life.

PRELUDE: THE MENSTRUAL CYCLE

All the ova that a woman will ever have were produced right at the beginning of her life when she herself was a fetus. They are stored in her ovaries until, at puberty, hormones released by the anterior pituitary (FSH and LH), begin the cycle of changes resulting in the final maturation of a single ovum each month and its release from the ovary (*ovulation*). Simultaneously other organs of the reproductive tract undergo cyclical changes in activity, preparing the tract for the implantation of a fertilised ovum and the nurturing of the developing embryo.

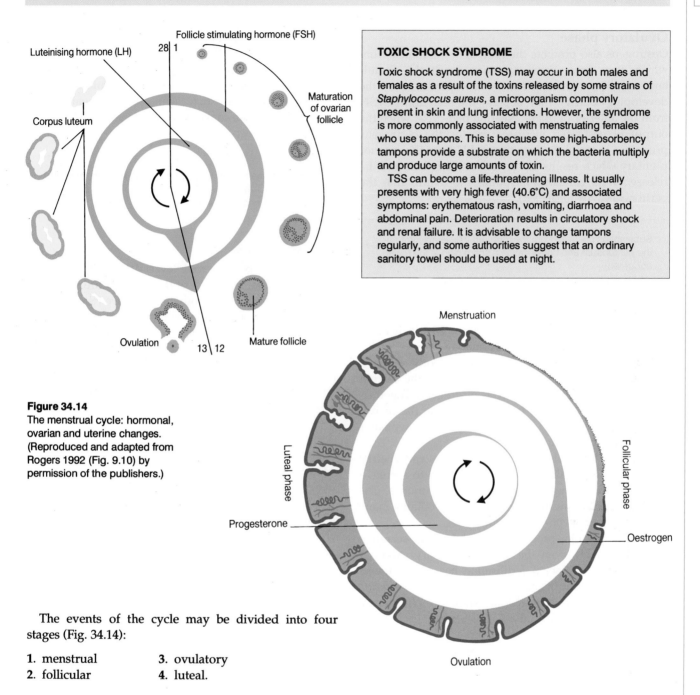

Figure 34.14
The menstrual cycle: hormonal, ovarian and uterine changes. (Reproduced and adapted from Rogers 1992 (Fig. 9.10) by permission of the publishers.)

TOXIC SHOCK SYNDROME

Toxic shock syndrome (TSS) may occur in both males and females as a result of the toxins released by some strains of *Staphylococcus aureus*, a microorganism commonly present in skin and lung infections. However, the syndrome is more commonly associated with menstruating females who use tampons. This is because some high-absorbency tampons provide a substrate on which the bacteria multiply and produce large amounts of toxin.

TSS can become a life-threatening illness. It usually presents with very high fever (40.6°C) and associated symptoms: erythematous rash, vomiting, diarrhoea and abdominal pain. Deterioration results in circulatory shock and renal failure. It is advisable to change tampons regularly, and some authorities suggest that an ordinary sanitary towel should be used at night.

The events of the cycle may be divided into four stages (Fig. 34.14):

1. menstrual
2. follicular
3. ovulatory
4. luteal.

Menstruation

The beginning of the menstrual cycle is by convention timed from the first day of menstruation. At this time the rich vascular lining of the uterus breaks down and bleeding occurs for about 3 to 5 days. Simultaneously the secretion of FSH and LH from the anterior pituitary begins to increase. These hormones promote the maturation of several ovarian follicles each of which contains a single ovum. ⑥

Follicular phase

On about the sixth day of the cycle one follicle overtakes the others in its development and continues to grow while the others regress. As the follicle enlarges it pro-duces increasing quantities of oestrogens. Oestrogens have widespread effects upon a woman's body (see p. 605). In the reproductive organs important changes occur in:

● the endometrium
● the cervical mucus
● the vaginal epithelium.

The endometrium grows thicker and the glands grow. The cervical mucus become thinner and more alkaline. These changes favour the survival of sperm and their movement through the female reproductive tract. The vaginal epithelium becomes cornified.

⑥
In everyday language, what names do women use to describe menstruation?

Ovulatory phase

Oestrogens also promote the growth of the follicle from which they have come (positive feedback). Simultaneously, together with *inhibin* (also produced by the developing follicle), they depress the secretion of FSH from the anterior pituitary. Nearing mid-cycle, when the output of oestrogen increases greatly, the oestrogens provoke a surge in the secretion of LH from the anterior pituitary which results in bursting of the follicle and the release of its contents, including the ovum, into the peritoneal cavity (*ovulation*).

> Substances released from the ruptured follicle may irritate the peritoneum and briefly cause a sharp pain in the lower abdomen.

Luteal phase

In the luteal phase the cells of the ruptured follicle begin to proliferate resulting in the formation of a yellowish looking body (*corpus luteum* – literally 'body yellow'). The cells of the corpus luteum produce the steroid hormone progesterone as well as oestrogens. Together, these hormones produce further changes in the uterus, cervix and vagina all of which prepare the woman's body for the possibility of pregnancy.

The blood vessels and glands of the endometrial lining develop further and the cells begin to secrete a fluid containing sugars, amino acids and mucus. The cervical mucus now becomes thick and contains many cells. The vaginal epithelium proliferates.

Oestrogens and progesterone inhibit the secretion of FSH and LH from the anterior pituitary. About 1 week after ovulation, if fertilisation has not occurred, the corpus luteum begins to regress, and the secretion of oestrogens and progesterone declines. Withdrawal of hormonal support affects the endometrial lining resulting in breakdown of some tissue. Release of prostaglandins from the necrotic tissue accelerates the process and promotes the flow of menstrual blood. ⑦

As the concentration of oestrogen and progesterone in the blood decreases, the secretion of FSH and LH from the anterior pituitary increases again and a new cycle begins.

⑦
What are prosta-glandins?

Associated changes

The cyclical change in hormone levels also brings about other changes including alterations in:

- breast tissue
- body temperature
- mood.

Breast tissue

During the proliferative phase of the cycle, the rising oestrogen concentration causes proliferation of the ducts of the mammary glands. When progesterone is added in the secretory phase then there is growth of the lobules and alveoli too. Blood flow to the mammary glands increases coupled with increased tissue fluid formation. All these changes cause some enlargement of the breasts, which can make them feel tender, and begin to prepare the breasts for lactation.

> In some women the enlargement is great enough for them to need two sizes of bras, one for the later stages of the luteal phase and one for the rest of the cycle.

Body temperature

The change in progesterone levels during the menstrual cycle alters the sensitivity of the temperature regulating systems such that core body temperature rises by about 0.5°C in the secretory phase of the cycle. If ovulation does not occur, the secretion of progesterone does not increase and body temperature does not rise.

> Recording body temperature each day at a regular time is one way of discovering if and when ovulation has occurred.

Mood

Many women experience changes in mood during the cycle, particularly in the days just prior to menstruation (*premenstrual tension*; Table 34.1). At this time the levels of oestrogens and progesterone are changing quite sharply. In some women the symptoms are associated with a relative lack of progesterone.

CONCEPTION

If the ovum is fertilised by a spermatozoon (Fig. 34.15), the fertilised egg (*zygote*) divides to form a growing mass of cells (Fig. 34.16) some of which will form the new embryo, and some the placenta. Cells within this mass begin to secrete the hormone HCG (*human chorionic gonadotrophin*), which maintains the corpus luteum so that it continues to secrete oestrogens and progesterone. As a result the various changes in the reproductive organs are maintained and breakdown of the uterine

Table 34.1   Features of the premenstrual syndrome*
Symptoms and signs
Feeling bloated Increased abdominal girth Breast tenderness Mood changes (e.g. irritability, depression, aggression)
* Compiled from Elder 1988.

Ovum

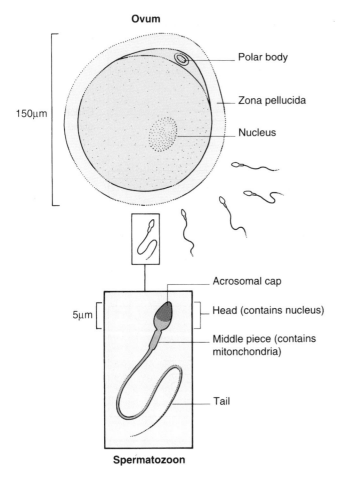

- Polar body
- Zona pellucida
- Nucleus

150μm

Spermatozoon

5μm

- Acrosomal cap
- Head (contains nucleus)
- Middle piece (contains mitonchondria)
- Tail

Figure 34.15
Ovum and spermatozoon.

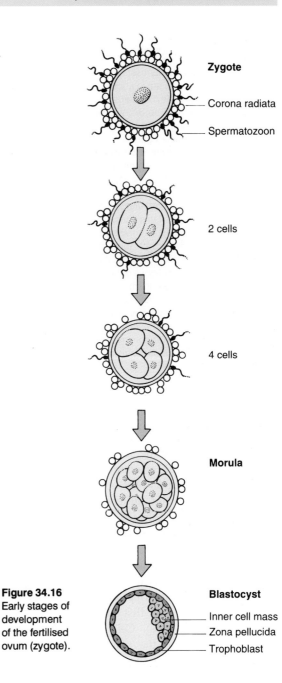

Zygote
- Corona radiata
- Spermatozoon

2 cells

4 cells

Morula

Figure 34.16
Early stages of development of the fertilised ovum (zygote).

Blastocyst
- Inner cell mass
- Zona pellucida
- Trophoblast

FEMALE INFERTILITY

The first questions to be answered when seeking the cause of female infertility are whether the ovum can reach the uterus and whether the sperm can reach the ovum. There may be obstruction of the uterine tubes due to infection or previous surgery, for example for tubal pregnancy (see p. 570) which may also cause adhesions of the fimbriae. The uterus may be tilted backwards (*retroverted*) preventing the collection of semen around the cervix. The cervix itself may be infected, the pus and infected mucus forming a barrier to sperm.

If regular normal ovulation does not occur, conception is less likely to take place. There are many causes of amenorrhoea: severe physical or mental illness; anorexia nervosa; obesity. Lack of, or infrequent, ovulation without amenorrhoea may be due to disorders of the ovaries caused by cysts, tumours or endometriosis. Endocrine disorders affecting the production of FSH and LH may also prevent ovulation.

Finally, it may not be possible for the fertilised ovum to implant in the uterus. The endometrium may not be receptive due to hormonal imbalance (oestrogen and progesterone), there may be congenital abnormalities such as a bicornuate uterus, fibroids may be present – or a forgotten IUCD (see p. 566) may still be in position!

---

lining does not occur. Instead the blastocyst burrows into the endometrium of the uterus and becomes fixed there (*implantation*) and both embryo and placenta develop from it.

The first days of development

The ovum released from the ovary is transported along the uterine tubes. It is here that fertilisation of the ovum by the spermatozoon normally occurs. Some of the sperm reaching the uterine tube adhere to the layer of glycoproteins enveloping the ovum (*zona pellucida*) to which some nutrient cells (*corona radiata*) are also attached. The binding of sperm to the glycoproteins triggers a reaction leading to the breakdown of the *acrosomal cap* in the spermatozoon (Fig. 34.15) and the

ECTOPIC IMPLANTATION

Under normal circumstances, the fertilised ovum embeds in the wall of the uterus, but in about 1 in 50 conceptions the ovum embeds outside the uterus, in a uterine tube, in the abdomen or, rarely, in an ovary. Ectopic implantation may be due to narrowing of the uterine tube as a result of infection or previous surgery.

Tubal pregnancies are not viable. If the implantation is at the end of the tube that is furthest from the uterus (i.e. the distal end), it is possible that a tubal abortion will occur; the developing trophoblast becomes separated from the wall and is extruded into the peritoneal cavity where it is eventually absorbed. If this does not happen, the pregnancy continues until either it is terminated surgically or the tube ruptures (a ruptured ectopic tubal pregnancy). The latter causes severe haemorrhage into the peritoneal cavity resulting in sudden collapse of the mother.

Viable abdominal pregnancy is rare because the fetus usually dies and is calcified. Occasionally the pregnancy reaches term and the baby is delivered by laparotomy. The placenta is not removed because it is attached to the outer wall of the uterus, the abdominal organs or an ovary. Removal would cause uncontrollable haemorrhage.

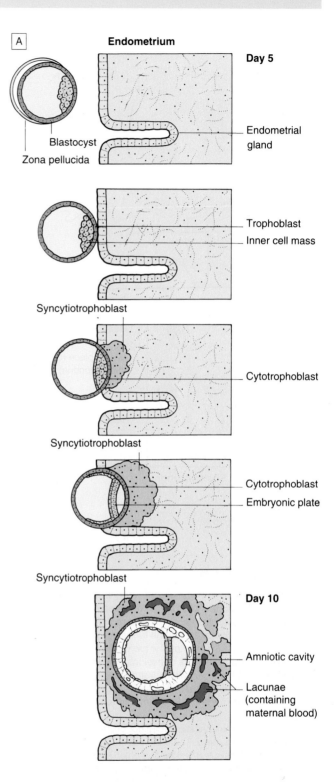

release of proteolytic enzymes contained within it. These enzymes digest the glycoproteins in the zona pellucida and enable the spermatozoon to penetrate to the cell membrane of the ovum itself.

The fertilised egg (*zygote*) now begins the process of cell proliferation and differentiation that continues throughout pregnancy as the new individual grows and develops. The zygote divides mitotically to form a clump of cells (*morula*). The morula develops into a *blastocyst* as fluid accumulates in the centre of the clump (Fig. 34.16). As cell division and differentiation proceed, an outer layer of cells (*trophoblast*) can be distinguished from a group of cells that bulge into the fluid-filled cavity (*inner cell mass*). Cells of the trophoblast are destined to become the placenta, whereas the inner clump of cells becomes the embryo. This stage of development is reached about 4 to 5 days after ovulation. By this time the mass of cells has usually reached the uterus.

Implantation

5 days after fertilisation the blastocyst 'hatches' from the zona pellucida, allowing the cells of the trophoblast to directly contact the endometrial wall. When this happens the cells of the trophoblast multiply, and work their way into the endometrium (*implantation*) (Fig. 34.17A). By about the tenth day after fertilisation the developing embryo is completely enclosed by endometrial tissue and the cells that will develop into the placenta are in place. At this stage the embryo is nourished by the transfer of materials across the cells of the trophoblast, by diffusion and pinocytosis. ⑧

THE PLACENTA

Development

During implantation, the cells of the trophoblast differentiate into two layers (Fig. 34.17):

- syncytiotrophoblast
- cytotrophoblast.

⑧
What is pinocytosis?

Figure 34.17
Implantation of the
conceptus and
development of
the placenta:
A Implantation (*left*)
B Early development
   of the placenta (*right*).

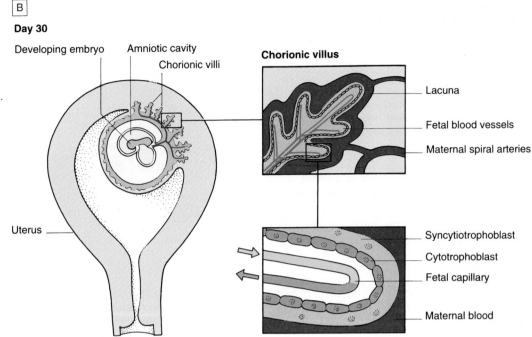

The syncytiotrophoblast burrows further into the endometrium, digesting maternal tissues and resulting in the formation of blood-filled spaces (*lacunae*) which will form part of the maternal circulation of the placenta (Fig. 34.17B). Extensions consisting of both syncytiotrophoblast and cytotrophoblast cells form and extend into the endometrium and into the spiral arteries which supply maternal blood.

Simultaneously some cells on the embryo side develop, and together with the cells of the trophoblast form the *chorionic villi* of the placenta which expand into the maternal blood-filled spaces created by the extra-villous trophoblast. Cells within the villi develop into blood vessels and join with other vessels originating from the embryonic cells to form the fetal circulation to the placenta. ⑨

Functions

The placenta is the life-support system for the developing embryo (Fig. 34.18). It:

- delivers oxygen and nutrients required for growth
- disposes of the waste products of embryonic metabolism
- is a protection against some constituents of maternal blood
- manufactures several hormones important in pregnancy.

Surprisingly, although the cells of the placenta are partly foreign to a woman's body they are not rejected by her immune system.

Transport and barrier functions

Oxygen and carbon dioxide passively diffuse across the placenta, whereas substances such as glucose, amino acids, electrolytes and minerals are taken across by specific transport mechanisms.

Most proteins cannot cross the barrier very easily because they are too large, but the IgG class of immunoglobulins is transferred by receptor-mediated endocytosis at one membrane of the syncytiotrophoblast

⑨
What is the name given to the structure containing blood vessels that links the fetus and the placenta?

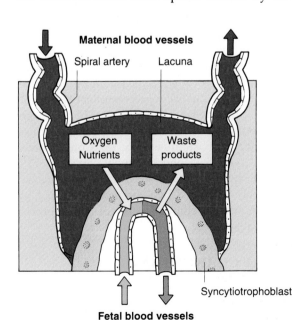

Figure 34.18 (*left*)
Functional organisation of the placenta.

and by exocytosis at the other (see Ch. 2). In the early stages of pregnancy the amounts transferred are small but by the third trimester concentrations in maternal and fetal blood are similar.

> Rhesus anti-D antibodies are of the IgG class (Ch. 15). They cross the placenta from mother to baby where they may cause destruction of fetal red cells if the baby's blood group is Rhesus positive (see Rhesus incompatibility, Ch. 4).

Liposoluble substances, such as alcohol, diffuse passively across the placenta from the mother to the baby. Similarly bilirubin, a waste product of haemoglobin breakdown, diffuses in the opposite direction from the fetal to the maternal blood. ⑩

Hormones

The cells of the syncytiotrophoblast manufacture several hormones and continue this function throughout pregnancy (Fig. 34.19). These hormones include:

- human chorionic gonadotrophin (HCG)
- human chorionic somatomammotrophin (HCS) (also known as human placental lactogen or HPL)
- progesterone
- oestrogens (principally oestriol).

HCG appears very early in pregnancy, secreted by the outer cells of the blastocyst even before implantation. Its identification by immunoassay (a method which allows very tiny amounts to be detected) in maternal blood is proof of pregnancy. HCG maintains the steroid-secreting function of the corpus luteum until this is taken over by the placenta itself after about the first 3 months of pregnancy.

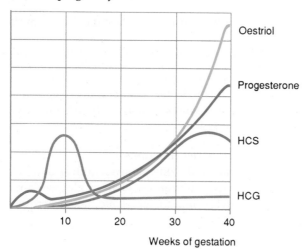

Figure 34.19
Pattern of hormone secretion during pregnancy. The scale used for oestriol and progesterone is the same, but differs from that for HCS and for HCG which are measured in i.u. (international units) instead of mmoles per litre. (Based on data in Hytten & Chamberlain 1991.)

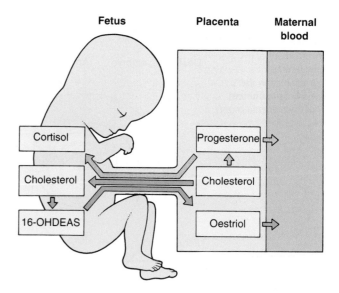

Figure 34.20
Formation of steroid hormones by the fetoplacental unit (16-OHDEAS – 16-hydroxydehydroepiandrosterone).

HCS, like HCG, is mainly secreted into the maternal circulation. It brings about many of the maternal adjustments necessary to support the growth of the fetus (see below).

Progesterone is synthesised by the placenta from cholesterol (see Ch. 10). The formation of oestrogens, however, is a cooperative process involving the fetus as well as the placenta (Fig. 34.20) (*fetoplacental unit*). Consequently, the urinary excretion of oestriol by the mother can be used as an index of fetal well-being. ⑪

Immune mechanisms

Placental and fetal cells are partly foreign to a woman's body because of the paternal component in their make-up. Yet they are not normally rejected but instead grow and develop alongside maternal cells and tissues.

The cells that ought to be in the front line for attack and destruction by maternal immune mechanisms are those of the syncytiotrophoblast that burrow into the uterine lining. However, these cells are unusual in that they lack proteins of the *major histocompatibility complex* (*MHC*). MHC proteins have to be present in the membrane of a targeted cell for many T cells to recognise them and swing into action (see Ch. 15). Consequently the cells of the syncytiotrophoblast are not attacked.

In addition, the growth and survival of the placental cells is probably promoted by substances produced by the endometrium that stimulate growth and suppress local immune responses.

MATERNAL CHANGES AND ADJUSTMENTS

During pregnancy, adjustments are made in many systems of the mother's body designed to prepare her to

⑩
What are the effects on the fetus of excessive alcohol consumption by the mother?

⑪
Where does cholesterol come from?

by the corpus luteum of the ovary under the action of HCG. Thereafter the placenta becomes the major source of the hormones involved. These are responsible for promoting the growth of maternal tissues, and for re-adjusting her physiological systems so that the mother can accommodate and maintain the fast growing fetus, whilst maintaining her own equilibrium. The systems involved include those determining:

- O_2 supplies and CO_2 disposal
- fluid and electrolyte balance
- nutrient balance
- defence and waste disposal
- temperature regulation.

In addition, there are changes in structural components of the body affecting posture and locomotion, and consequences for the nervous system affecting mood and behaviour.

Oxygen supplies and carbon dioxide disposal

The supply of oxygen to the growing fetus is protected by changes occurring in the mother in:

- ventilation
- numbers of red cells
- circulation.

Ventilation

The need for oxygen increases progressively during pregnancy with the growth of the fetus and of maternal tissues (uterus and breasts). At term, resting oxygen consumption is up by about 15% over non-pregnant levels.

More oxygen is needed also for the extra energy expended in daily activities because of the mother's weight gain (total 12.5 kg on average; approximately 20% of body weight).

Ventilation (see Ch. 7) increases progressively in pregnancy (Fig. 34.21). This is caused by progesterone increasing the sensitivity of the respiratory control system to CO_2 so that ventilation is greater at any particular level of arterial CO_2 than in the non-pregnant state. The depth of breathing increases but the number of breaths per minute does not change.

As a result of the increased ventilation, the partial pressure of oxygen in alveolar air increases and that of carbon dioxide decreases, with the result that maternal arterial PO_2 increases and PCO_2 falls by about 10 mmHg. These changes increase the rate of diffusion of gases across the placenta, facilitating fetal oxygen uptake as well as carbon dioxide excretion.

Red cell numbers

Production of red cells by the bone marrow is stimulated by erythropoietin and human chorionic soma-tomammotrophin leading to a 20% increase in the total

accommodate and support the growing fetus. In the first 2 months of pregnancy, when the fetus is relatively tiny and the placenta is at an early stage of development, the changes are largely produced by the hormones secreted

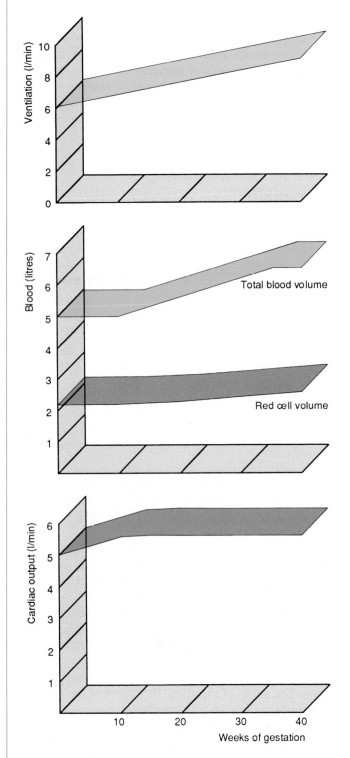

numbers of red cells in the circulation. However, as the volume of plasma increases as well by an even larger amount (Fig. 34.21), the numbers of red cells per litre of blood (*red cell count*; see Ch. 4) actually falls (*physiological anaemia of pregnancy*).

Circulation

The growth of maternal tissues causes an increase in the number of blood vessels in the circulation. In addition, hormonal changes cause relaxation of some vascular smooth muscle, leading to a fall in total peripheral resistance. For example, relaxation is produced by increased levels of progesterone and decreased responsiveness to angiotensin II. Circulatory pressure is maintained by:

- expanding blood volume (see Ch. 13 and below)
- increasing cardiac output (see Ch. 5).

The expansion in blood volume is made up of an increase in plasma volume of about 1 litre and by the progressive increase in total numbers of red cells which occurs throughout pregnancy (Fig. 34.21).

Cardiac output increases early in pregnancy reaching about 40% above the non-pregnant state by 3 months and remaining that way until term (Fig. 34.21). Heart rate and stroke volume both increase by about 15 to 20%.

As a result of all these changes in volume and cardiac output, arterial blood pressure normally hardly changes although there is usually a small decrease (about 10 mmHg) in diastolic pressure.

The expected weight gain during pregnancy is 2 kg in the first 20 weeks and 0.5 kg per week thereafter, amounting to approximately 12 kg in total. Increased blood volume accounts for about 1.5 kg and interstitial fluid for another 1 kg. The remaining weight increase is accounted for as follows:

- breasts 0.5 kg
- fat 3.5 kg
- placenta 0.6 kg
- fetus 3.4 kg
- amniotic fluid 0.6 kg
- uterus 0.9 kg.

(Bennett & Brown 1989)

Figure 34.21
Respiratory and circulatory changes in pregnancy. (Based on data in Hytten & Chamberlain 1991.)

Fluid and electrolyte balance

The expansion of blood volume in pregnancy is associated with an expansion also of interstitial fluid volume resulting in an increase of extracellular fluid volume by about 2 to 3 litres. The changes underlying this retention of salt and water are complex and involve:

- altered renal function
- altered sensitivity of control mechanisms. ⑫

⑫
What do you understand by 'interstitial fluid'?

Renal function

Many changes occur in renal function including alterations in:

- blood flow
- glomerular filtration rate (GFR)
- tubular transport.

Renal blood flow and GFR (see Ch. 8) both increase quite early on in pregnancy by about 50%. Consequently the renal tubules are presented with increased amounts of solutes to be recovered. Salt and water transport are both enhanced by the actions of aldosterone and ADH (see below) to more than match the increased load delivered but the transport of glucose and amino acids is not. Indeed the tubular transport maximum for both glucose and amino acids may decrease. Once the load of glucose and amino acids delivered to the tubules exceeds the tubular transport maximum (see Ch. 8) glucose and amino acids appear in the urine (*glycosuria and amino-aciduria of pregnancy*).

In the later stages of pregnancy when the fetal skeleton is growing at its fastest (see Ch. 35), absorption of calcium by the renal tubules increases and more calcium is recovered from the filtrate. Tubular reabsorption of calcium is stimulated by parathyrin which is secreted in increasing amounts by the parathyroid glands (see Ch. 10) as maternal blood calcium concentration falls.

Control mechanisms

The renin–angiotensin system (see Chs 10 and 13) is stimulated with the result that aldosterone secretion by the adrenal cortex increases. The secretion of aldosterone is also enhanced by increased secretion of ACTH by the anterior pituitary. This gland enlarges by about 40% during pregnancy. As aldosterone promotes the renal tubular absorption of sodium (see Chs 8 and 10), more sodium accumulates in the body.

Extra water is retained too as a result of the thirst-promoting effects of angiotensin II (and possibly prolactin) as well as by an increase in the sensitivity of the osmoreceptors in the hypothalamus to changes in osmotic pressure. This leads to a lowering of maternal plasma osmolality by about 10 mosmoles/kg H_2O after 3 months.

Nutrient balance

The fetus requires adequate supplies of all nutrients to support its growth relying chiefly on glucose for energy. Maternal dietary requirements are increased also by the growth of her reproductive tissues and the increased energy costs of her daily activities. The adjustments made to meet these demands include changes in:

- food intake
- metabolism.
- digestive function

Table 34.2 Increases recommended in daily dietary intake in pregnant women*	
Nutrient	% increase
Calcium	+140
Folate	+100
Zinc	+ 30
Iodine	+ 25
Protein	+ 11
Iron	+ 8

* Compiled from Truswell 1986.

Food intake

Appetite is stimulated early on in pregnancy probably by the effects of hormones such as progesterone on the feeding centres in the hypothalamus (see Ch. 31) as well as by the stimulus provided by the 10% decrease in fasting blood glucose concentrations that occurs in the first 3 months of pregnancy. Sometimes women experience cravings for unusual foods and substances (a condition known as *pica*), and distaste for other foods that were previously enjoyed.

In early pregnancy the intake of food exceeds immediate needs and consequently fat is laid down and provides an energy store for the mother in the later stages of pregnancy when the demands of the growing fetus reach their peak.

There is an increased requirement for various nutrients during pregnancy (Table 34.2). If these requirements are not met the fetus draws on the mother's reserves at her expense.

One still hears pregnant women being told that they must 'eat for two'. As with much traditional advice there is some sense in this recommendation. It means eating a well-balanced diet to provide the nutrients needed by the mother and the growing fetus, including adequate fibre and fluids to overcome any tendency to constipation. What it does not mean is frequent second helpings of gooey puddings, which are high in calories and low in nutrition!

Digestive function

The functioning of the digestive organs is affected by the change in hormonal balance during pregnancy. Chief among these is a reduction in tone and motility of the tract which is believed to contribute to:

- heartburn (see Ch. 6)
- feelings of nausea
- constipation.

Because of the reduction in motility it takes longer for food residues to pass through the gut. This does little to increase the absorption of nutrients such as glucose, amino acids and fats because these are already practically fully digested and absorbed in the non-pregnant state (see Ch. 6). However, it may enhance the absorption of water and salt in the colon, making the faeces harder.

The secretion of gastric acid decreases in the first half of pregnancy. This and the slower transit of food materials enhances the absorption of iron and calcium in the upper small intestine. Calcium absorption is also increased by calcitriol such that by 6 months calcium absorption is twice that of the non-pregnant state (see Ch. 13). ⑬

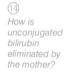

Why is increased calcium absorption necessary?

Metabolism

The mother's metabolism is readjusted so that energy stores in the form of fat are built up in the early stages of pregnancy and then drawn upon later. By using fatty acids in preference to glucose in the later stages of pregnancy, glucose is spared for the fetus. Extra glucose is also generated from amino acids by gluconeogenesis (see Ch. 14).

These metabolic effects are produced by the actions of several hormones including cortisol and the placental

⑭

How is unconjugated bilirubin eliminated by the mother?

SOME COMMON PROBLEMS OF PREGNANCY

Many women sail through pregnancy in the best of health; others are plagued by a variety of minor ailments, such as constipation and heartburn. To the mother, these ailments can be very distressing, for example the young woman who finds that her breasts and abdomen are covered in stretch marks (*striae gravidarum*). These marks are caused by the stretching and tearing of layers of tissue in the dermis. They are red at first when the mother's size increases, and they persist as silvery lines after the pregnancy. The application of creams and moisturisers during pregnancy does not always prove effective in preventing the appearance of stretch marks. If a woman values the perfection of her body, this type of disfigurement may cause her to resent her baby.

Constipation during pregnancy has two probable causes:

- progesterone-induced relaxation of the bowel
- pressure on the bowel from the growing fetus.

Change in eating habits may also be involved. Prevention should be the aim – more fibre-containing foods, more water to drink and more exercise such as walking. Apart from causing discomfort, constipation may aggravate small haemorrhoids which are already present.

Heartburn (see Ch. 6) may also be troublesome. Progesterone relaxes the oesophageal sphincter of the stomach and allows reflux of the stomach contents into the oesophagus. Later in pregnancy, the condition is exacerbated by the increasing size of the uterus and the baby, which displaces abdominal organs such as the stomach, making it easier for gastric contents to be squeezed into the oesophagus. An old wives' tale states that heartburn means that the baby will be born with a lot of hair!

Other ailments attributed to the relaxing effects of hormones and the increasing size of the baby are backache and varicose veins.

---

hormone human chorionic somatomammotrophin (HCS). HCS is secreted in increasing amounts during pregnancy (Fig. 34.19). It is similar in many ways to growth hormone and is therefore sometimes referred to as the 'maternal growth hormone of pregnancy'. Like growth hormone and cortisol, it has an anti-insulin effect which shifts metabolism towards the breakdown of fat stores (*lipolysis*) and the release of fatty acids into the bloodstream (see Ch. 14).

Waste disposal

The fetus produces many metabolic waste products including:

- CO_2
- urea, creatinine and uric acid
- unconjugated bilirubin.

All of these are eliminated via the placenta. In each case the substance diffuses across the barrier and is then eliminated via maternal excretory systems. Very little urea is formed by the fetus simply because the growing baby is in positive nitrogen balance (see Ch. 14). Bilirubin is formed from the turnover of red cells (see Ch. 4). Its production may increase if fetal red cells are destroyed by maternal antibodies. ⑭

Temperature regulation

A woman's body temperature rises by 0.5 to 1.0°C after ovulation (see p. 568) and remains elevated until mid-pregnancy if conception occurs. Thereafter it returns to its original level. Blood flow to the skin, particularly of the hands and feet, increases progressively during pregnancy and helps to dissipate heat. The increased blood flow may be caused by circulating vasodilator substances.

Women who have Raynaud's disease may find that their condition is less troublesome when they are pregnant. Circulating vasodilator substances help to preserve blood flow to their hands and feet.

Posture and movement

Posture is affected in two ways:

- altered weight distribution
- softening of ligaments.

The increasing weight carried abdominally by the woman has to be supported by a change in posture, and the spine becomes increasingly curved. Several hormones including progesterone and relaxin cause softening of the connective tissue linking bones at joints (*ligaments*; see Ch. 28), and therefore loosens the skeleton. This is important in making pelvic structures more flexible at the time of birth but can cause problems and discomfort in the later stages of pregnancy.

Mood

Along with the considerable physical changes occurring within a woman's body as a result of the altered secretion of many hormones come changes in mood and in sense of well-being. Some women in the middle stages of pregnancy can have a sense of never having felt so well before. There can be a heightened sense of awareness with many sensations appearing more vivid than hitherto. These passive changes in mood are intermingled with the normal anxieties and reactions associated with coming to terms with the new status of motherhood and the anticipation and fears associated with the imminent birth of a child.

PARTURITION

By convention, the length of gestation is timed from the first day of the last menstrual period prior to conception. Parturition occurs after an average of 40 weeks' gestation. During this time the uterus develops to accommodate the growing fetus but then, at term, it provides the muscle power to expel the new-born baby from the mother's body through the dilated cervix. The signals initiating the process of parturition in humans are not yet fully understood.

Uterine contraction

Like most other smooth muscle (see Ch. 22), uterine muscle can contract spontaneously. However, during most of pregnancy its contractile activity is held in check by the inhibitory action of progesterone. As pregnancy proceeds, ripples of contraction begin to occur once more (Braxton Hicks' contractions) causing very small changes in intrauterine pressure. As the levels of oestrogen rise towards the end of pregnancy (Fig. 34.19) these contractions become more frequent and more powerful.

The increasing level of oestrogen affects the uterine smooth muscle in two ways. It increases the number of:

- gap junctions between cells
- receptors for oxytocin.

The gap junctions (see Ch. 2) allow excitation to spread from cell to cell and therefore allow larger, concerted contractions to occur. Simultaneously, the increase in numbers of receptors to oxytocin allows the smooth muscle to become more sensitive to circulating levels of this hormone and more powerful contractions are produced that can raise intrauterine pressures to between 4 and 12 kPa (30–90 mmHg). These waves of contraction tend to begin at the top of the uterus, where some cells may act as a pacemaker, and sweep down towards the lower segment of the uterus (Fig. 34.22). These contractions, occurring during pregnancy before the cervix dilates, are usually painless but can be uncomfortable.

Cervical dilation

Towards the end of pregnancy the connective tissue of which the cervix is composed softens and the cervical opening dilates. The connective tissue softens probably under the action of several hormones such as oestrogens and relaxin. Dilation occurs under the pressure exerted by the fetus as it is squeezed towards the opening by uterine contractions (Fig. 34.22). Softening and dilation proceed fairly slowly.

As the cervix dilates, sensory receptors within it are excited. Some reflexly stimulate the secretion of oxytocin from the posterior pituitary; others give rise to the sensation of pain. The oxytocin secreted by the pituitary promotes further waves of contraction, which distends the cervix even more, and consequently even

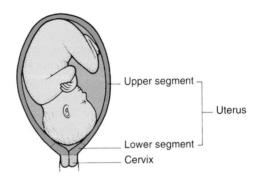

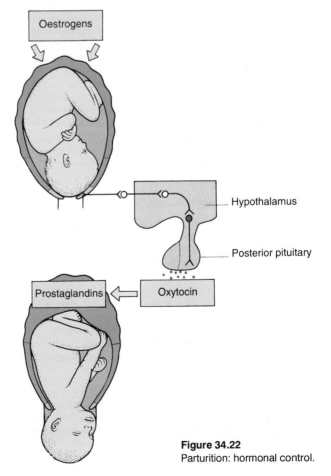

Figure 34.22
Parturition: hormonal control.

more oxytocin is secreted (positive feedback). Oxytocin increases uterine contractions by stimulating the formation of prostaglandins as well as by acting directly on its own receptors.

Delivery

Eventually the baby is expelled from the uterus which contracts down and the muscle fibres permanently shorten. This causes the placenta to be stripped away from the wall. Bleeding from the torn vessels is checked by contraction of the uterine muscle fibres around them. Further contractions of the uterus squeeze the placenta out into the vagina. The whole process from the beginning of labour to delivery of the placenta can take anything from a couple of hours to a couple of days. ⑮

PUERPERIUM

The puerperium is defined as the time from the end of the last stage of labour until most of the systems that changed as a result of pregnancy have reverted to their prior state. This takes about 6 weeks, at which time the first menstrual period postpartum may occur in a woman who is not breast feeding her child. Resumption of ovulation and menstrual periods is delayed, however, by lactation, which continues well beyond the end of the puerperium, from 4 to 18 months, or even longer.

Reproductive organs

At term, the uterus weighs about 1 kg. This reduces to the 50 to 100 g of the non-pregnant state by degeneration and shrinkage of cells and tissue. The muscle continues to contract spontaneously in response to oxytocin. This occurs particularly during breast feeding when oxytocin secretion is increased (see p. 580).

The degenerating lining tissues of the uterus, particularly around the placental site, are shed and leak out through the vagina for a few days after parturition. After a week the vaginal discharge (*lochia*) consists simply of mucus, leucocytes, epithelial cells and exudate. This secretion has a protective effect and guards against ascending infection.

A new endometrial lining then develops and, once ovulation occurs, undergoes the characteristic menstrual cycling of proliferation, secretion and shedding again (Fig. 34.14).

Body systems

The fluid retained during pregnancy is lost within a few days resulting in blood volume returning quickly to the non-pregnant state. Simultaneously cardiac output reverts too. With the sudden decrease in the concentration of vasodilator substances, such as progesterone, the tone of the muscle in the blood vessels increases.

⑮
Which hormone could be given by injection to stop bleeding after delivery of the placenta?

PLACENTA PRAEVIA

The placenta develops at the site of implantation of the trophoblast, which, ideally, takes place in the upper uterine segment (see Figs 34.7 and 34.22). Occasionally, the placenta develops either wholly or partially in the lower uterine segment (*placenta praevia*; see Figs 34.22 and 34.23). Depending on the area of the placenta attached to the lower segment, this is potentially a life-threatening condition. This is because, as the lower uterine segment grows and stretches after the 12th week of pregnancy, the placenta is likely to become separated from the uterine wall, causing bleeding from the maternal venous sinuses. Bleeding from the vagina after the 28th week of pregnancy is known as *antepartum haemorrhage*, and placenta praevia is one of the causes.

There are four types of placenta praevia:

- Type I is the least serious with only a small portion of the placenta attached in the lower segment. Normal delivery is possible and bleeding is usually minimal.
- Type II will allow normal delivery, but bleeding is likely to be moderate and the baby may suffer from hypoxia.
- Type III makes normal delivery impossible because the placenta is so placed that it would deliver first. Severe bleeding is likely to occur in late pregnancy.
- Type IV means that the placenta is attached centrally across the inner mouth of the cervix (*internal os*). Normal delivery is impossible and, when the placenta begins to separate, bleeding is torrential.

Placenta praevia can be diagnosed early for those women who attend antenatal clinics regularly and an elective caesarean section (see p. 579) can be planned. Those who do not have any antenatal care, for whatever reason, are at risk.

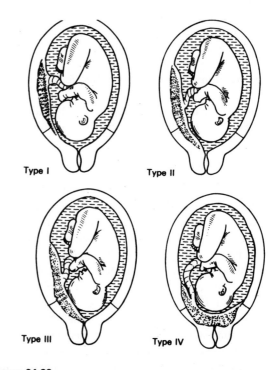

Figure 34.23
Types of placenta praevia. (Reproduced from Chamberlain & Dewhurst 1986 (Fig. 3.1) by permission of the publishers.)

Veins that became varicose during pregnancy, because of this loss of tone, gradually recover. Similarly there is recovery of tone in the smooth muscle of the gut and of the bladder, though, for the first few days, a woman may have some problems with constipation and retention of urine, exacerbated by the effects of childbirth on pelvic organs and muscles. Renal function (GFR, blood flow and structural changes) also gradually reverts to the non-pregnant state.

Newly delivered mothers are taught, and encouraged to continue, postnatal exercises. These exercises improve circulation in the legs, strengthen the pelvic floor muscles (to avoid future stress incontinence), ease backache and help return the abdominal muscles to the pre-pregnant condition. The exercises are beneficial to almost any woman, whether a mother or not, especially for easing backache and keeping the pelvic floor muscles in good condition. Full details of these exercises can be found in *Myles Textbook for Midwives* (Bennett & Brown 1993).

CAESAREAN SECTION

Sometimes a baby cannot be delivered per vagina. The alternative is to perform a caesarean section, an operation so named because Julius Caesar is said to have been delivered by that method. There are two types of caesarean section – classical and lower segment.

Caesarean section in the lower part of the uterus (lower uterine segment) is more commonly used because healing takes place more quickly and successfully. There is also less likelihood of rupture during future pregnancies because there is more fibrous tissue than muscle in this part of the uterus. The classical approach through the upper part of the uterus (upper uterine segment) is used before 32 weeks' gestation because there is not a clear division between the two segments at that stage of the pregnancy.

Caesarean sections are elective (i.e. planned before labour begins) for the following reasons:

● disproportion between the baby's head and the mother's pelvis
● types III and IV placenta praevia (possibly type II also) (see Fig. 34.23)
● three or more fetuses.

Depending on the mother's health during pregnancy and the condition of the fetus, caesarean section may also be planned if there is breech presentation (buttocks and feet in position to deliver first), hypertension due to pregnancy (*pre-eclampsia*), diabetes mellitus, antepartum haemorrhage or retarded growth of the fetus.

Emergency caesarean section would be performed during labour for the following reasons:

● prolapse of the umbilical cord
● eclampsia (untreated pregnancy-induced hypertension or rapid onset of hypertension)
● rupture of the uterus
● disproportion discovered during labour
● fetal distress
● failure of the labour to progress.

Mood

The sudden drop in the concentration of steroid hormones has a rebound effect on mood in many women and can result in a short period of depression just after the baby is born. If there were pre-existing tendencies to psychological disturbance then the effects may be more marked and more long lasting (*postnatal depression*).

LACTATION

Milk is formed by the mammary glands. The mammary glands grow at puberty (see Ch. 35). Further development and enlargement of the glands occurs during pregnancy. After parturition the formation of milk is stimulated and milk is expelled from the ducts of the gland in response to suckling.

Development of glands

The breasts develop during pregnancy under the combined action of several hormones including:

● oestrogens
● progesterone
● HCS (also termed HPL).

Some milk is formed during pregnancy but the amounts are small compared with the surge of production occurring after parturition. HPL (human placental lactogen) inhibits the production of prolactin (which promotes the formation of milk) and the fetoplacental steroids inhibit its milk-producing effects. Once the levels of these hormones have dropped dramatically postpartum, the action of prolactin is unrestrained.

Composition of milk

Human breast milk contains a mixture of nutrients and electrolytes. Its composition differs in a number of respects from cows' milk (Table 34.3). Notably it contains less sodium and calcium but is richer in vitamins C and D. Human breast milk also contains large quantities of IgG which are important in combating many microorganisms to which the baby will be

Table 34.3 Composition of milk (per litre)*		
	Human	*Cows'*
Energy (kcal)	700	670
Protein (g)	11	35
Fat (g)	40	37
Carbohydrate (g)	73	50
Sodium (mmol)	7	22
Calcium (mg)	350	1200
Vitamin C (mg)	38	15
Vitamin D (μg)	8	1.5

* Compiled from Truswell 1986.

exposed. After about a week, IgA (see Ch. 15) predominates in the milk and this confers some protection against microorganisms entering the baby's digestive system.

Suckling

The secretion of prolactin, which stimulates milk formation, and of oxytocin, which promotes milk ejection, are both stimulated by suckling (see Ch. 10). During pregnancy, the skin receptors around the nipples of the breasts, are not as sensitive as they are after the baby's birth. The stimulus of the baby's sucking reflexly excites the secretion of prolactin and oxytocin from the pituitary (Fig. 34.24). Prolactin secretion from the anterior pituitary is controlled by two hormones, prolactin releasing hormone (PRH) and prolactin inhibiting hormone (PIH) secreted by nerves of the hypothalamus into the portal hypophyseal blood vessels (see Ch. 10). Prolactin inhibits the action of LHRH on the secretion of FSH and LH by the pituitary as well as the actions of these hormones on the ovary. Consequently, ovulation and the return of menstrual cycles is inhibited. If suckling occurs frequently and regularly, ovulation does not reoccur in many women until breast feeding has ceased.⑯

What are your views on breast feeding?

BREAST FEEDING

Midwives and health visitors encourage a positive attitude to breast feeding because (briefly) breast milk is the correct food for a human baby and the activity of breast feeding helps to strengthen the bond between mother and baby. Breast feeding does not appeal to all mothers: some find the process embarrassing or 'messy'; some try to breast feed but give up easily; others may be discouraged by the unsuccessful attempts of friends or relatives.

Breast feeding is not easy for every mother. It has been likened to whistling – once you've got the knack, you enjoy it and want to keep on. The technique of suckling must be taught and supervised initially. The nipple is taken right into the baby's mouth, as far as the junction between the hard and soft palate (see Ch. 29); contact between the nipple and soft palate stimulates the sucking reflex. If the baby is allowed to chew, with his hard little gums, on the nipple, then it will become sore and cracked – and very painful. Breast-feeding mothers often find that milk is expelled from their breasts when they hear a baby cry or if they think about their baby. This can be managed by using adequate padding until the supply of milk and the baby's demands are coordinated. Breast milk can be expressed and stored, in a sterile bottle, in the fridge, so it is possible for parents to have an evening out, leaving the baby with granny or a baby sitter.

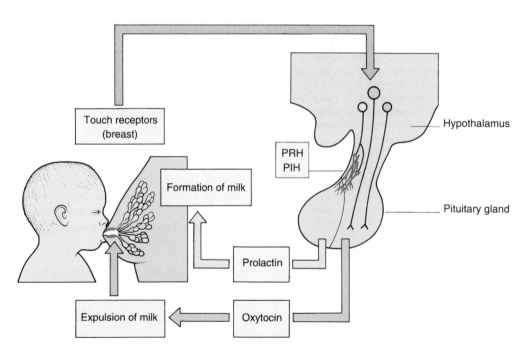

Figure 34.24
Hormonal control of milk secretion and ejection during breast feeding (PRH – prolactin releasing hormone; PIH – prolactin inhibiting hormone).

KEY POINTS

What you should now know and understand about sex, reproduction and pregnancy:

- the structure and function of the reproductive organs in men and women
- what physiological changes occur in men and women during sexual arousal and sexual intercourse, and how they are produced
- what the menstrual cycle is and how it affects a woman's body
- the anatomical and physiological basis of commonly used methods of contraception
- factors of importance in conception and how infertility may arise
- how conception normally arrests a woman's periods
- what the placenta is and what it does
- what changes normally occur in a woman's body during pregnancy and how they occur
- major events occurring at the time a woman goes into labour, gives birth, and recovers in the days immediately after
- the structure of the breasts and how the production and flow of milk is controlled.

REFERENCES AND FURTHER READING

Alberts B, Bray D, Lewis J, Raff M, Roberts K, Watson J D 1983 Molecular biology of the cell. Garland Publishing, New York

Bancroft J 1989 Human sexuality and its problems, 2nd edn. Churchill Livingstone, Edinburgh
(Covers all aspects of human sexuality, biological and psychological)

Bennett V R, Brown L K (eds) 1993 Myles Textbook for midwives, 12th edn. Churchill Livingstone, Edinburgh

Chamberlain G, Dewhurst J 1986 A practice of obstetrics and gynaecology, 2nd edn. Churchill Livingstone, Edinburgh, p 39

Edwards C R W, Bouchier I A D (eds) 1991 Davidson's Principles and practice of medicine, 16th edn. Churchill Livingstone, Edinburgh

Elder M G 1988 Reproduction, obstetrics and gynaecology. Heinemann Medical Books, Oxford
(Includes useful, and clearly presented anatomical and physiological background)

Emslie-Smith D, Paterson C, Scratcherd T, Read N W 1988 Textbook of physiology, 11th edn. Churchill Livingstone, Edinburgh

Filshie G M, Guillebeaud J 1990 Contraception: science and practice. Butterworth–Heinnemann, London
(Authoritative book for reference)

Hytten F, Chamberlain G 1991 Clinical physiology in obstetrics, 2nd edn. Blackwell, Oxford
(Very useful for further information on the changes occuring in a woman's body in pregnancy)

Koren G 1990 Maternal–fetal toxicology: a clinician's guide. Marcel Dekker, New York
(Useful reference work dealing with the effects on the fetus of drugs used in pregnancy, and other substances to which the mother may be exposed)

Larsen W J 1993 Human embryology. Churchill Livingstone, Edinburgh

Lincoln R 1991 Psychosexual medicine. Chapman & Hall, London

Mann T, Lutwak-Mann C 1981 Male reproductive function and semen. Springer, Berlin

Miller A W F, Callander R 1989 Obstetrics illustrated, 4th edn. Churchill Livingstone, Edinburgh

Page K R 1993 The physiology of the human placenta. UCL Press, London
(Advanced textbook providing an authoritative survey of current knowledge)

Rogers A W 1992 Textbook of anatomy. Churchill Livingstone, Edinburgh, p 121

Shaw R, Soutter P, Stanton S 1992 Gynaecology. Churchill Livingstone, Edinburgh
(Weighty but clearly presented book. Useful for reference)

Truswell A S 1986 ABC of nutrition. British Medical Association, London
(Collection of short interesting articles first published in the British Medical Journal. Includes one on pregnancy and one on infant feeding)

Wilkinson C 1992 Abnormal cervical smear test results: old dilemmas and new directions. British Journal of General Practice 42: 336–339

Williams P L, Warwick R, Dyson M, Bannister L H 1989 Gray's Anatomy, 37th edn. Churchill Livingstone, Edinburgh

Chapter 35
DEVELOPMENT FROM CONCEPTION TO ADULTHOOD

As you sit reading this book as a young adult or, not so young, mature student, you may marvel at the fact that all the information needed to direct your growth to the person you are now was once contained within a single cell (Fig. 35.1). Your personal development from conception to adulthood has been determined by the genetic blueprint contained within the nucleus of that cell. Expression of the genetic code led rapidly to differentiation of cell function in utero resulting in the baby that was born.

At birth, your environment changed abruptly. Within only a short space of time you adapted to totally new circumstances, leaving the wet, warm and sheltered environment of the uterus for a world in which you had to breathe air, adjust to hot and cold environments and begin to fend for yourself. After this momentous event you embarked upon roughly two decades of gradual, though no less important, change as you grew through infancy and childhood to maturity. The final burst of development taking you from childhood into adulthood was adolescence. During this period your reproductive system matured enabling you to pass on your genes to another generation.

FIRST STAGES OF LIFE

Your unique development plan was once tightly packed as 46 chromosomes (see Ch. 2) within a single cell. The expression of this genetic information played a major part in dictating the way you developed in utero from that cell to an embryo, a fetus and ultimately a newborn baby.

DEVELOPMENT AND FUSION OF THE GAMETES

Each new person is created by the fusion of one male and one female gamete (*spermatozoon* and *ovum*) (see Ch. 34). The primitive cells (*spermatogonia* and *oogonia*) that develop into mature spermatozoa and ova are produced in the fetal ovaries and testes (see Ch. 34). Each mature spermatozoon and ovum contains 23 chromosomes, only half the number present in other human cells. This halving of chromosomal number occurs as a result of *meiosis* during development of the gametes. When the gametes fuse, the resulting cell, the *zygote*, contains the full complement of 46 chromosomes. Spermatozoa and ova are both produced by meiosis but the staging of development differs between the two sexes.

If gametogenesis or fertilisation is impaired, zygotes may form containing a different number of chromosomes resulting in altered development.

Meiosis

Each human cell including the primitive gametes (spermatogonia and oogonia) contains 46 chromosomes (23 pairs). Each pair of chromosomes consists of two structurally similar chromosomes (*homologues*), one of maternal origin, the other paternal (Fig. 35.2).

The first event in the process of meiosis (Fig. 35.3) is the replication of DNA in each homologue to form *double-stranded DNA*. The two chromosomes of each pair come together and some reshuffling of genetic material occurs between them. When the first meiotic division begins, the 23 pairs of chromosomes line up around the middle of a spindle of microtubules formed between the two poles of the cell (compare with mitosis; Ch. 2). The members of each pair of chromosomes separate, 23 being drawn to one pole of the cell and 23 towards the other. The cell divides, forming two daughter cells each containing only 23 chromosomes, half the usual number (*haploid* cell).

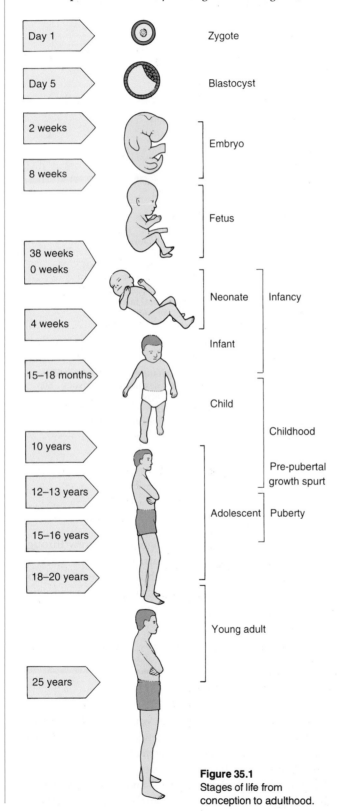

Figure 35.1
Stages of life from conception to adulthood.

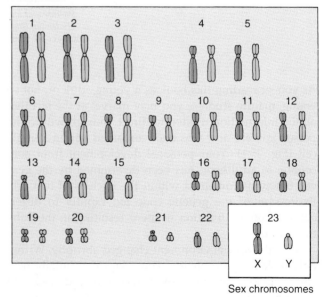

Figure 35.2
The 46 chromosomes of a human cell arranged in 23 pairs.
(Adapted from Williams et al 1989.)

The daughter cells divide for a second time (*second meiotic division*). The chromosomes again line up at the middle of the spindle of microtubules but this time the two strands of DNA in each chromosome separate and each is drawn to opposite poles of the cell along the spindle and the cell divides forming two daughter cells. The second meiotic division is similar to mitosis (see Ch. 2) but differs from it in that only 23 chromosomes are involved from start to finish instead of 46. The resulting daughter cells are the mature gametes (spermatozoa and ova).

Male

In the male, meiotic division of the spermatogonia begins in the testes at puberty (see p. 605) when the reproductive organs reach maturity. From then on, sperm production continues prolifically throughout life (see Chs 34 and 36).

Female

In the female, immature egg cells (*oocytes*) begin their first meiotic division whilst still in utero in the fetal ovaries. It is at this very early stage of life that reshuffling of genes inherited from parents occurs. Meiosis stops part way and the cells remain in this arrested state until they are stimulated by ovulation many years later to complete the process. Unlike the process in the male, when this first division occurs, the cell divides unequally yielding one large cell and a much smaller one, known as the *first polar body* (Fig. 35.4).

The second meiotic division takes place at fertilisation when a sperm penetrates the ovum. Division again occurs unequally yielding one large cell (the mature ovum) and a much smaller one (*second polar body*). Simultaneously the first polar body also divides creating a third polar body. The role of these polar bodies is unknown.

Altered development

The 46 chromosomes present in the fertilised ovum (*zygote*) consist of one pair of sex chromosomes, XX in the female and XY in the male, and 22 pairs of others (*autosomes*) (Fig. 35.2). Each pair of chromosomes and the genes within it, determine different characteristics of the maturing adult. If meiosis or fertilisation is disordered, zygotes that contain an abnormal number of chromosomes may form, resulting in altered development. Usually this precipitates spontaneous abortion at an early stage of pregnancy but sometimes the embryo may survive and a baby be born with congenital malformation. Abnormal numbers of chromosomes can result from:

- one or more chromosome pairs failing to separate during meiosis (*nondisjunction*)
- more than one sperm fertilising the ovum (*polyspermy*).

Nondisjunction

If a pair of homologous chromosomes fails to separate, the two gametes formed will contain 24 and 22 chromo-

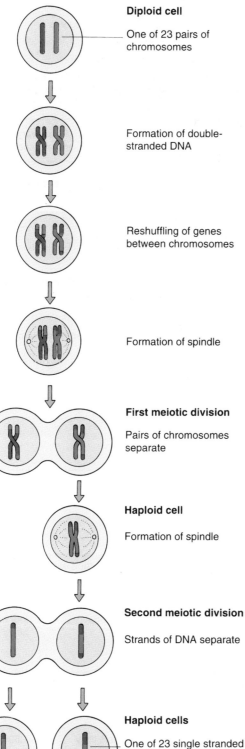

Figure 35.3
The process of meiosis.

Diploid cell

One of 23 pairs of chromosomes

Formation of double-stranded DNA

Reshuffling of genes between chromosomes

Formation of spindle

First meiotic division

Pairs of chromosomes separate

Haploid cell

Formation of spindle

Second meiotic division

Strands of DNA separate

Haploid cells

One of 23 single stranded chromosomes

somes respectively. When these aberrant gametes fuse with a normal gamete the resulting zygote will either possess 47 or 45 chromosomes.

If nondisjunction occurs with the sex chromosomes a variety of aberrant chromosomal patterns may result. For example, the pattern could be XXX if there was one sex chromosome too many or X alone (XO) if there was one missing (Table 35.1).

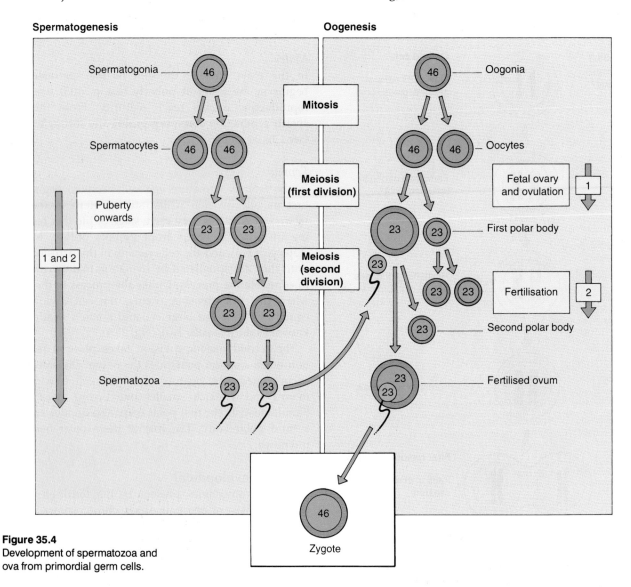

Figure 35.4
Development of spermatozoa and
ova from primordial germ cells.

Table 35.1   Examples of aberrant chromosomal patterns (karyotypes) resulting from nondisjunction of the sex chromosomes, and their consequences

Karyotype		Sex	Consequences	Name of syndrome	Incidence (per no. of live births of that sex)
Chromosome numbers	Sex chromosomes				
45	XO	Female	Impaired sexual development	Turner's	1:5000
47	XXX	Female	Minor		
47	XXY	Male	Impaired sexual development	Klinefelter's	1:500
47	XYY	Male	Minor		

An XO chromosomal pattern gives rise to *Turner's syndrome*, in which abnormalities are detectable at birth and there is abnormal maturation of the reproductive organs. An XXX pattern, however, tends not to give rise to observable abnormality until adolescence when the reproductive organs enter their final stage of maturation.

Nondisjunction can also occur with the autosomes. The most common is nondisjunction of chromosome 21 giving rise usually to an ovum with three (*trisomy*) rather than two chromosome 21s. The result is the development of *Down syndrome*.

Less common congenital abnormalities resulting in the development of grossly abnormal fetuses arise from nondisjunction of chromosomes 18 and 13.

Polyspermy

In the unlikely event that two sperm simultaneously penetrate the same ovum, the resulting zygote possesses a total of 69 rather than 46 chromosomes. This causes severe developmental disturbances, for example *partial hydatidiform mole*. Most result in early spontaneous abortion.

A *hydatidiform mole* is a conceptus consisting chiefly or entirely of placental tissue. A *complete hydatidiform mole* (all placental tissue and no embryo) results when the nucleus of the zygote consists entirely of paternal chromosomes, the maternal nucleus having disappeared before fertilisation. Complete hydatidiform mole occurs in about 1 in 500 pregnancies. A *partial mole* (some embryonic development) results when the nucleus contains twice the normal number of paternal chromosomes plus the normal number from the mother.

THE FIRST 2 WEEKS OF LIFE

Once fertilisation has occurred, the tiny developing ball of cells has just a fortnight to embed itself into the endometrium of the uterus and turn on the hormonal mechanisms that stop menstruation from occurring (see Ch. 34). If it fails, it will be aborted in the menstrual fluid.

Day 1

In the upper reaches of a uterine tube, a single spermatozoon penetrates an ovum (*fertilisation*) prompting the egg to undergo its second meiotic division (see p. 585 and Figs 35.3 and 35.4). The spermatozoon loses its tail, and its nuclear material is drawn towards the nucleus of the ovum. 12 hours after penetration of the ovum by the spermatozoon the maternal and paternal nuclei fuse and the genetic blueprint deciding the size, shape, sex and personality of the new individual is in place. 12 hours

later, at the end of the first day, the zygote divides forming two daughter cells and the process of development has begun.

Very soon after fertilisation, an immunosuppressant protein (*early pregnancy factor*) appears in the mother's blood. The detection of this protein is used as an early indicator of pregnancy.

Days 2 to 14

Cell division and differentiation

Cell division occurs every 12 to 15 hours with the result that 3 to 4 days after fertilisation the *conceptus* consists of a cluster of about 16 to 32 cells (*morula*) (Fig. 35.5). The

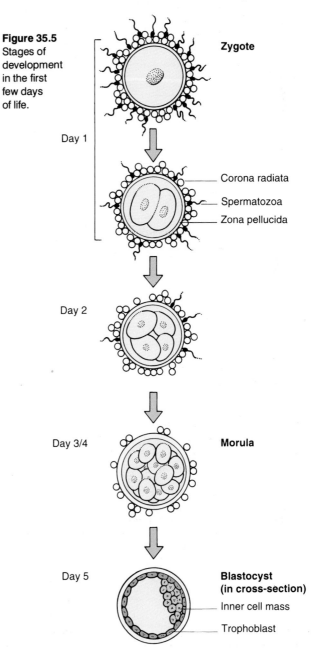

Figure 35.5 Stages of development in the first few days of life.

Day 1 — Zygote

Corona radiata
Spermatozoa
Zona pellucida

Day 2

Day 3/4 — Morula

Day 5 — Blastocyst (in cross-section)
Inner cell mass
Trophoblast

cells are still enclosed by the *zona pellucida* (see Ch. 34) and by some associated nutrient cells (*corona radiata*). The zona pellucida helps to prevent polyspermy by barring the entry of other sperm once the ovum has been fertilised. It also stops the conceptus attaching itself prematurely to neighbouring tissue such as the wall of the uterine tube.

① *What type of muscle is present in the wall of the uterine tube?*

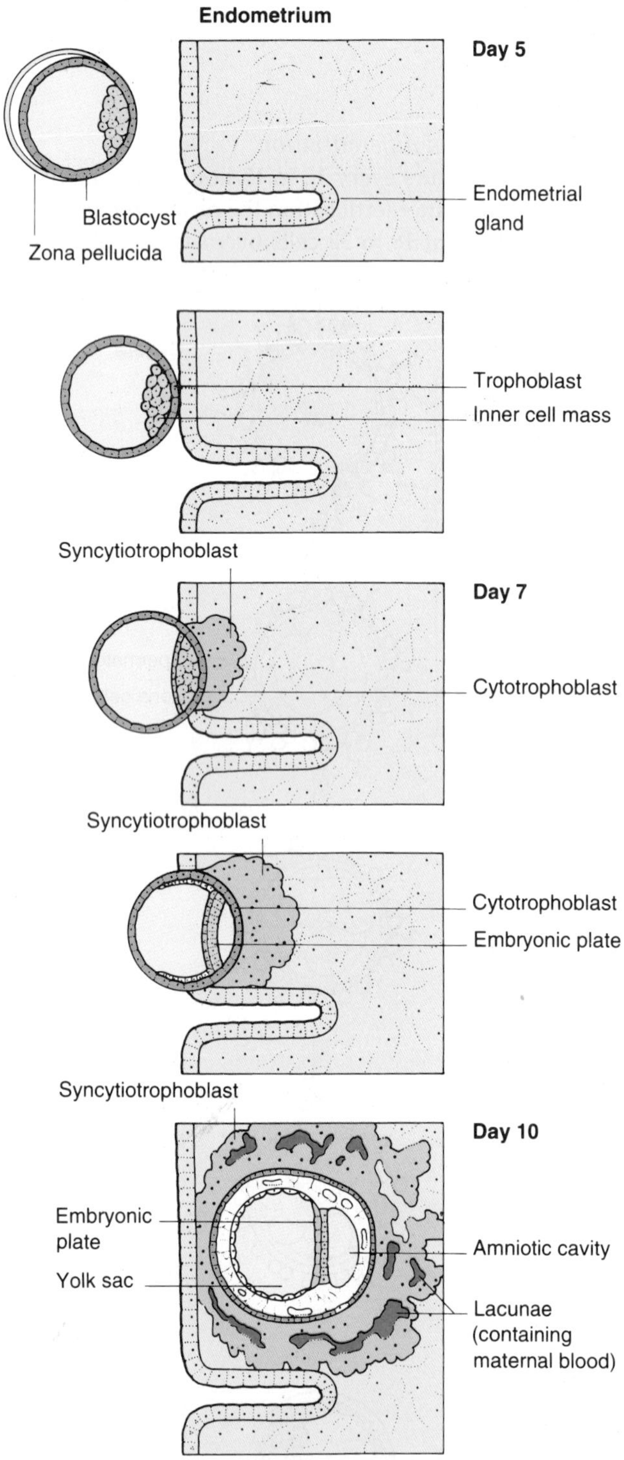

Figure 35.6
Implantation of the conceptus in the wall of the uterus.

② *Which other cells in the body store glycogen in large amounts?*

At about 4 days of life a space appears within the ball of cells. Simultaneously, the first signs of cell differentiation appear. Within the ball of cells and to one side is a small mass of cells (*inner cell mass*) destined to become the embryo (Fig. 35.5). At this stage, the ball of cells is termed a *blastocyst* and the cells forming its wall are referred to as the *trophoblast*. The blastocyst is swept into the uterine cavity by the action of cilia and the contraction of muscle of the uterine tubes. ①

TWINS

Twins may be identical or non-identical. Identical twins develop from the same fertilised ovum (*monozygotic twins*) whereas non-identical twins form as a result of the release and fertilisation of two ova (*dizygotic twins*).

Most monozygotic twins develop as a result of division of the inner cell mass into two parts at about the end of the first week of life. If division is incomplete, *Siamese twins* develop. These twins are joined together to a greater or lesser extent, and sometimes can be successfully separated by surgery after birth.

Some monozygotic twins develop as a result of the division of the cluster of primitive cells into two morulae, or two blastocysts, in the first few days of development.

Implantation

When the trophoblastic cells developing next to the inner cell mass make contact with the wall of the uterus (*endometrium*) they differentiate into two layers (Fig. 35.6):

● syncytiotrophoblast
● cytotrophoblast.

The cells of the *syncytiotrophoblast* burrow into the endometrium, *implanting* the blastocyst into the wall of the uterus. Implantation begins around day 6 or 7 and continues throughout the next few days so that the *conceptus* is completely embedded within the endometrium by the end of the first fortnight.

The syncytiotrophoblast digests its way through endometrial tissues, including blood vessels, secretory glands, and cells packed with stores of glycogen. Consequently at this very early stage the conceptus is surrounded by a highly nourishing environment. ②

Spaces (*lacunae*) appear within the syncytiotrophoblast, filled with maternal blood. These are the beginnings of the placental circulation.

Within the conceptus, differentiation and development is occurring. A space (*amniotic cavity*) develops between the inner cell mass and the cytotrophoblast. The original cavity of the blastocyst forms the *yolk sac* (Fig. 35.6).

The crucial events at this stage of development are those guaranteeing proper implantation of the conceptus. This depends on the endometrium and how it has developed under the action of hormones secreted by the corpus luteum (see Ch. 34). If development is deficient, implantation may not occur and the conceptus is aborted. At this very early stage of development the mother might only just be suspecting that something has happened. Her next menstrual period is due but should be arrested by the continued secretion of hormones from the corpus luteum.

EMBRYONIC LIFE

From the third week of life to the eighth, the conceptus is termed an *embryo*. Many crucial developments take place during this time.

Weeks 3 and 4

In weeks 3 and 4 there is an astonishingly rapid development of the cells of the *embryonic plate*. At the begin-

ning of the third week the embryonic plate differentiates into three layers (Fig. 35.7):

● ectoderm
● mesoderm
● endoderm.

The growth of this 'sandwich' of tissues accelerates, some parts overtaking others in their speed of expansion. As a result tissues fold lengthwise and horizontally so that the embryonic tissue is converted from a flat plate of cells into a C-shaped cylindrical body (Fig. 35.7). ③

By 4 to 5 weeks the flat plate has been transformed into a tiny embryo (Fig. 35.8) possessing:

● a primitive heart and circulation
● the beginnings of a nervous system
● embryonic eyes and ears
● the first suggestion of developing limbs.

All this is occurring at a time when the mother-to-be has only just realised that she may be pregnant. This and the month following are critical periods of development. So much is happening so very quickly. Any disturbances of development, caused by drugs, radiation or viruses, will at these early stages have profound effects and can lead to serious congenital malformations. ④

Weeks 5 to 8

During the second month of life the basic structure of each of the systems of the body is formed and by 8

③
What do the prefixes ecto-, meso- and endo- mean?

④
Which common virus can cause severe congenital abnormalities?

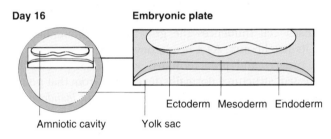

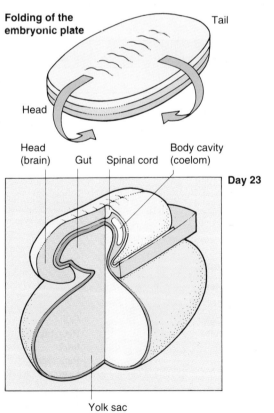

Figure 35.7
Folding of the embryonic plate.

Day 16

Embryonic plate

Amniotic cavity   Yolk sac

Ectoderm   Mesoderm   Endoderm

Folding of the embryonic plate

Tail

Head

Head (brain)   Gut   Spinal cord   Body cavity (coelom)

Day 23

Yolk sac

4–5 weeks   Lens pit (primitive eye)

Brain

Otic pit (primitive ear)

Heart

Upper limb bud

Spinal cord

Actual size

Lower limb bud

Connecting stalk

Yolk sac

Figure 35.8
Structure of the human embryo – 4 to 5 weeks of age (inset: actual size).

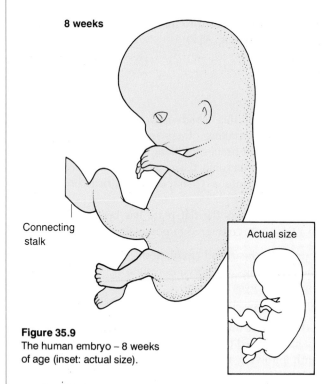

8 weeks

Connecting stalk

Actual size

Figure 35.9
The human embryo – 8 weeks of age (inset: actual size).

weeks of life the tiny embryo looks recognisably human (Fig. 35.9).

As a result of the folding of the embryonic plate, the amniotic cavity that was above the embryonic plate enfolds the embryo so that by 8 weeks the embryo is suspended in a fluid-filled cavity (Fig. 35.10A & B). A connecting stalk links the embryo with the developing placenta (see Ch. 34). The stalk becomes the umbilical cord containing:

- two umbilical arteries
- one umbilical vein.

Parts of the cavity of the yolk sac below the embryo (Fig. 35.7) develop into the digestive tract. Outpouchings from the yolk sac become the:

- lungs, trachea and larynx
- liver and digestive glands
- bladder and urethra of the urinary system.

The three distinct layers (*ectoderm*, *mesoderm* and *endoderm*) of the embryonic plate develop into different types of cells and tissues (Table 35.2). Organs usually consist of a mixture of these cell types. For example, the stomach is composed of neural, contractile, haemopoietic, epithelial and endocrine cells.

Each cell influences the growth and differentiation of its neighbours. As a result, development proceeds in an orderly and predetermined way. If the process is arrested, structures normally developing from that point may not form at all. For example the drug *thalidomide*, used in the 1960s as a sedative but now banned from use in pregnant women in some countries including the UK, critically arrests the development of the limbs and

Table 35.2 Embryonic origins of cells and tissues

Cell type	Germinal layer		
	Ectoderm	Mesoderm	Endoderm
Neural	CNS ANS Sensory receptors	–	–
Contractile	–	Muscle – skeletal – cardiac – smooth	–
Support cells	–	Cartilage Bone Skin – dermis	–
Haemopoietic	–	Erythrocytes Immune system	–
Epithelial	Skin – epidermis – glands – nails/hair Eye – lens	Blood vessels Renal tubules	Gut Respiratory tract Pancreas Liver
Endocrine	Pituitary gland Adrenal medulla	Adrenal cortex Ovaries Testes	Thyroid Parathyroids

Key: CNS = central nervous system; ANS = autonomic nervous system can affect the ear and the heart, structures that are forming simultaneously early in development (see Fig. 35.8).

FETAL LIFE

The *fetal period* is defined as that from the beginning of the ninth week of development to the time of birth (normally at 38 weeks). Considerable growth occurs during this period (see Fig. 35.16). The systems established in the first 2 months of life continue to mature, such that by about 6 months (26 weeks) the fetus is capable of independent existence, should it be born prematurely. In the last 3 months, further maturation occurs and stores of fat are built up in readiness for the transition from uterine to extrauterine life.

3 to 6 months

At about weeks 9 to 12 the fetal kidneys begin to produce urine. This is excreted into the amniotic cavity.

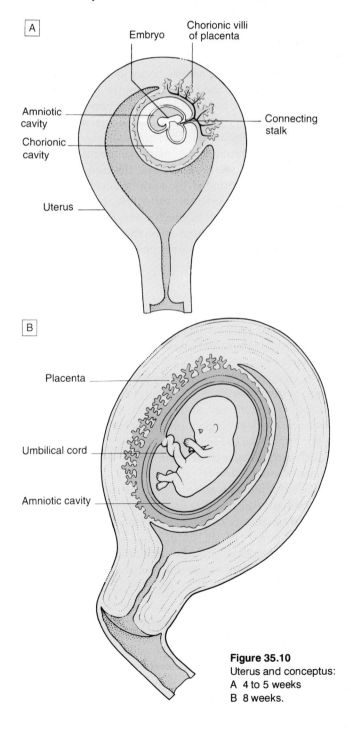

Figure 35.10
Uterus and conceptus:
A 4 to 5 weeks
B 8 weeks.

DETECTING ABNORMALITIES BEFORE BIRTH

'Is my baby normal?' is a question that many expectant mothers ask of the family doctor, midwife or obstetrician. Until the advent of specific blood tests, scanning, amniocentesis and other investigations, the only way to offer reassurance was by looking for normality in the mother's health, previous obstetric history (if appropriate) and that of female relatives.

Alphafetoprotein is present in maternal serum during pregnancy. Abnormally high levels indicate open defects of the fetus, for example open neural tube defects, because there is leakage of the protein into the amniotic fluid from where it reaches the mother's blood via the placenta. Some areas offer an MSAFP (maternal serum alphafetoprotein) screening programme to parents as part of the routine antenatal care.

Ultrasonic scanning (USS) is offered to many pregnant women. For those who are unsure of the date of their last menstrual period, because they have used an oral contraceptive, scanning provides an accurate assessment of gestational age. The mother requires little preparation other than having a moderately full bladder and being given an explanation of the procedure. Scanning at 6 weeks' gestation will show whether the pregnancy is intrauterine, whether there is more than one fetus and whether ovarian cysts or fibroids are present. Scanning at 16 to 18 weeks will show the presence of fetal abnormalities such as spina bifida and cardiac defects.

USS is also used in conjunction with amniocentesis so that the placenta can be avoided when a needle is inserted to withdraw amniotic fluid. Amniocentesis is usually performed between weeks 16 and 18 – prior to 16 weeks, there is insufficient fluid and, after 18 weeks, there may be insufficient time to arrange termination of the pregnancy should it be advised. This is because the amniotic fluid analysis may be not be completed within 5 weeks. The need for psychological support is probably greater than the physical preparation, which only requires the bladder to be empty so that it will not be punctured when the needle is inserted. It is possible to locate the placenta and obtain a suitable collection of amniotic fluid without the moderately full bladder needed when studying the fetus in detail.

Chromosomal analysis of cells from the amniotic fluid will confirm the presence of Down syndrome or the sex of the fetus when an X-linked disorder is a possibility. The detection of certain enzymes and metabolites in the amniotic fluid may indicate the presence of an inborn error of metabolism such as phenylketonuria. The presence of acetylcholinesterase in the amniotic fluid, together with a raised level of alphafetoprotein indicates the probability of a neural tube defect. It is possible to detect some genetic disorders, such as sickle cell anaemia and thalassaemia, by DNA analysis.

The fluid in the cavity (*amniotic fluid*) is ingested by the fetus, absorbed by the developing digestive system and then re-excreted.

Bones grow and ossification begins (see p. 602). As the nervous system develops, the fetus becomes active, makes movements and becomes capable of reflex responses. As the fetus becomes larger the mother usually becomes very aware of fetal movements.

Genitalia develop. In the female, the developing ovaries begin to produce primordial follicles ready for the next generation to be conceived (see Fig. 35.4). By the fifth month of life the fetal ovaries have manufactured all the 5 million ovarian follicles the woman-to-be will ever possess.

Also in the fifth month, the fetus becomes covered with soft downy hair (*lanugo*) and brown fat begins to form.

In the sixth month, the fetal lungs begin to produce surfactant, a substance extremely important in breathing (see Ch. 7) that must be present in sufficient quantities for the baby to be able to breathe easily after birth. Without surfactant the lungs are extremely difficult to expand.

Fetal movements are an important indication that the fetus is alive and not distressed. Patterns of movements vary; one fetus may be more active during the day and another may start exercising just as the mother is going to sleep! A change in pattern, reduced frequency or cessation of movements should be reported to the midwife immediately. Occasionally an active fetus will get the umbilical cord wound round its neck. Once the baby's head is born, the midwife always checks to make sure that the cord is not around the neck. If necessary, the cord is either loosened or clamped and cut before delivering the baby's body.

---

7 to 9 months

Maturation continues. Babies born from now on can survive, with assistance, but each remaining week in utero helps the fetus to build up its reserves (Table 35.3) and become more able to cope with the challenges it will meet at and immediately after birth. The nervous

⑤
How long does the neonatal period last?

Table 35.3 Growth of fetal energy stores towards the end of gestation

Stores	Weeks of gestation					
	20	28	31	33	34	38
Body fat content (%)*	1	3.5	—	—	8	15
Body carbohydrate content (g)*	—	—	—	9	—	34
Liver glycogen (%)†	—	—	1	—	—	4

* From Widdowson 1981.
† From Shelley 1964.

system is still developing. Each day that passes heralds the appearance of new responses, and better coordination of function and control.

The hair that had begun to grow all over the body in the fifth month is now well established and a head of hair is forming. As fat is laid down under the skin, the wrinkly 5-month-old fetus is transformed into the usually chubby looking full-term baby. By the time the baby is born, at about 38 weeks of age, body fat makes up 15 to 16% of its total body weight of 3.4 kg.

ADAPTING TO LIFE OUTSIDE THE WOMB

At birth, momentous changes occur in the functioning of different parts of the body. During the first few days and weeks of life the new-born baby (*neonate*) has to adapt to its completely new surroundings. Within the uterus it was supplied with oxygen, nutrients, minerals and vitamins through the placental circulation and waste materials were eliminated through the same route. It was surrounded by a warm cushion of fluid, protecting it from external variations in temperature and limiting the stimuli to which it was exposed.

Once the baby has been born the functions of the placenta are taken over by three major systems:

- respiratory
- digestive
- urinary.

Each of these systems began to function in utero, but each has to mature and adapt for the baby to survive after birth.

The changes in these systems, particularly the respiratory system, necessitate major changes also in the circulatory system and in its control. Relative sizes and positions of major organs of the thorax, abdomen and pelvis are shown in Figure 35.11A & B.

Although detached at birth from its mother, the human cannot survive independently of its parents, unlike some other creatures. This is because the nervous and musculoskeletal systems are very immature. Regulatory mechanisms maintaining internal stability in the face of external change, for example temperature regulatory mechanisms, are also immature. Consequently the neonate is more vulnerable to many external threats than the adult. ⑤

MAINTAINING OXYGEN SUPPLIES

In utero, oxygen and carbon dioxide were exchanged between maternal and fetal blood vessels of the placenta (see Ch. 34). Although breathing movements occur in the fetus no significant exchange of gases occurs across

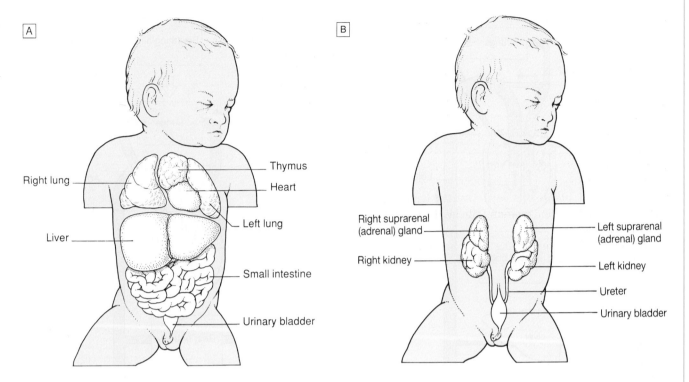

Figure 35.11
Major organs of the thorax and abdomen in the neonate:
A Thoracic and abdominal organs
B The urinary system and adrenal glands.
(Reproduced from Rogers 1992 (Figs 12.4 & 12.5) by permission of the publishers.)

the developing alveoli because it is amniotic fluid, not air, that is being moved into and out of the fetal lungs. At birth, when the baby takes its first breath, the lungs expand, the flow of blood through the lungs increases and the way the blood is routed through the heart changes. Change also occurs in the production of red cells and in the synthesis of haemoglobin.

> Normal, regular respirations are usually established within 60 seconds of delivery. Most midwives routinely clear the baby's mouth and nose of mucus, amniotic fluid etc., using a specially designed mucus extractor. This is usually sufficient intervention to encourage the baby to take his first breath; occasionally further steps have to be taken, for example to remove meconium from the airway. Holding the baby up by his ankles and slapping him is painful and dangerous – the spine is hyperextended, the intracranial pressure increased and the baby may be dropped.

Fetal and neonatal circulation

The main features of the fetal circulation are shown in Figure 35.12A. There are three pathways which are open in the fetal circulation and which begin to close at birth and normally remain closed in the adult. These are:

- foramen ovale
- ductus arteriosus
- ductus venosus.

Foramen ovale

The foramen ovale is a hole in the wall between the two atria. It is covered in the left atrium by a loose flap of tissue. Because the foramen ovale is directly opposite the openings of the veins, blood returning to the heart from the superior and inferior vena cava mostly passes straight through this hole into the left atrium. From there it is pumped into the left ventricle and then via the aorta to the organs and tissues of the body.

Relatively little blood passes from the right atrium through the right ventricle into the pulmonary circulation because the resistance to blood flow in the pulmonary vessels is high. This is partly because the lungs are not expanded, and the pulmonary blood vessels as well as the alveoli are relatively small in size, and partly because of the effects of local factors, such as oxygen and carbon dioxide concentrations, on smooth muscle in the pulmonary vessels (see Chs 5 & 7). ⑥

When the neonate takes its first breath, the pulmonary blood vessels expand because the pressure surrounding them (intrathoracic pressure; see Ch. 7) falls, and because local chemical conditions change. The resistance to blood flow drops and more blood passes through the pulmonary veins into the left atrium (Fig. 35.12B). This increases the blood pressure in the left atrium and forces the flap covering the foramen ovale tightly against the wall, closing off the opening. Continued pressure maintains this contact and eventually in most people the hole

⑥
What are the effects of low oxygen and high carbon dioxide concentrations on vascular smooth muscle of the lung?

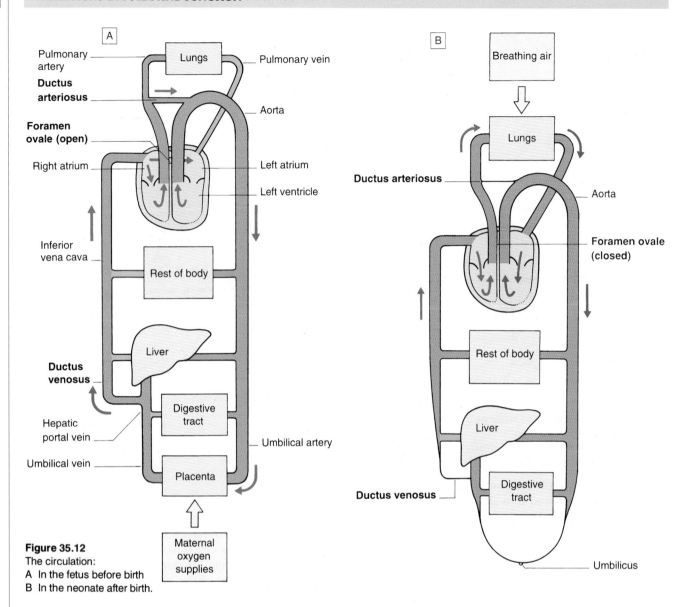

Figure 35.12
The circulation:
A In the fetus before birth
B In the neonate after birth.

is sealed off permanently by the growth of connective tissue.

Ductus arteriosus

The ductus arteriosus is a short vessel linking the pulmonary artery and the aorta (Fig. 35.12A). It is open in the fetus, diverting some of the blood pumped out of the right ventricle away from the lungs and into the systemic circulation.

The smooth muscle in the wall of the ductus arteriosus is very sensitive to the concentration of oxygen in the blood. When this rises (Fig. 35.13), after the baby has taken its first breath, the smooth muscle contracts and the vessel constricts. This reduces the flow of blood through the ductus arteriosus encouraging more blood to flow through the pulmonary circulation. Consequently, the pressure of blood in the left atrium increases pressing the flap covering the foramen ovale more tightly against the wall that separates the atria (*septum*).

NEONATAL HYPOXIA

If the baby should become hypoxic after birth, the muscle of the ductus arteriosus relaxes, the vessel dilates and blood is again diverted away from the pulmonary circulation. This is potentially serious because the fall in pressure in the left atrium may cause the foramen ovale to open up allowing deoxygenated blood back into the left side of the heart. The lowered oxygen concentration makes the ductus arteriosus dilate even more and the situation becomes even worse with even less blood going to the lungs.

Ductus venosus

The ductus venosus is a vessel taking blood from the hepatic portal vein directly to the inferior vena cava (Fig. 35.12A). It diverts some of the blood coming from the placenta away from the liver.

When the flow of blood through the placenta is reduced by uterine contractions of labour (see Ch. 34),

Table 35.4   Cardiorespiratory values compared

	Fetus (at term)	Neonate	Young adult
Heart rate (beats/min)	120–140	95–145	60–80
Blood pressure (systolic) (mmHg)	—	70–80	110–120
Respiratory frequency (breaths/min)	—	30–40* 40–80†	10–15

* Sleeping.
† Awake.

and later when the umbilical cord is cut, the quantity of blood flowing into the hepatic portal vein is reduced considerably and less blood passes through the ductus venosus (Fig. 35.12B). In due time the vessel shrinks, becoming just a small band of connective tissue (*ligamentum venosum*).

Lungs and breathing

After the first breath, the lungs grow very fast. The primitive conducting tubes sprout to form many more alveoli. In the first few months of life there is, as a result, a huge increase in the surface area of the lungs, vastly increasing the area available for gas exchange.

The respiratory rate in the neonate is higher than in the adult (Table 35.4). The baby breathes through its nose, cleverly managing to suckle and breath at the same time.

Red cells and haemoglobin

At the time of birth, the haemoglobin concentration is normally higher than that in the adult (Fig. 35.13 and Ch. 4), and rises for a day or two because of the loss of extracellular fluids (see below).

The sudden increase in the concentration of oxygen in the blood (Fig. 35.13) suppresses the secretion of erythropoietin. Consequently the production of red blood cells (see Ch. 11) decreases and the blood haemoglobin concentration falls over the first few weeks after birth. Simultaneously the type of haemoglobin synthesised changes from the fetal form (HbF), which avidly binds oxygen at low partial pressures of oxygen (Fig. 35.14), to the adult form (HbA) requiring higher pressures to become fully saturated (see also Ch. 7). ⑦

FLUID AND ELECTROLYTE BALANCE

In utero, the fetus was enveloped in amniotic fluid and its need for water and electrolytes was met by the mother via the placenta. For a few days after birth, the baby loses more fluid via the skin and the kidneys than it is able to replace from its feeds. Consequently it loses

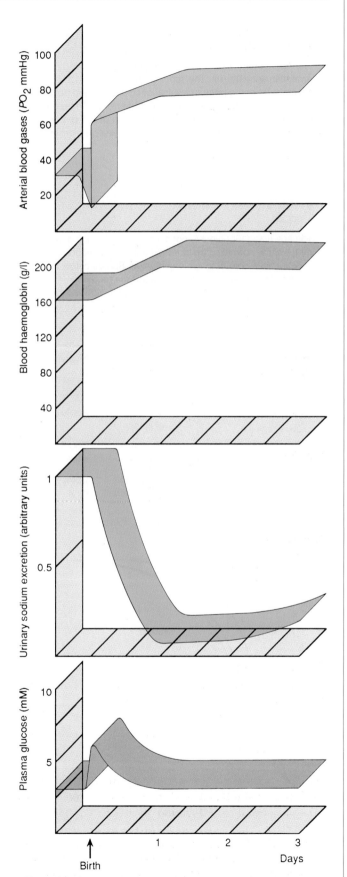

Figure 35.13
Some of the changes occurring at and after birth.
(Based on Case 1985.)

⑦
What is the difference in structure between adult and fetal haemoglobin?

APGAR SCORE

The Apgar score was devised by Virginia Apgar an American anaesthetist. The scoring system is an assessment of the baby's physical condition, carried out by the midwife at 1 minute and 5 minutes after birth. There are five signs, each of which is awarded a score of 0, 1 or 2. A normal baby scores 7 to 10. The signs assessed (in order of importance) are:

- heart rate
- respiratory effort
- muscle tone
- reflex response to stimulus
- colour.

The screening for colour is not always used, reducing the range of the normal score to from 6 to 8; this is recorded as 'Apgar minus colour' to avoid confusion. Scores below 7 (or 6) indicate a varying degree of asphyxia requiring resuscitation. The criteria used to score each sign are as follows:

Sign	0	1	2
Heart rate	Absent	< 100 beats/min	> 100 beats/min
Respiratory effort	Absent	Slow, irregular	Good or crying
Muscle tone	Limp	Some flexion of limbs	Active
Reflex response to stimulus	None	Minimal grimace	Cough or sneeze
Colour	Blue/pale	Body pink, extremities blue	Completely pink

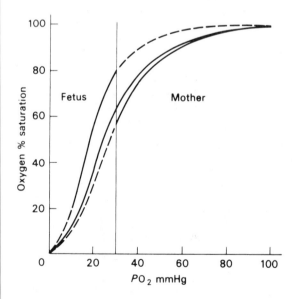

Figure 35.14
Oxygen–haemoglobin dissociation curves of fetal and maternal blood. The unbroken, continuous line in the centre is the curve for normal adult blood (see Ch. 7). (Reproduced from Hytten F, Chamberlain G 1991 Clinical physiology in obstetrics, 2nd edn, Figure 18.1, by permission of Blackwell Scientific Publications Ltd.)

weight. As the kidneys and regulatory mechanisms mature and as feeding becomes established, a securer balance is achieved between input and output of water and electrolytes.

Before birth

The fetus consists largely of water (more than 80% of body weight) (compare adult values; Ch. 13). During fetal development most of this fluid is extracellular, but by 38 weeks the ratio of extracellular to intracellular fluid is about 50:50.

The fetal kidneys produce urine from 9 to 12 weeks of life. The urine formed is excreted into the amniotic cavity contributing to the amniotic fluid enveloping the baby. The amniotic fluid also consists of fluid from the lungs and the skin. Amniotic fluid provides the baby with some freedom to exercise its growing limbs, which is important for proper development of the musculo-skeletal system.

Amniotic fluid is swallowed by the fetus, and its components are absorbed by the digestive tract and re-excreted.

At birth

At birth, the fluid present in the lungs is squeezed out as the fetus is pushed through the narrow birth canal. After the baby has been delivered, blood may drain from the placenta into the fetus (*placentofetal transfusion*). As about 33% of fetal blood volume is contained within the vessels of the placenta this transfusion may be quite large. The size of the transfusion depends on how quickly the cord is clamped. The volume transfused affects the neonate's blood pressure (pressure depends partly on blood volume; see Ch. 5) and the total number of red cells in the fetal circulation.

When the delivery of a baby is managed by a midwife, or doctor, the umbilical cord is clamped and cut sometime before the delivery of the placenta (third stage of labour). If the baby arrives quickly at home, or in a public place, without professional help, then it is safest not to tamper with the cord because the risk of infection and haemorrhage would be high. The baby (and the placenta if it has been expelled) should be wrapped warmly and professional help sought.

After birth

After birth, the baby loses water through its skin, which is much thinner than in the adult, and water and salts through the kidneys. As these losses are not immediately matched by an equivalent increase in fluid intake, the baby loses weight (up to 10% of its birth weight within the first few days). Most of this loss is from the extracellular fluid compartment (interstitial fluid and plasma).

As endocrine and renal systems (see Chs 10 and 8) adapt to new circumstances, the kidneys conserve more water and salt, and urinary losses decrease (Fig. 35.13). Simultaneously the intake of fluid increases as oral feeding begins and a new balance is established.

Over the first 2 to 3 years of life the power of the kidneys to conserve water and salts, and to excrete waste increases, with the result that the growing child is better able to tolerate disturbances in fluid and electrolyte balance. Until then, babies and young children are at greater risk of dehydration than an adult, especially during episodes of diarrhoea and vomiting. ⑧

NUTRIENT SUPPLIES

In the last few months of fetal life, stores are built up, providing the neonate with reserves to draw upon immediately after birth. After birth the digestive system (see Ch. 6) rapidly adapts to processing milk instead of amniotic fluid, and endocrine control systems gradually adapt to meet the challenges posed by intermittent feeding, increased activity and other stresses.

Before birth

In utero, all nutrients were supplied to the fetus through the placenta. Fetal glucose concentration is about half that in the mother and varies with her blood glucose concentration. Towards the end of fetal development stores of fat and carbohydrate build up (Table 35.3).

At birth

The stress of birth increases activity in the sympathetic nervous system, and large amounts of adrenal medullary hormones (adrenaline and noradrenaline) are secreted. These hormones promote the breakdown of glycogen to glucose, and fats to fatty acids (see Chs 10 and 19). This increases blood glucose concentration immediately after birth (Fig. 35.13), helping to maintain energy supplies when the supply of nutrients through the placenta ceases.

After birth

The neonatal digestive system rapidly adapts to processing a diet of milk. Digestive enzymes are synthesised and secreted to break down the constituents of milk. Of these, lactase is extremely important as it digests the main carbohydrate in milk, lactose. Movements of the gut propel the ingested milk through the digestive tract and push out accumulated waste materials. The first stool to be passed consists of epithelial cells, undigested mucus, and bile pigments (collectively referred to as *meconium*). The stool is black or dark green in colour due to the presence of bile pigments (see Ch. 9). In a few days the stools become greeny-brown. Eventually, as breast feeding is established and the digestive system develops, the soft stools become yellowish. Bowel motions occur very frequently, up to seven times a day in breast-fed babies, and evacuation occurs reflexly. ⑨

One of the major changes occurring after birth is increased secretion of many gastrointestinal hormones, including gastrin, CCK-PZ, motilin and GIP (see Ch. 6). These hormones:

● promote the growth of the digestive system
● stimulate digestive activity
● promote the secretion of insulin.

DEFENCE AND WASTE DISPOSAL

The new-born baby has to develop its ability to deal with bacteria, viruses, toxins and other environmental chemicals. As with the other systems, there are at first some short-term measures tiding the neonate over while its own systems of immunity and waste disposal develop.

Immunity

Before birth, some antibodies (IgG class; see Ch. 15) cross the placenta from mother to fetus, providing the

⑧
What might cause diarrhoea and vomiting?

⑨
How many other digestive enzymes can you name?

INFANT IMMUNISATION SCHEDULES

Prior to the introduction of wide-scale immunisation in the 1950s, the prevalence of childhood infectious diseases was responsible for the high infant mortality rate. In 1940 there were 46 281 cases of diphtheria with 2480 deaths; between 1979 and 1986 there were 26 cases and 1 death. The cases of paralytic polio were reduced from 4000 in 1955 to 35 between 1974 and 1978 – this included 25 cases in 1976–1977 when infection occurred in unvaccinated people. Since the introduction of immunisation against measles in 1968, the number of notified cases has dropped from hundreds of thousands each year to an average of less than 100 000 – but up to 1992 there was still an average of 13 deaths a year. The most recent immunisation to be introduced protects against Hib (*Haemophilus influenzae* type b) infection. This bacterium causes several illnesses, including one type of meningitis, severe croup, pneumonia, and joint, blood and bone infections. In 1992, Hib was the commonest cause of meningitis in children under 4 years old – about 65 died each year and about 150 were left with permanent brain damage (HEA 1992).

All children need help to fight against infectious diseases, the continuing death rate caused by measles is probably due to the reluctance of some parents to allow their children to be immunised. Unless there are contraindications specified by a doctor, all children should be immunised. The recognised schedule is as follows:

Vaccine	Age
Diphtheria/tetanus/pertussis, oral polio, Hib	lst dose: 2 months 2nd dose: 3 months 3rd dose: 4 months
Measles/mumps/rubella	12–18 months
Diphtheria/tetanus, oral polio	4–5 years

neonate with some protection against bacterial infection. After birth, the neonate acquires more maternal antibodies (IgG, IgA and IgM) from breast milk.

> The presence of maternal antibodies in breast milk is just one of the reasons why it is the most suitable nourishment for the human baby. Modified cows' milk contains all the nutrients required by the baby but does not provide any protection against early infections.

Lymphoid tissue forms early in development (from the fifth week of life) and develops through fetal, and neonatal life, infancy and childhood until puberty. Tonsils and adenoids reach their maximum size at about the age of 6 years, whereas the thymus, though already relatively large at birth (Fig. 35.11A), attains its maximum size around puberty. ⑩

⑩
What does the thymus do?

Disposal of liposoluble waste

One of the problems faced by the new-born is the elimination of liposoluble waste materials, such as bilirubin. In utero, these substances passed across the placenta by passive diffusion and were processed by the mother's liver, before being excreted in her urine (see Chs 9 and 15). At birth, the capacity of the neonatal liver to process such substances is low. This contributes to the jaundice occurring in some babies shortly after birth as a result of the breakdown of large numbers of red cells. After birth, enzyme systems, such as conjugases metabolising liposoluble substances, increase in activity, with the result that waste products such as bilirubin are processed more efficiently, and jaundice disappears, normally within a week.

TEMPERATURE REGULATION

At birth, the baby is expelled from the relatively stable environment of the mother's uterus, into one which may be hot or cold and which may suddenly change from one to the other. The neonate's ability to thermoregulate is very limited.

Before birth

The fetus produces heat through metabolism, and in the later stages of pregnancy from the exercise it has kicking and moving inside the uterus. Fetal temperature (38°C) is above that of the amniotic fluid (37°C). Surplus heat is carried away in the blood flowing through the placenta. In utero the danger to the fetus is usually one of overheating. If the mother's body temperature rises in a fever, fetal temperature rises too.

⑪
How does water move through the skin?

At birth

At birth, there is usually very rapid heat loss. There can be a fall of 1°C every 5 minutes in some circumstances,

for example in an exposed, very low birth weight (1 kg) baby, resulting rapidly in hypothermia. In a cold environment the baby loses heat by:

- conduction and convection to the cooler air
- evaporation of water from its skin
- radiation to colder objects such as windows and walls.

> It is important that the delivery room is comfortably warm, that the baby is dried, and is insulated from the cooler environment by clothing, or by nestling against its mother.

After birth

Temperature regulating mechanisms (see Ch. 16) gradually mature in the first few years of life but during this time the infant or young child is especially vulnerable to extremes of temperature, and depends on the caregiver for protection.

Heat production

The neonate generates heat in several ways:

- basal metabolism
- assimilation and metabolism of food
- physical activity
- metabolism of brown adipose tissue (BAT).

Of these, the main source of extra heat in a cold environment is BAT. There is brown adipose tissue over the shoulders, around the kidneys and over the heart. BAT is a useful source of energy but it is only an emergency mechanism. Energy from the diet which is used to generate heat reduces that available to power growth.

Heat loss

New-born babies lose heat relatively easily because of:

- large surface:volume ratio
- transepidermal water loss.

For its mass, a baby has a proportionately larger skin surface area than an adult and consequently loses relatively more heat by convection, conduction and radiation. Also the skin of the new-born is very thin particularly in premature infants. A lot of water is lost through it and heat is used up in evaporating this water from the skin surface. However, adaptation of the skin occurs rapidly in the weeks after birth and water losses decrease. ⑪

Maintaining body temperature

The thermoneutral zone (see Ch. 16) for babies is about 32 to 36°C. Below this range of environmental temperatures, the naked baby maintains core temperature chiefly by increased metabolism of brown fat (*nonshivering thermogenesis*; see Ch. 16 and Fig. 35.15). Blood flow to the skin, and therefore heat loss, is reduced by

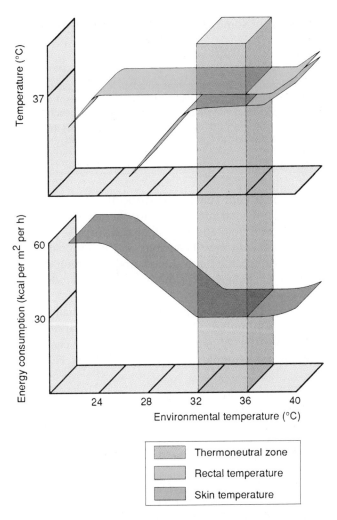

Figure 35.15
Maintenance of core body temperature in the naked neonate by cutaneous vasoconstriction and non-shivering thermogenesis. (Adapted from Rutter 1992 and Turner 1988.)

vasoconstriction. However, the best insulation for a baby in a cold environment is suitable clothing and bedding.

> If a baby's rectal temperature is normal but its skin feels cool, the baby is probably maintaining its body temperature by metabolising brown fat and is therefore using up extra calories to stay warm.

Losing heat in a hot environment is also a problem for the new-born in that sweating mechanisms are not yet very effective. The number of active sweat glands increases steadily up to the age of about 2 years.

REFLEXES, AWARENESS AND ABILITIES

Although considerable development of the nervous system occurs before birth, maturation of the nervous system continues for many years afterwards. Maturation

is visible to parents and friends in the almost daily changes occurring in the baby's and young child's awareness, behaviour and abilities. The new-born baby responds to the stimuli of light and sound and touch by simple reflexes. As maturation occurs during the first year of life, the infant develops the ability to make more complex movements and begins to make sense of the stimuli around it. Skills and understanding develop further in the second year of life when the infant begins to talk and to take charge of its own behaviour. ⑫

The first few months
The new-born baby responds reflexly to many different stimuli. In response to:

- bright light – it blinks
- a sudden sound – it startles
- oral stimuli – it sucks
- an object pressed against its palm – it grasps
- backward movement of its head – it extends its arms (*Moro reflex*).

These are just a few of the many simple reflexes that can be elicited. The presence of the reflexes shows that the sense organs are functioning and that simple neural links have been established between sensory and motor systems.

As the baby grows older, and the nervous system matures, behaviour and capabilities change as reflex responses become more complicated. Whereas the new-born baby is simply startled in response to a sudden sound, the 3- to 4-month-old baby turns its head to face the source of the sound. Whereas a new-born baby simply gazes at a face, following every movement with its eyes, a 4- to 6-week-old baby responds to a familiar face (such as its mother's) by smiling.

Coordinated reflex activity of different muscle groups develops enabling the baby to sit up, stay sitting and keep his head erect. What the baby lacks in his first few months of life and develops later is the careful control exercised by higher centres in the brain (cerebrum and cerebellum) over spinal and brain stem mechanisms (see Chs 27 and 28). For example, when a baby of 3 to 4 months old reaches out for an object he usually misjudges where it is, rather like an adult with cerebellar dysfunction (see Chs 27 and 28). A 6-month-old infant can voluntarily grasp an object in his hand but he has yet to develop the skill of picking things up with his fingers. He makes sounds but cannot yet form them into words. These skills of manipulation and speech rely on the maturation of function of the motor areas of the cerebral cortex and adjacent association areas, as well as the stimulation provided by the infant's environment.

The first year (infancy)
In the second 6 months of life the cerebellum and the cerebral cortex develop more control over posture and

⑫
What sort of stimuli interest a young baby?

⑬

How might you help an infant of 9 to 12 months learn the meaning of words?

movement, and many neural links are forged within the association areas of the cerebral cortex (see Chs 30 and 33).

Posture and movement

The infant progressively develops the ability to raise his head, sit, stand and then to walk, albeit in a tottering way. Control over head movements develops first, followed by control over arms and hands and then legs, the same sequence of maturation as in utero. As manipulative skills develop, the clumsy grasp is replaced by 1 year of age by a careful picking up of objects between finger and thumb. Coordination develops too so that the 9-month-old infant can, with some success, use a spoon to feed himself.

Understanding

At 7 months of age an infant usually responds to his name. Sufficient learning of the sound and the associated stimuli has occurred for him to respond appropriately. By 9 to 12 months of age he is able to imitate sounds and has understanding of the associations

(meanings) of some of the complex sounds (words) he hears. ⑬

Occasionally, an infant becomes so adept at using gestures instead of sounds/words, and his parents equally adept at interpreting the gestures, that the development of speech is delayed. The infant knows the correct words and can say them, but pointing and grunting are often quicker and easier!

The second year (early childhood)

The developmental programme for the nervous system continues to unfold and to delight and surprise parents and friends with new behaviour and communication. Movements become more skilled, understanding develops, and the infant takes more control over what he does.

By about 13 months of age the infant can usually walk unaided but, rather like someone with Parkinson's disease (see Chs 27 and 28), he has difficulty changing direction, for example when turning corners. He uses

---

DEVELOPMENTAL ASSESSMENTS

The health visitor carries out a series of developmental assessments until the child reaches school age. These assessments are usually carried out at home because a truer picture of the child's abilities is seen when he is in his own, familiar environment. Some assessments, such as hearing tests, may be performed at the health clinic because two experienced people are needed to test hearing accurately; all children have a hearing test when 8 to 9 months old. Health visitors receive special training in this skill.

Children can be assessed using the following broad headings:

- *Infant stimulation/motor (gross and fine)* – how a baby responds to his environment and progresses through sitting, crawling and walking, at the same time developing more precise skills, such as doing up buttons.
- *Cognitive* – general understanding, for example plays pat-a-cake, stacks blocks.
- *Development of language* – which is closely associated with hearing and vision.
- *Self-help* – how the child learns to feed, dress and wash himself.
- *Socialisation* – how the child responds to others, parents, siblings, strangers.

These areas of development are all interrelated and must be used to form a whole picture of the child's development. For example, if a child has not developed the appropriate motor skills to stack blocks, it doest not mean that he is lacking in understanding; similarly, a deaf or blind baby will not be able to respond in the normal way but is not necessarily lacking in intelligence.

Parents and those associated with child care look for essential developmental milestones, for example the first

smile at 4 to 6 weeks, and if these are not attained at the appropriate age further investigations may be necessary.

The following is a brief list of the main milestones:

4 to 6 weeks	Smiles – usually at mother
12 to 16 weeks	Turns head to sound
	Holds object placed in hand
12 to 20 weeks	Watches own hands – hand regard
20 weeks	Reaches for and grabs objects
26 weeks	Transfers objects from hand to hand
	Sits – supported by hands
	Chews and feeds self with a biscuit
	Lifts head when supine
9 to 10 months	Uses index finger to investigate objects
	Uses thumb and forefinger to pick up small objects
	Crawls/creeps
	Plays pat-a-cake, waves bye-bye
	Holds out arm for coat etc. when being dressed
13 months	Casting – throwing toys from cot, high chair
	Walks unaided
	Two to three single words
15 months	Stops casting
	Feeds self
	Stops putting objects in mouth (mouthing)
15 to 18 months	Mimics household tasks (e.g. dusting)
18 months	Becomes aware of toilet needs
21 to 24 months	Joining two to three words
2 years	Dry by day – occasional 'accident'
3 years	Dry by night
	Able to dress self except for difficult fastenings
	Able to stand, briefly, on one foot.

his hands a lot to build, pick up objects, and feed himself. He imitates his mother's actions. Sounds that he makes become strung together into language, at first unintelligible (to parents, that is) but then forming simple sentences. These new behaviours reflect the development of Wernicke's and Broca's areas (see Ch. 30).

By the age of 2 years, the child develops some understanding of the sensations associated with defaecation and urination and begins to take deliberate action in response to them. This and other similar behaviours represent the beginnings of purposeful voluntary activity. More and more control is exercised over primitive reflex behaviours as the cerebrum increasingly dominates the activities of the brain stem and spinal cord.

GROWTH

Growth has been defined as 'the progressive development of a living being or part of an organism from its earliest stage to maturity, including the attendant increase in size' (Butterworths Medical Dictionary 1978). It includes therefore the changes occurring in the structure and properties of different cells as well as overall increases in the size of the body and its constituent parts. These changes follow a genetically determined pattern but are influenced by other factors including nutrition and hormones.

BODY SIZE

The most rapid period of growth occurs in utero (Fig. 35.16). Thereafter, there is steady growth in height and weight until the adolescent growth spurt preceding adulthood.

Height
97 to 98% of the height of the body is due to the bones of the skeleton and the intervening fibrocartilaginous discs. Growth in height therefore represents growth of bones and joints. Height depends also on posture and muscle strength.

Weight
The weight of the body depends largely on three tissues:

- bone
- muscle
- adipose tissue.

Body weight increases more or less in line with the increase in height, but whereas linear growth stops in adulthood because bones stop increasing in size, weight can continue to increase as a result of physical training, which develops muscle tissue (see Chs 17 and 22), or of overeating, which increases fat stores (see Ch. 14).

THE PORTAGE HOME TEACHING SCHEME

Sadly, some children do not follow the normal pattern of mental development, and remain retarded throughout their lives. Early in the twentieth century these children were admitted to special hospitals for the mentally deficient where they received little, if any, stimulation. The Mental Health Act of 1960 abolished from legal usage the term 'mental deficiency' together with the classifications of idiot, imbecile and feeble minded. Since then, the terms 'mental subnormality' followed by 'mental handicap' have been used. More recently, the study of learning theories has increased the understanding of the problem, and affected children are referred to as having specific learning disabilities – in other words, they are no longer graded and labelled. Most people with learning disabilities are not physically ill and whenever possible they are cared for in the community, preferably at home. There are various schemes for helping the pre-school child who has a learning disability; one is known as the Portage Home Teaching Scheme.

Portage is the name of a town in Wisconsin USA where the model was first developed by David and Martha Shearer and their colleagues. It is a home teaching service for pre-school children with specific learning disabilities. To qualify for home teaching, the child has to be at least 1 year behind the normal development expected for his age, except in the case of babies born with known handicapping disorders such as Down syndrome. For Down syndrome babies, the teaching is commenced as soon as the diagnosis is confirmed; for example the mother is shown how to provide extra stimulation of all the senses and to note the baby's responses. This helps to identify areas where the baby's learning may be particularly slow.

The home teaching team is usually led by a senior clinical psychologist and the teachers may be professional people, for example health visitors, social workers or others trained to use the system. After assessment of the child by the psychologist, the teacher visits on a weekly basis, setting precise tasks for the mother (or carer) to carry out with the child each day. The teacher assesses the child's ability to achieve the task and sets criteria for attainment; for example 'Ben will pull off socks', to be carried out four times a day, success criterion – three times out of four. Ben will have had previous tasks where he has pulled off his socks with help; now he is expected to manage unaided. These tasks cover all areas of development – socialisation, language, self-help, cognitive and motor ability. The children's progress is discussed with the team at weekly meetings, ideas are exchanged and the psychologist gives advice.

Opinions vary regarding the efficacy of this type of teaching. It is not possible to have a control group because learning disabilities in children cannot be matched, for example no two children with Down syndrome are alike in their abilities. Undoubtedly there are remarkable improvements in some children, but the exact reason cannot be defined; is it the teaching, the intensive visiting, the support for the carers, or a bit of each? Some find the form of teaching unacceptable – it is based on operant conditioning (see Ch. 30) which can be seen as learning tricks for rewards. Whatever the opinions of normal people, many children with specific learning disabilities have been helped to reach their full potential and to integrate well into the school environment.

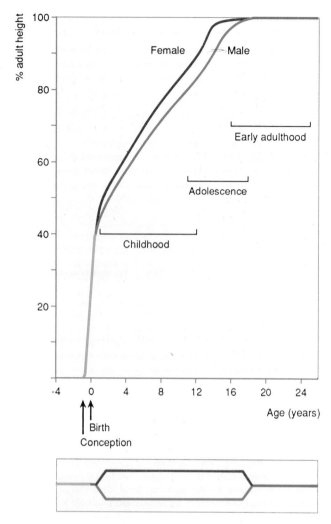

Figure 35.16
Growth in height from conception to maturity: boys and girls in the UK. (Based on Moore 1988 and Tanner 1989.)

Development of bones and teeth

Process

The connective tissue that is ultimately transformed into bone makes its appearance during the fifth week of life. It forms a model for the bone formation (*ossification*) beginning in the succeeding weeks.

The first centres of ossification to become established are termed primary centres. These are followed by secondary centres (*epiphyses*) (Fig. 35.17). In each developing bone the epiphyses are separated from the primary centres by a layer of cartilage termed the *epiphyseal plate*.

As growth proceeds the cartilage is gradually replaced by bone, including that between the primary and secondary centres. The latter event is termed *fusion of the epiphyses*. When it occurs in the long bones (of the legs and arms) at 16 to 21 years of age it marks the end of their longitudinal growth. The stage of development of the bones can be used to assess the developmental stage a child has reached (Figs 35.18 and 35.19).

Rates of growth

When bones grow, they do not grow at a uniform rate all over. In the limb bones for example, more growth usually occurs at one end than the other. This can be important in deciding management of a fracture in a child. Also different bones mature at different rates. The development of the bones of the pelvis and lower limbs lags behind that of the upper limbs and shoulder girdle. Some of the last bones to complete development are those of the vertebral column and those of the base of the skull which continue to mature until about the age of 25 years.

Skull

In the infant, the bones of the skull are not fused together. There are gaps between them (the largest termed *fontanelles*) filled with fibrous connective tissue (Fig. 35.20). These gaps allow movement, which is important especially at the time of birth. The largest gap, the *anterior fontanelle*, is filled in by the end of the second year of life.

The shape of the skull changes greatly from infancy to adulthood (see Ch. 29), largely because of the growth still occurring at the base of the skull and the development of the teeth. This is one of the reasons why facial features change so much during childhood, adolescence and early adulthood.

Teeth

The primary teeth begin to calcify at 4 to 6 months of fetal life. In the infant, the first teeth to erupt are usually the mandibular incisors. The secondary teeth develop inside the jaw bones and begin to push through and displace the primary teeth at about 6 years of age (Fig. 35.21). Whereas the second permanent molar erupts consistently at about 12 years of age (apparently used in the UK at one time to indicate when a child could be put

> Care of a child's teeth should begin as soon as the teeth erupt. A small, soft toothbrush moistened with water is usually sufficient until the child is able to cooperate with spitting out toothpaste – an activity enjoyed by most children. Initially the aim is for the child to get used to having the brush put in his mouth. If the gums are sore because more teeth are erupting, then it might be necessary to stop using the brush for a day or two. Conservation of primary teeth, apart from maintaining the normal function of biting and chewing, helps the growing jaw to retain a good shape and may avoid crooked eruption of the permanent teeth.

Figure 35.20 (*right*)
Structure of the skull in the neonate:
A From the front (anterior view)
B From the side (lateral view).
(Reproduced from Rogers 1992 (Fig. 12.2) by permission of the publishers.)

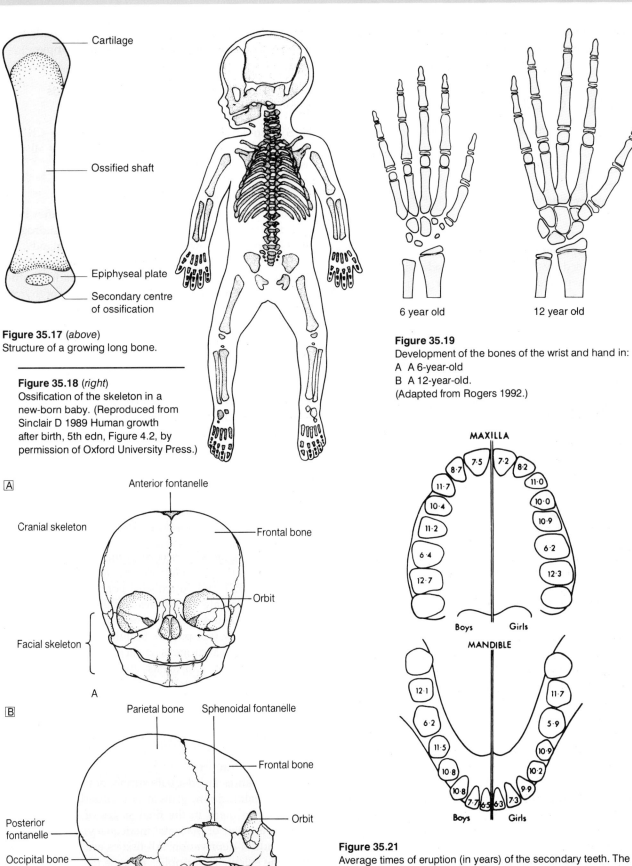

Figure 35.17 (*above*)
Structure of a growing long bone.

Figure 35.18 (*right*)
Ossification of the skeleton in a
new-born baby. (Reproduced from
Sinclair D 1989 Human growth
after birth, 5th edn, Figure 4.2, by
permission of Oxford University Press.)

Figure 35.19
Development of the bones of the wrist and hand in:
A A 6-year-old
B A 12-year-old.
(Adapted from Rogers 1992.)

Figure 35.21
Average times of eruption (in years) of the secondary teeth. The
times of eruption of the third molars (wisdom teeth) are not shown
because they are so variable. (Reproduced from Sinclair D 1989
Human growth after birth, 5th edn, Figure 5.2, by permission of
Oxford University Press.)

to work!) the third molars (wisdom teeth) come through at any age from 18 years onwards or may not erupt at all. ⑭

⑭

How many primary molars does a child normally have?

CONTROL OF GROWTH

The main factors influencing growth are:

- genetic
- hormonal
- nutritional
- environmental.

Genetic factors

The developmental sequence and its expression is predetermined by the instructions coded in our DNA. There are separate genes coding for different aspects of body shape and form, and a huge variety of genes leading to differences in features between different individuals. For example there are different genes responsible for determining the growth of the long bones as compared with other parts of the body.

> A defect in the gene controlling the length of the long bones gives rise to *achondroplasia*, a form of dwarfism in which only growth of the limbs is deficient. Other parts of the body grow normally.

The unique combination of genes each person possesses (identical twins excepted) leads to individual differences between people. An obvious difference in the genetic blueprint is that between males and females. Differences in only 240 bases in a molecule of DNA (see Ch. 2) give rise to the different characteristics of male and female persons including the different timescale of development between the sexes (see p. 602) as well as ultimate differences in height, body composition and form.

Hormonal factors

Hormonal factors of importance include:

- human chorionic somatomammotrophin (HCS)
- androgens (fetal, adrenal and gonadal)
- thyroxine
- somatotrophin.

The importance of each of these varies at different stages of life from that in utero, through childhood and into adolescence.

In utero

The factors controlling growth at this stage are not well understood. It is probable that at very early stages of life, growth and development are determined by substances secreted locally by all cells. As tissues differenti-

ate, regulators of growth produced by specific endocrine glands and tissues become important, for example:

- HCS secreted by the placenta
- androgens secreted by the fetal adrenal glands
- thyroid hormones.

HCS (also known as placental lactogen; see Ch. 34) stimulates the production of somatomedins by all fetal tissues. These hormones promote growth.

Infancy and childhood

The fetal adrenal glands (Fig. 35.11B) regress after birth and the zone in the cortex that secretes androgens shrinks in size. However other endocrine glands, including the pituitary and the thyroid, grow steadily. Thyroid hormones (see Ch. 10) are important for maturation of bones, teeth and the brain. Deficiency of thyroid hormones in childhood leads to *cretinism*.

Somatotrophin (growth hormone) secreted by the anterior pituitary (see Ch. 10) has a major role in determining growth after birth. It:

- stimulates cell division
- stimulates the formation of DNA
- maintains protein synthesis
- stimulates somatomedin production by liver and kidney.

Somatomedins stimulate the proliferation of cartilage and therefore affect the linear growth of bones (see p. 602 and Ch. 28).

Adolescence

The beginning of adolescence is marked by increased secretion of the gonadotrophins, follicle stimulating hormone (FSH) and luteinising hormone (LH). These hormones stimulate the ovaries and the testes to mature and increase their secretion of oestrogens and testosterone respectively (see p. 605). Simultaneously, the secretion of adrenal androgens is increased in both sexes. The secretion of androgens stimulates growth, and the secretion of gonadal hormones leads to the different characteristics expressed in male and female individuals, including differences in height and build (see p. 606).

Nutritional factors

Growth requires an adequate supply of raw materials. If there is malnutrition, growth is retarded. Malnutrition can occur in utero in the final stages of fetal development as a result of placental inadequacy, or, after birth, as a result of deprivation. All tissues are not affected to the same extent. The supplies to some tissues seem to be protected at the expense of supplies to others. In childhood, catch-up growth of height and weight usually occurs once adequate food is provided, but deprivation early in life may permanently affect development by limiting supplies at critical periods of growth.

Environmental factors

Before birth (*antenatally*) the baby's environment is dictated by the conditions in utero, and the mother's state of health and well-being. After birth (*postnatally*), environment in its widest sense can include any external stimuli affecting the baby whether these be opportunities to run and play, disturbances of family life affecting the infant's emotional development, or other physical factors such as time of year.

Antenatal

Babies that are 'small for dates' may have experienced retardation of growth because of impaired nutrition or because of the toxic effects of substances present in the mother's bloodstream. It is now well known that mothers who smoke or who drink regularly tend to give birth to babies that are smaller than expected.

Postnatal

Children who experience emotional upset may not grow as well as those who grow up in a secure environment. This is likely to be mediated via the hypothalamus and limbic system (see Ch. 31).

Interestingly children grow at different rates at different times during the year. The rate of growth in height tends to be greatest in the springtime whereas the rate of growth in weight is greatest in the autumn. These annual changes in growth rate may be related to the changes in length of daylight during the year. Light and dark is known to affect various body systems (see Ch. 18).

ADOLESCENCE AND PUBERTY

Adolescence is the period of time during which the developing human undergoes his/her final stages of physical maturation. *Puberty* is that time during adolescence when secondary sexual characteristics appear and the reproductive system matures sufficiently for reproduction to be possible. These changes are triggered by increased secretion of the gonadotrophins by the anterior pituitary gland. The gonadotrophins excite the gonads to secrete steroid hormones, such as oestradiol and testosterone, that have widespread effects on many body cells and tissues including the reproductive organs.

The timing of development varies between individuals with the result that, during the teenage years, individuals of exactly the same age may have attained very different stages of development.

HORMONAL CHANGES AND EFFECTS

During childhood, the pituitary gland secretes small amounts of the gonadotrophins. The beginning of adolescence is marked by the start of pulsatile secretion of gonadotrophin releasing hormone (GnRH – also known as LHRH) from the hypothalamus (Fig. 35.22), which brings about pulsatile secretion of the gonadotrophins, FSH and LH. These hormones in turn promote the development of the gonads, increasing their secretion of oestrogens in girls and testosterone in boys. Simultaneously the secretion of androgens by the adrenal gland

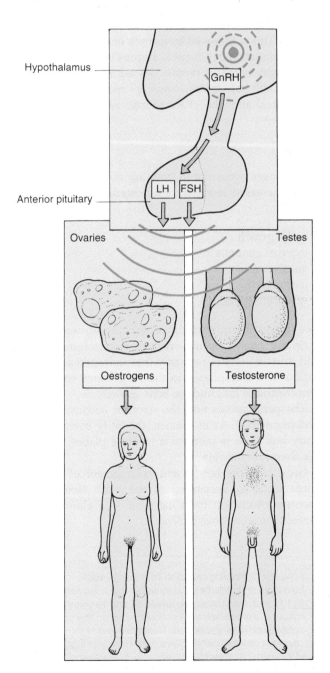

Figure 35.22
Hormonal control of puberty.

⑮
What do you
understand by
pulsatile
secretion?

increases, due possibly to another, as yet unidentified, pituitary hormone. ⑮

Together these hormones affect cellular function in many different tissues resulting in:

- development of the secondary sexual characteristics
- maturation of the reproductive organs
- changes in psyche and behaviour.

Secondary sexual characteristics

Female

In girls, the first external evidence of the radical changes that are about the take place is the development of the breasts. This is followed by growth of pubic and axillary hair. Simultaneously there is a spurt in the growth rate, and height increases rapidly. As adolescence proceeds, the growth of bones, muscle and adipose tissue accelerates, and the characteristic female proportions develop.

⑯
How can it be
recognised
that ovulation
is occurring?

Male

The changes occurring in boys are more extensive. The vastly increased secretion of testosterone from the testes affects:

- body growth
- external genitalia
- vocal cords
- hair growth
- sebaceous glands.

The broad-shouldered, muscular proportions of the male are caused by the effect of testosterone on bone and muscle tissue. Eventually this androgen also causes fusion of the epiphyses in the long bones resulting in termination of longitudinal bone growth.

The penis grows and the scrotum becomes wrinkly and pigmented. As in women, the body becomes more hairy but there is more of it in more places, including the chest and the chin.

Growth of the larynx and enlargement of the vocal cords leads to deepening of the voice (see Ch. 29). Increased secretion from the sebaceous glands predisposes adolescent boys to acne.

Acne is a distressing condition for the adolescent. It affects both boys and girls, being at its worst in girls between 16 and 17 years, and in boys between 17 and 19 years. It occurs at a time when self-confidence is often low and one's appearance is very important. Understanding of the misery it causes is needed, rather than a dismissive 'you'll grow out of it'. There are a variety of treatments available, including locally applied gels, antibiotic therapy, the drug isotretinoin which reduces sebum secretion, and hormonal treatment.

Reproductive organs

Female

Internally, oestrogens facilitate growth of the ovarian follicles and promote the development of the muscle, blood vessels and secretory lining of the uterus. The fact of this maturation becomes evident at the first menstrual bleed (*menarche*) when the lining, built up under the action of oestrogens, breaks down. Initially, menstrual cycles are not accompanied by ovulation (*anovulatory cycles*) but, after 12 to 18 months, ovulation becomes a regular feature, progesterone is secreted, and the adult pattern of hormonal change and events in the menstrual cycle is established (see Ch. 34). From this time on, the woman is fertile and reproduction is possible. ⑯

The time at which puberty begins may be linked to the attainment of a predetermined weight for height. As nutrition and health care has improved enormously in the western world over the last 150 years, that weight has been attained at ever earlier ages. It is believed that this is the reason that the average age of puberty has declined over the last 150 years in the UK and USA from about 17 to 13 years. Menarche does not occur in girls until after the peak spurt of growth in height is over.

Male

At the start of adolescence, the testes begin to enlarge. Within them, the primitive germ cells, *spermatogonia*, are stimulated by FSH and testosterone to mature into fully fledged spermatozoa. Simultaneously the glands of the male reproductive system enlarge and secrete increased amounts of the fluids supporting the sperm. The seminal glands for example begin to secrete fructose, a sugar which sperm cells use for nourishment.

Psyche

At puberty the divergent physical development in young men and women is paralleled by divergence in behaviour. Young men tend to be more aggressive than women and this appears to be related to the level of secretion of testosterone. During adolescence the interaction between the sexes alters. Most young men begin to find a developing interest in young women and vice versa. These changes in behaviour are complex and depend on the social context as well as changing levels of hormones.

Some people do not develop heterosexual attractions and instead find people of the same sex to be sexually attractive (*homosexuality*). The reasons for this are still unclear. Genetic, psychological and social factors may all be involved, the particular blend of influential factors probably differing from one person to another.

Another significant change in adolescence is in socialisation – the growth in understanding of interactions between people and the ability to communicate in more subtle ways. One disorder of mental develop-

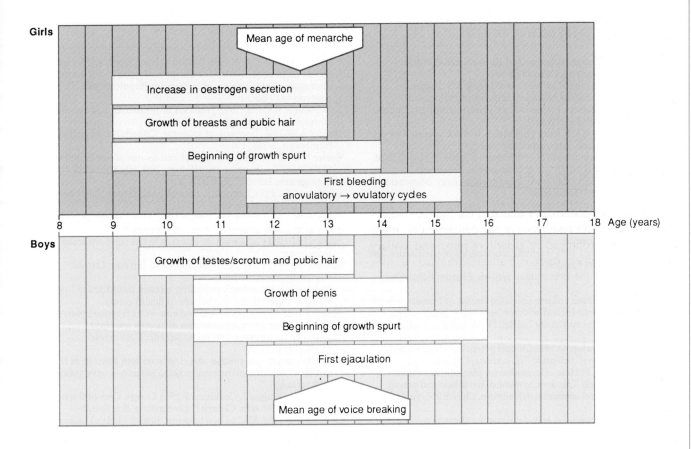

Figure 35.23
Timing of onset of various events during adolescence in girls and boys showing the wide range in age of onset.
(Based on Bancroft 1989.)

ment that may emerge in a small minority of people in their late teens is *schizophrenia*. It may be due to abnormality in the development of neural pathways involved in social interaction.

EARLY AND LATE DEVELOPERS

The onset of puberty in boys and girls varies considerably between individuals (Fig. 35.23) with the result that teenagers of the same age may be at very different stages of sexual development. In a group of 14-year-olds there will be some who have barely begun pubertal change as well as those who have fully matured sexually. Those who are quick to mature physically tend also to score better on intelligence tests than those of the same age who have not reached the same stage of physical development.

These temporary biological differences can give rise to many psychological problems ranging from an unwarranted sense of inferiority in the late developer, to a feeling of frustration in the early developer, mature in body but constrained by society's definitions of 'age of maturity'.

KEY POINTS

What you should now know and understand about growth and development from conception to adulthood:

- how, when and where spermatozoa and ova develop
- crucial events of the first 2 weeks of life
- what major developments are taking place in the first weeks and months of life and their timing
- how some common forms of altered development may arise, such as monozygotic twins, Down syndrome, and short stature
- differences between premature and full-term babies and likely consequences for care of the neonate
- how the cardiorespiratory system alters at birth
- why the neonate's internal environment is not as stable as that of the adult and the implications for care
- major developmental changes occurring in infancy and childhood
- factors affecting growth and their relative effects at different periods of development
- what is happening to a young person's body during puberty and how these changes occur.

REFERENCES AND FURTHER READING

Bancroft J 1989 Human sexuality and its problems, 2nd edn. Churchill Livingstone, Edinburgh
(Very useful authoritative book on all aspects of human sexuality, including its biological basis and development)

Behrman R E, Kleigman R 1990 Nelson's Essentials of paediatrics. W B Saunders, Philadelphia

Bennett V R, Brown L K (eds) 1993 Myles Textbook for midwives, 12th edn. Churchill Livingstone, Edinburgh

Campbell A G M, McIntosh N 1992 Forfar & Arneil's Textbook of paediatrics, 4th edn. Churchill Livingstone, Edinburgh

Case R M (ed) 1985 Variations in human physiology. Manchester University Press, Manchester
(Contains a useful chapter giving more detailed information about physiological changes before and after birth)

Critchley M (ed) 1978 Butterworths medical dictionary, 2nd edn. Butterworths, London

Davis J A, Dobbing J 1981 Scientific foundations of paediatrics, 2nd edn. Heinemann, London

Falkner F, Tanner J M 1986 Human growth. Plenum Publishing, New York
(Authoritative three volume specialist review of human growth)

HEA 1992 Protect your child with the new Hib immunisation. Health Education Authority Leaflet, Department of Health, London

Hytten F, Chamberlain G 1991 Clinical physiology in obstetrics, 2nd edn. Blackwell Scientific Publications, Oxford
(Reference text. Further information on placental function)

Illingworth R S 1987 The development of the infant and young child: normal and abnormal, 9th edition. Churchill Livingstone, Edinburgh
(Authoritative specialist text, detailing the characteristics of the developing child and what the paediatrician looks for and why. Useful for reference)

Illingworth R S 1991 The normal child, 10th edn. Churchill Livingstone, Edinburgh

Larsen W J 1993 Human embryology. Churchill Livingstone, Edinburgh
(Well illustrated detailed text, written for medical students. Useful source of further information)

Leaflet MM/005/889/A200a A parent's guide to immunisation, 2nd edn. Merieux UK

Miller G A 1992 Psychology. The science of mental life. Pelican Books, London

Moore K L 1988 The developing human, 4th edn. W B Saunders, Philadelphia
(Clinically oriented textbook of embryology written for medical students. Provides an overview of development, as well as detailed descriptions of the development of each system)

Nillson L, Hamberger L 1990 A child is born. Doubleday, London
(A beautiful book written for the general public with astonishing photographs of all stages of human development from conception to birth)

Robertson N R C (ed) 1992 Textbook of neonatology. Churchill Livingstone, Edinburgh

Rogers A W 1992 Textbook of anatomy. Churchill Livingstone, Edinburgh, p 148, 150

Rutter N 1992 Temperature control and its disorders. In: Robertson N R C (ed) Textbook of neonatology, 2nd edn. Churchill Livingstone, Edinburgh, p 217–231

Scharden J L 1993 Chemically induced birth defects, 2nd edn. Marcel Dekker, New York
(Valuable reference work, cataloguing over 3300 drugs and chemicals with respect to their teratogenicity)

Shelley H J 1964 Carbohydrate reserves in the newborn infant. British Medical Journal i: 273–275

Sinclair D 1989 Human growth after birth, 5th edn. Oxford University Press, Oxford
(A lucidly written book providing a broad introduction to all aspects of growth for all students of health care)

Singer S 1985 Human genetics, 2nd edn. W H Freeman, New York
(Clearly presented fundamentals of human genetics)

Tanner J M 1989 Foetus into man, 2nd edn. Castlemead Publications, Ware
(Authoritative, yet concise and clearly written account of the results of research on human growth. Includes a very good bibliography)

Turner T L, Douglas J, Cockburn F 1988 Craig's Care of the newly born infant, 8th edn. Churchill Livingstone, Edinburgh

Valman H B 1988 ABC of one to seven. British Medical Journal, London
(Collection of short articles reprinted from the British Medical Journal)

Valman H B 1989 The first years of life, 3rd edn. British Medical Journal, London
(Collection of short articles reprinted from the British Medical Journal)

Widdowson E M 1981 Nutrition. In: Davis J A, Dobbins J (eds) Scientific foundations of paediatrics, 2nd edn. Heinemann, London, p 41–43

Williams P L, Warwick R, Dyson M, Bannister L H 1989 Gray's Anatomy, 37th edn. Churchill Livingstone, Edinburgh

Chapter 36
GROWING OLDER

We grow older from the moment of conception. Our bodies change. Some capacities develop and others wane so that at different stages of life we can do some things and not others. Some of the changes occurring in our bodies once we have reached physical maturity, such as the menopause in women, are a continuation of the developmental process programmed into us from the start of our lives. But added to that developmental programme are the many challenges sustained throughout our lives that injure cells and tissues and progressively derange and weaken body systems.

The developmental programme and the cumulative effects of injury combine to produce many changes in our bodies as we age, ranging from obvious alterations to our appearance to the declining ability to run a mile, fend off a threatening infection, or remember the name of a new acquaintance. The extent of the changes vary from person to person. Some people become chronically ill or very frail as they grow older, but others continue to enjoy a fit and active life, even into their nineties.

BASIC CONCEPTS, CHANGES AND CONSEQUENCES

CONCEPTS

The changes occurring in our bodies as we grow older are partly a natural process programmed into our cells from the moment of conception (*age-related changes*), and partly the result of the cumulative damage sustained by our bodies throughout life (*age-associated changes*). Present evidence suggests that the majority of changes in humans are age associated rather than age related. Studies of ageing seek to distinguish one from the other and to determine the factors that prolong or curtail the life span.

Programmed development

Growing older is part of normal development. As children we expect to grow, and welcome the changes occurring in our bodies. However, once adulthood is reached many resent the further unfolding of the developmental programme as we pass the so-called prime of early adulthood. Once we have fulfilled our reproductive function, passed on our genes to the next generation and nurtured them into independence, our biological function has, in a sense, been fulfilled.

Cumulative damage

The longer we live the more challenges we encounter and the greater is the likelihood of injury to cells and tissues. Although our bodies are equipped with many means of defence to protect us against external and internal threats (see Ch. 15), defence is not perfect.

Drugs and environmental agents, for example UV light (see Ch. 15) and constituents of cigarette smoke (see Ch. 7), damage molecules and cells of our bodies. Also in the process of metabolism we manufacture substances, such as *free radicals* and *nitric oxide*, which, if not properly controlled, could cause harm.

> *Free radicals* are very reactive chemical species formed as a result of oxidative reactions within cells. They can damage DNA, proteins, and the lipid in cell membranes. *Nitric oxide* (NO) is made by many cells and is used in low concentrations as a cellular regulator. However, it is also manufactured in large quantities by macrophages and is highly toxic. The macrophages use it to kill microorganisms.

Studies of ageing

What is 'normal'?

Studies of ageing are hampered by the difficulty in distinguishing the natural preset programme from cumulative damage. It is not easy to define normal ageing. Is the person who survives for 100 years normal or exceptional? Are changes such as atherosclerosis part of the ageing process or symptomatic of disease? People differ from one another in their genes and in their catalogue of life experiences making each person's growth and development unique. In some people change occurs rapidly whereas in others it is slower. Different body systems change at different rates so that it becomes impossible to predict age-related changes in one system from observations made on another. ①

① What is atherosclerosis?

Strategies

Studies of ageing in humans may be either 'cross-sectional' or 'longitudinal'. In a *cross-sectional study*

comparisons are made simultaneously of groups of people of different ages (e.g. 20–29, 30–39, 40–49 etc.). In a *longitudinal study*, the changes occurring in the same person or group of people are observed and documented at different times during their lives.

The results obtained using each of these strategies are not necessarily identical. The trend may be similar (Fig. 36.1) or different (Fig. 36.2). The results of studies are now beginning to show that normal deterioration in

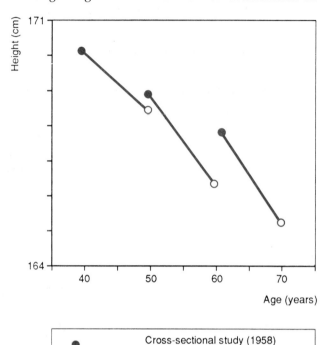

Figure 36.1
Cross-sectional (●) and longitudinal (●——o) data of height in men from the Rhondda in Wales. (Adapted from Wood & Badley 1983.)

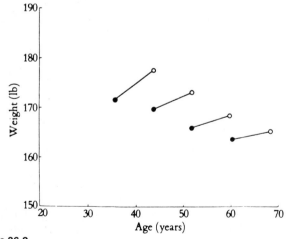

Figure 36.2
Cross-sectional (●) and longitudinal data (●——o) of weight in men in the USA. (Reprinted with permission from Rowe J W, Besdine R W Geriatric medicine, 2nd edition, Little, Brown and Company, copyright 1988.)

function in many body systems is not as great as was once believed and that some changes, once thought to be inevitable in old age, are actually a consequence of injury or disease (age associated) rather than development (age related).

CHANGES IN TISSUES

For a person who has reached adulthood to remain exactly the same as he grows older there would need to be continual and perfect:

- replacement of old cells by new ones
- maintenance of molecules inside and outside cells.

Neither of these occurs. Some cells die and are not replaced, and some molecules change.

Cells

In the adult, some cells, such as epithelial cells, go on reproducing and replacing lost cells, whereas others,

such as neurones, lose the ability to reproduce as they become highly specialised. As we grow older, most cells that go on reproducing do this more slowly. However, other cells, for example some epithelial cells of the skin, may be stimulated to proliferate, forming abnormal growths such as senile warts as well as cancers. ②

Renewal

Cells that go on reproducing in the body, such as liver cells and epithelial cells, are relatively unspecialised (see Ch. 2). Cells lost through injury are usually replaced. However, there is a limit to the number of times that a precursor cell may divide and this sets an upper limit to the life span of the organ or tissue which they form. This upper limit may be programmed into the genetic code by longevity genes, though this theory is still controversial.

As cells age, the time it takes for a cell to complete the cell cycle (Fig. 36.3 and Ch. 2) takes longer. The first part (G₁) becomes longer. Consequently the older you are the

②
What other cells lose the ability to reproduce?

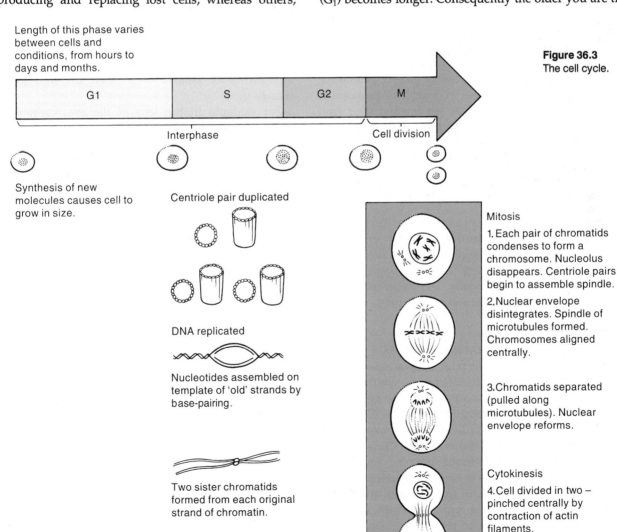

Figure 36.3
The cell cycle.

Length of this phase varies between cells and conditions, from hours to days and months.

G1 S G2 M

Interphase Cell division

Synthesis of new molecules causes cell to grow in size.

Centriole pair duplicated

DNA replicated

Nucleotides assembled on template of 'old' strands by base-pairing.

Two sister chromatids formed from each original strand of chromatin.

Mitosis

1. Each pair of chromatids condenses to form a chromosome. Nucleolus disappears. Centriole pairs begin to assemble spindle.

2. Nuclear envelope disintegrates. Spindle of microtubules formed. Chromosomes aligned centrally.

3. Chromatids separated (pulled along microtubules). Nuclear envelope reforms.

Cytokinesis

4. Cell divided in two – pinched centrally by contraction of actin filaments.

longer it takes for injuries to heal. Eventually the cycle is completely arrested by a protein produced by ageing cells which inhibits the transition from the G₁ to the S phase. Ageing cells also become less responsive to growth factors.

Losses

Cells which can no longer reproduce once they have become fully specialised include muscle cells and neurones. If these are damaged and die they cannot be replaced and the functions they support are lost. Many of these cells require growth factors to maintain their specialised state and regress if these decrease.

Cells singled out by the immune system for destruction may include the body's own cells. Autoimmune disorders become more common as we grow older. Inflammation accompanies cell destruction (see Ch. 15) resulting in the discomforting symptoms of rheumatoid arthritis for example, which is particularly troublesome in middle age.

Proliferation

Cells proliferate either if they escape from normal controls over their growth, as tumours do (see Ch. 2), or if they are stimulated to grow by growth-promoting factors released for example in injury. Consequently, although most cells slow up as we age and their total numbers fall, other cells may grow unchecked and reproduce more vigorously. Systems that police the body, distinguishing normal and abnormal cells, become less effective (see p. 618) and the growth of tumour cells, benign or malignant, may be unchecked.

Molecules

The chemistry of the body does not stay exactly the same as we get older. Some molecules are produced in increasing amounts, others in less. Some macromolecules change in structure and other substances gradually accumulate inside and outside cells.

Synthesis and breakdown

When faults occur in DNA (see Ch. 2) as a result of mutation or damage and the fault escapes repair, abnormal amounts and types of proteins are synthesised. In general, the rate at which most proteins are synthesised decreases with age. Lysosomal function (see Ch. 2) also alters resulting in some proteins being broken down more quickly and others more slowly. Consequently, the concentrations of different proteins inside and outside cells alter and this in turn affects cell and tissue function. For example, there are changes in the concentration of some plasma proteins which are associated with the formation of protein deposits (termed *amyloid*) in the blood vessels and joints. Whether this is a consequence of growing older or a reflection of pathological change is uncertain.

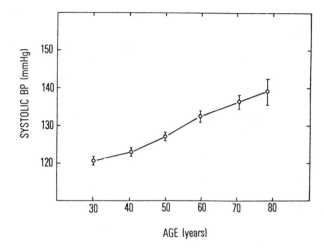

Figure 36.4
Effects of age on systolic blood pressure. (Reproduced from Thompson M K 1990 Commonsense geriatrics, Figure 3.2, by permission of the author and Clinical Press Ltd.)

Structure

Some macromolecules, such as the proteins in the lens of the eye, remain in the body for life once they have been formed. They are not broken down and replaced by new ones. Instead they often undergo gradual change. ③

For example in the lens of the eye, carbohydrate molecules become attached to proteins (*glycosylation*). This alters the crystalline structure of the proteins which, in turn, affects the ability of the lens to transmit and refract light. The result can be a worsening myopia (see Ch. 26) and the development of opacities (*cataracts*) that blur vision.

Similarly, proteins of the extracellular matrix (see Ch. 2), such as collagen and elastin, and glycoproteins such as hyaluronic acid also change in structure. More cross-linkages are formed. As a result, less water is held in the matrix and its properties alter. The connective tissue becomes less distensible. This is one of the reasons why the walls of blood vessels stiffen with age (*arteriosclerosis*), causing systolic blood pressure to rise (Fig. 36.4) and why intervertebral discs (see Ch. 28) become less good as shock absorbers.

Deposits

Although we possess many means of removing and eliminating waste substances (see Ch. 15) some substances inevitably accumulate in cells and tissues as the years go by. For example, substances such as silica dust, breathed in air, and asbestos remain within the body passed on from macrophage to macrophage. Metals such as aluminium and lead may accumulate too. Deposits of lipids (*atherosclerotic plaques*), as well as protein (*amyloid*), build up in blood vessels, and other deposits, such as *lipofuscin* a pigment, accumulate inside many cells. ④

③
What are macro-molecules? Can you give some examples?

④
How do aluminium and lead enter the body?

PHYSIOLOGICAL CONSEQUENCES

The various changes occurring in cells and tissues progressively alter the function of organs and systems and lead to changes in homeostasis (see Ch. 3) by affecting:

- the circulation
- control systems.

Circulation

The health of the circulatory system is crucial for the function of all parts of the body. Once its ability to supply adequate amounts of oxygen and nutrients to all tissues and remove waste products is reduced, the environment of all cells and tissues throughout the body is disturbed and this inevitably affects their activity (see Chs 3 and 5).

Hardening of the walls of blood vessels (*arteriosclerosis*), and the accumulation of fatty deposits within them (*atherosclerosis*) progressively limit the blood supply and affect the nutrition of cells and tissues. The consequences depend on the tissue affected.

Muscle tissue

Lack of blood supply to muscle cells affects their ability to contract and to sustain a contraction (see Chs 17 and 22). This is particularly serious when it occurs in the coronary vessels as it affects cardiac output, and as a result all other tissues of the body. ⑤

Nervous tissue

Supply of blood to the brain is vital. Only a few minutes' deprivation leads to cell death (see Ch. 11). Deprivation may result from deposits blocking the vessels or from weakened vessels that rupture (*cerebral*

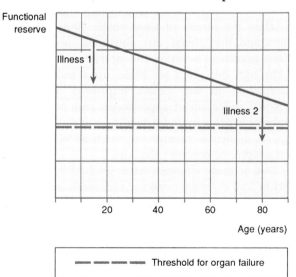

Figure 36.5
How decline in reserves with age threatens someone's ability to cope with the challenge of illness. (Adapted from Allen S C 1988 How respiratory and cardiac reserves decline in old age, Figure 1, by permission of Findlay Publications Ltd.)

haemorrhage). In either case cell death results in loss of neural function, the symptoms of which depend upon the parts of the brain affected. For example, in a stroke occurring in the right cerebral hemisphere, a person may lose sensation and motor control of the whole of the left-hand side of the body (see Chs 27 and 28). ⑥

Fortunately the nervous system possesses an enormous reserve of cells, such that some cell loss can occur without function necessarily becoming obviously disordered. Cells that remain may sprout (see Ch. 21), forming new connections in place of those that have been lost.

Renal tissue

Reduction in blood flow to the kidneys reduces glomerular filtration rate (see Ch. 8), damages renal tubules and results in progressive loss of renal function.

Control systems

Loss of cells, such as neurones, and changes in membrane proteins, such as receptors for hormones and neurotransmitters, affect the sensitivity and responsiveness of control systems (see Ch. 3). Variables such as body temperature that were previously well stabilised (see Chs 11–16) are not as well controlled, and actions that were once very adeptly performed become less slick. As we grow older we become less able to tolerate:

- variation in supply of nutrients and fluids
- changes in metabolism
- extremes of temperature.

Changes in control systems begin to occur long before any problems become apparent. This is because most systems have a considerable reserve of function under normal circumstances. Only when the system is stressed (as for example in illness) or reserves fall below a critical level, may the inadequacy of the system become apparent (Fig. 36.5).

Sensitivity and responses

Loss of cells in the nervous system and reduced sensitivity to transmitters makes reflex responses less powerful and less quick. For example, stretch reflexes (see Ch. 27), are less easy to elicit in the elderly. Also, sensations tend to be dulled and responses are not as rapid. The very old are not as sensitive to changes in environmental temperature and may therefore not take appropriate action when they become chilled (see Ch. 16).

Similarly, cells become less sensitive to hormones. One example of this is the insulin resistance that develops as we age (see p. 616). Sometimes a consequence of the decreased effect of a hormone on its target cells is a compensatory increase in its secretion by endocrine cells. For example, the concentration of gastrin in blood (see Ch. 6) increases as gastric secretion declines with age.

⑤
Lack of blood supply to which muscles causes intermittent claudication?

⑥
What is the name given to a weakness of an artery wall?

Many elderly people ask about the environmental temperature. For example, on a bitterly cold day you may be asked: 'Is it cold?' This sometimes indicates that the elderly person is recognising visual clues, such as frost or snow, but is not actually appreciating temperature change. It is important to make sure that the person is adequately clothed and that there is sufficient indoor heating.

Reserves

For day-to-day activities, most systems operate well below their maximum capacity. For example, in a healthy young person cardiac output at rest can be increased by 3 to 4 times when exercising (see Ch. 17), the liver has more than enough cells to process all the nutrients and waste products that it receives (see Ch. 9), and the brain has many more cells than we need to use. As control systems consist of many interrelated parts a deficiency in one organ or system may be compensated by adjustments made in others. However, the size of these reserves, and the capacity for compensation, declines with age as cells and tissues change.

A decline in reserves is usually not apparent under ordinary conditions but becomes so if systems are stressed as in exercise, or by injury or illness. For example, loss of cells from the substantia nigra (part of the brain involved in the control of movement; see Chs 27 and 28) occurs as we grow older without giving rise

to any symptoms. However, if the number of cells drops below a critical number, features of Parkinson's disease appear. In most people the critical number of cells is never reached and so symptoms of this loss do not develop. However, if there is neurological disease, or if there has been an acute loss of cells earlier in life, for example through drug-induced injury, the chances of cell numbers falling below the level required for normal function is increased (Fig. 36.6).

Cases of drug-related Parkinson's disease are known. Some people have developed the disease earlier rather than later in life through having taken or been given drugs contaminated with neurotoxic substances. Examples include LSD and improperly prepared pethidine.

CHARACTERISTIC CHANGES WITH AGE

As we grow older many changes occur in our:

- appearance
- level of physical fitness
- digestion, defence and metabolism
- abilities
- reproductive function and sexuality.

However much use is made of cosmetic products to retain a youthful complexion, a person of 50 does not look like a 25-year-old, and a person of 75 looks different again.

As we grow older our capacity for physical activity decreases. Even athletes who train regularly do not maintain the fitness of their youth. Body metabolism alters and this affects our nutritional needs and our ability to combat infection and injury.

Through the years we build up a unique fund of information in our brains imprinted by our own personal collection of experiences, and as a result we continue to grow in understanding and skill. Some other aspects of neural functioning, such as vision, hearing and adeptness, however, decline.

Most of these changes occur gradually but one, the decline and eventual cessation of reproductive functioning in women, is more abrupt. After the age of about 50 years, women can no longer conceive and bear children. Nevertheless sexual intercourse can still be enjoyed by women as well as men well into old age.

APPEARANCE

Older people look different from younger people because of changes in:

- skin, hair and nails
- body build.

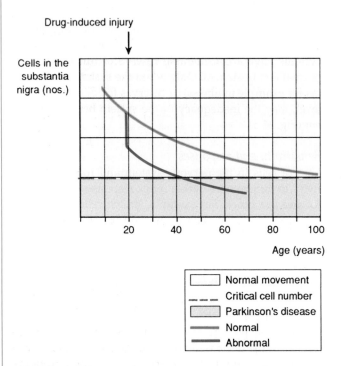

Figure 36.6
How symptoms of disease may arise in middle age as a result of injury sustained in young adulthood. (Adapted with permission from a diagram of M Horan, personal communication.)

LIFE AT 92 YEARS – A CASE STUDY

Mrs A has lived alone for 30 years. Her husband died suddenly, in his sixties. One day he walked up the street after tea, collapsed and died. During the past 30 years, Mrs A has grown older; she has developed many of the signs and symptoms which indicate to others that she is an old lady. In spite of her disabilities, she manages remarkably well.

The rented cottage in which she lives has two bedrooms which she hasn't seen for years, a large kitchen, a small bathroom, and 'the room'. 'The room' now contains her bed, a sideboard, a settee and several chairs all placed along the walls. Mrs A's upright wooden chair is in the middle of the room, within reach of the sideboard, which serves as a table.

Mrs A is cheerful, alert and without any bitterness at her circumstances. She occasionally expresses frustration when she cannot do things for herself, but more often she says, 'Aren't I lucky to have so many friends to help me?' Anyone who has time to stop for a chat or do a small job for her is a 'friend'.

Mrs A is grey haired, her skin is wrinkled and very thin on her lower legs. As well as arthritis in knees and hips, necessitating the use of a walking frame, she has arthritis in her finger joints and a 'dowager's hump'. Her finger- and toenails have thickened and are difficult to cut; a domiciliary chiropodist attends to her feet at 3-monthly intervals. Mrs A is fairly deaf but does not use a hearing aid. Her left eye is blind due to cataract formation and opacity of the cornea. The sight in her right eye has been prolonged by a lens implant but the retina is now failing. She has had full dentures for many years and finds soft food easiest to eat. Mrs A suffers from mild heart failure, controlled by her heart tablets (digoxin) and her water tablets (frusemide and amiloride). She has a tendency to be breathless and to wheeze, so she has a supply of 'wheezy' tablets (long-acting salbutamol) to take when necessary. Her legs and feet are very discoloured due to poor circulation and the skin on her heels tends to split. On her left thigh is a large purple scar, caused by a burn when she set her clothes on fire a few years ago. Mrs A is no longer allowed to have an open fire but has been provided with two 'portable' gas fires – with guards. All this makes depressing reading but Mrs A is content. She appreciates any help given and would hate to be separated from her home and her two cats.

So how does Mrs A manage? A home help visits every weekday, and at weekends if necessary. Mrs A's great nieces collect her washing once a week. Her 'bath nurse', as Mrs A calls her, visits once a week, and Mrs A puts the immersion and bathroom heaters on in readiness. A selection of frozen meals is provided; these are somewhat boring – 'always carrots and custard' she says! A Lifeline telephone is provided by the village – one member is in

charge of the funds – and Mrs A occasionally expresses concern that she never receives a bill. A cat flap allows the cats to come and go at will – she used to leave the back door open at night!

How does Mrs A spend her days? She does her own baking and makes marmalade for charity events. She enjoys reading large-print books and the mobile library calls fortnightly. She also reads a daily newspaper (using a magnifying glass) and the local weekly paper, keeping in touch with local events. The radio and television provide Mrs A with some entertainment, although she is very selective in her listening and viewing. When she was 90 she knitted a pram cover for an expected great grandchild. Visitors are the highlight of her days; she loves to talk and is very interested in people – long conversations can become very tiring for the visitor because of Mrs A's deafness. Villagers take her to church and she always attends the fundraising events held in the village hall – she needs a companion to help her cross the road. In the summer she walks down the long back garden, which is maintained by her landlord who lives in the adjoining cottage. Few are willing to take her out because of her disabilities but, provided that there are two people with her, she enjoys car rides over the moors, to the sea and through the forests. Mrs A likes to visit local churches but the light is usually a bit too dim for her to see well. A meal in a carefully chosen pub (no steps and a 'disabled' toilet) makes a welcome change from carrots and custard – with a glass of wine of course! Mrs A is always positive about her disabilities. She says, 'I'll try,' never 'I can't.'

Sadly, following a recent attack of bronchitis, Mrs A's sight has deteriorated further. She says that newsprint is blurred these days and that her electric light bulbs are becoming dim. Making her marmalade is now difficult because she can't see well enough to weigh the sugar or to get the marmalade into the jars – sensibly, she waits for it to cool before carefully spooning it in.

The eye specialist confirmed that the cornea of her right eye is becoming cloudy and that nothing more can be done to improve her sight. The village charity fund has provided a more powerful magnifying glass and a spotlight concentrates light where she needs it so Mrs A can still read the newspapers. After the visit to the eye specialist she said, 'I'm not going to give up – I'll make my son a birthday cake next week,' and she did.

In the future it may be necessary to consider alternative accommodation for Mrs A, but, at the present, she knows exactly where all her possessions are and is in a relatively safe environment. This is a good example of how a positive approach to growing older on the part of the individual and his or her friends and neighbours can maintain an acceptable quality of life.

Skin, hair and nails

Skin

Skin becomes thinner and more wrinkled because of thinning of the dermis and losses of subcutaneous fat (Fig. 36.7). These and other changes, such as:

- decreases in numbers of melanocytes and Langerhans' cells
- atrophy of glands (apocrine, eccrine and sebaceous)
- alterations in structure of sensory receptors

make the skin and underlying tissues much more vulnerable to injury. Bruising occurs more readily even though there are fewer blood vessels in the dermis. As the rate of renewal of cells slows down (decreased by 50% between the third and seventh decades), injuries take progressively longer to heal. ⑦

⑦ *What is the difference between apocrine, eccrine and sebaceous glands?*

Young

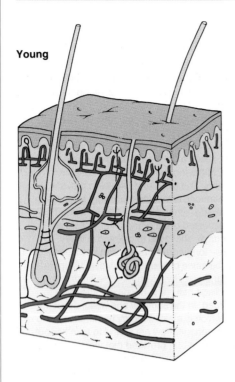

Old

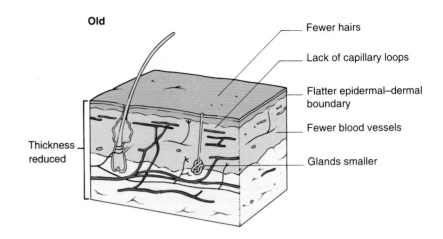

Fewer hairs

Lack of capillary loops

Flatter epidermal–dermal boundary

Fewer blood vessels

Glands smaller

Thickness reduced

Figure 36.7
Changes in the structure of the skin with age.

Hair

Hair becomes grey and then white because of the gradual loss of melanocytes at the base of each hair. The number of hair follicles decreases with the years, and the rate at which hair grows becomes slower with the result that hair of the scalp, the axilla and the pubic region becomes sparse in old age.

The baldness occurring in some men is due to an androgen-induced conversion of dark thick scalp hairs into lightly pigmented, short fine ones.

Nails

Nails grow more slowly. The rate of growth of fingernails in a centenarian (0.5 mm/week) is only half that of a 30-year-old (0.9 mm/week). Thickening of nails occurs wherever there is friction (as in poorly fitting shoes) or a poor blood supply. ⑧

Body build

Body build alters due to changes in:

- muscle and adipose tissue
- joints and bones.

Muscle and adipose tissue

Lean body mass decreases chiefly due to loss of skeletal muscle. This is coupled with an increase in the proportion of body fat. Whereas in a young adult 45% of body weight is contributed by muscle, by the age of 70 years this has fallen to about 27%. Although fat is lost from subcutaneous tissue in many parts of the body, it accumulates elsewhere, around abdominal organs for example, even in those who do not actually put on weight as they age.

⑧
What are nails made of? How does poor blood supply cause thickening?

⑨
What does Figure 36.2 reveal about trends towards obesity in the USA?

The reasons for this shift in the relative proportions of fat and muscle, and for the redistribution of fat stores are not entirely clear, but may be related to the changing proportions of sex steroids and glucocorticoids. Although some loss of muscle mass is due to a decrease in physical activity, it cannot all be explained in that way. The changing sensitivity to hormones such as insulin may also be involved. *Glucose tolerance* decreases (Fig. 36.8; see also Ch. 19, Fig. 19.2) resulting in higher plasma concentrations of glucose after meals. As a result relatively more glucose is available to be taken up into adipose tissue and converted into fat.

Not surprisingly in societies where there is no shortage of food, the incidence of obesity increases in all but the very old. The need for calories decreases with age through the reduction in metabolic rate caused chiefly by the loss of skeletal muscle. If dietary habits are not adjusted, and if less and less exercise is taken, obesity is inevitable. ⑨

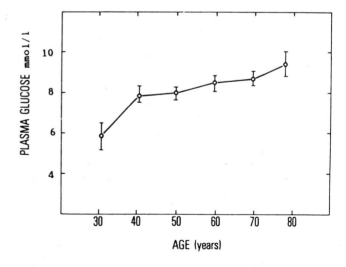

Figure 36.8
Plasma glucose concentration 2 hours after oral glucose, showing decline in glucose tolerance with age. (Reproduced from Thompson M K 1990 Commonsense geriatrics, Figure 2.2, by permission of the author and Clinical Press Ltd.)

Joints and bones

As we grow older we gradually lose height (up to 2–3 cm per decade) (Fig. 36.1). This is partly due to changes in the skeleton, such as narrowing of the vertebral discs and compression of the vertebrae, and partly to postural adaptations resulting from changes in the composition and structure of ligaments and muscles.

PHYSICAL FITNESS AND STRENGTH

Gold medal winners in swimming at the Olympic Games are in their teens and twenties, not their sixties. However active a person has been and however regularly he or she takes exercise, there is an inevitable decrease in physical performance with age. This is due in part to decreased:

- muscle mass
- circulatory efficiency
- respiratory efficiency.

Muscle mass

Growth of muscles depends on:

- usage
- metabolism.

Usage

Muscles grow and adapt according to the use that is made of them (see Chs 17 and 22). Some of the deterioration in physical fitness experienced by people in their middle years is due to the adoption of a more sedentary lifestyle. If exercise is continued the same loss of fitness does not occur. Fortunately, if exercise is gradually resumed after a period of inactivity, much muscle mass can be recovered.

However, as neurones begin to degenerate in later years of life, some muscle cells lose their motoneurones. Once this has happened the muscle cells cannot be excited and consequently they atrophy, again from disuse.

Metabolism

The growth and maintenance of muscle tissue relies also upon an adequate supply of nutrients via the circulation and on the hormonal regulation of cell metabolism.

Changes occurring in the vascular system with age (see below) can limit the delivery of nutrients to muscle tissue and restrict growth. Also changes in the sensitivity of cells and tissues to hormones, including insulin and androgens, influence muscle metabolism.

Circulation

A general hardening of tissues within the cardiovascular system makes both the vessels and the heart stiffer. This increases the work the heart has to do to drive the blood around the circulation. Changes also occur in the effectiveness of neural and hormonal control systems. ⑩

Vessels

Blood vessel walls thicken and stiffen (*arteriosclerosis*) as the connective tissue alters (see p. 612) and the amount of calcium within them increases. Stiffer vessels are less expansible and offer more resistance to blood flow (see Ch. 5). As a result the supply of blood to organs and tissues is progressively reduced and arterial blood pressure increases (Fig. 36.4).

Narrowing of blood vessels through *atherosclerosis* (fatty thickenings bulging into the lumen of the vessel) restricts flow even more.

Heart

Similar changes in cardiac tissue make the heart less distensible. Consequently the ventricles cannot fill as easily, and this affects the pumping action of the heart (Fig. 36.9). Calcification and sclerosis of heart valves contributes also to reduced cardiac performance.

The number of pacemaker cells also decreases, especially after the age of 60 years. In a 75-year-old person the numbers may be reduced to 10% of that in a young adult.

Control

The baroreceptor reflex (see Ch. 5) works less efficiently, with the result that elderly people are more likely to experience dizziness when they stand up quickly. Cells and tissues of the cardiovascular system become less sensitive to adrenaline and noradrenaline. One result of this is a decrease in the maximum achievable heart rate from about 200 beats per minute to less than 160 beats

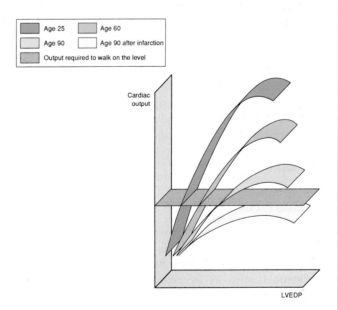

Age 25　Age 60
Age 90　Age 90 after infarction
Output required to walk on the level

Cardiac output

LVEDP

Figure 36.9
Change in cardiac performance with age: LVEDP – left ventricular end-diastolic pressure (see Ch. 5 – Starling's law of the heart). (Adapted from Allen S C 1988 How respiratory and cardiac reserves decline in old age, Figure 3, by permssion of Findlay Publications Ltd.)

⑩
If the heart has to work harder, what effect does this often have on it?

per minute. The general level of activity within the sympathetic nervous system increases however, possibly in compensation. ⑪

⑪
What would you expect to happen to the concentrations of adrenaline and noradrenaline in the blood?

Respiration

Stiffening of tissues in the respiratory system and loss of some elastic recoil in the lungs increases the effort needed for breathing, and losses of alveolar and vascular tissue reduce the capacity of the lungs to take up oxygen (see Ch. 7). These changes do not limit oxygen uptake at rest but become limiting as more demanding activities are attempted.

Breathing

The power of recoil of the lungs decreases as we age with the result that the volume of air left in the lungs at the end of a gentle expiration (*residual volume*; see Ch. 7) increases. Simultaneously structures in the chest wall begin to stiffen limiting the extent to which the lungs can be filled. Consequently vital capacity declines slightly.

As the force with which air can be expelled depends on muscle power as well as elastic recoil, and as both of these decrease, the rate at which air can be expelled from the lungs (FEV_1) declines also (from 83% to about 68% by the age of 70 years).

These changes in respiratory function hardly have any noticeable effect on an elderly person who is seated, or who is strolling along a road, but effects become apparent on exertion, such as climbing stairs. Whereas someone who is 20 years old may, when exercising, increase the ventilation of his lungs by 10 times, an 80-year-old person can only increase it by 4- to 5-fold.

Oxygen uptake

The deterioration occurring in ventilation of the lungs alters the balance between ventilation and perfusion (see Ch. 7). Some parts of the lung, predominantly the basal regions, become increasingly badly ventilated, and therefore the blood from these areas does not become fully oxygenated, resulting in a gradual decline in arterial PO_2 (Fig. 36.10).

DIGESTION, DEFENCE AND METABOLISM

Nutritional requirements change as levels of physical activity decrease and as decline occurs in digestive function and body metabolism. As the processing of many substances, such as microorganisms and xenobiotics, declines the individual becomes more susceptible to infection and to the toxic effects of drugs. ⑫

⑫
What are xenobiotics?

Nutrition and metabolism

Appetite

The desire to eat depends on the smell and taste of food as well as on changing levels of nutrients in the blood (see Ch. 14). The number of taste buds and olfactory neurones decreases in old age, leading to a loss of some of the sensations contributing to the pleasure of eating.

Digestion

The secretory and absorptive capacity of the digestive tract declines with age. Reduced secretion of acid by the parietal cells of the stomach contributes to reduced absorption of calcium (see Ch. 6) and decreases protection against bacterial infection. The number of villi in the small intestine decreases, with the result that the surface area available for absorption also decreases, but this does not usually significantly limit the absorption of nutrients.

Assimilation of nutrients

Glucose is taken up into cells and metabolised less efficiently. The glucose concentration reached in plasma after ingesting a standard dose (*glucose tolerance test*) increases (Fig. 36.8). Plasma insulin concentrations also increase more than usual (*hyperinsulinaemia*). The degree to which these changes occur depends on a variety of factors including the regular diet and exercise. If regular exercise is taken, glucose tolerance tends not to change as much.

> As glucose tolerance worsens, the number of people who develop diabetes mellitus increases. In western Europe and the USA about I in 10 people over the age of 65 years are diabetic (Kesson & Knight 1990).

Temperature regulation

A variety of different changes contribute to impaired thermoregulation in the elderly including *decreased*:

- mobility
- sensitivity to environmental temperature
- ability to sweat and to shiver.
- vasoconstrictor responses.

As a result elderly people are less able to tolerate extremes of environmental temperature and may in cold climates be prone to *hypothermia* (see Ch. 16).

Defence and waste disposal

The elderly are more susceptible to infections and are more likely to develop some cancers than younger adults. This may be due to a decline in the effectiveness of the immune system. Getting rid of waste materials is also more difficult as liver size decreases and renal function declines.

Immune system

From puberty, the thymus decreases in size (see Chs 4 and 35) and goes on doing so throughout life (*invol-

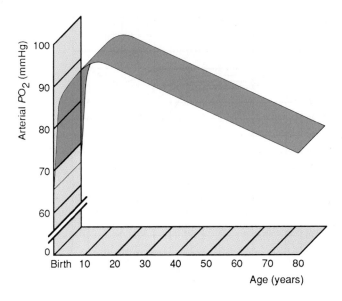

Figure 36.10
Arterial PO_2 as a function of age. (Adapted from Murray 1976, incorporating data of Mansell et al 1972, Nelson 1966, and Sarbini et al 1968 by permission of W B Saunders.)

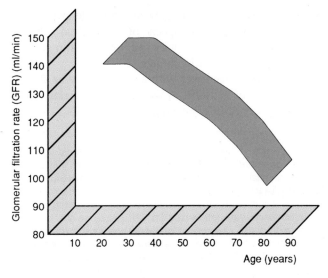

Figure 36.11
Change in glomerular filtration rate with age as measured by creatinine clearance. (Adapted from Rowe 1976, as quoted in Rowe & Besdine 1988.)

ution). Although the numbers and proportions of leucocytes in the blood do not change with age there are changes in the number of defence cells in the tissues. For example, as we grow older there are fewer Langerhans' cells in the skin and fewer and smaller clumps of lymphoid tissue (Peyer's patches) in the gastrointestinal tract (see Ch. 15).

The responses of the immune system to challenge (see Chs 4 and 15), both humoral and cellular, become less vigorous. There are decreases in:

- antibody production
- T cell response and replication
- secretion and effects of interleukin 2 (IL2).

The formation of autoantibodies however does not decrease; in contrast the incidence of antibodies targeted against the body's own cells increases with age. ⑬

Liver function

The liver gradually becomes smaller in size, paralleling the decline in skeletal muscle mass, and the amount of fibrous tissue within it increases. As the liver's total capacity to process materials declines, the clearance of drugs from the body becomes less efficient.

Renal function

The number of functional nephrons (see Ch. 8) decreases and those that remain become less sensitive to hormones. The consequences of this include *decreased*:

- glomerular filtration rate (GFR)
- concentrating power
- ability to produce H^+ and ammonia
- responsiveness to diuretics.

The decrease in glomerular filtration rate (GFR) (about 10 ml/min/decade; Fig. 36.11) results in a reduction in the clearance of water-soluble waste substances, which also affects the clearance of drugs, for example digoxin. Drug doses that are safe in younger people may therefore easily reach toxic levels in the elderly.

The reduced power of the countercurrent system leads to a reduced ability to concentrate urine and conserve water. Consequently, an elderly person cannot cope with fluid deprivation as well as someone younger. Similarly, the reduced capacity of the kidneys to generate and excrete hydrogen ions makes the older person less able to tolerate acid–base disturbances. ⑭

All these changes make it more difficult for stability to be maintained in fluid, electrolyte and acid–base balance. Challenges presenting no problems in the young (see Chs 12 and 13) cannot be tolerated as easily by the elderly. Consequently diuretics and intravenous fluids have to be given with even greater care.

> Nurses caring for elderly people who are receiving any form of medication should be able to recognise possible adverse reactions to the drugs. The most common reactions are mental confusion, constipation, postural hypotension and unexplained falls. It is not unknown for drug-induced mental confusion to be mistaken for senile dementia. Any change in the normal pattern of bodily function should be reported. Adverse reactions often occur during or after a period of stress, such as bronchitis or a bereavement.

ABILITIES

Changes in the nervous system with age influence many aspects of perception, intellect and activity. Deterior-

⑬
What may be the effect of body cells being targeted by antibodies?

⑭
What affects the amounts of acid and base in body fluids?

ation in vision and hearing occurs and sleep patterns alter. Although many aspects of intellectual activity remain intact even in the very old, responses in general tend to become slower in old age.

Brain weight decreases with age. This may be due in part to losses of neurones as well as to a reduction in the number of dendritic connections between cells.

> The number of dendritic connections retained into old age may be related in part to the level of mental activity. Just as we can retain a better level of physical activity by exercising our muscles, we may retain connections between neurones for longer in environments that are mentally stimulating and which encourage activity (see Ch. 33). Just as we are encouraged to save money for our old age we should also develop hobbies or interests which will provide stimulation during retirement or after the children have left home. Nurses as health educators have the opportunity to help people grow old in a positive way, maintaining physical and mental activity suited to the individual.

Vision

Vision deteriorates with age because of multiple changes occurring in the optical system and in the retina of the eye.

Optics

Changes occur in the chemistry of the fluids of the eye and the substance of the cornea and lens that alter their light transmitting properties. For example, the lens becomes yellowed and areas of opacity may develop. As a result less light is transmitted to the retina, and focusing is not as good causing vision to become less sharp. Gradual narrowing of the pupil (*mydriasis*) also reduces the amount of light transmitted. ⑮

⑮
What fluids are there in the eye?

> More than 90% of people over the age of 65 years have regions of opacity in the lens (*cataracts*).

The lens stiffens with age (see p. 612) resulting in a progressive loss of ability to accommodate for near vision (*presbyopia*; see Ch. 26), with the result that many people in their forties find they need to start wearing glasses for reading.

Retina

More blood vessels grow into the retina. Rupture and ischaemia become more likely leading to areas of retinal damage and consequent loss of vision. Other changes include decreased ability to adapt to darkness when moving from bright to dim surroundings, and to discriminate colours, particularly green and blue. ⑯

⑯
Why might discriminating green and blue colours be difficult?

Hearing

More than 50% of people over the age of 75 years have

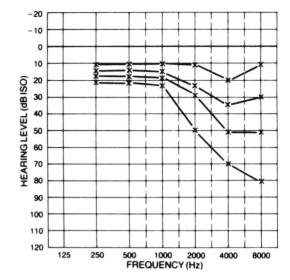

Figure 36.12
Progressive loss of sensitivity to sounds of high frequency with years of exposure to dangerous noise. Compare this figure with those in Chapter 25. (Reproduced with permission from Freeland A 1989 Deafness: the facts, Figure 21, by permission of the author and Oxford University Press.)

problems with hearing. This is commonly due to degeneration of nerve cells, leading to deafness for sounds of high frequency (see Ch. 25). This is made worse by exposure, during one's lifetime, to excessive noise (Fig. 36.12). The high frequency sounds that are heard less well include those giving us the consonants such as s, t, k etc., that are important in distinguishing different words (see Ch. 25). Consequently an elderly person may have especial difficulty with conversation.

> ### SENSORY DETERIORATION – A CASE STUDY
>
> Our attention in the practice was directed towards a 74-year-old widower who had moved into a block of council flats but appeared to be on no doctor's list. The reason for being asked to see him was that he appeared mentally disturbed and was constantly made fun of by groups of children who gathered to jeer at him as he returned from the shops. The cause of their merriment was that he doffed his hat with great politeness and greeted a bush standing ouside the entrance. Examination showed that he had bilateral cataract so advanced that he could not distinguish the bush from the human figure which had become familiar to him. In one way, it was fortunate that inspissated wax and sensorineural deafness had made him very deaf, so that he did not hear the mockery, but it had completed his isolation from sensory stimuli. After cleaning his ears, supplying a hearing aid, and having the cataracts extracted, he was able to laugh at his misfortune, and join a working man's club where he was respected as a fine darts player. He was poorly nourished, and temporarily impaired by sensory deprivation, but recovered well.
>
> Reproduced from Thompson M K 1990 Commonsense geriatrics, p. 72, by permission of the author and Clinical Press Ltd.

Shouting louder does not help but speaking face to face in a deeper voice, and using gestures intelligently, will.

Other changes occurring in the ears include stiffening of various tissues including the tympanic membrane and the basilar membrane. Both affect the transmission of vibrations from the air to the hair cells.

Another difficulty that may develop in some people is difficulty in localising the source of a sound. Sound localisation depends on the comparisons made within the brain of information received from each ear (see Ch. 25), and is therefore affected by deafness developing in either ear.

Intellect

Loss of intellectual ability with age is not an inevitable part of growing older. It is truer to say that intellect changes. We go on learning throughout life and therefore the store of vocabulary and other information in our brains goes on increasing (see Ch. 33). However, we become less good at memorising unrelated facts although we retain the ability to learn ideas. Consequently it is quite normal for someone over the age of 35 years to become more forgetful of some information such as the names of new friends and acquaintances.

Over the age of 60 to 65 years, it is usual for the learning of new information and skills to take a little longer. Information is not registered and processed quite as quickly, and responses are less quick also.

Movement

Joints

Inflammatory changes occurring at joints (*arthritis*) occur universally with increasing frequency as we age. Over the age of 65 years, arthritis is very common. Arthritis restricts mobility, sometimes severely, and can cause considerable discomfort. ⑰

Reflexes

Losses of neurones and diminished neural function affect motor control in several ways. Reflexes (see Ch. 27) are not elicited as easily. For example ankle jerks (reflex response similar to the knee jerk) can be elicited in only 5% of the elderly. Also altered function in the dorsal (posterior) columns changes the perception of position and may give rise to more problems with balance in old age.

Sleep

The pattern of circadian rhythms (see Ch. 18) change as we grow older. One consequence is altered sleep. From our thirties onwards sleep tends to become shallower and does not last as long. The time spent at the deepest level of sleep (stage IV; see Ch. 31) is markedly reduced (from about 20% at age 16–18 years to about 3% between 50 and 60 years). This brings relief to some from sleepwalking and nightmares, but also makes it more likely that we will awaken during the night. As we grow older, stage IV sleep disappears entirely and it becomes the norm to awaken more than once during the night, have difficulty getting back to sleep, and to awake in the morning feeling less than refreshed. The total number of hours spent asleep at night gradually declines from around 8 hours on average in young adulthood to about 7 hours at the age of 60 years and goes on declining.

SEXUALITY AND REPRODUCTION

A marked reduction occurs in the secretion of ovarian hormones in women in their late forties and early fifties, resulting in atrophy of reproductive organs and tissues as well as affecting other systems and structures including the cardiovascular system and the skeleton. The years over which major changes occur in the structure and function of the reproductive organs are known as the *climacteric*. One event occurring during this time is the cessation of menstruation (*menopause*).

Corresponding changes in testicular function occur in men as they grow older, but much more gradually, and these contribute to loss of physical power and change in body build as well as to a decline in reproductive capacity and sexual drive.

Women

From the age of about 35 years the ovaries begin to decrease in weight and size. Primordial follicles are lost throughout life but between the ages of 40 and 50 years the rate of loss increases sharply with the result that by the age of 50 years few if any are left (Fig. 36.13).

The decline in ovarian function during the climacteric leads to decreased secretion of ovarian hormones, such as oestrogens, and results in a variety of changes in many organs and tissues including (Fig. 36.14):

- genitourinary system
- hypothalamus and pituitary gland
- oestrogen-sensitive tissues (such as bone, brain and the cardiovascular system).

These changes give rise to a variety of symptoms including irregular periods, 'hot flushes' and psychological effects, which vary considerably in their intensity between women. For most women symptoms are mild and the menopause approaches and is passed uneventfully, but for a minority (about 10%) the experience is disabling.

Some hormones continue to be produced by the ovary in very much smaller amounts once all the primordial follicles have disappeared.

Genitourinary system

Reproductive organs and tissues atrophy. The uterus and external genitalia shrink in size, and there are

⑰
Which type of arthritis occurs as a result of wear and tear?

18

Why do you think the average age for the onset of the menopause has risen?

19

What is the vaginal pH prior to the menopause?

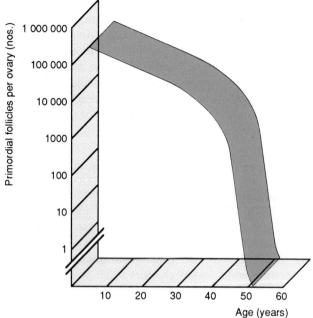

Figure 36.13
Decline in the number of primordial follicles with age. (Adapted from Richardson, Senikas, & Nelson 1987, incorporating data of Block 1952.)

atrophic changes in the vagina and cervix. Changes also occur in adjacent tissues including the bladder and the urethra, which may contribute to urgency in passing urine and to stress incontinence.

As ovarian function declines, there is a gradual decrease in the amount of monthly blood loss and periods become irregular before finally stopping altogether at the menopause. The average age at which this occurs (in Britain and the USA) is currently 51 years

(range 45–55 years), having risen from 47 years in the last century. Ovulation can still occur for a few months or even a couple of years after periods have stopped. The date of the menopause therefore does not mark the exact end of a woman's reproductive capability even though the possibility of conception becomes increasingly remote. 18

Atrophy of the vaginal epithelium leads to a decrease in the amount of glycogen available for bacterial metabolism (see Ch. 34) and consequently the production of lactic acid declines and the vaginal pH rises to about 7. This increases a woman's susceptibility to infection and atrophic vaginitis can occur. 19

Hypothalamo-pituitary function

The decline in the secretion of gonadal steroids affects hypothalamic and pituitary function (see Ch. 34). When the concentration of oestrogens in blood falls the secretion of FSH and LH increases. LH is characteristically secreted in bursts (see Ch. 10, Fig. 10.6) and the size of these bursts increases as ovarian function declines.

During the menstrual cycle the cycling of hormone levels produces regular changes in body temperature. As menstruation becomes irregular and the menopause approaches, disturbances of temperature regulation are experienced by most women (85%). A woman may suddenly feel very hot, have a flushed skin, and begin to sweat (*hot flushes*). As this is followed by vasoconstriction she may then feel chilled. Symptoms continue for a while after the menopause as tissues continue to adapt to the changing levels of hormones (Fig. 36.14).

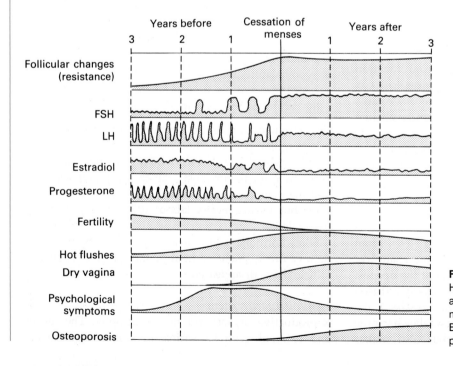

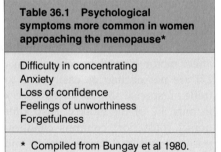

Table 36.1 Psychological symptoms more common in women approaching the menopause*		
Difficulty in concentrating
Anxiety
Loss of confidence
Feelings of unworthiness
Forgetfulness
* Compiled from Bungay et al 1980.

Figure 36.14
Hormonal changes and symptoms associated with the menopause. (Reproduced from Bancroft 1989 (Fig. 5.6) by permission of the publishers.)

Oestrogen replacement therapy (one form of HRT; see below) has been found to be helpful in controlling hot flushes, which suggests that changing levels of oestrogens are indeed involved in producing these symptoms.

Bone

Bone undergoes continual renewal and remodelling throughout life (see Ch. 28). In both men and women the amount of mineral in bones decreases from about the age of 30 years onwards, but in women the rate of loss increases sharply during the climacteric (Fig. 36.15). The amount of bone tissue present depends on the balance between formation by osteoblasts and its breakdown by osteoclasts (see Ch. 28). Oestrogens restrain the activity of the osteoclasts, so that once oestrogen levels begin to fall, more bone is broken down than is replaced and the density of bone tissue in women decreases.

As the turnover of tissue is greater in spongy bone (cancellous bone) than compact bone these effects are most rapid in spongy bone. Vertebrae contain a lot of spongy bone and there are significant amounts in the femur and the radius. Loss of bone from vertebrae adds to the decrease in height with age and can lead to progressive curvature of the spine (*dowager's hump*). The loss of tissue from the femur and radius makes these bones particularly susceptible to fracture.

Losses of bone tissue are not so great in those who remain physically active. Growth of bone tissue, like that of muscle, is promoted by the stresses and strains of physical activity.

Hormone replacement therapy (HRT), in which oestrogens are given with or without other hormones such as progestogens and testosterone, is now widely available. Women who are at risk from osteoporosis, either having a family history of the disorder or showing reduced bone density, may be advised to accept the treatment. However, any history of cardiovascular disease precludes the use of HRT. Women receiving HRT normally have regular health checks – blood pressure, weight and height are recorded, urinalysis is carried out, the breasts are examined and enquiries made regarding any side effects. A vaginal examination to palpate the uterus and ovaries should be carried out annually.

Brain

Changes in steroidal levels are associated with alterations in mood (see Ch. 34). During the climacteric, when the secretion of steroid hormones declines, and levels becomes less predictable, a woman may experience a variety of psychological symptoms (Table 36.1). These symptoms continue for a short while after the menopause as the brain adapts to the new steroid status,

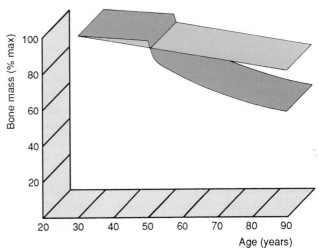

Figure 36.15
Losses of bone with age in men (blue) and women (purple). (Constructed from data in Rowe & Besdine 1988, and Hukins & Nelson 1987.)

LIFE BEGINS AT 92 FOR ACCIDENT-PRONE LES

Ninety-two-year-old Australian Leslie Colley is short-sighted and deaf. But the former gold miner who was declared unfit for service in the first world war has become a father for the ninth time.

Les, whose oldest child is a 71-year-old great-grandfather, said the new arrival came as a complete surprise. 'It just happened. I would have been happy enough chopping up wood, but now I'll have to be a father all over again.'

Les and his 38-year-old Fijian wife Patty were married two years ago. 'This was an accident,' he said. 'I don't really think I could manage another one.'

Les has lived a fairly robust life working as a docker, farmer and miner. He spends much of his retirement chopping wood and growing vegetables on a small farm in Ararat, 100 miles north of Melbourne.

He put his virility down to good food and life in the bush. 'I don't feel any different than when I was 22. I go to bed early, wake up early and don't eat junk food.'

Despite the pressures of coping with fatherhood in his twilight years, Les said he had been more nervous about breaking the news to his oldest son Norman. 'I didn't know how he would react.'

Norman, who has five children, 26 grandchildren and 12 great-grandchildren, admitted that he was shocked to learn he had a new half-brother.

'I haven't seen dad for a couple of years. I heard rumours his wife was pregnant, but never knew whether to believe it. He's fitter than me and has never been afraid of hard work, but I bet this was the hardest job he's done for a while.' Young Oswald's other living siblings Doreen, aged 68, Max, aged 63, Nancy, aged 60, and Bill, aged 58, are looking forward to meeting their half-brother.

But Norman and his wife won't be hurrying over to see the new arrival just yet. 'We can't rush over, we're both on walking sticks,' he said.

Les is not the oldest-ever dad in the world. That honour apparently goes to a Brazilian aged 112 who had a daughter with a 27-year-old woman.

Reproduced from a report by Angella Johnson (c) The Guardian 1991.

possibly in the way that withdrawal symptoms accompany the cessation of some drugs (see Ch. 19).

Cardiovascular system

Oestrogens in women have a protective effect against atherosclerosis in that they alter lipid metabolism and lower the plasma concentration of cholesterol. After the menopause the risk of atherosclerosis developing becomes the same in both sexes.

Men

In contrast to women, there is no age at which reproductive function naturally ceases. There are well-attested instances of men fathering children even in their nineties (see p. 623). However, changes do occur in reproductive function albeit very gradually and to differing extents between individuals.

Hormones

It is common, though not universal, for there to be some decline in testicular function as men grow older resulting in decreased secretion of testosterone. Simultaneously, concentrations of FSH and LH in blood increase. ⑳

⑳
What are FSH and LH?

Sexual function

Sperm continue to be produced throughout life as does the capacity to engage in sexual intercourse. However, the speed and intensity of responses to sexual stimulation and the frequency of sexual activity decrease with age, and nocturnal erections and emissions occur less often.

KEY POINTS

What you should now know and understand about growing older:

- some of the molecular and cellular changes occurring with age
- consequences of molecular and cellular change for the physiology and anatomy of the human body
- the difference between age-related and age-associated change
- how sexual and reproductive capacities change in men and women
- differences in women before, during and after the menopause
- why physical appearance changes as we grow older
- why the old are not as strong physically as the young
- how and why nutritional and environmental needs change
- why the elderly usually cannot see or hear or sleep as well as the young
- why the treatment and management of illness in the elderly may differ from that in younger people
- reasons why there may be considerable variation in health and fitness between people of the same age.

REFERENCES AND FURTHER READING

Allen S C 1988 How respiratory and cardiac reserves decline in old age. Geriatric Medicine 18(April): 23–24

Bancroft J 1989 Human sexuality and its problems, 2nd edn. Churchill Livingstone, Edinburgh, p 290

Bennett G J, Ebrahim S 1992 The essentials of health care of the elderly. Edward Arnold, Sevenoaks
(Comprehensive coverage of all the issues involved in caring for the elderly. Includes a useful section on the biology of ageing)

Block E 1952 Quantitative morphological investigation of the follicular system in women. Acta Anatomica 14: 108

Brocklehurst J C, Allen S C 1987 Geriatric medicine for students. Churchill Livingstone, Edinburgh
(Concise small book focusing on diseases and disorders common in the elderly and their treatment)

Brookbank J W 1990 Biology of ageing. Harper Collins College, New York

Bungay G, Vessey M, Thom M, Studd J 1980 Study of symptoms in middle life, with special reference to the menopause. British Medical Journal 281: 181–183

Coni N, Davison W, Webster S 1992 Ageing: the facts. Oxford University Press, Oxford
(Readable book containing lots of information. Describes what happens in ageing as well as providing a guide for the general reader)

Evered D, Whelan J 1988 Research and the ageing population: Ciba Foundation symposium, 134. John Wiley & Sons, Chichester

Freeland A 1989 Deafness: the facts. Oxford University Press, Oxford, p 96

Hukins D W L, Nelson M A 1987 The ageing spine. Manchester University Press, Manchester

Johnson A 1991 Life begins at 92. The Guardian, 3rd August

Kesson C M, Knight P V (eds) 1990 Diabetes in elderly people: a guide for the health care team. Chapman & Hall, London
(Concise, straightforward, useful small book)

Macheath J 1983 Activity, health and fitness in old age. Croom Helm, Beckenham
('Promotion of health in old age through exercise')

Maddox G L 1987 Encyclopedia of aging. Springer Publishing, New York
(Reference work including much information on relevant topics and explaining hundreds of terms and concepts relating to the life of the elderly and the ageing process)

Mansell A, Bryan C, Levison H 1972 Airway closure in children. Journal of Applied Physiology 33: 711–714

Murray J F 1976 The normal lung. W B Saunders, Philadelphia

Nelson N M 1966 Neonatal pulmonary function. Pediatric Clinics of North America 13: 769–799

Richardson S J, Senikas V, Nelson J F 1987 Follicular depletion during the menopausal transition: evidence for accelerated loss and ultimate exhaustion. Journal of Clinical Endocrinology and Metabolism 65: 1231–1237

Rowe J W 1976 The effect of age on creatinine clearance in man: a cross sectional study. Journal of Gerontology 31: 155

Rowe J W, Besdine R W 1988 Geriatric medicine, 2nd edn. Little Brown, Boston, p 515

Sarbini C A, Brassi V, Solinas E, Muiesan G 1968 Arterial oxygen tension in relation to age in healthy subjects. Respiration 25: 3–13

Shaw M W 1984 The challenge of ageing: a multidisciplinary approach to extended care. Churchill Livingstone, Edinburgh
(User-friendly book. Excellent practical application of facts about ageing for all those concerned with planning and providing support and care)

Thompson M K 1990 Commonsense geriatrics. Clinical Press, Bristol, p 65, 72, 107

Wood P H N, Badley E M 1983 An epidemiological appraisal of bone and joint disease in the elderly. In: Wright V (ed) Bone and joint disease in the elderly. Churchill Livingstone, Edinburgh, p 1–22

Chapter 37
DEATH AND DYING

People die as a result of the failure of one or more body systems through injury, disease or ageing. The principal causes of death differ at different stages of life. After death, characteristic changes occur in the body, altering its appearance.

Personal experiences of dying depend upon its cause, its circumstances and the support provided.

DEATH

CAUSES

The principal causes of death differ in different parts of the world and have changed over the years in places such as Britain (Fig. 37.1) and other European countries. In Britain at the turn of the century, infectious diseases were the biggest killer, but since then there has been a dramatic fall in deaths from infections, largely because of improved water supplies and better hygiene as well as the discovery and use of antibiotics. However, infectious diseases remain a major cause of death in some Third World countries, especially amongst children. In 1990 in countries such as England and Wales major causes of death by age (Fig. 37.2A & B) include:

- developmental abnormalities in the very young
- accidents and injury in young adults
- circulatory diseases and cancer (*neoplasia*) in older persons.

Age at death
Several different measurements are used to describe the patterns of life and death within a population:

- mortality index
- survival curves
- life expectancy.

Mortality index
The mortality index is the number of people, per thousand of population, dying in a given year. Mortality is highest at the beginning and the end of our lives, times when we are most vulnerable either because of the immaturity of our body systems (see Ch. 35) or because of their deterioration (see Ch. 36).

Survival curves
Survival curves (Fig. 37.3) show the percentages of people in a population who have survived to different

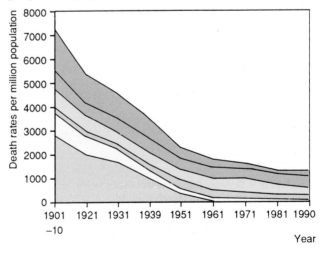

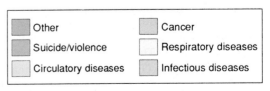

Figure 37.1
Mean annual death rates by major cause of death among males aged 25 to 44 years in England and Wales from 1901 to 1990. (Courtesy of S. Donnan, Department of Public Health and Epidemiology, University of Manchester. Source: OPCS.)

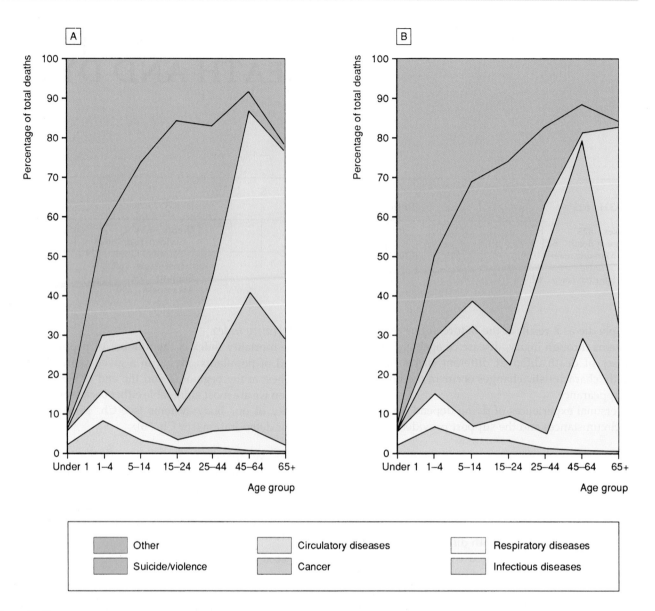

Figure 37.2
Principal causes of death at different ages in England and Wales, 1990:
A Males
B Females.
(Courtesy of S. Donnan, Department of Public Health and Epidemiology, University of Manchester. Source: OPCS.)

ages. The differences in the shapes of the curves in countries such as England and Wales at the beginning and the end of the twentieth century, and between western and Third World countries reveal the effects of different social conditions including water supplies, housing and diet. In Third World countries many deaths occur in childhood (Table 37.1) through malnutrition and infectious disease, whereas in other countries over 75% of the population can anticipate a long life of 70 years or more. ①

However, better social conditions seem not to have had much effect on the maximum life span, which in all communities of the world is still about 100 to 110 years of age.

Life expectancy
Average life expectancies are estimated from the data for mortality and survival. In most communities, average life expectancy is increasing, although there are still considerable differences between different countries of the world (Table 37.1).

DEFINITIONS

Throughout our lives, cells die within our bodies either because they have come to the end of their natural life span or because they have been fatally injured. In that sense, death is a natural part of the process of living. Cells that die are usually replaced by others. Consequently the life of the body continues. As we age, the

① *Many children in the Third World who are malnourished do not look thin. Why is this? What is the condition called?*

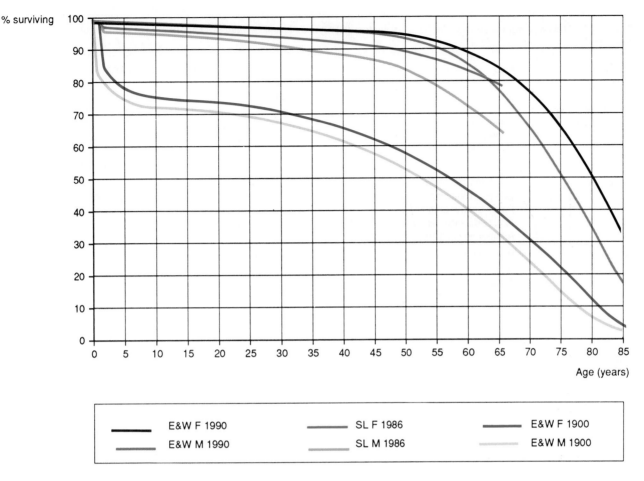

Figure 37.3
Survival curves for men (M) and women (F) in England and Wales (E&W) in 1900 and in 1990, and in Sri Lanka (SL) in 1986.
(Courtesy of S. Donnan, Department of Public Health and Epidemiology, University of Manchester. Sources: OPCS and World Health Statistics Annual 1991.)

replacement of cells occurs more slowly and, as a result, different aspects of body function deteriorate (see Ch. 36).

The body continues to live as long as internal stability is maintained (see Ch. 3). Individual organs and tissues contribute to homeostasis (see Chs 4–16) and their failure upsets one or more key constituents of the interstitial fluid, altering the internal environment and impairing the function of other organs and tissues. Once this leads to failure of cardiac function and circulation of the blood stops, the life of the body as a cooperative society of organs and tissues ceases. As the internal environment deteriorates even further all the cells of the body gradually cease to function too.

Death therefore is a process beginning with the failure of one part of the body which leads to failure of the life of the body as a whole.

Difficulties arise in deciding the stage in this process at which a person can be declared to be 'dead' particularly when there is loss of brain function. Loss of cerebral function results in loss of personality leading

Table 37.1 Childhood mortality and life expectancy in different countries*

	Under-5 mortality (per 1000 live births)	Life expectancy (years)
Afghanistan	292	43
Guinea Bisseau	246	43
Bangladesh	180	52
Kenya	108	60
Colombia	50	69
United Kingdom	9	76
USA	11	76
Australia	10	77
Switzerland	9	77
Iceland	5	78
Japan	6	79

* Compiled from Third World Guide 93/94.

to the circumstances in which someone's body may continue to live, or to be maintained on a respirator, although awareness and purposeful activity no longer

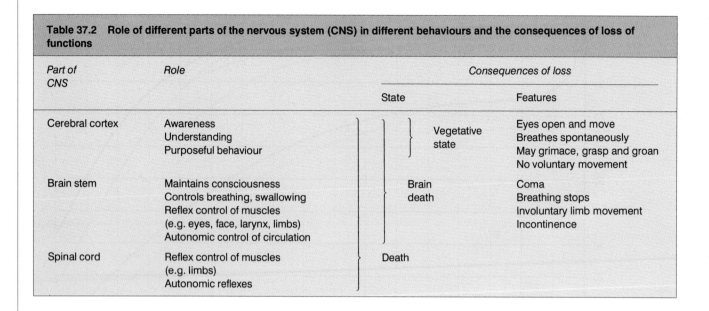

Table 37.2   Role of different parts of the nervous system (CNS) in different behaviours and the consequences of loss of functions

Part of CNS	Role	Consequences of loss		
			State	Features
Cerebral cortex	Awareness Understanding Purposeful behaviour	Vegetative state		Eyes open and move Breathes spontaneously May grimace, grasp and groan No voluntary movement
Brain stem	Maintains consciousness Controls breathing, swallowing Reflex control of muscles (e.g. eyes, face, larynx, limbs) Autonomic control of circulation	Brain death		Coma Breathing stops Involuntary limb movement Incontinence
Spinal cord	Reflex control of muscles (e.g. limbs) Autonomic reflexes	Death		

exist. Medically, distinctions are made between three states (Table 37.2):

- the vegetative state
- brain death
- certified death.

Vegetative state

Someone whose cerebral cortex is irreversibly damaged, but whose brain stem is intact, may live for many years in a state in which any awareness of the surrounding environment and purposeful activity (see Chs 30–33) is totally absent even though most of the body remains alive. Breathing occurs spontaneously, the heart beats, blood circulates and reflex movements occur but there is no understanding, communication or voluntary activity.

In this state, someone's personality has been irretrievably lost, with the result that it can be said that the 'person' has died even though the body remains alive. The fact that eyes open and many reflexes remain intact, especially those affecting hands, face, and eyes (see Chs 27–29) can falsely give the impression that conscious awareness still exists.

> The relatives and friends of a patient whose brain is permanently damaged may find it difficult to accept that recovery is impossible. This is particularly so when reflexes persist, especially the reflex grasping of a hand. When a grieving relative says, 'But nurse, he knows I'm here – he squeezed my hand,' it takes courage and empathy to explain the situation.

Brain death

Someone whose brain stem is irreversibly damaged will be in coma (see Ch. 23) and breathing stops (see Ch. 7). Life can be maintained by artificial ventilation as the heart continues to beat. Absence of detectable activity in the EEG (see Ch. 23) suggests brain death but is not proof of it.

Brain death is confirmed if it is impossible to elicit any brain stem reflexes and if all factors that could temporarily depress brain stem function, such as drugs and hypothermia, have been excluded. Reflexes tested include:

- pupillary and corneal reflexes (see Ch. 26)
- cough reflex and CO_2-induced respiratory movements (see Ch. 7).

COPING WITH DEATH

No nurse finds caring for a dying patient easy. Each death is different and courage, empathy and skills in communication are needed. Without these, a nurse may feel inadequate and frightened – 'I felt so helpless, I just didn't know what to say.' When nursing a dying patient it is often easy to think, 'This could be my young sister,' or 'my Dad'. Thoughts such as these may make it difficult for the nurse to carry out her nursing care without becoming more distressed. If a decision has been made to discontinue a life support system, the nurse may find that her emotions are at variance with the medical decision and, even, with what seems logical.

There are many such ethical issues relating to death which nurses have to understand and consider, making up their own minds about what they believe to be right. Classroom discussions about death and dying are helpful but some nurses, and other members of the caring team, find that they need more individual help. Many hospitals employ counsellors, or there is a local counselling service available to the staff. The hospital chaplain and visiting clergy are always willing to help. Also, organisations such as the Samaritans and Compassionate Friends (support for bereaved parents) can help by putting someone in touch with specialist counsellors.

When someone is brain dead it is still possible to elicit spinal reflexes (see Ch. 27) as the spinal cord is still functioning.

Certified death

Legally, a person is certified as dead once circulatory and respiratory function has ceased irreversibly. Loss of circulatory function is judged to be irreversible once the ECG (see Ch. 5) has shown no sign of activity for at least 5 minutes. If there is uncertainty over whether the heart has stopped beating, artificial ventilation is maintained for at least 2 hours after signs of life have ceased. ②

CHANGES POST-MORTEM

Once the circulation has ceased, the internal environment deteriorates rapidly affecting cells and tissues and leading to alterations in a person's body and appearance. For example stiffening of the body (*rigor mortis*) occurs a few hours after death. Discolouration and softening occur later as decomposition begins to occur. ③

TRANSPLANTS

Organs should be removed as soon as possible after circulation and respiration have ceased, and death has been confirmed. Cells and tissues remain viable for a short time after death and therefore can be transplanted successfully into another body. Cooling arrests deterioration and helps to preserve normal function.

Rigor mortis

Stiffening of the body is caused by the binding of actin to myosin in muscles as a result of a gradual increase in intracellular calcium concentration and depletion of ATP (see Ch. 22). As muscle cells die after death, ions such as sodium and calcium leak into the cytoplasm from the extracellular fluid and from intracellular organelles. These ions cannot be evicted and relaxation cannot occur because the ATP needed for these processes (see Ch. 22) is depleted.

Rigor mortis begins 2 to 4 hours after death, the face stiffening before the hands and feet. Maximal stiffness develops between 12 and 48 hours depending on the environmental temperature, but then wears off over the next day or two as lysosomal enzymes (see Ch. 2) digest cellular proteins. These changes in the body are used by the pathologist and coroner as indicators of the probable time of death, should this not be known, for example if someone dies alone, or in unusual circumstances. ④

Decomposition

Blood drains from the surface structures of the body to accumulate in the parts below (*dependent parts*) in the hour or two after death. As cells die, lysosomal enzymes begin the process of digestion that eventually disrupts

red cells (*haemolysis*) and softens and finally liquefies the tissue. Bacterial contamination hastens the digestive process and produces iron sulphide which stains the tissues green and black. However, if the body is kept in a cold environment discolouration and decomposition are considerably delayed.

In preparing the body for burial or cremation undertakers replace the blood with an embalming fluid that destroys bacteria and preserves the tissues. As a result the corpse of a non-coloured person usually has a waxy white appearance unless make-up has been applied.

DYING

An individual's personal experience of dying will depend on a number of factors including the:

- events of death
- support given
- level of awareness.

EVENTS

Death may occur suddenly, or gradually in the case of a terminal illness.

Sudden death

Sudden death is due to lack of blood flow to the brain (*cerebral ischaemia*). This can be caused in several ways, for example by cerebral haemorrhage (*stroke*) or by a cardiac arrest. In each case the person rapidly loses consciousness because of the loss of blood supply to the brain. Someone who has a heart attack may also experience a sharp crushing pain in the chest as a result of ischaemia of the cardiac tissues (see Ch. 32).

Terminal illness

Death occurs gradually when there is failure of one or more of the organs and systems that maintain the composition of the internal environment (see Chs 3–16). The quality of the internal environment gradually deteriorates leading to malfunction of other cells and tissues too. For example, in respiratory failure hypoxia and hypercarbia develop (see Chs 7 and 11) leading to the failure of other organs such as the brain and heart. In renal failure (see Ch. 8), plasma potassium and hydrogen ion concentrations increase (see Chs 13 and 12) disturbing cardiac function. In liver failure (see Ch. 9) toxic substances such as ammonia and bilirubin accumulate poisoning other tissues including the brain.

In terminal illness, the specific symptoms experienced and the problems faced (Table 37.3) are partly related to the original illness and partly to its secondary effects including the individual's increasing inability to care for

② *What is the main risk involved if the circulation re-starts after 4 to 5 minutes?*

③ *What is the name given to decomposition of tissues in a living person?*

④ *What differences are there between the work of a pathologist, a microbiologist and a haematologist?*

Table 37.3   Some of the clinical features that may be present in terminal illness
Anorexia
Weakness/immobility
Pain
Dyspnoea
Cough
Insomnia
Constipation
Nausea

CARING FOR THE DYING PERSON

Basic nursing care should not be neglected when a person is dying, even when to provide care seems an unnecessary disturbance of the person's peace. None of us know exactly when death will occur, nor how much discomfort the semi-conscious patient can still appreciate. Neglect of care may, in time, inflict more discomfort. 'It is unpardonable to subject him to unnecessary discomforts which simple nursing procedures can so easily prevent. An alteration of position and the provision of clean bed linen may relieve distress and help to prevent the additional pain which would accompany pressure sores' (Chilman & Thomas 1987).

Individual carers have the responsibility of deciding what care is appropriate and how often it should be provided. Apart from assuming that the patient, if semi-conscious or unable to communicate, still feels discomfort, one should also take the feelings of relatives and friends into account. It is a distressing time for relatives, waiting for a loved one to die. Many things not mentioned or not consciously noticed at the time are remembered later, sometimes adding to feelings of guilt, for example 'She was my mother, why didn't I say something?' A recently bereaved daughter said, 'Her mouth looked so dry and sore, it must have been uncomfortable.' And a son said, 'He didn't have a pressure sore when he went into hospital but they wouldn't use a sheepskin so he got sore. They didn't use his denture cleaning tablets either.' The nurse should spare time to talk to the patient and his relatives, to answer questions as honestly as possible and not be afraid of saying 'I don't know.' When a person is dying, as well as providing care for that person, the nurse is also caring for the relatives; helping them to feel that their loved one is approaching death peacefully and comfortably.

himself. In malignant disease of the digestive tract for example, disease-related symptoms may include nausea and vomiting, whereas in diseases of the cardiorespiratory system problems may include difficulty in breathing (*dyspnoea*). In renal failure, someone may be confused and behave abnormally because of the accumulation of toxic substances, such as urea and potassium, in the body and their effects on the nervous system. In terminal malignant disease there may be pain, although this is not inevitable. ⑤

The immobility and nutritional problems of terminally ill patients are factors leading easily to secondary problems such as constipation and pressure sores. Drying of the mouth is another common problem due in part to mouth-breathing as well as to difficulties in maintaining proper fluid balance. ⑥

Last stages

Some people slip away uneventfully and peacefully but for others the last stages of life may be marked by symptoms that can be very distressing to relatives and friends, though not necessarily to the dying person who may have lost consciousness.

If renal failure occurs, the build-up of waste products such as urea and potassium in the blood may affect the brain, causing confusion, restlessness and sometimes hiccups. Weakening of muscles and confusion may result in incontinence, and secretions which can no longer be coughed up may accumulate in the airways making breathing very noisy. Breathing patterns alter as circulation fails and brain stem function deteriorates. For example breathing may become intermittent (referred to as *Cheyne–Stokes respiration*).

People who almost die but recover sometimes describe having experienced a variety of phenomena such as feeling disembodied, hearing music or seeing visions. These experiences may be the result of hallucinations associated with altered brain function.

SUPPORT

Through the pioneering work of Dame Cicely Saunders (who was first a hospital social worker and then a nurse before becoming a doctor) it is now recognised medi-

⑤
If someone is suffering from dyspnoea, what position may be most comfortable for him and why?

⑥
What measures can be taken to prevent the development of pressure sores in the terminally ill patient?

cally that much can be done to ease the process of dying. If the disease process results in chronic pain, drugs such as morphine can be given to alleviate discomfort. Anticholinergic drugs (see Ch. 3) such as hyoscine can be used to reduce secretions as well as relieve nausea. In addition, the comfort of another person, their presence and sensitive care can also do much to give psychological support and reduce anxiety.

Pain relief in the form of medication should not be denied the patient who is terminally ill. The tablets or injection should be given at regular intervals before the pain returns (not after is has caused the patient anxiety and distress). In this way the patient seldom experiences pain and is more able to face the remainder of his life with courage.

AWARENESS

Once someone has lost consciousness he will not be aware of what is happening, and so symptoms of the last stages of death, which can be distressing to family and friends, may not actually be sensed by the patient himself.

However, it should never be glibly assumed that a

person is unaware of his environment simply because he does not respond to conversation or touch. Changes in brain function can make it impossible for someone to speak or to respond although he may still be able to sense much of what is going on around him (see Chs 23, 28 and 29). It is therefore always best for the nurse to assume that a patient can hear, and for her to speak and act accordingly, maintaining respect at all times for the living and the dying.

KEY POINTS

What you should now know and understand about death and dying:

- why death is regarded as a process rather than an event
- the distinctions made between different states of life and death including brain death and the vegetative state
- how death of the body results from homeostatic failure
- the basis of some of the clinical features associated with dying
- changes occurring in the body post-mortem.

REFERENCES AND FURTHER READING

Charles-Edwards A 1983 The nursing care of the dying patient. Beaconsfield Publishers, Beaconsfield

Chilman A M, Thomas M 1987 Understanding nursing care, 3rd edn. Churchill Livingstone, Edinburgh.

Jennett B 1987 Brain death and the vegetative state. In: Weatherall D J, Ledingham J G G, Warrell D A (eds) Oxford textbook of medicine, 2nd edn. Oxford University Press, Oxford, p 21.48–21.51
(Clear description of distinctions made between different states)

Lamb D 1985 Death, brain death and ethics. Croom Helm, Beckenham

OPCS: Office of Population Censuses and Surveys, London

Ogilvie C (ed) 1981 Birch's Emergencies in medical practice, 11th edn. Churchill Livingstone, Edinburgh

Pallis C 1983 ABC of brain stem death. British Medical Journal, London
(Collection of short articles from the British Medical Journal)

Ritchie A C 1990 Boyd's Textbook of pathology, 9th edn. Lea & Febiger, Philadelphia

Saunders C, Baines M 1989 Living with dying: the management of terminal disease, 2nd edn. Oxford University Press, Oxford
(Second edition of the acclaimed short book that has helped many health care staff to improve the quality of life for very many terminally ill patients)

Thomas M 1988 Coping with distressing symptoms. In: Wilson-Barnett J, Raiman J 1988 (eds) Nursing issues and research in terminal care. John Wiley & Sons, Chichester
(One of several useful chapters reviewing the basis of different aspects of nursing care of the dying)

Third World guide 93/94. Instituto del Tercer Mundo, Montevideo
(A mine of useful information about different countries of the world including some data on health)

Wilson J D, Braunwald E, Isselbacher K J, Petersdorf R G, Martin J B, Fauci A S, Root R K 1991 Harrison's Principles of internal medicine, 12th edn. McGraw-Hill, New York

World Health Statistics Annual 1991. World Health Organization, Geneva

Index

To make the index more useful for the reader, the following conventions have been used:

bold page numbers = main discussion of a subject
italic page numbers = application boxes

Where a reference refers to either a table or a figure, this has been noted (in parentheses) after the page number.

Abbreviations used in the index include:

CSF = cerebrospinal fluid
CO_2 = carbon dioxide
ECF = extracellular fluid
H^+ = hydrogen ions
O_2 = oxygen

B

C

Dear Reader,

We would welcome your comments on this text, and would also be very pleased to hear from you with any suggestions you may have for new publications.

Do write to me at the following address:

Ellen Green
Commissioning Editor
Churchill Livingstone
1–3 Baxter's Place
Leith Walk
Edinburgh EH1 3AF